4e

Understanding the
Australian Health Care System

4e

Understanding the
Australian Health Care System

Eileen Willis PhD, MEd, BEd

Emeritus Professor, College of Nursing and Health Sciences,
Flinders University, Adelaide, South Australia

Louise Reynolds PhD, GradCertEd, BHSc (PHC), FPA

Senior Lecturer in Paramedic Science, Faculty of Health,
Education, Medicine and Social Care,
Anglia Ruskin University, UK

Trudy Rudge RN, PhD, BA(Hons)

Adjunct Professor, Susan Wakil School of Nursing and Midwifery,
Sydney University, Sydney, New South Wales

ELSEVIER

ELSEVIER

Elsevier Australia. ACN 001 002 357
(a division of Reed International Books Australia Pty Ltd)
Tower 1, 475 Victoria Avenue, Chatswood, NSW 2067

4th edition © 2020 Elsevier Australia. 3rd edition © 2016; 2nd edition © 2012; Reprinted 2013. 1st edition © 2008 Elsevier Australia.

ISBN: 978-0-7295-4328-6

Notice

National Library of Australia Cataloguing-in-Publication Data

---

A catalogue record for this book is available from the National Library of Australia

---

Content Strategist: Melinda McEvoy
Content Project Manager: Shruti Raj
Edited by Chris Wyard
Proofread by Melissa Faulkner
Permissions Editing and Photo Research: Regina Lavanya Remigius
Cover and internal design by Georgette Hall
Index by Innodata Indexing
Typeset by Toppan Best-set Premedia Limited
Printed in China by 1010 Printing International Limited

Last digit is the print number: 9 8 7 6 5 4 3 2 1

Contents

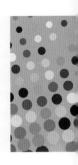

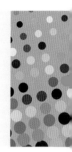

Video Table of Contents

A suite of video interviews with practitioners and thought leaders have been created for this edition and are available on the Evolve site: http://evolve.elsevier.com/AU/Willis/understanding/

The videos further explore the themes and content within the chapters, as well as outlining challenges of the profession and advice for new graduates.

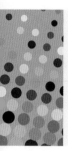

Dedication

This edition is dedicated to our colleague the late Dr Luisa Toffoli, three-time contributor to the nursing profession chapter who passed away before final publication of this edition.

Acknowledgements

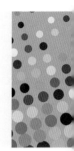

Understanding the Australian Health Care System is the fourth edition of this book. It has involved collaborative effort, plus the skills, knowledge and resources of many people to whom we offer our gratitude.

We are again indebted to our contributors, some of whom are new and many of whom have stayed with us for this fourth edition. We thank them for sharing their expert knowledge from their fields of practice and the special insights that they bring to their chapters. The manuscript is enhanced by the thoughtful comments provided by anonymous reviewers whom we also thank and acknowledge.

We thank and are indebted as always to the Elsevier team – Melinda McEvoy, Shruti Raj Srivastava and Chris Wyard and others behind the scenes. Their continued interest in this book and its development, and their skilled and patient management that has helped us meet deadlines amid the busy lives of both editors and contributors, is much appreciated.

We wish to acknowledge with special thanks Emeritus Professor Helen Keleher who worked with us on the first three editions. We welcome Professor Trudy Rudge as co-editor.

We also thank those nearest and dearest to us for their forbearance, especially on long evenings and weekends when we were distracted by the manuscript. We deeply appreciate your support and encouragement.

We have again enjoyed working together on this book, and we trust that readers enjoy the book as much as we have enjoyed our collaborations during its preparation and production.

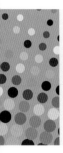

Contributors

Jane Bickford PhD
Senior Lecturer, College of Nursing and Health Sciences, Flinders University, Adelaide, South Australia

Chris Brebner PhD, BAppSc (Speech Path)
Associate Professor, College of Nursing and Health Sciences, Flinders University, Adelaide, South Australia

Anne Cahill Lambert AM, MPubAdmin, BHA, FCHSM, CHM
Consumer Advocate; Chief Executive Officer (retired)

Lisa Callahan MPH, MAud, BBehSc
Lecturer, College of Nursing and Health Sciences, Flinders University, Adelaide, South Australia

Melainie Cameron PhD, MHSc, BAppSc (Ost)
Associate Professor, School of Health and Wellbeing, University of Southern Queensland;
Extraordinary Professor, Research entity for Physical Activity, Sport, and Recreation (PhASRec), North-West
University, Potchefstroom, South Africa

Stephen Carter PhD, MSc, BPharm
Lecturer, Faculty of Pharmacy, University of Sydney, Sydney, New South Wales

Alex Collie PhD, BAppSc(Hons), BA
Professor, School of Public Health and Preventive Medicine, Monash University, Melbourne, Victoria

Fran Collyer PhD (Sociology)
Associate Professor, Department of Sociology and Social Policy, School of Social and Policy Sciences, Faculty of
Arts and Social Sciences, University of Sydney, Sydney, New South Wales

Judith Daire PhD
Lecturer, School of Public Health, Faculty of Health Sciences, Curtin University, Bentley Campus, Bentley,
Western Australia

Judith Dwyer AM, PhD, MBA, BA, FCHSM, FAICD
Adjunct Professor, Southgate Institute, College of Medicine and Public Health Flinders University, Adelaide,
South Australia

Caroline Ellison PhD
Crossing the Horizon Associate Professor of Ageing and Disability, School of Psychology, Social Work and
Social Policy, University of South Australia, Adelaide, South Australia

Jenny Gamble SFHEA; CF

Professor and Head of Midwifery, School of Nursing and Midwifery, Faculty of Griffith Health, Griffith University, Brisbane, Queensland

Elizabeth Goble RN, PhD(c), MMedSc, BSc (Hons)

Associate Lecturer, College of Nursing and Health Sciences, Flinders University, Adelaide, South Australia

Adam Govier MPhysio, BAppSc (Physio)

Director of Physiotherapy, Central Adelaide Local Health Network, South Australia

Colleen Hayes GradCert Remote Health, Anangu Teacher Education Diploma

Indigenous Health Lecturer, Poche Centre, College of Medicine and Public Health, Flinders University, Alice Springs, Northern Territory

Julie Henderson PhD, GradDip (Info Stud), BA(Hons)

Adjunct Senior Research Fellow, College of Medicine and Public Health, Flinders University, Adelaide, South Australia

Suzanne Hodgkin PhD

Associate Professor, John Richards Centre for Rural Ageing, La Trobe University, Melbourne, Victoria

Helen M Keleher PhD, MA(HlthSt), BA, RN

Professor (Adj), School of Rural Health, Monash University, Melbourne, Victoria

Brenton Kortman MHSc (OT), BAppSc (OT), OTD

Adjunct Senior Lecturer, College of Nursing and Health Sciences, Flinders University, Adelaide, South Australia

Lindsay Krassnitzer MIPH, GradCert (Public Sector Management), BHS, BHlthSc, BSc(Hons)

Associate Lecturer, School of Health Sciences, Flinders University, Adelaide, South Australia

Tyler Lane DPhil, MSc, BA

Research Fellow, School of Public Health and Preventive Medicine, Monash University, Melbourne, Victoria

Christopher Lind PhD

Associate Professor in Audiology, College of Nursing and Health Sciences Flinders University, Adelaide, South Australia

Iris Lindemann MEd, BNutDiet, BSc, EdD(c)

Education Consultant, Adelaide University, South Australia

Marian McAllister APD, MND, BSc(Hons)

Lecturer, College of Nursing and Health Science, Flinders University, Adelaide, South Australia

Janny Maddern EdD, MBA, BAppSc(SpPath), LMACHSM, AFIML

Adjunct Associate Professor, Department of Health Care Management, College of Medicine and Public Health, Flinders University, South Australia

Anne-Marie Mahoney EdD, MTrngDev, BNurs

Lecturer, Rural Department of Nursing and Midwifery, College of Science, Health and Engineering, La Trobe University, Wodonga, Victoria

Louisa Matwiejczyk Adv. APD, PhD(c), GradDip (NutDiet), BA(Hons)

Lecturer, College of Nursing and Health Sciences, Flinders University, Adelaide, South Australia

Sandra Mortimer PhD (c), GradCert (Mgt), BAppSc (OT)

Lecturer in Occupational Therapy, College of Nursing and Health Sciences, Flinders University, Adelaide, South Australia

Kirsty Rawlings BAppSc(ExSpSc), Hons HMS, B Ed Studies, GAICD, AEP

Lecturer, Clinical Exercise Physiology, School of Health Sciences, University of South Australia, Adelaide, South Australia

Sandeep Reddy PhD, MMgmt, MSc, MBBS, DPH

Associate Professor, School of Medicine, Deakin University, Burwood, Victoria

Louise Roberts PhD

Lecturer, College of Medicine and Public Health, Flinders University, Adelaide, South Australia

Suzanne Robinson PhD, MSc, BSc

Professor, Health Systems and Health Economics, School of Public Health, Faculty of Health Sciences, Curtin University, Bentley, Western Australia

Erica Sainsbury PhD, MSc, Grad Dip EdStud (Higher Ed), BPharm (Hons), MPS, MSHP, MACE

Senior Lecturer, School of Pharmacy, Faculty of Medicine and Health, University of Sydney, Sydney, New South Wales

Julie Satur PhD, MHSc (Hlth Prom), DipApplSc (Dent Ther)

Professor, Oral Health, Melbourne Dental School, University of Melbourne, Melbourne, Victoria

Steve Selig PhD, BSc(Hons), AES, AEP, ESSAF

Chair, Clinical Exercise Science (retired), School of Exercise and Nutrition Sciences, Deakin University, Burwood, Victoria

E Michael Shanahan PhD, MPH, MHPE, BMBS, FAFOEM, FRACP

Head, Department of Rheumatology, Flinders Medical Centre, College of Medicine and Public Health, Flinders University, Adelaide, South Australia

Anthony Smith PhD, MSc, BSc, DipAppSci(MedRad), FASMIRT

Associate Professor, Academic Lead – Research, University of Newcastle Department of Rural Health, Faculty of Health and Medicine, University of Newcastle, New South Wales;
Adjunct Associate Professor, Medical Imaging and Radiation Sciences, Faculty of Medicine, Nursing and Health Sciences, Monash University, Melbourne, Victoria

Keith Sutton PhD, BNurs

Lecturer in Rural Mental Health, Monash University Department of Rural Health, Warragul, Victoria

Matthew Sutton MMusc&SportPhty, BPhty

Senior Lecturer, College of Nursing and Health Sciences, Flinders University, Adelaide, South Australia

Kerry Taylor PhD, MPHC, BNg, GradDip (Hlth Ed), DipTch

Adjunct Associate Professor, Poche Centre for Indigenous Health and Wellbeing, College of Medicine and Public Health, Flinders University, Alice Springs, Northern Territory

Rachel Tham PhD, MHSc, MPH, BDS

Research Fellow, Mary MacKillop Institute for Health Research, Faculty of Health Science, Australian Catholic University, Melbourne, Victoria

Luisa Toffoli RN, PhD(USyd), MN(UniSA)

Senior Lecturer, School of Nursing and Midwifery, University of South Australia, Adelaide, South Australia

Julia Twohig PhD (c), BAdult&VocEduc(Hons), AdvDip (Homoeopathy)

Lecturer and Homoeopathic Private Practice, Endeavour College of Natural Medicine, Adelaide, South Australia

Susan Waller PhD, MPhty, APAM

Senior Lecturer, Monash University Department of Rural Health, Warragul, Victoria

Bernadette Ward PhD

Senior Lecturer, School of Rural Health, Faculty of Medicine, Nursing and Health Sciences, Monash University, Melbourne, Victoria

Karen Willis PhD, MA, GradDip (HP), BA

Professor, Allied Health Research, Chair, Academic and Research Collaborative in Health, La Trobe University / Royal Melbourne Hospital, Melbourne, Victoria

Caroline Yates RN, RCN, MA, GradCert (Tertiary Teaching), BSc(Hons)

Lecturer, School of Health Systems and Health Economics, Faculty of Health Sciences, Curtin University, Bentley, Western Australia;
Health Information Management/Teaching Academic, School of Health Systems and Health Economics, Faculty of Health Sciences, Curtin University, Bentley, Western Australia

Reviewers

Melissa Carey, RN, PhD, MN, MAP, BN

Senior Lecturer in Nursing, University of Sothern Queensland, University Darling Heights QLD, Australia

Susan Crowther, RM, PhD, MSc, PGCertED, BSc (Hons)

Professor of Midwifery, Robert Gordon University, Garthdee House, Garthdee Road, Aberdeen AB10 7AQ, United Kingdom

Gretel Jones, MBA, BAppSc(Physiotherapy)

Unit Assessor Australian Health Care System CMM10580, School of Health and Human Sciences, Southern Cross University, GOLD COAST CAMPUS, Southern Cross Drive, Bilinga, QLD, 4225, Australia

Jane Mulcahy, PhD, MAPS, BA

Lecturer and Unit Coordinator, Research Supervisor, Victoria University, PO Box 14428, Melbourne, Vic 8001, Australia

Penny Roe, PhD, BSocWk (Hons)

Lecturer, Flinders University, College of Nursing & Health Sciences, Sturt Campus, Bedford Park, South Australia, Australia

Angela Sheedy, MPH, GradCert (University Teaching & Learning), BHSc(Nursing)

Lecturer in Health, Course Coordinator Health Science, College of Health and Human Sciences, Charles Darwin University Ellengowan Dr, Casuarina NT 0810, Australia

Max Sully, PhD, MA (Psychology)

College of Science, Health, Engineering and Education (SHEE), Murdoch University, 90 South St, Murdoch WA 6150, Australia

CHAPTER 1

Understanding the Australian health care system: how to use this book

Eileen Willis, Louise Reynolds and Trudy Rudge[a]

Key learning outcomes

When you finish this chapter you should be able to:

- understand the structure of this book
- identify the main drivers for health system reform and key conceptual ideas that underpin those drivers
- be familiar with the three main types of health care systems across the developed world
- recognise major ideas impacting on health care reform arising from economic rationalism and neoliberalism
- have an idea of the outcomes of any health reform using Tuohy's theories of institutional mix and structural power
- understand the key questions to ask using Bacchi's framework of 'what's the problem represented to be?'
- have a clear idea of what is understood as interprofessional practice
- be aware of the impact of the safety and quality movement in health care.

Key terms and abbreviations

activity-based funding (ABF)	casemix
acute care	community and public health
adverse events	Council of Australian Governments (COAG)
antimicrobial stewardship	Diagnosis Related Groups (DRG)
Australian Health Practitioner Regulation Agency (AHPRA)	economic rationalism
	effectiveness
Australian Medical Association (AMA)	efficiency
autonomy of practice	equity

[a]We acknowledge the contribution by Helen Keleher to the chapter in the 3rd edition of this book.

evidence-based medicine (EBM)
general practice / general practitioner (GP)
global financial crisis (GFC)
hospital-acquired conditions (HACs)
hospital-acquired infections (HAIs)
Independent Hospital Pricing Authority (IHPA)
institutional mix
interprofessional education (IPE)
interprofessional practice (IPP)
medical dominance
Medicare
mixed system
neoliberalism
new public management (NPM)
Organisation for Economic Co-operation and
    Development (OECD)

Pharmaceutical Benefit Scheme (PBS)
professional closure
professional monopoly
public–private partnership (PPP)
private for profit
productivity
regulation
self-regulate
sentinel event
systematic literature review (SLR)
structural balance / power
the market
the State
welfare state
What's the problem? (WPR)
World Health Organization (WHO)

Introduction to the structure of this book

Welcome to the fourth edition of *Understanding Australian Health Care Systems.* This book introduces you to some of the core issues and theoretical concepts that provide insight into the way various Australian health care systems are organised. All health professionals work within these systems, so having a grasp of how they are organised will ease your pathway into professional life. The contributing authors have all been selected for their grasp of health research, their first-hand knowledge of these systems, and their experience in teaching undergraduate and postgraduate health professionals.

How the book works

Section One

The book is divided into two sections. Section One includes 16 chapters in which we introduce you to the range of Australian health care systems These include the mental health, worker's compensation, Indigenous, complementary and the private health care systems, along with the organisation of social services for those with a disability or chronic illness. This section also touches on the role of **Medicare**, the **Pharmaceutical Benefit Scheme (PBS)**, and concepts such as public health, primary health care, digital health, and rural health. Many of these systems continue to change, as a result of government attempts to make them more efficient and productive. To assist you in understanding what drives these changes and reforms we provide a comparison with the public and private health care systems in the United Kingdom (UK) and the United States of America (USA). Health care reform in these countries has influenced the direction of change in Australia in both the public and the private sectors. Importantly we throw light on some of the major changes occurring around quality, safety and risk.

Section Two

Section Two of the book has 12 chapters covering a range of health professions. The authors of these chapters were tasked with writing about their profession and the work that is performed by professionals from the fields of: nursing, midwifery, speech pathology, audiology, health management, paramedics, dentistry and oral health, pharmacy, sports science, exercise physiology, nutrition and diet, medicine, occupational therapy and physiotherapy. In our brief to the authors of these chapters we asked them to:

◆ outline what impact the various health reforms have had on their key quality and safety issues of relevance to their professional practice

◆ explore how their profession works interprofessionally particularly with people who have chronic conditions.

Thinking about professionals

Not all occupations call themselves professionals, so what do we mean when we talk about the health professions? When sociologists answer this question, they invariably draw on the ideas of an American sociologist, Eliot Freidson (1923–2005), who framed the answer by asking 'Who controls the work?' He argued that work in capitalist societies could be controlled by **the market** (for-profit sector), or by **the State** (governments), or by a specialised highly skilled group of workers or professionals. He suggested that where the knowledge and skills required to do a task is highly specialised, control is in the hands of a **profession**.

In Freidson's (1970a, 1970b) classic study of the professions, he positioned medicine as the most ideal typical profession and in doing so outlined the key characteristics that all professions aspire to. These are:

◆ a strong service ethic with set standards and ideals that sets it apart from other occupations

◆ specialised training and a science orientation that forms a unique body of knowledge that gives it a **professional monopoly** in this area. This monopoly is often achieved through accreditation of its educational course, and formal registration that restricts access so that other occupational groups cannot perform many of the procedures, such as prescribing drugs. This is called **professional closure**. In some instance the use of the title will be protected, such as 'nurse' or 'midwife', and

◆ **autonomy of practice** over this work, with the capacity to set their own price and **self-regulate** (Freidson 1970a, p. 2).

The power of particular health professions (such as medicine) comes from the fact that illness and disease are so unique and full of uncertainty that only this expert group has the specialist skills and knowledge to cure. Both the State and the individual patient put their trust in the professional's capacity to use their discretionary judgement to determine what is the best treatment for the patient. This trust is given to professionals by the State and the patient because it is assumed that they work in the best interest of their patients with a high level of skill underpinned by a high level of education (Freidson 1970a, 1970b). This gives the profession considerable esteem in the eyes of patients and in some instances power over the work of other health professionals. This power over other professions is described as **medical dominance** (Kenny 2004; Willis 1983).

As governments have increasingly strived to control costs through imposing health care reforms, they have moved to negotiate with the health professions, particularly medicine. Ultimately, these negotiations are over the control that the medical profession has within the health care system and attempts to curb that power through reforms, as well as control of costs.

One way that governments impose control over the health professions is through **regulation**. To this end, in 2009, the Australian federal government established the **Australian Health Practitioner Regulation Agency (AHPRA)** as it was concerned with the maldistribution of health professionals, the lack of flexibility in gaining registration across state borders and the limited access to services for some population groups. This agency has centralised the registration process of 16 health professions under 15 separate professional boards, including students. The various professional boards still manage the registration and accreditation of their members, as well as formal complaints about malpractice, but it is done under the watchful eye and with the assistance of the agency (Australian Health Practitioner Regulation Agency (AHPRA) 2018). The APRHA is currently reviewing the process of accreditation and may move to a system where an accrediting body will need to tender for the process as a result of the **Council of Australian Governments** (COAG's) Accreditation of Review (AHPRA 2018).

> **PAUSE** *for* **REFLECTION** ... As a student in a health care study program, have you noticed a hierarchy or difference in status and prestige within the various health degree programs at your university? If so, how would you organise this hierarchy of professional health degrees? Is it based on a student's score? Is it based on the number of years students must study to gain accreditation, or is it based on some other factors?

The establishment of AHPRA extends government control into the management of professions and their associations. Another control mechanism is the attempt to contain rising costs. Examples include the introduction of **Diagnosis Related Groups (DRG)** or **casemix** and **activity-based funding (ABF)** in the late 1990s and more recently the announcement by the **Independent Hospital Pricing Authority (IHPA)** to change the funding for **sentinel** and **adverse events** (Independent Hospital Pricing Authority (IHPA) 2017a, 2017b). These government-directed processes impact on the way health professionals, particularly doctors and nurses, organise care and as a consequence challenge professional autonomy (see Chapter 3 for a discussion on these reforms).

So far we have suggested that there are three major players in health care: the professions, the government (which we sometimes refer to as **the State**), and the **private for-profit** sector (which we will sometimes refer to as **the market**). Of course there is also the consumer movement representing patients (sometimes called a client, or a consumer), but there is debate and indeed, uncertainty, about how powerful they actually are in the business of health care reform (Tuohy 1999).

In the next section we provide a theoretical discussion on the factors behind health care reform. We have taken two approaches to this. Firstly, we outline what we find theoretically helpful and what we think is happening in the health care sector here in Australia, but also in many other developed nations. Secondly, we provide you with some questions for tackling health reform and health policy wherever you see it, in the hospital, in residential aged care, or in your profession's registration board.

Tuohy's theory of health care systems change

Our own theory is based on the work of Tuohy, a Canadian political scientist and her book *Accidental Logics*. Before you read our interpretation of her work, bear in mind that it is a *theory*. You should read it as a political and sociological interpretation, rather than the 'facts' or evidence-based. Theories help us to shape both what we see and how we understand the world, but they are not the truth, just a theory, although Tuohy uses case studies to support her theory. Secondly, we suggest that health care reform is driven by a series of economic philosophies and practices. They are also driven by values-based arguments about equity and the costs of inaction on equity and **effectiveness**. **Efficiency**, **effectiveness** and **equity** are core drivers for health system performance, so the theorists we have selected address these outputs in some way.

Fundamental to any theory of health care reform is the question of who pays for the services that are provided. Tuohy (1999) argues that health care reform has been high on the policy agenda in most developed nations since the early 1980s and that in all cases the debate has been couched in the following way – *given that health is central to the well-being of a nation, what role should the state play, and what role should the market play in providing health care* (Tuohy 1999, p. 3)? Behind Tuohy's question is the tension between three types of systems (Docteur & Oxley 2003). These are the public-integrated model, the public-contracted model (see Chapter 2) and the private insurance model (see Chapter 3). In the *public-integrated model*, hospitals and health services are funded directly by the government as part of the **welfare state** through levies and taxation. **Medicare** funding for public hospitals fits this model (public-integrated model). Medicare funds are also used to fund **general practice** and medical specialist services. This is an example of a *public-contracted service delivery model* provided by private providers (Docteur & Oxley 2003). The third model, the *private insurance model*, is a system where citizens pay for their health care directly to an insurer, or the professional such as you do when you go to your physiotherapist who is in private practice. Australia is a **mixed system** of all three models of service provision. We can summarise the first two models as welfare state-based or public systems (with some patient co-payments), while the third model is a market-driven system.

You can see from this three-cornered model that there are three players: the government or state, the professionals and the private for-profit sector (insurance companies, private hospitals, private professionals, medical device and pharmaceutical industries, consultants). Tuohy suggests that health reform rises or falls on who has the power between these three players. The group that holds the balance of power holds the **structural balance** (Tuohy 1999). For example power might reside in the government with its authority to freeze Medicare reimbursements for **general practitioners (GPs)** (Australian Government 2018) (Case study 1.1), or in the professions (particularly medicine) with their highly sophisticated skills, or in the private sector with its wealth and political capacity to influence decisions. As a consequence the patient is either portrayed in health policy as a citizen of the State with the right to free health care, or as a patient to whom the doctor provides the best possible care, or a consumer purchasing a health product in a competitive market.

Case Study 1.1

Shifts in the balance of power: the Medicare rebate freeze 2014–20

In the 2016 federal election the Australian Labor Party announced it would lift the freeze on GP rebates if it won the election. The irony of this was not lost of the federal Coalition Government, given it was the Labor Party that introduced this freeze on GP rebates in 2013 in order to reel the budget back in. In 2014 in the May budget the Coalition Government attempted to deal with the cost blow-outs in Medicare in other ways; one proposal was a (AU)$7 co-payment made by the patient for GP consultations, and pathology and imagining services that would be offset by a $5 reduction in the Medicare rebate the doctor received. The government quickly retracted this proposal, given the strong campaign by the **Australian Medical Association (AMA)**, the Labor party, the Greens, the Independents and other health groups and also because the freeze proposed till 2020 on GP rebates saved more money than the $7 co-payment. However, at the 2016 election the Coalition agreed to review the medical benefits schedule, and to introduce a Practice Incentive Program (Caruso et al. 2008). It also established the Health Care Homes Program (Department of Health 2018). Health Care Homes funds GP services independently of Medicare reimbursement and is not based on the time spent with a patient (as Medicare rebates currently are), but on the quality of the outcome.

As Tuohy reminds us, the political party in power must have the will to bring about particular changes, but it must also be able to mobilise support across government, the private sector and the professions to bring about change. In the case of the $7 co-payment, the Coalition Government lacked political support from within its own party and from the cross-bench members[a] whom it needed to support the legislation. It was also opposed by the medical profession and a number of health advocacy groups who ran very successful campaigns focusing on the high cost to vulnerable patients. Opposition also came from private providers of pathology services such as Sonic Health Care claiming they had had a drop in services even though the legislation was not passed. In their case, this would also have led to a drop in share price.

Tuohy (1999) refers to the idea that all the conditions for change must be right before it can be achieved as the **institutional mix** and this case study demonstrates that the medical profession was able to mobilise **structural power.**

[a]These are members of parliament who come from minor parties or are independent.

What's new in the 21st century?

In the past these three groups (professions, the State and the private sector) were presumed to use very different tactics. However, this is no longer so. Over the last 30 years all three groups have moved to use similar tactics and strategies (Tuohy 1999). The State may employ market mechanisms, or take control of the collegial system, or the private system might enter into arrangements with the State to the point that these systems are now radically changed. The classic example of this is the way in which the State has introduced market measures into the welfare state forms of health care provision. This is called **new public management** and it is driven by a philosophy called **neoliberalism** and the practices of **economic rationalism** (Stanton et al. 2003).

Philosophies and practices driving change

Economic rationalism, or microeconomic reform, is a philosophical approach, emerging from neoliberalism, to the way governments manage that part of the economy known as the welfare state or the range of services it provides for citizens. The use of the word *rationalism* suggests that all economic decisions should first focus on productivity, profits and efficiency of practices, over questions of equity and social justice. However, it is important to note that governments do not reject equity and social justice in providing welfare services such as health and education to its citizens; however, they do put **productivity** and efficiency higher on the agenda and argue for strategies to achieve efficiency and productivity in spending tax-payers' money.

Proponents of economic rationalism also argue that the best way to ensure a robust economy and prosperity for the majority of people in any society is for the economy to be under the control of the private sector, rather than governments. Behind the philosophy is the idea that freedom in the economic sphere of society will generate wealth, productivity and efficiency across society (Stanton et al. 2005). Neoliberals also hold the view that individuals tend to act in their own self-interest. As a consequence they believe that, in a robust democracy, there should be maximum freedom of choice for the individual and limited interference by governments in citizens' lives or in their business dealings, in the belief that individuals will strive to achieve the best outcomes for themselves.

New public management (NPM)

NPM suggests that the public service and the welfare state, funded by government through tax-payers' money, can be made more efficient and productive if it is run like a private company operating through competitive practices. Examples include paying public hospitals bonuses if they see more patients, or keeping back a percentage of the budget until a service meets a target. Activity-based funding is another example. NPM can also include outsourcing non-essential services in the public sector such as cleaning and catering to a private company, or turning a public hospital pathology and radiology service into a business that must make a profit. It also means that when governments want a particular task done they must put it out to competitive tender allowing private companies to compete for the job, and in some cases the government and a private company may run a service such as a hospital together in what is known as a **public–private partnership (PPP).**

As a set of practices, NPM is not limited to health care or to Australia. NPM practices can be found in many other parts of the welfare state such as education, Indigenous affairs and provisions for the unemployed (outsourcing of funds to private companies to help the unemployed find work), and in many other countries. For example, following the **global financial crisis (GFC)** the International Monetary Fund and World Bank insisted that countries that needed to borrow funds to bail out their economies introduce the practices of NPM into their health care systems (van Gool & Pearson 2014).

Is new public management dead?

Some political scientists argue that new public management is dead (Crouch 2011). We would argue that it is alive and well, and takes new forms with each decade. One new approach deals with patient quality, safety and risk. Throughout this book, various authors will discuss the impact of the Australian Commission for Safety and Quality in Health Care on their profession (Australian Commission for Safety and Quality in Health Care (ACSQHC) 2017). The Commission publishes a number of standards that clinicians, hospitals, and health organisations need to meet in order to be accredited. This brings the control down to the level of the professional doctor, nurse or manager. Accreditation of hospitals is linked to the capacity to abide by the national standards. While it is important to keep Australian patients safe and to provide them with quality health care, many clinical standards and practices are now set by regulatory agencies such as the ACSQHC. You may like to return to an earlier section of this chapter where we discussed the key characteristics of professions and the role of the AHPRA, another regulatory agency. If the Commission sets standards that must be met by hospitals, and AHPRA accredits the professions, do health professions continue to have autonomy of practice?

PAUSE
for
REFLECTION
...

As of July 2018, the Independent Hospital Pricing Authority has indicated the federal government will not reimburse state and territory health departments at the same rate for **hospital-acquired conditions (HACs)** such as **hospital-acquired infections (HAIs)**. According to research by Mitchell et al. (2017), about 165,000 Australians contract an infection while in hospital every year. They report that Australia is the only **Organisation for Economic Co-operation and Development (OECD)** country that does not undertake regular surveys on the prevalence of infections or collect data on the exact number of HAIs.

At the same time one of the National Standards promulgated by the ACSQHC is **antimicrobial stewardship**. This requires all hospitals to have governance committees in place to ensure judicious use of antibiotics, given the dangers of over-use (ACSQHC 2018)

Some doctors in the past have used antibiotics *prophylactically* to ensure their patients do not get an infection post-surgery.

What dilemma can you now see facing these doctors given the two regulations above?

How to ask questions about health care reform

As you progress through your studies it will be useful to have a set of strategies for examining all health care reforms. There will certainly be many over the life of your career. Tuohy (1999) asks who has the balance of power at that particular time. Another approach is to examine the policy problem and to ask questions about how the problem is described. A political scientist who has done much work in this area is Carol Bacchi. She has developed a set of questions and bundled them together under the heading '*What's the problem represented to be*? (Bacchi 2012, 2016). **What's the problem (WPR)** argues that, when governments (or private companies) decide on a particular policy action, what is proposed tells us what they think the problem is. WPR provides six questions you can use when reading each chapter for your program of study. These six questions are presented in Table 1.1, along with Tuohy's question as no. 7.

TABLE 1.1 BACCHI AND TUOHY POLICY KEY QUESTIONS

1 What's the 'problem' represented to be in a specific policy proposal?	In the example of the $7 co-payment, it would appear the government saw the problem as a blow-out of the Medicare budget.
2 What presuppositions or assumptions underpin this representation of the 'problem'?	A co-payment would send a price signal to patients that each visit is costly. Behind this is the assumption that Australian citizens go to the doctor too often, and at times these visits are unnecessary. If we were aware of the costs we would go less often. There is an assumption that health expenditure must 'fit' within the current budget. An alternative policy direction could have been to increase the Medicare levy (taxing everyone, not just those who go to the doctor).
3 How has this representation of the 'problem' come about?	There is an assumption that citizens will abuse anything that is free, and be more careful when they have to pay for a service.
4 What is left unproblematic in this problem representation? Where are the silences? Can the problem be thought about differently?	The problem with this assumption is that we do not know whether or not people go to the doctor unnecessarily. There are no data to suggest this either way. But it is clear that this behaviour is what the policy set out to change.

Continued

TABLE 1.1 BACCHI AND TUOHY POLICY KEY QUESTIONS—cont'd	
5 What effects are produced by this representation of the 'problem'?	Well before the legislation was dropped by the Coalition Government many people stopped going to the doctor, and went to Accident and Emergency Departments instead. Private providers of pathology services claimed there was a drop in services even though the legislation had not passed.
6 How/where has this representation of the 'problem' been produced, disseminated and defended? How has it been (or could it be) questioned, disrupted and replaced? (Bacchi 2012).	Another way of defining the problem might be to suggest that paying doctors by the quantity of patients they treat, rather than the quality or effectiveness of their treatment, might be a fundamental flaw of Medicare. While it is true that health care costs have spiralled, it is also true that there has been little debate within the political arena about how much money we could spend, or want to spend on health care, or where such escalation of costs come from within the system. The co-payment focuses only on the user component rather than many aspects of demand in the system that could be considered as part of 'the problem'.
7 What do the three interest groups say about this problem, and what assumptions do they make?	The medical profession argued that it was inequitable and would mean poorer people would go without health care. They successfully lobbied for the policy to be dropped. Other consumer-led groups such as Save Our Medicare and GetUp had local campaigns and rallies, petition signing, phone calling and pamphlet campaigns to voice consumer concerns. Even within the government, politicians on the cross-bench argued against the co-payment.

Source: Bacchi C (2012) Introducing the 'What's the problem represented to be?' approach, in: Bletas A, Beasely C (Eds.) Engaging with Carol Bacchi: Strategic Interventions and Exchanges, University of Adelaide Press, Adelaide, pp. 21–24, https://www.adelaide.edu.au/carst/docs/wpr/wpr-summary.pdf

We have taken the proposed $7 co-payment as an example of how we analysed the policy. We suggest you might like to use this framework when you come to each chapter and consider the issues raised by the authors.

Interprofessional practice or navigator

Many attempts at health reform have been efforts to overcome fragmentation and duplication of health service delivery. Dealing with the fragmentation of how health professionals work has given rise to the concept of **interprofessional practice (IPP)**, which is the intended outcome from **interprofessional education (IPE)**. If you are studying health systems with students from a range of other professions, this is the first step in understanding their practice, in order that you might eventually work together. To summarise: *interprofessional education is defined as an intervention where the members of more than one health or social care profession, or both, learn interactively together, for the explicit purpose of improving interprofessional collaboration or the health / well-being of patients / clients, or both* (Reeves et al. 2013, p. 2).

The champions of IPP suggest it is required because it promotes efficiencies through teamwork and collaboration. IPP is seen as a strategy to help ameliorate the worldwide shortage of health professionals, estimated to be around 4.3 million (**World Health Organization (WHO)** 2010). Given the high costs associated with health care, including the cost of educating professionals, there is an argument for stronger team and collaborative approaches to patient care. This argument extends across the health spectrum from **community and public health** to **acute care** and from the developed world with its highly technological health systems to countries with low levels of health infrastructure. A genuine team approach provides opportunities quality time spent in patient assessment, and referrals and may even reduce the number of tests ordered. IPE that leads to IPP is also seen to reduce adverse events and to have higher patient satisfaction (WHO 2010).

If, as professionals, our work is based on the best scientific evidence it is important to test the evidence of those who champion IPP given its claims that it can improve the way professionals work. This can be done through examining **evidence-based medicine (EBM)**, particularly what is provided through the Cochrane database for **systematic literature review (SLR)**. A Cochrane SLR published in 2013 by Reeves et al., which updated their previous study (Laurant et al. 2005), examined IPP research published between 2006 and 2011. All these studies asked whether IPP had a positive impact on patient outcomes.

Reeves et al. (2013, p. 16) note that in 1999 when they did their first review they could find no eligible studies. However, they agree IPP is a growing area of health care reform that focuses on the very way health professionals work. This puts you and your profession smack in the middle of exciting and dynamic reform processes that promise to improve treatment for patients, to make work more interesting for clinicians and to provide a service that saves money. However, they write that what is still required are 'studies that assess the effectiveness of IPP interventions compared to separate, profession-specific interventions; second, RCT, CBA or ITS studies with qualitative strands examining processes relating to the IPP and practice changes; third, cost-benefit analyses' (p. 2). In support of this they did a further review in 2017 (Reeves et al. 2017), where once again they were cautiously in support of IPP, grading the evidence as low. This is a strange outcome, given the difficulties health professional (and patients) experience in communicating and that many **adverse events** are thought to originate in poor communication.

Another approach being taken in some Australian states, given the poor communication between health professionals, is the appointment of nurse navigators, midwife navigators or patient navigators (Queensland Government 2015). These health professionals take a patient focus, rather than a professional focus, and navigate the system for the person with a chronic illness, or a women who is vulnerable following the birth of a child (Dick 2017). Case study 1.2 outlines some initiatives being taken in rural New South Wales (NSW) by either nurse or midwife navigators to ensure women have greater access to care. It demonstrates the shift in the navigator model from an interprofessional focus to a patient focus.

Case Study 1.2

In Australia publicly funded, comprehensive and universal maternity services are available to all women. On leaving hospital with their baby, women transition to publicly funded child and family health services until their child reaches 5 years. Despite what looks like a seamless service, there are many issues in ensuring all women are able to access this care. In 2010 the CHoRUS study set out to discover what were the barriers to transition to care within NSW, and what were best practice models. All the usual barriers were present – lack of communication and failure of health professionals to talk or consult with each other. In several rural general practices and community health services, nurses or midwives have been appointed who meet with the women while they are in hospital and then assist them to navigate taking their baby home and contacting the child health services. While the women are in hospital these navigators have access to the multidisciplinary team, but they are also part of the team meetings within the community health services. These nurses or midwives are able to assess if the women or her baby need additional intervention from a wider multidisciplinary team and escalate the appointments with the appropriate service. Interestingly, the research reports that for these nurses and midwives their interprofessional practice is primarily with allied health professionals, rather than with medical professionals (Psaila et al. 2014a, 2014b).

What else have we provided?

To assist you in thinking about these questions, this book provides a number of resources. These include cross-references to other chapters that refer to similar topics, **Further Reading** lists useful for following up the issues, a **Glossary** of concepts and acronyms, and a list of **Abbreviations**. Remembering these terms is one strategy for coming to grips with all the complex systems. All chapters provide a list of **Review Questions** and **Online Resources**. If you are doing a tutorial these questions and the additional readings will be a useful guide. The chapters also provide you with a **Case study** that illustrates some of the issues pertinent to the topic. These are mainly patient or consumer focused. The **Pause for Reflection boxes** provide you with opportunity to reflect on the material. Throughout the book, the term 'patient' is generally used to refer to someone in an acute setting and 'client' as someone in a community setting.

Summary

In this introduction we have provided background on the following;

- The organisation of the book – it is divided into two sections with the first section covering a number of Australian health care systems and the second section dealing with 11 health professional groups.
- Key theoretical ideas proposed by Tuohy (1999) suggest that serious health reform occurs only at particular moments in history when all the necessary factors are in place for the group/s with the balance of power. These groups are the State, the market and the professions.
- We also suggested that you apply the questions raised by Bacchi (2012) to any health policy reform you encounter.
- The reform process of new public management was also discussed. We suggested it is still in use.
- Among new directions for clinical reform are interprofessional education and interprofessional practice. While these are being enthusiastically supported, to date there is insufficient evidence to suggest that they will revolutionise health care. An alternative approach is to use navigators.

Review Questions

1. What three groups have the balance of power in any health care system?
2. If a country has a national health service, what group would you presume has the balance of power?
3. Besides the balance of power, Tuohy (1999) suggests reform is shaped by a particular institutional mix. Can you identify particular political, historical or cultural factors that might influence the kinds of reforms introduced in Australia in the next few years?
4. Given that the federal government has established a number of regulatory agencies to oversee health care such as the Independent Hospital Pricing Authority (which sets the price paid for care) and the Commission for Safety and Quality in Health Care, how much autonomy do health professionals have when they work within a hospital or GP clinic?
5. In our view, nurses, midwives and allied health professionals have more to gain from IPP than doctors. Do you agree with this statement and, if so, why?

References

Australian Commission for Safety and Quality in Health Care (ACSQHC), 2017. Australian safety and quality framework for health care: putting the framework into action. ACSQHC, Sydney. https://www. safetyandquality.gov.au/wp-content/uploads/2011/01/ASQFHC-Guide-Healthcare-team.pdf.

Australian Commission for Safety and Quality in Health Care (ACSQHC), 2018. Antimicrobial Stewardship in Australian Health Care 2018. ACSQHC, Sydney.

Australian Government, 2018. Medicare indexation schedule. https://www.humanservices.gov.au/ individuals/services/medicare/medicare-safety-net.

Australian Health Practitioner Regulation Agency (AHPRA), 2018. Home page. https://www.ahpra. gov.au/.

Bacchi, C., 2012. Introducing the 'What's the problem represented to be?' approach. In: Bletsas, A., Beasley, C. (Eds.), Engaging With Carol Bacchi: Strategic Interventions and Exchanges. University of Adelaide Press, Adelaide, pp. 21–24. https://www.adelaide.edu.au/carst/docs/wpr/wpr-summary.pdf.

Bacchi, C., 2016. Problematizations in health policy: questioning how "problems" are constituted in policies. Paper presented at the ASSA (Academy of the Social Sciences)-funded Workshop on Understanding Australian Policies on Public Health, Flinders University.

Caruso, E., Cisar, N., Pipe, T., 2008. Creating a healing environment: an innovative educational approach for adopting Jean Watson's theory of human caring. Nurs. Adm. Q. 32 (2), 126–132.

Crouch, C., 2011. The Strange Non-Death of Neo-Liberalism. Polity Press, Cambridge.

Department of Health (DOH), 2018. Health Care Homes' updates and factsheets. DOH, Canberra. http:// www.health.gov.au/internet/main/publishing.nsf/Content/health-care-homes-information.

Dick, C., 2017. Vulnerable women to receive specialised midwifery care. http://statements.qld.gov.au/ Statement/2017/8/2/vulnerable-women-to-receive-specialised-midwifery-care.

Docteur, E., Oxley, H., 2003. Health-care systems: lessons from the reform experience. OECD, Paris. www. oecd.org/dataoecd/5/53/22364122.pdf.

Freidson, E., 1970a. Professional Dominance. Atherton Press, New York.

Freidson, E., 1970b. Profession of Medicine: A Study of the Sociology of Applied Knowledge. University of Chicago Press, Chicago.

Independent Hospital Pricing Authority (IHPA), 2017a. Pricing framework for Australian public hospital services 2017–2018. IHPA, Sydney. https://www.ihpa.gov.au/consultation/ pricing-framework-australian-public-hospital-services-2017-18.

Independent Hospital Pricing Authority (IHPA), 2017b. Risk adjustment model for hospital acquired complications: technical specifications – version 1.0. IHPA, Sydney. https://www.ihpa.gov.au/sites/g/ files/net636/f/risk_adjustment_model_for_hospital_acquired_complications_-_technical_ specifications_v1.0_july_2017_pdf.pdf.

Kenny, A., 2004. Medical dominance and power: a rural perspective. Health Sociol. Rev. 13, 158–165.

Laurant, M., Reeves, D., Hermanns, R., et al., 2005. Substitution of doctors by nurses in primary care. Cochrane Database Syst. Rev. (2), CD001271.

Mitchell, B., Shaban, R., MacBeth, D., et al., 2017. The burden of healthcare-associated infections in Australian hospitals: a systematic review of the literature. Infect. Dis. Health 22, 117–128.

Psaila, K., Fowler, C., Kruske, S., et al., 2014a. A qualitative study of innovations implemented to improve transition of care from maternity to child and family health (CFH) services in Australia. Women Birth 27, e51–e60. doi:10.1016/j.wombi.2014.08.004.

Psaila, K., Schmied, V., Fowler, C., et al., 2014b. Interprofessional collaboration at transition of care: perspectives of child and family health nurses and midwives. J. Clin. Nurs. 24, 160–172. doi:10.1111/jocn.12635.

Queensland Government, 2015. Nurse navigators. https://www.health.qld.gov.au/ocnmo/nursing/nurse-navigators.

Reeves, S., Perrier, L., Goldman, J., et al., 2013. Interprofessional education: effects on professional practice and healthcare outcomes (update). Cochrane Database Syst. Rev. (3), CD002213.

Reeves, S., Peline, F., Harrison, R., et al., 2017. Interprofessional collaboration to improve professional practice and healthcare outcomes (reveiw). Cochrane Database Syst. Rev. (6), CD000072.

Stanton, P., Willis, E., White, S., 2005. Workplace Reform in the Healthcare Sector: The Australian Experience. Palgrave Macmillan, London.

Stanton, P., Young, S., Willis, E.M., 2003. Financial restraint, budget cuts and outsourcing: impact of the new public management of health care in Victoria. Contemp. Nurse 14 (2), 115–122.

Tuohy, C., 1999. Accidental Logics: The Dynamics of Change in the Health Care Arena in the United States, Britan and Canada. OUP, New York.

van Gool, K., Pearson, M., 2014. Health, austerity and economic crisis: assessing the short-term impact in OECD countries. OECD working paper 76. OECD, Paris. https://www.oecd-ilibrary.org/docserver/5jxx71lt1zg6-en.pdf?expires=1556038444&id=id&accname=guest&checksum=B51ED36DA7B4FAC4D7F6B2395926F786.

Willis, E., 1983. Medical Dominance: the division of labour in Australian health care. Allan and Unwin, Sydney.

World Health Organization (WHO), 2010. Framework for action on interprofessional education and collaborative practice (WHO/HRH/HPN/10.3). WHO, Geneva. https://apps.who.int/iris/bitstream/handle/10665/70185/WHO_HRH_HPN_10.3_eng.pdf;jsessionid=A6E1F14B1A6E48045764A7505BBF87F9?sequence=1.

Further Reading

Alford, R., 1975. Health Care Politics: Ideological and Interest Group Barriers to Reform. University of Chicago Press, Chicago.

Mody, L., Meddings, J., Edson, B., et al., 2015. Enhancing resident safety by preventing healthcare-associated infection: a national initiative to reduce catheter-associated urinary tract infections in nursing homes. Clin. Infect. Dis. 1 (61), 86–94.

Tuohy, C., 1999. Accidental Logics: The Dynamics of Change in the Health Care Arena in the United States, Britain and Canada. OUP, New York.

Willis, E., 1989. Medical Dominance. Allen and Unwin, Sydney.

Online Resources

Keep up with all the major reforms in Australian Health at: http://www.health.gov.au/internet/main/publishing.nsf/Content/Home.

Keep up with the latest digital health innovations at: http://www.pulseitmagazine.com.au/.

Learn what is happening in your professions at AHPRA home page at: https://www.ahpra.gov.au/.

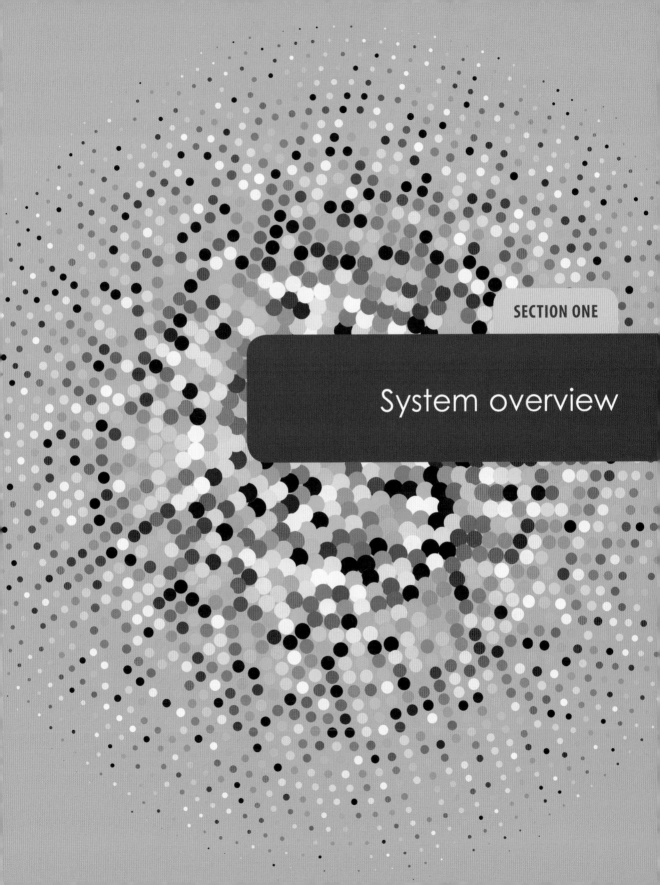

SECTION ONE

System overview

CHAPTER 2

The public health sector and Medicare

Lindsay Krassnitzer

Key learning outcomes

When you finish this chapter you should be able to:

- ◆ understand how the public health care sector in Australia is organised, funded and delivered
- ◆ describe the purpose and function of Medicare and its role in the Australian health care system
- ◆ recognise the role of public hospitals within the Australian health care system, and how they are funded and administered
- ◆ articulate and critique the roles of local, state and federal governments in funding and managing the public health care sector in Australia.

Key terms and abbreviations

activity-based funding
bed block
blame game
bulk-billing
co-payment/gap payment
Council of Australian Governments (COAG)
elective surgery
gate-keepers
general practitioners (GPs)
Gross Domestic Product (GDP)
hospital separation
inpatient
Local Hospital Network/Local Health Network (LHN)
market-based
market failure
Medicare
Medicare Benefits Schedule (MBS)
Medicare levy surcharge (MLS)
National Disability Insurance Scheme (NDIS)
outpatient
perverse financial incentives
Pharmaceutical Benefits Scheme (PBS)
progressive tax
universal access
welfare state

Introduction to the public health sector in Australia

The Australian health care system operates under a mixed model of public and private services. This chapter addresses the major components of the public health care sector: **Medicare** and public hospital services. The Australian public health care system is based on the principle of **universal access**; this means that all citizens (and permanent residents) have equal *access* to medical services. A universal health care system is one feature of a **welfare state**; 'welfare state' means a society in which the government provides for the welfare of citizens in terms of health care and other social services. In general terms, Australian society can be described as a modern **market-based** economy, with the country supporting the welfare state in many forms. The dual forces of the welfare state and market-based economy cause perpetual tensions in how the Australian health care system is administered and between stakeholders; some of these tensions are explored in this chapter. Similarly, the relationship between the private health and public health sectors has been described as an 'uneasy compromise' (Gray 2004), and Boxall and Gillespie state that 'attempts to find a sustainable balance between the two sectors have been a major driver of reform' (2013, p. 182). The mixed model system creates problems owing to the undefined roles of each sector (Boxall 2010; Boxall & Gillespie 2013), as we will explore in this chapter.

Health is considered a fundamental human right and every country of the world supports this notion, although achieving it is another question (World Health Organization (WHO) 2008). Health is also highly political (Duckett & Willcox 2015) – with the health system, its funding and outcomes being prominent throughout political debates. One of the driving forces for a universal access system is the idea that a market-based economy will not provide for those unable to purchase health services for themselves. This is known as **market failure** and in market-based societies this is a legitimate instance where government intervention is required to ensure all citizens have access to a service such as health care (Duckett & Willcox 2015; Podger & Hagan 1999).

Prior to 1975, Australians needed to purchase health insurance to provide for their own health care needs. Many people could not afford to do so and were disadvantaged by the failure of both the market and the government to provide health services for them. In 1975, the Whitlam Labor Government established an Australian health insurance scheme known as Medibank. In 1984, Medibank was re-introduced by the Hawke Labor Government as Medicare, which, with modifications, operates today. Australia is joined by countries such as Canada, Sweden, Singapore, New Zealand and the United Kingdom in providing a taxpayer-funded national health system accessible by all (Organisation for Economic Co-operation and Development (OECD) 2013).

The Australian health care system delivers some of the best health outcomes in the world, with one of the highest life expectancies and one of the lowest mortality rates under competitive expenditure levels in comparison with other similar countries (Australian Institute of Health and Welfare (AIHW) 2018a). It is important to remember this when discussing and debating the problems within the health care system: the system is not perfect but performs well when compared globally, although we should remember that the health care system is not the only contributor to health status. Current challenges facing the health system include ongoing tensions within the mixed model system, between levels of government and between policy-makers about the best way to organise the system

(Hall 2015; Macri 2016); population health challenges associated with the proliferation of chronic diseases and modifiable behavioural risk factors (AIHW 2016); and debates regarding health care costs (Eckermann et al. 2016).

PAUSE *for* REFLECTION ...   Fig. 2.1 from the AIHW provides data on a range of population health indicators amongst OECD countries. Were you surprised by these figures? Where Australia is performing below the OECD average, what could be done to improve these indicators?

Australian health care system administration and reform

Administration of the Australian health care system is complex and involves all (three) levels of government and other stakeholders, including private and public service providers. This leaves the system vulnerable to tensions between levels of government, and between external stakeholders who have varying levels of interest and influence in how the system functions. For example, Chapter 1 of this book introduced the concept of medical dominance – the medical profession is a powerful interest group and exerts considerable influence over how the health system is organised and funded (Palmer & Short 2014). Multiple stakeholders have vested interests in the Australian health care system. Gray (2004) puts it this way:

◆ Service providers are concerned with profit, income and clinical autonomy.
◆ Citizens are concerned with affordable access to quality services.
◆ Governments are concerned with ideology, electoral popularity and budgets.

Gray (2004) argues that these competing demands cannot all be addressed at the same time and, as Tuohy (1999) has noted, reform is contingent on the balance of power between these competing groups. Hall (2015, p. 493) describes the layers of government involvement in the Australian health care system as a 'strife of interests'.

The federal government does not directly provide health services, but is responsible for major funding programs such as universal medical services, the **Pharmaceutical Benefits Scheme (PBS)** and funding to state and territory governments to assist in the provision of public hospital services. The federal government is also responsible for the national administration of the health system and regulation of health care practitioners through the Australian Health Practitioner Regulation Agency, and it subsidises the uptake of private health insurance. The **Council of Australian Governments (COAG)** – made up of the state and territory premiers, the Prime Minister and the President of the Australian Local Government Association – through the COAG Health Council and its various committees provides national directions for health reform.

State and territory governments are responsible for financing (with assistance from the federal government) and managing public hospital services and other services such as public ambulance

FIGURE 2.1 OECD POPULATION HEALTH INDICATORS

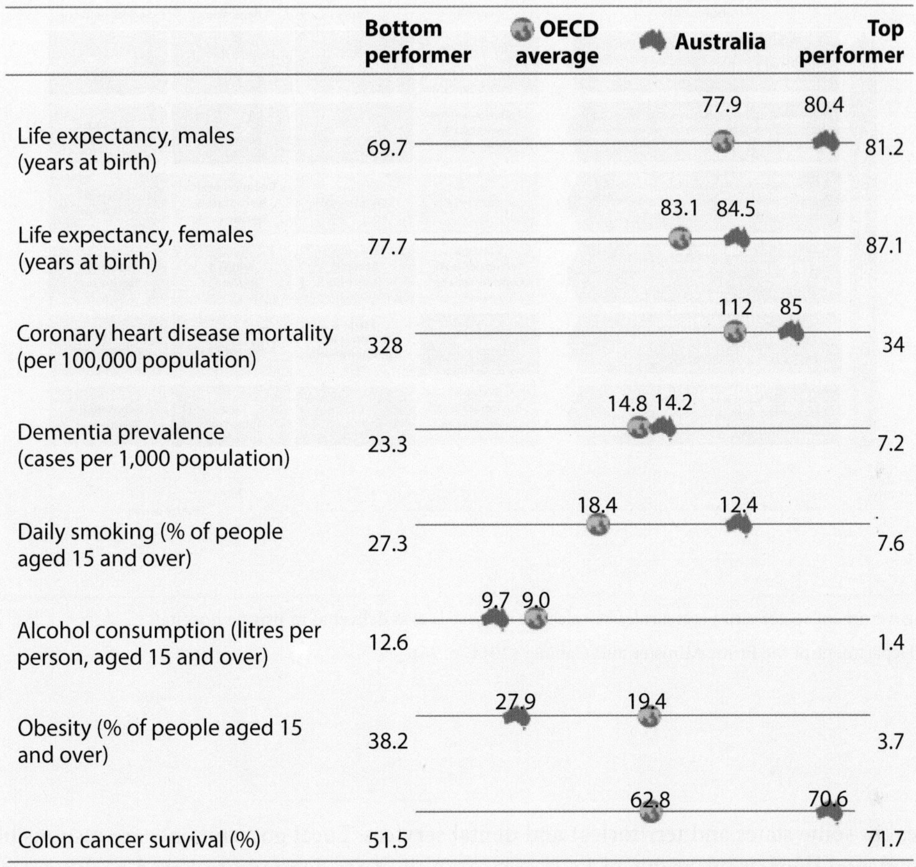

	Bottom performer	OECD average	Australia	Top performer
Life expectancy, males (years at birth)	69.7	77.9		80.4 / 81.2
Life expectancy, females (years at birth)	77.7	83.1	84.5	87.1
Coronary heart disease mortality (per 100,000 population)	328	112	85	34
Dementia prevalence (cases per 1,000 population)	23.3	14.8	14.2	7.2
Daily smoking (% of people aged 15 and over)	27.3	18.4	12.4	7.6
Alcohol consumption (litres per person, aged 15 and over)	12.6	9.7 / 9.0		1.4
Obesity (% of people aged 15 and over)	38.2	27.9	19.4	3.7
Colon cancer survival (%)	51.5	62.8	70.6	71.7

Note: Data for Australia reflect those in the OECD Statistics database and may differ from data presented elsewhere in this report due to the potential for slight variation in data definitions and calculation methodologies.

Sources: Australian Institute of Health and Welfare (2018a). Australia's health 2018, p. 30; Organisation for Economic Co-operation and Development (2017). Health at a Glance 2017: OECD Indicators. OECD, Paris.

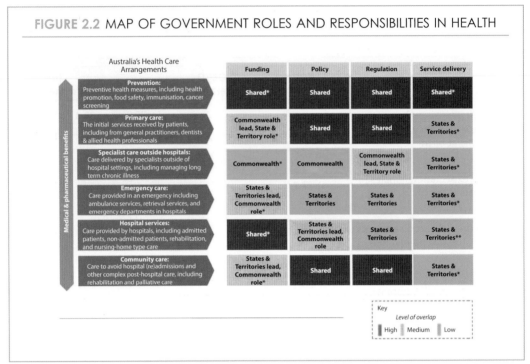

FIGURE 2.2 MAP OF GOVERNMENT ROLES AND RESPONSIBILITIES IN HEALTH

*=non-government sector also plays a role; **=elective surgery is also delivered in private hospitals

Source: Department of the Prime Minister and Cabinet (2014, p. 26)

services (in some states and territories) and dental services. Local governments are responsible for environmental impacts on health in local areas as well as for community-based health programs, food safety and physical environment impacts on health (such as public space). In addition to government involvement, private for-profit and not-for-profit agencies offer health services and private health insurance for purchase by individuals. Figs 2.2 and 2.3 provide detailed overviews of the roles and responsibilities of the different levels of government in funding, policy, regulation and service delivery, and where these overlap.

The organisation of the Australian health care system is complex, with multiple layers of administration, service delivery and financing. It is considered fragmented and bureaucratic (Hall 2015; National Health and Hospitals Reform Commission 2009). One of the outcomes of this fragmented health care system is the phenomenon of cost-shifting (see Box 2.1). Dwyer and Eagar (2008, p. 5) suggest that 'The current split of responsibilities sets up **perverse financial incentives** for governments and other providers, whereby one level can "win" financially through measures that cause the other

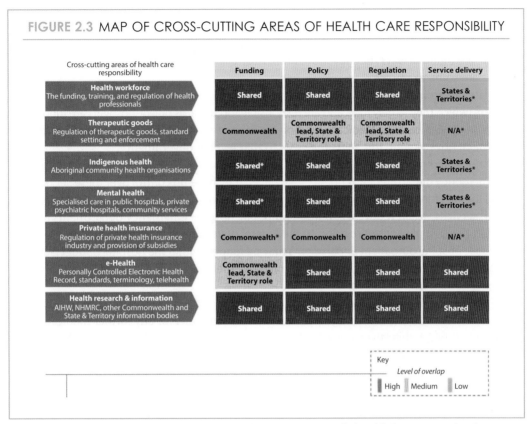

FIGURE 2.3 MAP OF CROSS-CUTTING AREAS OF HEALTH CARE RESPONSIBILITY

Cross-cutting areas of health care responsibility	Funding	Policy	Regulation	Service delivery
Health workforce The funding, training, and regulation of health professionals	Shared	Shared	Shared	States & Territories*
Therapeutic goods Regulation of therapeutic goods, standard setting and enforcement	Commonwealth	Commonwealth lead, State & Territory role	Commonwealth lead, State & Territory role	N/A*
Indigenous health Aboriginal community health organisations	Shared*	Shared	Shared	States & Territories*
Mental health Specialised care in public hospitals, private psychiatric hospitals, community services	Shared*	Shared	Shared	States & Territories*
Private health insurance Regulation of private health insurance industry and provision of subsidies	Commonwealth*	Commonwealth	Commonwealth	N/A*
e-Health Personally Controlled Electronic Health Record, standards, terminology, telehealth	Commonwealth lead, State & Territory role	Shared	Shared	Shared
Health research & information AIHW, NHMRC, other Commonwealth and State & Territory information bodies	Shared	Shared	Shared	Shared

Key
Level of overlap
High   Medium   Low

*=non-government sector also plays a role; **=Aboriginal Community Controlled Health Organisations also play a significant role

Source: Department of the Prime Minister and Cabinet (2014, p. 27)

level to "lose" financially.' If we explore Bacchi's (2012) 'What's the problem represented to be?' (WPR) framework (see Chapter 1), it is evident that the ways the health system is organised and funded are presented as *fundamental problems* and reform is the strategy used to attempt to resolve these problems.

Australian health reform generally focuses on two main issues: the relationship and responsibilities of the different levels of government in the health system, and the relationship between the private and the public health sectors (Palmer & Short 2014). Analysing the role of government in the Australian health care system is not new; however, Duckett (1999) suggests that the status quo may suit both levels of government as each can blame the other for deficiencies in the system.

BOX 2.1 COST-SHIFTING IN PRACTICE

There are multiple ways that governments in Australia can shift costs between each other. Here are some examples:

- State governments have an incentive to shift people away from expensive in-hospital care (which they largely fund and are responsible for) towards out-of-hospital care funded through Medicare. As Medicare funding for GP and specialist services comes from the federal government, this shifts the costs to that level of government.
- State governments have an interest in improving out-of-hours GP services to reduce emergency department attendances; however, they have no control over these services as they are funded by the federal government. Increasing access to affordable out-of-hours GP services would reduce the burden on public hospital emergency departments and shift the cost of service provision to the federal government.
- Public hospital outpatient departments may be funded within the hospital budget (state government responsibility) or may be billed as medical services to Medicare (federal government responsibility).
- Public hospitals provide medications to inpatients during their stay as part of their package of care, but will often discharge patients with prescriptions for any further medication required, which shifts the costs to the federal government-funded Pharmaceutical Benefits Scheme.

   This constant shifting between the two levels of government is referred to as the **'blame game'**.

PAUSE
for
REFLECTION
...

This section has briefly introduced you to the bureaucracy behind the Australian health care system. There are many levels of government involved in administering and funding this system and this mixed involvement can result in tensions, blame and cost-shifting. Drawing on the ideas outlined by Bacchi (2012) in Chapter 1, reflect on how the Australian health system is represented in the media. Does this representation accurately reflect the status of the Australian health system? Using Bacchi's questions, note down why you think the health system is represented the way it is.

Financing the Australian health care system

Within the Australian health care system, some medical care (such as public hospital care) is provided free of charge, whereas in other cases the health consumers are expected to contribute to the cost of the services they receive, which is known as a **co-payment** or **gap payment**. The government does not control the fees charged by private health practitioners (such as **general practitioners (GPs)**, private medical specialists and allied health professionals); they are able to set their own fees. Constitutionally, the government cannot force doctors to charge certain prices (you can read more about this in Chapter 21) (Elliot 2003). Medical practitioner fees and gap payments attract significant interest and were explored in the Senate Community Affairs Reference Committee review 'The value and affordability of private health insurance and out-of-pocket medical costs' (Parliament of Australia Senate Community Affairs References Committee 2017). Although most of the Senate Inquiry recommendations focused on private health insurance, one of the recommendations (5.23) was that the Australian Government should 'publish the fees of individual medical practitioners in a searchable database' (Department of Health, 2018a, p. ix). The Australian Government subsequently announced a Ministerial Advisory Committee on out-of-pocket costs, partly to investigate legal barriers to the publishing of medical practitioner fees.

Funding for the Australian health care system receives constant and intense scrutiny. Government health expenditure has been increasing over the past decade at approximately 5% per annum (AIHW 2018a). Governments have a vested interest in containing costs for political and budgetary reasons; however, it is argued that health service providers naturally resist government efforts to contain costs (and by default constrain their incomes), and there is 'an absence of sufficient political will to confront a powerful medical establishment' in relation to capping fees and gap payments (Gray 2004, p. 22). At present there is no systemic cap on funding available through Medicare benefits and therefore expenditure increases as service use increases (Duckett & Willcox 2015). One outcome of this approach is that 'supplier-induced demand' can influence the use of health services (Eckermann et al. 2016).

Overall health expenditure in Australia in 2015–16 was approximately (AU)\$170 billion, of which two-thirds was funded by governments and one-third was funded by non-government sources, including individuals (AIHW 2018a). Fig. 2.4 demonstrates how this funding was spent in 2015–16. In 2015–16, the Australian government provided 41% of the total health expenditure; state governments funded 26% of total health expenditure and individuals funded 17% of total health expenditure (AIHW 2018a). In 2018–19, total funding for health services by the Australian government comprised 16% of its overall budget, at almost \$79 billion (Commonwealth of Australia 2018). Although the health sector consumes considerable resources, it is also an important component of the Australian economy as the largest employing industry, with over 13% of the total Australian workforce. Over 1.6 million Australians are employed in the health and social assistance industry overall (Australian Bureau of Statistics 2018), including over 670,000 registered health practitioners (Australian Health Practitioner Regulation Agency 2017).

Health expenditure in Australia represents 9.6% of **Gross Domestic Product (GDP)** (AIHW 2018a), which is comparable to other OECD countries (Hall 2015). The country with the highest health expenditure in relation to GDP is the USA, where health expenditure consumes over 17% of GDP – markedly higher than any other OECD country (although the quality of health outcomes achieved for this level of expenditure is certainly questionable – see Chapter 3 for more details). In the 10-year period 2006–07 to 2015–16, total health expenditure in Australia increased by 50%.

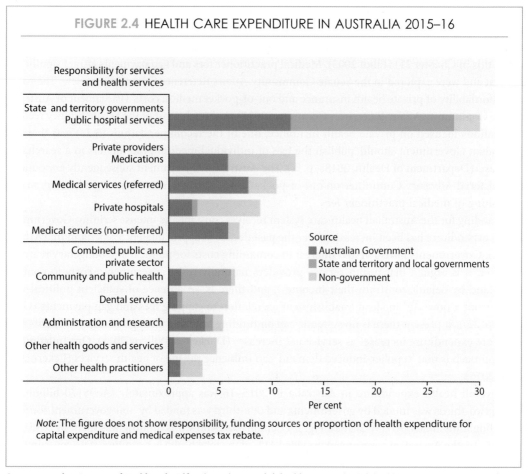

FIGURE 2.4 HEALTH CARE EXPENDITURE IN AUSTRALIA 2015–16

Note: The figure does not show responsibility, funding sources or proportion of health expenditure for capital expenditure and medical expenses tax rebate.

Source: Australian Institute of Health and Welfare (2018a). Australia's health 2018, Australia's health series no. 16. AUS221. AIHW, Canberra, p. 44. https://www.aihw.gov.au/getmedia/7c42913d-295f-4bc9-9c24-4e44eff4a04a/aihw-aus-221.pdf.aspx?inline=true

Medicare

Medicare is Australia's major health funding program, comprising a universal health insurance scheme that is administered (since 2011) by the Department of Human Services and legislated under the *Health Insurance Act 1973*. Medicare is based on the principle of universal access and ensures that all Australian citizens and permanent residents have access to medical and hospital services which are either paid in full or subsidised by government. One of the important aspects of Medicare is that treatment provided in public hospitals is always provided free of charge to the patient. Medicare also funds a limited range of non-medical services, including eye tests through optometrists and some referred allied health services. In addition to free or subsidised medical services, Australia also provides subsidised access to pharmaceuticals through the Pharmaceutical Benefits Scheme (see Chapter 7) as well as reciprocal health care agreements so that Australians can access health care in a number of other countries.

In 2016–17, almost 25 million people were covered by Medicare in Australia, 399 million services were provided through Medicare, and over $22 billion in medical benefits were paid (Department of Human Services 2017). The most common services provided (by volume) in 2016–17 were professional attendances (193 million services, 122 million of which were GP attendances), followed by pathology services (144 million services provided) (Department of Human Services 2018a). In financial terms, professional attendances received the most resources (at over $10 billion, with GP reimbursements accounting for half of this amount), followed by therapeutic procedures ($3.7 billion) (Department of Human Services 2018b).

Medicare is partly funded by taxpayers through the **Medicare levy**, which is a **progressive tax**; individuals contribute according to their (presumed) capacity to pay. Low-income earners and a limited number of others are exempt from paying the levy and assistance with meeting health care costs is provided through higher benefits to those with significant medical expenses under the Medicare Safety Nets (Extended and Original), and the Health Care Card; holders of this card pay lower amounts for health care and some other services.

In 2018–19, the Medicare levy rate was 2.0% of taxable income. In 2014 the levy had increased on from 1.5% to 2.0% in order to contribute funds to the **National Disability Insurance Scheme (NDIS)**. The levy was scheduled to increase further to 2.5% in 2019; however, this policy decision was reversed in the 2018–19 budget (see Chapter 12). In the 2018–19 budget it was estimated that the Medicare levy would raise approximately $17 billion in revenue for the Australian Government (Commonwealth of Australia 2018). A **Medicare levy surcharge (MLS)** also exists to encourage higher-income individuals to purchase private health insurance by applying a taxation penalty if they earn above a certain amount and do not have private health insurance. The MLS is added to the base Medicare levy rate of 2%. At the highest level of surcharge, individuals pay 3.5% of their taxable income through the Medicare levy and the MLS (see Table 2.1 for how this is calculated).

TABLE 2.1 MEDICARE LEVY SURCHARGE RATES BASED ON INCOME LEVEL, 2018–19

		Tier 1	Tier 2	Tier 3
Singles	$90,000 or less	$90,001–105,000	$105,001–140,000	$140,001 or more
Families	$180,000 or less	$180,00–210,000	$210,001–280,000	$280,001 or more
Medicare levy surcharge (in addition to standard 2% Medicare levy)	0%	1%	1.25%	1.5%

Sources: Australian Taxation Office (2018). Income thresholds and rates for the Medicare levy surcharge. https://www.ato.gov.au/individuals/medicare-levy/medicare-levy-surcharge/income-thresholds-and-rates-for-the-medicare-levy-surcharge/; Bartlett, C., Butler, S., Haines, L. (2016). Reimagining health reform in Australia: taking a systems approach to health and wellness. https://www.strategyand.pwc.com/media/file/Reimagining-health-reform-in-Australia.pdf

Payments for medical services delivered outside of hospitals are provided on a 'fee-for-service' model and are detailed in the **Medicare Benefits Schedule (MBS)** (Department of Health 2018b). This schedule, containing several thousand items, lists how much the government (through Medicare) will pay the service provider (e.g. the GP or specialist doctor) for each type of medical service; this is known as the 'schedule fee'. However, private service providers (e.g. GPs) can choose how much they will charge for a service. Medicare pays a rebate (also known as a benefit) of 85% of the schedule fee for most services; therefore a health consumer must pay the remaining 15% gap fee. Where the provider accepts the scheduled fee and does not charge the patient the gap fee, this is known as **bulk-billing**. Service providers can charge well above the scheduled fee and if they choose to do so the health consumer must pay the gap between the rebate and the amount charged. Bulk-billing rates fluctuate over time; in 2016–17, 78.5% of Medicare services were bulk-billed across Australia (Department of Human Services 2017). Despite this, in 2016–17 50% of patients reported out-of-pocket costs for Medicare-funded services, leading to 7% of Australian adults delaying or avoiding seeking health care (AIHW 2018b). The fee-for-service model has been criticised as inhibiting holistic health care, as it is focused on paying for a specific episode of (often acute) care rather than ongoing management of chronic or complex conditions (Boxall & Gillespie 2013; Duckett & Willcox 2015), which are now found to make up approximately 40% of GP encounters (Britt et al. 2016).

Medicare benefits are only payable for services that are deemed to be *clinically relevant*. If a patient requests a service that is *not* considered clinically relevant, then no benefit is paid towards that service; an example would be cosmetic surgery. In addition, under the *Health Insurance Amendment (Compliance) Act 2011*, Medicare uses a number of strategies to monitor the billing practices of practitioners to ensure that 'over-servicing' or fraudulent activities are minimised. However, the level of scrutiny applied here has been criticised (Palmer & Short 2014; Webber 2012) and the Healthier Medicare initiative is also focused on improving compliance (Department of Health 2016).

PAUSE
for
REFLECTION
...

Visit the Medicare Benefits Schedule website (www.mbsonline.gov.au) and explore some of the several thousand services funded and the rebates provided for these services.

Medical practitioners working in public hospitals providing public services are employed as salaried medical officers (i.e. they receive a specified income) and therefore are not paid on a fee-for-service basis. However, public hospitals themselves are currently funded on a fee-for-service basis known as **activity-based funding**. Public hospital services operate differently to out-of-hospital health services and are always provided at no cost to the health consumer. In addition to rebates for medical practitioner services, Medicare also provides a rebate of 75% of the schedule fee for services provided by a doctor in hospital to private patients. Those with private health insurance may have the remaining 25% cost of the service covered by their health insurance.

As you can see from Leanne's story in Case study 2.1, GPs are the most common first point of contact with the health system – in 2014–15, over 85% of Australians visited a GP (Australian Bureau of Statistics 2017). Access to more-specialised medical care is highly regulated in Australia. Patients cannot access the services of a specialist except through a referral from their GP, and a non-emergency hospital admission can be sanctioned only by a doctor. Hence GPs serve as **'gate-keepers'** for access to specialists. The only other freely accessible source of medical care is through hospital emergency departments. Individuals are able to choose and freely access other private forms of health care such as physiotherapy, dental services, etc., but they must pay for these services.

Australia's public hospital system

Public hospitals provided almost 6.6 million separations in 2016–17 (AIHW 2018c); a **hospital separation** is an episode of specific care which ends at discharge, death or transfer to another service / care type. Over 7.5 million public hospital emergency department attendances occurred in 2016–17 (AIHW 2017) and there were over 2.5 million admissions to Australian hospitals for surgery, of which only 340,000 were considered emergencies (required within 24 hours), with the remainder being considered **elective surgery**, which is surgery that needs to occur but not within 24 hours (AIHW 2018c). The use of the term 'elective' may imply the surgery is not necessary; however, this is not the case (Duckett & Willcox 2015). All medical conditions requiring surgery are categorised into categories of urgency. Although these differ from state to state, generally they are organised around the time the patient can wait before the condition deteriorates (AIHW 2013). The majority of elective surgery (67%) occurs in the private hospital system rather than in public hospitals (AIHW 2018c). In 2016–17, almost half of all admissions to public hospitals involved admission overnight or longer, whereas in private hospitals less than 40% of admissions required overnight admission, indicating a different service mix (a higher rate of day procedures) (AIHW 2018c).

PAUSE
for
REFLECTION
...

To understand the relationship between waiting times for elective surgery and categories of urgency, go to the MyHospitals website, provided in the Online Resources section of this chapter, and search for your closest public hospital. Review the waiting times for elective surgery by surgical specialty and by procedures. How does your hospital compare to the 'peer group median' (this refers to how the hospital compares with similar hospitals)?

Over $67 billion was provided to Australian public hospitals in 2016–17, and the sector employed an estimated 369,000 full-time equivalent positions with the largest employee group being nursing staff (AIHW 2018d). Demand for hospital services is continually increasing and between 2012–13 and 2016–17 public hospital separations increased by 4.5% every year, 2.8 times higher than population growth over the same period (AIHW 2018c). Challenges currently facing public hospitals include elective surgery waiting times, emergency department waiting times, **'bed block'** (where patients in

Case Study 2.1

Joining the dots of public and private health insurance

Leanne is 45 years old, single, and earns $95,000 a year. She pays the Medicare levy of 2% of her taxable income, which is $1900 per year. Leanne has private health insurance; otherwise she would have to pay the Medicare levy surcharge of an additional 1% of her taxable income (an extra $950 in tax per year), as she earns over $90,001. Her private health insurance costs $1600 per year and provides private hospital cover and 'extras' cover for services such as travel vaccinations, dental services, physiotherapy and massage. Leanne must pay a $500 excess if she goes to hospital; she chose to include this in her policy to reduce the cost of her premiums.

Leanne visits her GP as she has been experiencing chronic gastric reflux. She has a 15-minute consultation and her GP bulk-bills her for this. The Medicare Benefits Schedule (September 2018) pays a GP $37.60 for a standard consultation up to 20 minutes (not inclusive of any bulk-billing incentive payments that are in operation). At the end of this consultation, Leanne does not have to pay anything; she signs a form and her GP receives the payment of $37.60 from Medicare. If Leanne's GP chose to charge more than $37.60 for a standard consultation, then Leanne would need to pay the difference between $37.60 and the fee charged – the gap fee, or co-payment. This gap is not covered by private health insurance.

Leanne's GP refers her to a private gastroenterologist for further investigation. She visits the gastroenterologist's consulting rooms 3 weeks later. The gastroenterologist charges $168.50 for this consultation. The Medicare schedule fee is $86.85; however, Medicare covers only 85% of this cost (which equals $73.85). Leanne has to pay the difference of $94.65 ($168.50 consultation charge minus $73.85 Medicare rebate). Even though Leanne is accessing a private medical service, this gap fee is not covered by her private health insurance as it is not provided in hospital.

The gastroenterologist suggests Leanne needs to have an endoscopy for further investigation of her gastric problems and books her in for this in a private hospital the following week. Leanne's private health insurance covers the cost of this procedure; however, she must pay the $500 excess on her health insurance as well as a small gap payment for the assisting anaesthetist.

Leanne's GP could have referred her to a public gastroenterologist at the local public hospital outpatient clinic as a public patient. This service would have been provided to Leanne at no charge; however, she might have had to wait several months for an appointment and she would have had no choice about which doctor she would see. If it had then been decided that Leanne needed an endoscopy, she would have been placed on an elective surgery waiting list and could have waited several months or longer for the procedure to be done. The procedure would have been carried out in the public hospital and Leanne would have received no bill for the procedure.

emergency cannot be admitted to a ward owing to lack of beds) and ambulance bypass and ramping issues when emergency departments are overloaded.

In 2011, as part of the National Health Reform Agreement, Australia moved to a nationalised system of activity-based funding for public hospital services. Activity-based funding means that hospitals are paid for the specific services and procedures they provide and each service and procedure has a set price based on its characteristics (Eagar 2010). It is assumed that activity-based funding promotes efficiency because service providers are paid a set price – if a procedure payment includes a 3-day hospital stay and the patient is discharged at 2 days, then the service provider makes a 'profit' on this service (Solomon 2014). In 2017 the Australian Health Minister announced a major change to public hospital funding whereby, from 1 July 2018, hospitals would be financially penalised for certain patient complications (termed 'hospital-acquired complications') that are considered preventable (Independent Hospital Pricing Authority 2017).

Public hospitals provide services to **inpatients** who are admitted to hospital for surgery, investigations, medical management and other issues, and they also provide services on an **outpatient** basis to people who need medical treatment but do not require admission to hospital. An outpatient service might be where, after being discharged from an acute episode (e.g. heart surgery), a patient would need to visit a public hospital several times a year to see a specialist (in this case a cardiologist) to manage their condition on an ongoing basis). In 2016–17, there were almost 37 million non-admitted patient services provided to public patients in Australia (AIHW 2018e). Reducing the average length of stay is one mechanism used to reduce the cost of public hospital services, as each day in hospital can be very costly. In 2016–17 the average length of stay for patients admitted overnight in public hospitals declined to 5.3 days (AIHW 2018c).

All public hospitals across Australia are governed through entities known as **Local Hospital Networks** (LHNs), sometimes referred to as **Local Health Networks**. LHNs were established in 2011–12 under the National Health Reform Agreement as part of the national health reform process that commenced in 2008. The establishment of LHNs was designed to increase local accountability to improve public hospital services (Council of Australian Governments (COAG) 2011). Governance of local hospitals is provided through each LHN and its Governing Council, which is responsible for the budget and overall performance of all hospitals within the LHN. LHNs have relationships with the federal government as well as the relevant state government and consumers.

PAUSE
for
REFLECTION
…

Visit the National Health Funding Pool Administrator website and access the directory of Local Hospital Networks https://www.publichospitalfunding.gov.au/Directory. Find the LHN closest to you and click on the link, then access its most recent financial statement. How much funding has the LHN received this year? Is this figure surprising? Consider this figure in relation to total health expenditure and government health expenditure in Australia to put it into some context.

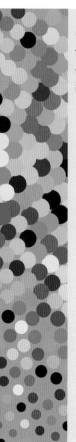

Summary

This chapter has introduced you to the basics of the Australian health care system. As you will have read, the system is complex and beset with problems, but still provides high-quality services. Major issues discussed include the following:

- Governance of the Australian health care system is shared across federal, state and local governments, with each sector of government responsible for different aspects in isolation or through shared ventures. This shared system contributes to tensions and issues such as cost-shifting and blame-shifting between sectors of government.
- There are tensions between the private and the public health sectors, and debates about which model of service delivery is optimal and equitable.
- Health expenditure in Australia has been rising year on year, which presents concerns and challenges for health policy-makers. Despite this, the level of expenditure in Australia is competitive when compared with similar countries.
- The Australian health care system performs well in comparison to health care systems in similar countries. Australia has enviable health outcomes and high life expectancy.
- Continual reform of the health care system places strain on all components of the system for ambiguous outcomes.
- Medicare provides universal access to free public hospital care for all Australian citizens and subsidised access to other medical services. A range of measures has been explored and/or implemented to contain the cost of providing Medicare; however, the principle of universal access remains.
- Public hospitals provide a large amount of high-quality specialist medical care in Australia, and are also vulnerable to funding and governance reform.

Review Questions

1 Describe how cost-shifting might impact on public hospitals.
2 Considering the perpetual state of reform in the Australian health care system, what are some of the potential impacts on the health professional workforce?
3 Given the overlap in funding and responsibility for the management of various parts of the Australian health care system, what do you see as the potential problems arising here?
4 Following on from identifying the problems in question 3, what do you think is the appropriate role for different levels of governments in this space?
5 The COAG Health Council and its advisory body the Australian Health Ministers Advisory Council are responsible at a national level for the operation of the health system. What difficulties might arise based on the membership of these groups?

References

Australian Bureau of Statistics, 2017. Health service usage and health related action, Australia, 2014–15. Cat. no. 4364.0.55.002. http://www.abs.gov.au/ausstats/abs@.nsf/Lookup/by%20Subject/ 4364.0.55.002~2014-15~Main%20Features~Consultations%20with%20health%20professionals~2.

Australian Bureau of Statistics, 2018. Labour force, Australia, detailed, quarterly, May 2018. Cat. no. 6291.0.55.003. Time series spreadsheet table 04: employed persons by industry division of main job (ANZSIC) – trend, seasonally adjusted, and original. http://www.abs.gov.au/AUSSTATS/abs@.nsf/ DetailsPage/6291.0.55.003May%202018?OpenDocument.

Australian Health Practitioner Regulation Agency, 2017. Annual report 2016/17. AHPRA and National Boards. http://www.ahpra.gov.au/documents/default.aspx?record=WD17%2f24009&dbid=AP&chksum =1y%2bEzMMIk59bKaFGykGADA%3d%3d.

Australian Institute of Health and Welfare (AIHW), 2013. National definitions for elective surgery urgency categories: proposal for the Standing Council on Health. AIHW, Canberra. https://www.aihw.gov.au/ reports/hospitals/national-definitions-for-elective-surgery-urgency/contents/summary.

Australian Institute of Health and Welfare (AIHW), 2016. Australian Burden of Disease Study: impact and causes of illness and death in Australia 2011. Australian Burden of Disease Study series no. 3. BOD 4. AIHW, Canberra. https://www.aihw.gov.au/getmedia/d4df9251-c4b6-452f-a877-8370b6124219/ 19663.pdf.aspx?inline=true.

Australian Institute of Health and Welfare (AIHW), 2017. Emergency department care 2016–17: Australian hospital statistics. Health services series no. 80. Cat. no. HSE 194. AIHW, Canberra. https://www.aihw .gov.au/getmedia/981140ee-3957-4d47-9032-18ca89b519b0/aihw-hse-194.pdf.aspx?inline=true.

Australian Institute of Health and Welfare (AIHW), 2018a. Australia's health 2018. Australia's health series no. 16. AUS221. AIHW, Canberra. https://www.aihw.gov.au/getmedia/7c42913d-295f-4bc9-9c24 -4e44eff4a04a/aihw-aus-221.pdf.aspx?inline=true.

Australian Institute of Health and Welfare (AIHW), 2018b. Patients' out-of-pocket spending on Medicare services, 2016–17. AIHW, Canberra. https://www.myhealthycommunities.gov.au/our-reports/ out-of-pocket-spending/august-2018.

Australian Institute of Health and Welfare (AIHW), 2018c. Admitted patient care 2016–17: Australian hospital statistics. Health services series no. 84. Cat. no. HSE 201. Canberra: AIHW. Available from: https://www.aihw.gov.au/getmedia/acee86da-d98e-4286-85a4-52840836706f/aihw-hse-201.pdf.aspx ?inline=true.

Australian Institute of Health and Welfare (AIHW), 2018d. Hospital resources 2016–17: Australian Hospital statistics. Health Services series no. 86, Cat. no. HSW 205. AIHW, Canberra. https://www.aihw.gov.au/ getmedia/c5fd554a-3356-474a-808a-5aab43d24708/aihw-hse-205.pdf.aspx?inline=true.

Australian Institute of Health and Welfare (AIHW), 2018e. Non-admitted patient care 2016–17: Australian hospital statistics. Health services series no. 87. Cat. no. HSE 206. AIHW, Canberra. https://www.aihw.gov.au/getmedia/a6c9c592-4e8b-4b53-b7f6-3a01d91ed801/aihw-hse-206.pdf.aspx ?inline=true.

Australian Taxation Office, 2018. Income thresholds and rates for the Medicare levy surcharge. https://www.ato.gov.au/individuals/medicare-levy/medicare-levy-surcharge/income-thresholds-and-rates-for-the-medicare-levy-surcharge/. Commonwealth of Australia, Canberra.

Bacchi, C., 2012. Introducing the 'What's the problem represented to be?' approach. In: Bletsas, A., Beasley, C. (Eds.), Engaging With Carol Bacchi: Strategic Interventions and Exchanges. University of Adelaide Press, Adelaide. https://www.adelaide.edu.au/carst/docs/wpr/wpr-summary.pdf.

Bartlett, C., Butler, S., Haines, L., 2016. Reimagining health reform in Australia: taking a systems approach to health and wellness. https://www.strategyand.pwc.com/media/file/Reimagining-health-reform-in-Australia.pdf.

Boxall, A.M., 2010. Reforming Australia's health system, again. Med. J. Aust. 192, 528–530.

Boxall, A.M., Gillespie, J.A., 2013. Making Medicare: The Politics of Universal Health Care in Australia. University of New South Wales Press, Sydney NSW.

Britt, H., Miller, G.C., Henderson, J., et al., 2016. General practice activity in Australia 2015–16. General practice series no. 40. Sydney University Press, Sydney. https://ses.library.usyd.edu.au/handle/2123/15514.

Commonwealth of Australia, 2018. Budget paper no. 1: Budget strategy and outlook 2018–19. https://budget.gov.au/2018-19/bp1/bp1.pdf.

Council of Australian Governments (COAG), 2011. National Health Reform Agreement, https://www.publichospitalfunding.gov.au/national-health-reform/agreement.

Department of Health, 2016. Healthier Medicare. http://www.health.gov.au/internet/main/publishing.nsf/Content/healthiermedicare.

Department of Health, 2018a. Ministerial Advisory Committee on out-of-pocket costs. http://www.health.gov.au/internet/main/publishing.nsf/Content/min-advisory-comm-out-of-pocket.

Department of Health, 2018b. Medicare Benefits Schedule online. http://www.mbsonline.gov.au/internet/mbsonline/publishing.nsf/Content/Home.

Department of Human Services, 2017. Annual report 2016–17. https://www.humanservices.gov.au/sites/default/files/2017/10/8802-1710-annual-report-2016-17.pdf.

Department of Human Services, 2018a. All Medicare by MBS category processed from July 2017 to June 2018 (services). http://medicarestatistics.humanservices.gov.au/statistics/do.jsp?_PROGRAM=%2Fstatistics%2Fmbs_group_standard_report&DRILL=on&GROUP=all+Medicare+by+MBS+categories&VAR=services&STAT=count&RPT_FMT=by+state&PTYPE=finyear&START_DT=201707&END_DT=201806.

Department of Human Services, 2018b. All Medicare by MBS category processed from July 2017 to June 2018 (benefits). http://medicarestatistics.humanservices.gov.au/statistics/do.jsp?_PROGRAM=%2Fstatistics%2Fmbs_group_standard_report&DRILL=on&GROUP=all+Medicare+by+MBS+categories&VAR=benefit&STAT=count&RPT_FMT=by+state&PTYPE=finyear&START_DT=201707&END_DT=201806.

Duckett, S., 1999. Commonwealth / state relations in health. In: Hancock, L. (Ed.), Health Policy in the Market State. Allen and Unwin, St Leonards, NSW.

Duckett, S., Willcox, S., 2015. The Australian Health Care System, fifth ed. OUP, Victoria.

Dwyer, J., Eagar, K., 2008. Options for reform of Commonwealth and state governance responsibilities for the Australian health system. Paper commissioned by the National Health and Hospitals Reform Commission (NHHRC), August. NHHRC, Canberra.

Eagar, K., 2010. ABF Information Series no. 1. What is activity based funding? Centre for Health Service Development, University of Wollongong.

Eckermann, S., Sheridan, L., Ivers, R., 2016. Which direction should Australian health system reform be heading? Aust. N. Z. J. Public Health 40 (1), 7–9.

Elliot, A., 2003. Is Medicare universal? Department of the Parliamentary Library, Canberra.

Gray, G., 2004. The Politics of Medicare: Who Gets What, When and How. University of New South Wales Press, Sydney NSW.

Hall, J., 2015. Australian health care – the challenge of reform in a fragmented system. N. Engl. J. Med. 373, 493–497.

Health Insurance Act 1973 (current version). Australian Government, Canberra. https://www.legislation.gov.au/Details/C2017C00255.

Health Insurance Amendment (Compliance) Act 2011. Australian Government, Canberra. https://www.legislation.gov.au/Details/C2011A00010.

Independent Hospital Pricing Authority, 2017. Risk adjustment model for hospital acquired complications – technical specifications version 1.0. https://www.ihpa.gov.au/sites/g/files/net636/f/risk_adjustment _model_for_hospital_acquired_complications_-_technical_specifications_v1.0_july_2017_pdf.pdf.

Macri, J., 2016. Australia's health system: some issues and challenges. J. Health Med. Econ. 2, 2.

National Health and Hospitals Reform Commission, 2009. A healthier future for all Australians – final report of the National Health and Hospitals Reform Commission June 2009. COAG, Canberra. http://www.federalfinancialrelations.gov.au/content/npa/health/_archive/national-agreement.pdf.

Organization for Economic Cooperation and Development (OECD), 2017. Health at a Glance 2017: OECD Indicators. OECD Publishing, Paris. https://www.oecd-ilibrary.org/docserver/health_glance-2017-en .pdf?expires=1536461521&id=id&accname=ocid177318a&checksum=018BA9C6CC6F7A8D60B36E848 417FB1C.

Palmer, G., Short, S., 2014. Health Care and Public Policy: An Australian Analysis, fifth ed. Palgrave Macmillan, South Yarra.

Parliament of Australia Senate Community Affairs References Committee, 2017. Value and affordability of private health insurance and out-of-pocket medical costs. https://www.aph.gov.au/Parliamentary_ Business/Committees/Senate/Community_Affairs/Privatehealthinsurance/~/media/Committees/ clac_ctte/Privatehealthinsurance/Report/report.pdf.

Podger, A., Hagan, P., 1999. Reforming the Australian health care system: the role of government. Occasional papers: new series no. 1. Department of Health and Aged Care, Canberra.

Solomon, S., 2014. Health reform and activity based funding. Med. J. Aust. 200, 564.

Tuohy, C., 1999. Accidental Logics: The Dynamics of Change in the Health Care Area in United States, Britain and Canada. OUP, New York.

Webber, T.D., 2012. What is wrong with Medicare? Med. J. Aust. 196, 18–19.

World Health Organization, 2008. The right to health. Office of the United Nations High Commissioner for Human Rights and World Health Organization, Geneva.

Further Reading

Australian Institute of Health and Welfare, 2018a. Australia's health 2018. Australia's health series no. 16. AUS221. AIHW, Canberra. https://www.aihw.gov.au/getmedia/7c42913d-295f-4bc9-9c24 -4e44eff4a04a/aihw-aus-221.pdf.aspx?inline=true.

Bartlett, C., Butler, S., Haines, L., 2016. Reimagining health reform in Australia: taking a systems approach to health and wellness. https://www.strategyand.pwc.com/media/file/Reimagining-health-reform-in -Australia.pdf.

Department of Health, 2017. History of the Department. http://www.health.gov.au/internet/main/ publishing.nsf/Content/health-history.htm.

Duckett, S., Willcox, S., 2015. The Australian Health Care System, fifth ed. OUP, Victoria.

Hall, J., Viney, R., 2000. The political economy of health sector reform. In: Bloom, A. (Ed.), Health Reform in Australia and New Zealand. OUP, South Melbourne.

National Health Reform Agreement, 2011. Council of Australian Governments. http:// www.federalfinancialrelations.gov.au/content/npa/health/_archive/national-agreement.pdf.

Palmer, G., Short, S., 2014. Health Care and Public Policy: An Australian Analysis, fifth ed. Palgrave Macmillan, South Yarra.

Online Resources

Australian Institute of Health and Welfare – provides comprehensive information, publications and statistics about most aspects of the Australian health care system, population groups and specific diseases: www.aihw.gov.au.

COAG Health Council: http://www.coaghealthcouncil.gov.au/.

Department of Human Services – administers Medicare Australia: www.humanservices.gov.au.

Medicare Benefits Schedule: www.mbsonline.gov.au.

MyHospitals: https://www.myhospitals.gov.au/. Search for any hospital and review the waiting times for surgery. You can also compare hospitals, download data and review additional measures such as length of stay, emergency department attendances and safety and quality performance.

National Health Funding Pool Administrator: https://www.publichospitalfunding.gov.au/.

CHAPTER 3

The private health sector and private health insurance

Fran Collyer, Karen Willis and Helen Keleher

Key learning outcomes

When you finish this chapter you should be able to:

- explain the scope of the private health sector within the Australian health care system and how it is organised, funded and delivered
- discuss current debates about private health insurance in Australia and implications for equity and access
- describe the tensions between advocates for universal access via Medicare and advocates for a strong private sector.

Key terms and abbreviations

Australian Bureau of Statistics (ABS)

Australian Prudential Regulation Authority (APRA)

contracting out

day hospital

information asymmetry

moral hazard

private health insurance (PHI)

privatisation

private health insurance rebate

private hospitals

public–private partnerships (PPPs)

sentinel events

Introduction

This chapter is about the private health care sector in Australia. As noted earlier in this book, Australia has a hybrid, public–private health system. Rather than an integrated system, the health sector tends to operate within two parallel arenas – a public one and a private one. This offers many challenges to government and to patients navigating services. The provision of public medical services and the funding of the universal health insurance system, Medicare, are discussed in Chapter 2, while other aspects of Australian health care with a significant private component, such as the aged care sector, complementary health care and dental care, are discussed in Chapters

8, 14 and 15 respectively. In recent years, Australians have been encouraged to contribute to the financing of their health needs by purchasing **private health insurance (PHI)** in addition to the universal tax-based insurance coverage provided by Medicare. This has substantially changed the health care system in Australia. This chapter will concentrate on PHI and **private hospitals**, as these are the two most prominent and influential aspects of the private health care system in Australia.

Private health insurance

PHI in Australia began with the Friendly Society movements of the 1840s. These were mutual associations, established to assist members during sickness or unemployment by providing them with health or welfare insurance. Individuals were able to join a Friendly Society for an annual fee, and subscription gave its members access to a Friendly Society doctor and to medicine dispensed by a Friendly Society dispensary. Subscription enabled members to offset their medical costs, although the amounts paid rarely covered the full costs of a private hospital or doctor.

Collyer et al. (2015) explain the origins of Australia's two-tier insurance system and its various iterations through the 20th century, making the point that the medical profession has historically maintained a system of charging patients via a fee-for-service model, with higher fees for those who could afford to pay. The rights of doctors to private practice have continued and are guaranteed in the Australian constitution, and this has been important in entrenching the power of the medical profession, often referred to as medical dominance (see Willis 1989 and Chapter 21). Political parties and political ideology in Australia have influenced the health care field. Social democratic parties – such as the Australian Labor Party – focus on a collective approach to health care, ensuring equitable access in a publicly funded system. Conservative parties, such as the Liberal and National parties, take an individualistic approach and promote the private market as best able to deliver health care. Collyer et al. (2015) discuss the battles fought by the Australian Labor Party to establish a universal health insurance system – one that protected those rights while assuring affordable services for all citizens. This was accomplished with the commencement of Medibank from 1975, but was undermined a few years later by the Fraser Liberal-Coalition Government, which abolished Medibank in favour of building up the private health insurance industry. Medibank and universal health insurance were then restored by the Hawke Labor Government in 1984 and renamed 'Medicare'.

The contemporary PHI environment

By offering care that is free at the point of service, in all public hospitals, Medibank and later Medicare lowered the membership rates of PHI. This was not considered particularly problematic until the election of the Howard Liberal-Coalition Government in 1996. In 1997, major changes were introduced to address what the Government perceived as the 'problem' of low PHI membership. It was claimed that Australia needed a 'dual system' of both public and private provision, one argument being that having a vibrant private system would take the pressure off the public system (Elliott 2006). The government took the position that the public system should be available primarily for those who needed it, with people able to afford PHI encouraged to use the private system. Incentives were provided (also known as 'carrots') for people to purchase PHI, and penalties (also known as 'sticks') if they did not do so. The policy 'carrots' were:

♦ the Private Health Insurance Incentive Scheme: a rebate on the cost of PHI premiums, initially set at 30% of the cost to individuals, but subsequently means tested to ensure higher income earners receive a lower or no rebate, and

♦ community rating: a guarantee that premiums are not based on a person's medical history, health risks or age.

The policy 'sticks' were:

♦ the Medicare Levy Surcharge: tax penalties for people over a certain income without PHI, and

♦ Lifetime Health Cover: a 2% loading on top of the PHI premium for every year individuals aged over 30 delay buying PHI for hospital cover (with the loading removed after 10 years of continuous cover).

The percentage of the population covered by PHI has risen from 31% in 1999 to approximately 47% in 2017 for hospital insurance, and to 55% for those holding ancillaries or extras insurance (covering dental, optical and other non-hospital related benefits) (Australian Institute of Health and Welfare (AIHW) 2018a). Because the number of people with PHI has expanded, the annual cost of the **PHI rebate** for taxpayers has also risen, from (AU)$1.4 billion in 1999–2000 to $5.7 billion in 2015–16, and is projected to increase to $6.7 billion in 2019–20 (Cheng 2018). This money has been provided to the private sector and withdrawn from the public health system. Harris (2013) also makes the point that the effect of this subsidy erodes Medicare's equity-of-access principle. The subsidy, mostly, goes to people who are financially better off, enabling them to have better access to hospital care, particularly elective surgery.

When Medibank Private – Australia's government-owned and largest private insurance provider – was privatised in 2014, the insurance landscape shifted significantly. From that point, PHI in Australia became a primarily for-profit enterprise. As of 16 May 2018, there were 37 private health insurers listed with the government regulator the **Australian Prudential Regulation Authority** (APRA 2018), with 11 smaller organisations having restricted membership to their own member base (similar to the Friendly Societies). Two of the companies, Medibank Private and BUPA, are for-profit organisations and have 54.6% of the market share (Finder, Advice Evolution 2018).

Case study 3.1 highlights the experience of Australians with and without PHI. While initially PHI could be regarded merely as an additional 'choice' for Australians, the 'sticks and carrots' policy mechanisms have altered the landscape, increasing the number of people with PHI, shifting peoples' perceptions and practices about how best to meet their health needs, and expanding the number of private-sector services as new opportunities open up for health professionals to work in the private sector. Alongside the continued under-resourcing of public-sector medicine and the increasing difficulty in accessing timely public care, these changes have made it more difficult for people to 'choose public'.

Case Study 3.1

'Choosing' to go private

Given that Australia has universal access for all citizens to be treated without cost in public hospitals, and a Medicare system, which citizens contribute to through the taxation system, why has the government been able to convince approximately 50% of the population they should have private health insurance? In our interviews with 78 Australians (Lewis & Willis 2018; Willis et al. 2016), the main reasons given for having PHI were:

- to avoid the Medicare Levy Surcharge
- to enable choice of doctor and hospital
- to avoid lengthy waiting periods in the public system (particularly for elective procedures)
- concern that the public system will not meet their health needs
- perception of high quality of health care in the private system.

The following examples from our study illustrate the dominance of positive views about the private sector, as well as the challenges people have in navigating between public and private.

Consider the cases of Penny, Ahn and Jin, and Paul. As you read through these examples, make a list of what you believe their story highlights about health care:

- Does the system work in the ways they discuss?
- Are their experiences indicative of a health policy problem?
- What does their experience tell us about the health care system in Australia?

Penny is aged 21 years and has two children, both with multiple, ongoing health problems. Penny is on a low income and does not have private health insurance. She wishes she could afford it:

> If I knew my children and I were going to be so sick, I would've got private health insurance because we would've been well a lot quicker I think.

With no experience of the private system, Penny believes the private system would be better than the public:

> I think in the private system they might get more choice than in the public … With private you're paying for your own health instead of public so you should get more when you pay for it. You might get looked after quicker and there might be a waiting time still but not as long, more comfortable – if you have surgery or something more comfortable, maybe more space in a room. I'm not 100% sure but maybe those are the things that are better.

Ahn (aged 65) and **Jin** (aged 61) migrated to Australia from China 30 years ago. They have two adult daughters. Ahn is a hospital porter and Jin works in a supermarket. They purchased PHI in 2000:

> … because that year I think the government push the people to join the Medibank Private. That's why we joined the private. They're talking about when you're old you will pay more money. *That's why we go to join.*

Additionally, they worry about waiting lists for surgery in the public system:

> I think they told me if you go to private it's faster. If not, you need to wait long periods, maybe two months, *three months. If you go to private, maybe couple of weeks.*

As PHI has become more expensive, the pair have contemplated dropping their cover and relying on the public. However, as they are ageing, they worry about doing this:

> You see when you get older your problem will come up you see. You need more health care. Maybe now we don't need to go to the hospital, or maybe later you need to go to the hospital to do the operation or do something, so I think if no, I don't have the private fund I think its not secure.

Ahn and Jin draw on their experience from a time when their daughter needed surgery, and how the specialist persuaded them they should use the private system:

> Then the doctor say, 'If you go to public I only watch. You see, my assistant do the operation' … But on that occasion, my daughter is different. He has to do it. So he told me that I'm doing the operation and then we'll change to private. I think, oh you are good doctor, so I better rely on you *to do it.*

Paul, aged 34, is university educated and has a managerial position in local government. Married with two children, his family has had many encounters with the health care system. He discusses how important PHI is to him, and how he has navigated between public and private health care systems. When discussing the decision to 'go private' Paul says:

> I've been a private patient for having diagnostic scopes done. And I did those as a private patient obviously, because as a private patient I can get in and get them done, which is the absolute benefit of having private cover, I can choose my treating specialist and I can say I'm available on these days, how does that work for you, rather than sitting on the waitlist.

Paul says that the private system:

> Is nicer, not so much that the staff are nicer, but the staff are under a lot less pressure is the perception of it. Because you are going into the private hospital to have very specific treatments, they are not dealing with the emergency cases and the ambulances and that sort of dynamic workflow. They have a roster of what's on for the day and they work to that roster and they leave, and it's done so there's a lot less stress in that environment and as a result they are nicer about it … Even though some of the procedures that people are going for can be reasonably heavy, they have spoken to their specialist they've chosen, and they have chosen this date, everything is a lot more planned for and structured. It's just that more 'nicer' environment to be in.

Paul discusses his use of the public system:

> In emergency situations I have to go to the public hospital, but I definitely notify them that I am a private patient and use whatever perks and privileges that might bring with them, because I have paid for them I suppose. For elective surgery I will always go private where I can afford the opportunity to do so.

Paul highly values having PHI:

> There have been times in our life where you know, we have thought of dropping the private health insurance because the bills were tight and you know the family had to come first, but we always managed to find a way to keep the private health cover, because if something happened to go wrong for us and touch wood nothing's gone too wrong for us ... But had anything come up we could get to the top of the waitlist, we could pick our specialist, pick our hospital, basically pick from a choice of treatment dates. Which is always preferable to going on the waitlist.

This brief case study of PHI tells us quite a bit about people's views. One strong theme emerging from these interviews is that people feel they 'get something extra' if they have PHI, though they are not always sure of what this might be. Another is the level of concern raised about not being treated quickly if they have to rely on the public system. Quite notable is that very few participants suggest their choices are drawn from lived experience of differences between public and private forms of care. This raises questions about the extent to which their choices are 'free', or perhaps have been shaped by the higher premiums that will be imposed if they fail to join by a certain age, or by prevailing discourses in the media and elsewhere that systematically encourage them to be fearful about the public system and which emphasise the benefits of the private system.

PAUSE
for
REFLECTION
...

- Why have low numbers of people purchasing PHI come to be regarded as a 'policy problem'?

One controversial topic is the use of public hospitals by privately insured patients. The Commonwealth and states have an agreement that people can choose to be a private patient in a public hospital, and that the public hospitals can charge for these private patients at a fee set by each state. Importantly, however, there is no requirement for people to declare their PHI status (Seah et al. 2013). Some argue that this compromises one of the objectives of subsidising PHI in the first place, which was to 'take the pressure off the public system'. However, patients with PHI are also paying for access to the public system through the taxation-based Medicare levy. In our research, we found that when people with PHI enter a public hospital they may be asked if they have PHI and whether they would like to 'help out the hospital' by using their PHI. If they do so, some of the costs of care are shifted to the private sector. We found those patients with greater understanding of the health care system were less likely to declare their PHI status, a major reason being to avoid out-of-pocket costs incurred when using PHI.

PAUSE *for* REFLECTION ...

Do you think people should use their PHI when admitted to a public hospital?
Give reasons for your answer.

The private health care sector in Australia

The private sector comprises private hospitals, most medical, dental and allied health services, pharmacies, much of the aged care sector, most radiology and pathology services, PHI and companies engaged in the manufacturing or sale of medical devices and e-health technologies. The health care sector in Australia has a unique history, distinctly different from that of Europe or America, where religious organisations were the forerunners in the former, and corporations in the latter.

Private hospitals in Australia

The first hospitals in Australia were funded by the British Navy, for treating naval personnel and convicts. In 1848, after the transportation of convicts had slowed, the Naval hospitals were formally handed over to the civilian government, and began to cater for individuals who were neither convicts nor serving in the Navy. These 19th-century hospitals were subsidised by government, but were increasingly associated with religious orders. Eventually many became integrated into the public hospital system and largely paid for by the state (Hicks 1981). The early hospitals were associated with death and disease, and attended only by the poor, with the wealthy being treated in their own homes. Over time, hospital care and health outcomes improved and began to attract a broader public. Fully private hospitals (i.e. hospitals owned and managed by private individuals or organisations (AIHW 2017)) emerged only in the second half of the 19th century. Public hospitals dominated the provision of hospital care in Australia until the late 20th century. Since then the market share of private hospitals has grown substantially.

The **Australian Bureau of Statistics (ABS)** annually collects information on the structure and performance of the private hospital industry, which is published in Private Hospitals, Australia (Australian Bureau of Statistics (ABS) 2014, 2015). Broadly, the private sector runs three types of hospitals: acute, psychiatric and freestanding **day hospital** facilities, providing services in endoscopy, gastroenterology, ophthalmic surgery, plastic and cosmetic surgery, gynaecology, fertility treatment and family planning (ABS 2015).

In 2016–17, there were 1325 hospitals in Australia, of which 695 were public hospitals, and 630 private. These figures indicate a small decrease in public hospitals (there were 746 in 2012–13) and a larger increase in private hospitals (there were 592 in 2011–12). Of all the admissions, 6.6 million occurred in public hospitals and 4.4 in private (AIHW 2018b). Public and private hospitals differ significantly in the kind of medicine provided, with public hospitals undertaking 92% of all emergency admissions, and private hospitals accounting for 59% of all elective admissions (AIHW 2018b). They also differ in the source of funding they receive. In general terms, the state and territory governments and the Australian Government provide most of the funds for public hospitals, while private hospitals are largely funded by PHI and out-of-pocket payments by patients.

Both private and public hospitals are subject to National Safety and Quality Health Service Standards of care. The states and territories also have their own legislation to regulate private health facilities and enforce licensing standards. State and territory licensing provisions for private hospitals mandate compliance with a range of operational and quality requirements. Private and public hospitals are required by legislation to submit episode-level data to state and territory governments as well as to report **sentinel events** and adverse outcomes data. The collection of such data contributes to the transparency of consumer information about the two sectors, although in reality most consumers are unlikely to know how to access this information.

In most jurisdictions, legislation incorporates controls on the number and geographical location of private hospital beds (Productivity Commission 1999). For example, the New South Wales government legislation (NSW Health 2018) is designed to plan and provide for a wide range of health services across the state, and maintain the standards of these services.

However, such decisions are open to legal challenge from the private sector, and courts have at times determined that the private sector has the right to strategically place its hospitals in areas which maximise patient input and therefore profit – even though the geographical area may be already well supplied with hospitals (White & Collyer 1998, p. 19). Legislation also sets the requirements for licensing, including the minimum standards for the provision of safe, appropriate and high-quality health care for patients in private health facilities.

Implementation of such regulations is made particularly difficult in the Australian case by **information asymmetry**. Publicly available information about public hospitals and the public health care system is more readily available than information about private hospitals and private medicine (Lewis et al. 2018). With little or no data about the way patients move between private and public services (Collyer et al. 2017), little is also known about how doctors combine their work across the two sectors (Cheng et al. 2013). This is also the case for primary medical care, which, in most cases, is part of the private sector. As Duckett (2017) argues, 'the Commonwealth government collects little information on what happens in general practice' and thus designing a health system that rewards good patient management is difficult.

Ownership of private hospitals

Private hospitals vary in terms of categories of ownership and funding, and in size from small facilities with a few beds to major facilities with several hundred beds. Unlike the United States, with its multiple, privately owned, large teaching and research hospitals, private hospitals in Australia primarily offer little in the way of emergency medicine, tend not to be involved in research or teaching and conduct only elective (planned) surgical services. Industry ownership of private hospitals ranges from for-profit hospitals through religious/charitable hospitals to not-for-profit hospitals. Only a quarter of the private hospitals operate as not-for-profit entities. Ramsay Health Care is Australia's largest operator of for-profit private hospitals in Australia, with 73 hospitals and day surgery units, and is ranked in the top five globally. Healthscope is Australia's second largest operator of for-profit private hospitals, with 43 hospitals, and is a leading provider of pathology services in New Zealand, Malaysia and Singapore. The Catholic Church is the largest provider of not-for-profit private hospital services. Its company, Catholic Health Australia, has 20 public hospitals, 36 private hospitals and 130 nursing homes and hostels. Other not-for-profit hospital owners include the Sisters of Charity, Mercy Health, Mater Health Services and Uniting Care.

In the 1990s, the Productivity Commission (1999, p. xii) found that 'private hospitals were increasingly co-locating with public hospitals to allow for the sharing of facilities and equipment and to provide greater convenience for doctors and patients'. Co-location provides hospital owners with multiple business opportunities, as it 'funnels' patients into the private hospital from the nearby emergency departments, enables specialists, nurses and other health care workers to work in both environments and allows the private hospital operator to focus on the most profitable areas of medicine. Brown and Barnett (2004, p. 429) identify four variants of co-located public–private hospitals in Australia:

(1) the traditional model of locating a for-profit hospital in close proximity to a public hospital;
(2) a shared campus where a private and a public hospital occupy the same site;
(3) a shared building with the two hospitals occupying different space within the building; and
(4) where the public hospital, under contract to a state government, is operated and owned by the corporate hospital chain in return for patient payments from the state concerned.

It has been an explicit strategy of recent governments, both federal and state/territory, to consistently deregulate the health sector and encourage private providers to fund and operate hospitals. Thus, Brown and Barnett (2004, p. 432) state that, like other Western nations, the Australian government – at both Commonwealth and state levels – has sought corporate investment in hospital services to shift health care costs from the public sector to the private sector. As with many other government services, there is an increasing trend towards the **privatisation** of health services. Of course, the private hospital sector is dependent on the rates of PHI in the population (as discussed above), and the growth in PHI membership over the past two decades has boosted revenue for both the for-profit and the not-for-profit private hospitals.

There have been questions about the discrepancies in charges between private and public hospitals. Seah et al. (2013) for instance, explain that a public hospital can only charge the fixed rate that is set by the federal government, which is less than the fee that most private hospitals charge for the same services. Through this loophole, the government further subsidises the care of privately insured patients. However, public hospitals gain revenue from treating privately insured patients. In 2010–11, 10.0% of all patients in public hospitals were private patients, compared with 7.8% in 2005–6 (Independent Hospital Pricing Authority 2017), and 6.2% in 1999–2000. By 2015, this had grown to 14% of all public hospital bed days (Australian Private Hospitals Association 2017). This brings public hospitals a significant boost to their finances. Another way of putting this is to say that, according to the Australian Institute of Health and Welfare, private health insurers spent $1.136 billion on public hospital services in 2015–16, or 7.6% of their total outlays. Five years earlier, it was $671 million or 6.8% (see Parnell 2017). While this provides public hospitals with much needed revenue, it is not a trend welcomed by the private hospital owners, as it significantly reduces potential income in the private hospitals (Australian Private Hospitals Association 2017). Nor is it an efficient way to fund public hospitals, because government subsidies for private insurance do not reduce demand on the public hospitals, but rather increase them, encouraging hospital usage rather than community-based solutions to ill-health (Duckett 2018).

Public–private partnerships

Since the 1990s, private-sector financing has increasingly been sought for the construction and operation of health care facilities for treating public patients (Collyer & White 2001; Collyer et al. 2001). Under such arrangements, the private sector builds and finances new hospital facilities, and may also enter into a contract to manage the facility (Productivity Commission 1999). Duckett (2013) explains that under some of these **public–private partnerships (PPPs)** a private company will take responsibility for both building the new hospital and providing the maintenance on the building for a 20- or 50-year period – known as a design, build, finance and maintain arrangement. The costs of the building and the maintenance are paid for through regular facility payments over the life of the building. This means that the state government does not have to pay the full capital costs up front and the immediate debt burden for governments is thereby reduced.

However, there is a need for caution against any enthusiasm that may be generated by such arrangements. Davidson (2011) queries the argument that PPPs represent better value for money than financing the project with government borrowings. Duckett (2013) cites the many hospitals around Australia built under such arrangements that have been returned to the public sector at considerable cost to governments and the public purse. Collyer et al. (2001) analyse the case of the Port Macquarie Base Hospital, a PPP, which cost government 30% more than equivalent publicly funded hospitals. Despite firm evidence about the higher cost of PPPs over the longer term (e.g. McKell Institute 2014), they remain a popular option with governments.

In 2016, there were nine privately owned and/or operated hospitals providing public hospital services which were predominantly or substantially funded by state governments (AIHW 2018c). In 2018 the Northern Beaches Hospital in French's Forest, Sydney was added to this list. Table 3.1 provides a list of these hospitals, indicating that four are owned by for-profit enterprises (Healthscope and Ramsay Health Care), four by the Catholic Church, and two by community-owned, not-for-profit organisations.

Other forms of private medicine

PPPs to manage public hospitals are only one aspect of private medicine in Australia. Fee-for-service medicine in the primary health care sector (Chapter 6), privately delivered services in aged care (Chapter 8) and dentistry (Chapter 15) are primarily private-sector services. Moreover, privately delivered services increasingly occur within public hospitals, even within the public hospitals that are owned by the state and managed by public-sector employees. **Contracting out** has become a common phenomenon in many businesses and government departments over recent decades. Within Australian hospitals, cleaning and security services were initially targeted, eventually followed by many health and medical services such as hospital pharmacies and laboratory/diagnostic facilities.

TABLE 3.1 PRIVATELY OWNED / MANAGED PUBLIC HOSPITALS		
State / territory	**Hospital**	**Ownership**
New South Wales	Hawksbury District Health Service Northern Beaches Hospital	St John of God (Catholic Church) Healthscope Ltd (for-profit)
Victoria	Mildura Base Hospital	Ramsay Health Care (for-profit)
Queensland	Mater Adult Hospital Mater Mother's Hospital	Mater Private Hospitals (Catholic Church) Mater Private Hospitals (Catholic Church)
Western Australia	Joondalup Health Campus Peel Health Campus St John of God Midland Public Hospital	Ramsay Health Care (for-profit) Ramsay Health Care (for-profit) St John of God (Catholic Church)
South Australia	McLaren Vale and Districts War Memorial Private Hospital	(Community owned, not-for-profit)
Tasmania	May Shaw District Nursing Centre	May Shaw Health Centre Inc. (community owned, not-for-profit)

In New South Wales, the closure of many outpatient clinics – which forces patients to see specialists as private patients in their own businesses – is part of the same trend of 'hollowing out' the public hospitals by 'contracting within' to companies, trusts and not-for-profit organisations. No systematic statistics are collected by the AIHW on these practices, or the extent to which these have intensified over past decades, even though they have significantly increased out-of-pocket costs to patients.

Tensions in the public–private health space

If we wish to understand the Australian health care system, questions need to be asked about whether the public and private systems in Australia are successfully complementary or in competition, whether the private sector actually creates capacity in the public sector, and how PHI membership levels might have an effect on public hospital waiting lists (and whether this is a positive or negative effect). The divergent positions about the health care system are described as:

> On the 'left' are those who stand up for Medicare as a universal, free, tax funded system, while on the 'right' are those who would see private insurance take over the dominant role in funding healthcare.
> *(Doggett & McAuley 2013, p. 1)*

This polarisation of views about the health care system has played out historically, with conservative governments tending to support private health insurance and Labor governments supporting universal care paid for through the taxation system (Collyer et al. 2015). Yet, at the same time, there has been an overall political convergence on the existence of, and support for, private-sector medicine in Australia. This is evidenced by the PPP arrangements that both sides of government (Liberal and Labor) have negotiated at both federal and state levels, and is reflected in the lack of real debate about the consequences of the steady growth of the private health sector, especially since the 1990s.

It is not difficult to find evidence of a direct relationship between the growth of private sector medicine and the growth of the PHI industry. The private sector has been given enormous material support by governments through the **private health insurance rebate**. Yet, Doggett and McAuley (2013, p. 3) argue 'shifting health expenditure from public insurance to private insurance is simply shifting from one re-distributive mechanism (the tax and expenditure system) to another (the health insurance system), which can properly be described as a "privatised tax"'. Further, they argue, the dynamics of the health market, which is now characterised by medical interventions not possible previously, along with patients' and professionals' demands for such interventions, are distorted by the presence of insurance – because insurance of any kind, public or private, carries what economists refer to as '**moral hazard**'. They explain this as:

> ... the tendency for people to use more of a service when it is free or subsidised at the point of delivery than they would if they were paying from their own pockets. It applies both to patients and to doctors suggesting services, and is amplified in healthcare by consumers' tendency to over-estimate the effectiveness of therapies while under-estimating their non-financial costs, such as the risk of infection or long periods of convalescence.
>
> *(Doggett & McAuley 2013, p. 3)*

So increased spending on PHI adds to the cost of health care overall, without necessarily getting better health outcomes. The PHI rebate, in particular, must be analysed as a 'propping up' of an industry by government at the expense of increased funding into the public system. The rebate also works against the principles of universal access and equity of funding for those most in need. It has been argued it would be cheaper for government to remove the PHI subsidy and treat those people who drop their PHI and become reliant solely on the public system (Cheng 2018).

PAUSE
for
REFLECTION
...

1 Given the cost of the PHI subsidy, and its effects on the health care system, why do you think governments on both sides of politics continue to support it?

2 What effects might there be on the health system if the PHI rebate is removed and funds reallocated to public hospitals?

(Consider the article by Duckett, published in *The Australian* on 7 January 2015, about the effects of redirecting the rebate: http://grattan.edu.au/news/redirect-the-subsidy-to-cure-insurance-headache).

Summary

This chapter has provided an overview of the private health care sector in Australia and some of the tensions between its growth and issues of cost, quality health care, access and equity. Despite the existence of Medicare, a universal health insurance scheme that provides free public-hospital care and subsidises care for all patients in private hospitals as well as visits to private practitioners (including allied health services), there has been growing alarm within the community about rising 'out-of-pocket' costs, difficulties in accessing timely care, and the need for, and costs of, PHI. These issues are, as we have discussed in this chapter, fundamentally connected with the growth of private medicine.

Review Questions

1 What are some of the benefits, and the drawbacks, of a hybrid private–public health care system?

2 Does private health insurance provide meaningful choice?

3 Why do you think governments intervene in the private health insurance market?

4 Consider the arguments in Chapter 2 about the viability of Medicare. What do you think would be the effect on Medicare if people with private health insurance were able to opt out of paying the Medicare levy on condition that they used private health insurance or self-financed their care in public hospitals?

5 Name some of the information asymmetries discussed in this chapter. Who benefits from these asymmetries?

References

Australian Bureau of Statistics (ABS), 2014. Private hospitals, Australia, 2012–13. Commonwealth of Australia. Cat. no. 4390.0. http://www.abs.gov.au/AUSSTATS/abs@.nsf/Lookup/439 0.0Main+Features12012-13?OpenDocument.

Australian Bureau of Statistics (ABS), 2015. Private hospitals, Australia, 2013–14. Commonwealth of Australia. Cat. no. 4390.0. http://www.abs.gov.au/AUSSTATS/abs@.nsf/Lookup/4390.0Explanatory%20 Notes12013-14?OpenDocument.

Australian Institute of Health and Welfare (AIHW), 2017. Australia's hospitals 2016–17 at a glance, AIHW, Canberra.

Australian Institute of Health and Welfare, 2018a. Private health insurance expenditure, 2015–2016, AIHW, Canberra. https://www.aihw.gov.au/getmedia/08320d6a-4ceb-4c75-a16b-aa1a4c9f6d15/aihw-20592- private-health-insurance-expenditure.pdf.aspx.

Australian Institute of Health and Welfare (AIHW), 2018b. Australia's health 2018, AIHW, Canberra. Cat. no. AUS 221, https://www.aihw.gov.au/reports/australias-health/australias-health-2018/contents/ table-of-contents.

Australian Institute of Health and Welfare (AIHW), 2018c. Hospital resources 2016–17: Australian Hospital Statistics Cat. no. 205. AIHW, Canberra.

Australian Private Hospitals Association, 2017. Private patients in public hospitals. Department of Health options paper. http://www.apha.org.au/wp-content/uploads/2017/09/Private-Patients-in-Public-Hospitals-August-2017.pdf.

Australian Prudential Regulation Authority, 2018. Register of private insurers. https://www.apra.gov.au/register-private-health-insurers.

Brown, L., Barnett, J.R., 2004. Is the corporate transformation of hospitals creating a new hybrid health care space? A case study of the impact of co-location of public and private hospitals in Australia. Soc. Sci. Med. 58, 427–444.

Cheng, T., 2018. Private health rebates cost taxpayers billions work well – is it time they were scrapped? The Conversation. http://www.abc.net.au/news/2018-02-07/private-health-insurance-is-it-time-to-scrap-rebates/9405542.

Cheng, T.C., Joyce, C.M., Scott, A., 2013. An empirical analysis of public and private medical practice in Australia. Health Policy (New York) 111 (1), 43–51.

Collyer, F.M., McMaster, J., Wettenhall, R.W., 2001. Public enterprise divestment: Australian Case Studies. University of South Pacific Press, Fiji.

Collyer, F.M., White, K.N., 2001. Corporate control of healthcare in Australia. Discussion paper no. 42, Australia Institute, Australian National University, Canberra.

Collyer, F.M., Harley, K., Short, S.D., 2015. Money and markets in Australia's healthcare system. In: Meagher, G., Goodwin, S. (Eds.), Markets, Rights and Power in Australian Social Policy. Sydney University Press, Sydney, pp. 257–291.

Collyer, F.M., Willis, K., Lewis, S., 2017. Gatekeepers in the healthcare sector: knowledge and Bourdieu's concept of field. Soc. Sci. Med. 186, 96–103.

Davidson, K., 2011. Hospital PPPs show no signs of good health. Sydney Morning Herald. http://www.smh.com.au/federal-politics/political-opinion/hospital-ppps-show-no-signs-of-good-health-20110626-1gln4.html. 27 June.

Doggett, J., McAuley, I., 2013. A new approach to health funding. D!ssent no. 42. http://www.ianmcauley.com/academic/dissent/healthfund2013.pdf.

Duckett, S., 2013. Public–private hospital partnerships are risky business. The Conversation, 30 July. https://theconversation.com/public-private-hospital-partnerships-are-risky-business-16421.

Duckett, S., 2015. Redirect the subsidy to cure insurance headache. The Australian, 7 January. http://grattan.edu.au/news/redirect-the-subsidy-to-cure-insurance-headache.

Duckett, S., 2017. Australia's health system is enviable, but there is room for improvement', The Conversation, 22 September. https://theconversation.com/australias-health-system-is-enviable-but-theres-room-for-improvement-81332.

Duckett, S., 2018. Coercing, subsidising and encouraging: two decades of support for private health insurance. In: Cahill, D., Toner, P. (Eds.), Wrong Way: How Privatisation and Economic Reform Backfired. La Trobe University Press, Carlton, pp. 40–58.

Elliot, A., 2006. 'The best friend Medicare ever had?' Policy narratives and changes in Coalition health policy. Health Sociol. Rev. 15 (2), 132–143.

Finder, Advice Evolution, 2018. Health insurance statistics 2019. https://www.finder.com.au/health-insurance-statistics.

Harris, A., 2013. Things you should know about private health insurance rebates. The Conversation, 1 July. https://theconversation.com/things-you-should-know-about-private-health-insurance-rebates-15560.

Hicks, R., 1981. Rum Regulation and Riches. RT Kelly P/L, Sydney.

Independent Hospital Pricing Authority, 2017. Private patients in public hospitals, final report. IHPA, Canberra. https://www.ihpa.gov.au/sites/g/files/net636/f/publications/final_report_-_ihpa_-_private_patient_public_hospital_utilisation.pdf.

Lewis, S., Willis, K., 2018. Do you really need private health insurance? Here's what you need to know before deciding. The Conversation, 28 March. https://theconversation.com/do-you-really-need-private-health-insurance-heres-what-you-need-to-know-before-deciding-93661.

Lewis, S., Willis, K., Collyer, F.M., 2018. Navigating and making choices about healthcare: the role of place. Health Place 52, 215–220.

McKell Institute, 2014. Risky business: the pitfalls and missteps of hospital privatization. https://mckellinstitute.org.au/app/uploads/McKell-Institute-Risky-Business-Nov-2014.pdf.

NSW Health, 2018. Private health facilities. Regulation and Compliance Unit, NSW Government, Sydney. https://www.health.nsw.gov.au/hospitals/privatehealth/pages/default.aspx.

Parnell, S., 2017. States urging hospitals to bill health insurers is pushing up premiums, analysis shows. The Australian, 6 October. https://www.theaustralian.com.au/national-affairs/health/states-urging-hospitals-to-bill-health-insurers-is-pushing-up-premiums-analysis-shows/news-story/1f33d52ac125ed ca2ffabead65ab82c3.

Productivity Commission, 1999. Private hospitals in Australia, Commission research paper. AusInfo, Canberra. https://www.pc.gov.au/research/completed/private-hospitals/privatehospitals.pdf.

Seah, D., Cheong, T., Anstey, M., 2013. The hidden cost of private health insurance in Australia. Aust. Health Rev. 37 (1), 1–3.

White, K.N., Collyer, F.M., 1998. Health care markets in Australia: ownership of the private hospital sector. Int. J. Health Serv. 28 (3), 487–510.

Willis, E., 1989. Medical Dominance. Allen and Unwin, Sydney.

Willis, K., Collyer, F., Lewis, S., et al., 2016. Knowledge matters: producing and using knowledge to navigate healthcare systems. Health Sociol. Rev. 25 (2), 202–216.

Further Reading

Australian Institute of Health and Welfare (AIHW). Australia's health 2018. Cat. no. AUS 221. AIHW, Canberra. https://www.aihw.gov.au/reports/australias-health/australias-health-2018/contents/table-of-contents.

Jericho, G., 2018. Is private health insurance a con? The answer is in the graphs. The Guardian, 6 February. https://www.theguardian.com/business/grogonomics/2018/feb/06/is-private-health-insurance-a-con-the-answer-is-in-the-graphs.

Online Resources

Australian Prudential Regulation Authority (APRA; formerly Private Health Insurance Administration Council, PHIAC) – regulates (from July 2015) the private health insurance industry in Australia; the site includes reports and statistics on PHI in Australia: www.apra.gov.au.

Australia's health 2018 – the website of the biennial publication Australia's health: https://www.aihw.gov.au/reports/australias-health/australias-health-2018/contents/table-of-contents/.

CHAPTER 4

International health care systems

Judith Daire, Caroline Yates and Suzanne Robinson

Key learning outcomes

When you finish this chapter you should be able to:

- ◆ define the key concepts related to international health care systems
- ◆ identify the significant features and elements of a health care system
- ◆ compare and contrast types and performance of health care system models
- ◆ identify key driving factors for the current changes in health care systems or health sector reforms.
- ◆ understand future challenges for health care systems.

Key terms and abbreviations

activity-based funding (ABF)

bipartisan agreement

block-funding

electronic health record (EHR)

Health Care Home (HCH)

health care system

health care system performance

health determinants

health sector reforms

health system

market-driven and welfare health care systems

national health insurance (NHI) model

national health model

national health systems

out-of-pocket model

Patient Centered Medical Home (PCMH)

Patient Protection and Affordable Care Act (PPACA)

payment for performance

private health insurance (PHI) model

social insurance model

Introduction

Good health is fundamental to human welfare and sustained socio-economic development; however, this cannot be achieved without a well-functioning health system that promotes good health (World Health Organization (WHO) 2010). A well-functioning health system is described as one that 'delivers quality services to all people, when and where they need them' (WHO 2018). Given the central role of promoting a population's well-being, health systems are an integral part of the society and its development.

The aim of this chapter is to give an overview of the key concepts related to health care systems and to consider the characteristics of health systems from an international perspective. The chapter will then explore the performance of health systems with a particular focus on different health models, including the US system, which predominantly takes a market-based approach to health care, and the UK system, which takes a predominantly public-based approach. It will compare the UK and US models with the Australian context and consider the potential learning for Australia. It will finally consider future challenges and policy directions for health systems in Australia and beyond.

Definitions of key concepts

As you start studying health system or health care system, you will realise from the literature that the terms such as health system, health care system, health care delivery system, health care service system, medical care system, health sector, health services organisation and many others are used interchangeably (van Rensburg 2012). Although they all have characteristics of a system, they are different in that some have more inclusive or have wider connotations than others.

A system generally refers to a collection of parts that interact together and function as a whole (Ackoff & Rovin 2003). In a narrower sense, a **health system** is seen as an institution of 'health care', where *health care* refers to the organised social actions in response to the occurrence of disease and disability and for averting the risks to health (van Rensburg 2012). In other words, a **health care system** comprises the actions and institutions that strive to promote, protect or restore the health of individuals and populations. In a broader sense, the health system is viewed as including more than just health services, encompassing activities falling beyond the general scope of the health sector (sanitation, nutrition, housing, transport, education, etc.), which in the broadest sense affect the health of the population. It is this more inclusive approach that the WHO promotes (see Chapters 5 and 6). Accordingly, WHO (2000, p. 2) suggests that:

> A health system consists of all organisations, people and actions whose primary intent is to promote, restore or maintain health. This includes efforts to influence determinants of health as well as more direct health-improving activities.

Often when referring to the health system, the literature takes a more focused definition that relates to provision and investment in health services (i.e. primary, secondary and tertiary care), whether it be in the public or private sector, that is, the health care system. For example, Quadagno (2010, p. 126) defines health care systems as consisting 'of organisations that both deliver care and medical services (hospitals, physicians' practices, clinics) and that arrange for the financing of care (governments, agencies, states, local communities, and private insurance companies)'. See Box 4.1 for a summary of the clarifications for the concept 'health system' and related concepts.

What all definitions have in common is that health care systems are complex and involve a number of different institutions, organisations and professions. This reflects the nature of health as a fundamental outcome that health systems pursue. Though some view health as the absence of disease or medically measured risk factors, the WHO (1946) definition is broad and dynamic, namely 'a state of complete physical, mental and social well-being and not merely the absence of disease or infirmity'. It reflects the complex interactions of a person's genetics, lifestyle and environment. The Australian Institute of Health and Welfare (AIHW) reports that a person's health generally depends on two things: determinants (factors that influence health) and interventions (actions taken to improve health, and the resources required for these interventions) (AIHW 2018).

Health determinants are multifaceted, interrelated factors that influence health, which are categorised into social, economic, political, cultural and environmental determinants. Essentially, these are the conditions into which people are born, grow, live, work and age (WHO 2013, 2018).

PAUSE *for* REFLECTION ...

In consideration of the World Health Organization's definition of health systems, what are the main objectives of a health care system, and why? Who are the key actors in the Australian health care system?

BOX 4.1 DEFINITION OF A HEALTH SYSTEM AND THE RELATED CONCEPTS

- **Health care system:** activities and institutions in a society that deliver health care services to the population. These comprise health departments, hospitals, clinics and services (medical, nursing, dental, traditional health care, homeopathy), etc. – all being distinguishable systems of health care or parts thereof.
- **National health care system:** health sector of a society or country, encompasses policies, programs, institutions and actors that provide health care – organised efforts to treat and prevent disease (Berman). Note that, beyond the official or mainstream health care, the non-official, unorthodox health practices and care traditions also constitute part of a country's health care system.
- **Health system** includes the entire national health care system as well as all those extraneous matters which are either directly or indirectly associated with health especially the surrounding environment of the health care system and the population served.

Source: Adapted from van Rensburg, H. (2012). Health and Health Care in South Africa. Van Schaik Publishers, Pretoria

Health care system goals, elements and characteristics

Health systems, as noted by Gilson (2012), can be defined either by what they seek to do and achieve or by their elements and characteristics. The primary or defining goal of a health care system is to improve health. However, the goals of health care systems go beyond just improving health to include wider goals around quality, safety, and equity or fairness in the distribution of health care funding that meet the expectations of society. The WHO suggests that the goals of health care systems include promoting good health for citizens, responsiveness to the needs and expectations of the population and a fair means of funding operations. Hence progress in relation to these goals rest on four elements: (1) provision of efficient and equitable health care services, (2) resource generation, (3) financing and (4) stewardship (Frenk 2010; WHO 2007). A number of conceptual frameworks useful for understanding and analysing the nature of health systems in terms of their goals and elements exist (Smith & Hanson 2012), of which the WHO health system building blocks system remains dominant. This breaks down the health system into six essential building blocks; see Fig. 4.1.

It is believed that, to achieve their goals, health systems have to provide services, develop health workers and other key resources, mobilise and allocate finances and ensure health system leadership and governance. The building blocks are, however, not stand-alone but rather interconnected; hence the building blocks have to work together for the health system to be effective.

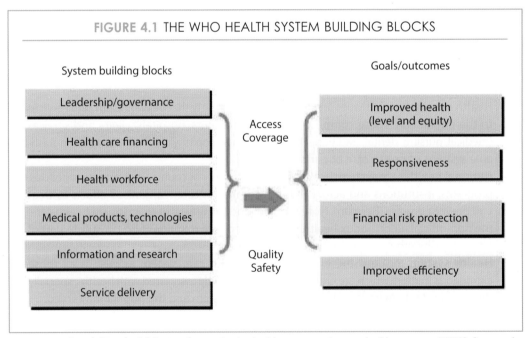

FIGURE 4.1 THE WHO HEALTH SYSTEM BUILDING BLOCKS

Source: WHO (2007). 'Everybody's business', strengthening health systems to improve health outcomes: WHO's framework for action. WHO, Geneva, p. 3.

Others have critiqued the WHO health system framework as a 'reductionist' view. For example, in an attempt to expand the view of health systems, Frenk (2010) suggested that health systems should be understood not only in terms of their component elements or parts (human resources, finances, hospitals, clinics, technologies, etc.). Rather, in addition to the elements, health systems also consist of the interactions and interrelations between these elements as well as the environment external to the system. Furthermore, viewing a 'health system' as comprising elements represents only the institutional or supply-side of the health system. Health systems also include the population both as an external beneficiary and as an integral part of the system (Frenk 2010).

PAUSE
for
REFLECTION
...

Consider how well the Australian health system performs in relation to the WHO building blocks. Which health system elements that are not included in these building blocks have been key in determining health system performance in Australia? Why do you think they are not included in the WHO building blocks?

National health care system models or typologies

Health care systems are quite different in each country and society, resulting from a process that Tuohy (1999a, 1999b) describes as essentially 'accidental', a product of a specific time and particular circumstances. The variation in national health care systems is strongly influenced by the economic and political systems as well as the underlying norms and values prevailing in the respective societies (Van Olmen et al. 2012). As noted by Stevens and Van der Zee (2007), health care systems are not only organised around social structures and political institutions; they also incorporate values and ideologies from the larger culture. Consequently, national health care systems often reflect political institutions, deeply rooted social values, ideologies from larger society and cultural norms, and expectations of the citizenry (Lameire et al. 1999). As a result, health care systems vary considerably in how they are funded and administered and in how medical services are distributed. Generally, health care systems may be thought of as being either:

- welfare based – a public system where the government provides the health care system for all citizens, or
- market driven – a private system where the services are run by private providers, and citizens pay for their own health care.

Welfare-based health care systems are predominantly underpinned by the principles of solidarity, where the cost of care in a country is subsidised across population age groups and levels of income. In welfare-based health care systems, health care is primarily viewed as a social or collective good, and all citizens benefit, irrespective of health care needs and costs. Other societies are influenced by the growing market-oriented ideas of perceiving health care as a commodity accessed through the open market like all other goods and services.

A great variety of health system models can be distinguished in developed and developing countries. These can broadly be categorised into five models (Kulesher & Forrestal 2014):

- **National health model:** also known as the Beveridge model, this is characterised by universal health care coverage of all citizens by a central government and financed through general tax revenues. Service distribution and provider payments are controlled by governments. Examples of the national health model include Denmark, Ireland, New Zealand and the United Kingdom.

- **Social insurance model:** also known as the Bismarck model, this is characterised by compulsory coverage that is funded by employer, individual and private insurance funds. Factors of production are controlled and owned by government or private entities. It is also referred to as tax-based insurance. Funding is derived from employment taxes and held in separate funds specifically for the national health program. Examples of the social insurance model include Austria, Belgium, France, Germany, Luxemburg and the Netherlands.

- **National health insurance (NHI) model:** this system has elements of both Beveridge and Bismarck. It uses private-sector providers, but payment comes from a government-run insurance program that every citizen pays into. The classic NHI system is found in Canada, but some newly industrialised countries – Taiwan and South Korea, for example – have also adopted the NHI model.

- **Private health insurance (PHI) model:** this model is characterised by employment-based or individual purchase of private health insurance financed by individual and employer contributions. Service delivery and financing are owned and managed by the private entities operating in an open market economy. Examples of the private insurance model include Switzerland and the United States.

- **Out-of-pocket model:** though not formally recognised, this model is prevalent in countries which are still developing their national health care systems towards an organised mass medical care health care system. For example, in many developing countries, consumers tend to pay for services out of pocket, which is associated with catastrophic health expenditure. If they cannot pay, they do not get medical care.

PAUSE
for
REFLECTION
...

Consider the different health care system models. How do you think each of these impacts on the health care access for the disadvantaged population groups and what this might mean for their health care outcomes?

No country has a pure form of one health system model; instead, most countries have mixed models where two or more models may coexist. **National health systems** are therefore characterised by the dominant model at one time. It is also important to note that health systems are not static but are continuously changing in response to the changes in both the internal and the external environment (i.e. changing roles of providers, breakthroughs in medical knowledge occurring within health). More recently, governments have deliberately implemented changes in the health care system as a response to prevailing organisational and contextual changes, which have collectively been referred to as **health sector reforms**.

Health sector reforms and the driving factors

Health systems are not static, but rather adjust and change to accommodate demographic, social, economic, environmental and technological changes (AIHW 2018). Health care systems of most countries are evolving and evidently significant changes and transitions have been observed over many years. The main driving factors include ageing populations, changing disease patterns, scientific and technological developments, growing public demand, a quest for greater efficiency, fairness and responsiveness to the expectations of the people, nurturing of health rights and entitlements, rising costs and growing consumer consciousness (van Rensburg 2012). Logically, these issues give rise to general dissatisfaction among governments, providers and consumers alike – due to the overall performance of the health systems, inefficiencies in the use of resources, neglect of primary and preventive care and lack of responsiveness of services to users' needs and demands. Consequently, most countries are consistently subjected to health sector reforms with a view to improving equity, access, efficiency, effectiveness and responsiveness to population's health needs. See Table 4.1 for examples of health care reforms in different countries based on their health care system models.

Generally, health sector reforms are aimed at universal access to care, cost containment, enhanced quality of care, increased patient choice and satisfaction and securing public accountability as well as public participation in organising and managing health services. Often reforms are achieved by refining the role of government, shifting emphasis towards primary health care (see Chapter 5 and 6) and cutting back on sophisticated, high-tech specialised medicine and hospitalisation in order to render health care more affordable, accessible and preventive in nature. Likewise, reforms are also associated with increased emphasis on health promotion and healthy lifestyles. As part of these reforms, the performance of a national health care system is constantly under review in comparison with other countries to assess how it is faring in achieving the ultimate goal of health as well as equity, access, responsiveness and quality of health care (Collins et al. 1999). See Table 4.1 for examples.

PAUSE
for
REFLECTION
...

Consider the mixed health care system model in Australia as outlined in Chapters 2 and 3. What sort of health sector reforms have taken place in Australia? What have been the major driving factors?

TABLE 4.1 EXAMPLES OF HEALTH CARE REFORMS IN DIFFERENT COUNTRIES BASED ON HEALTH CARE SYSTEM MODELS

Country	Predominant health care system model	Health sector issues	Reform aims
USA	Free market system where the private health insurance is prevalent	Unequal access due to a big uninsured population Dissatisfaction with fee-for service model	Creating more universal health insurance coverage for the uninsured population
Poland and Czech Republic	Socialist model of health care systems	Centralised system with heavy government control of decision-making and resource allocation	Decentralisation of responsibilities in decision making to lower levels of the health system Introduction of private or mixed public–private Privatisation of public services
Sweden and German	Bismark model of national health insurance	Rising costs of health care, growing inequality and declining access to health care.	Introduced private health insurance and providers to give consumers choice to supplement the national health insurance Decentralisation and privatisation
UK	National Health Service	Rising health care costs, growing inequality in access to health care services	Privatisation Decentralisation of health policy Separation of purchasing and provider role of health care services

Health care system performance

A key concern of governments and others who invest in health systems is how to tell whether and when the desired improvements in **health care system performance** are being achieved. It is not easy to compare health system performance – the reasons for this relate to the different processes, structures, institutions and organisation of health care systems. A recent survey undertaken by the Commonwealth Fund explored the performance of health care systems across 11 Organisation for

Economic Co-Operation and Development countries (OECD 2018; Schneider et al. 2017). The key performance areas of interest related to quality, access, efficiency, equity and healthy lives. See Table 4.2 for the health care system performance rankings in OECD countries.

Overall, the United Kingdom, Australia and the Netherlands were reported as the top performing health systems; see Table 4.2. The UK is ranked first compared with other countries in all areas except Health Care Outcomes, where it ranks 10th. Australia is second, ranking highest on Administrative Efficiency and Health Care Outcomes, Care Process and Access, but low on Equity. The Netherlands is among the top performers on Care Process, Access and Equity; its performance on Administrative Efficiency stands out as an area for improvement. New Zealand performs well on measures of Care Process and Administrative Efficiency, but is below the 11-country average on other indicators.

Surprising, even though the US has the highest per capita health expenditures, performance of its health care system ranks last among the 11 high-income countries. It is important to note, however, that it is the only high-income country lacking universal health insurance coverage. Over the last 10 years, the US has taken significant efforts to expand coverage through the ***Patient Protection and Affordable Care Act*** (**PPACA**) (United States Congress 2009–10). The 2017 Commonwealth Fund report shows that the PPACA has catalysed remarkable gains in access to care across the US (Schneider et al. 2017).

Comparing countries' health care system performance using standardised performance data offers benchmarks on how to improve care providing useful insights. The main difference between the USA and the UK relates to the differences around **market-driven and welfare health care systems**. That is, the USA system is founded on market-driven values and a culture that has been characterised by a respect for individualism and entrepreneurship (Trompenaars &

TABLE 4.2 HEALTH CARE SYSTEM PERFORMANCE RANKINGS IN OECD COUNTRIES

	AUS	CAN	FRA	GER	NETH	NZ	NOR	SWE	SWIZ	UK	US
Overall ranking	2	9	10	8	3	4	4	6	6	1	11
Care process	2	6	9	8	4	3	10	11	7	1	5
Access	4	10	9	2	1	7	5	6	8	3	11
Administrative Efficiency	1	6	11	6	9	2	4	5	8	3	10
Equity	7	9	10	6	2	8	5	3	4	1	11
Health care Outcomes	1	9	5	8	6	7	3	2	4	10	11

Source: Schneider, E.C., Sarnak, D.O., Squires, D., Shah, A. and Doty, M.M. et al. (2017). Mirror, mirror 2017: international comparison reflects flaws and opportunities for better U.S. health care. http://commonwealthfund.org/~/media/files/publications/fund-report/2017/jul/schneider_mirror_mirror_2017.pdf

Hampden-Turner 1998). The UK health care system was shaped by notions of equality and equity – quite different values to those that underpinned the US health care system. However, in recent times the UK system has moved towards more market-based principles around competition- and incentive-driven provision of care in line with the ideas of new public management outlined in Chapter 1. The UK system remains underpinned by the principle of universal access to health care with a mixture of market-based approaches to ensure efficient administrative health system performance.

Described as a complex 'web' of services, providers, recipients and organisational structures (WHO 2018), the Australia's health care system falls somewhere in the middle, combining features similar to the US and the UK health care systems. For example, when Australia introduced a universal health insurance system in the 1970s, it followed the same principles that underpinned the UK NHS but funded practitioners on a fee-for-service basis and allowed people the freedom to select their provider without needing to register with any particular gate-keeper. It appears, however, that the UK and the US are now taking on a number of elements from the Australian health care system. Both countries are moving towards health care systems characterised by a public–private mix such as that of Australia. The question then becomes: how public or how private should the system be?

PAUSE *for* **REFLECTION** ...

Consider the following:
- What do you consider to be the major contributing factors to health system performance?
- In comparing the UK system and the USA to Australia, what are the key differences in both funding and government involvement?
- What relationship does health expenditure in UK, US and Australia have on health status and outcomes?
- How well do the health systems of these countries perform in terms of life expectancy or morbidity or mortality rates?
- What organisations portray these statistics and why do we need to know this information?
- How should health expenditure be controlled?

What are the factors that impact on health system performance?

The performance of health systems is affected by a number of aspects relating to the *hardware* and *software* of the system (Gilson 2012). The hardware relates to organisational and structural aspects (legal, financing structures) as well as clinical and service delivery aspects. The software areas include the norms, values, culture and traditions of institutions. As noted above, the US health system has a much more individualistic and market-based perspective on health care than the UK – the NHS encompasses a more egalitarian perspective that provides universal access and a notion that health care should be available to all regardless of wealth. These different perspectives underpin both the hardware and the software elements of the USA and UK health systems and are interlinked. Whereas the UK system is funded by taxation, the funding distribution mechanisms have taken on a more market-based approach and have moved from **block-funding** (which tends to be based on historical patterns of funding) to **activity-based funding (ABF)** (which focuses on **payment for performance**). This approach has been adopted by a number of countries and is aimed at increasing efficiencies in the health system (O'Reilly et al. 2012). However, evidence for its effectiveness relating to efficiency and other aspects is mixed. What we do know is that ABF, along with other efficiency measures, seems to have increased awareness of the cost of health interventions. However, ABF can limit system reform, especially when such reform means that services may need to change or reduce activity. The limiting factor of payment for performance is that it rewards activity without consideration for equity and effectiveness (Wranik 2012). In Australia, we have seen a shift in focus to include ABF in the hospital setting; although this could go some way to increasing the awareness of costs and potential efficiency savings, it does need to be considered alongside other policies that reward effectiveness and equity considerations.

Another difference between Australia and the UK is in the government structure. The UK has a single, centralised government system while Australia has two tiers of government concerned with health: the Commonwealth and state governments. In Australia, the health services (hospitals) are the business of state governments, with different hardware and software dimensions existing across them, while the business of primary care, such as GP services, tends to sit with the Commonwealth government. This adds even more complexity to the system and can make system integration even more problematic. (See Chapter 2 for an example of this problem, sometimes referred to as the 'blame game'.) Internationally, evidence shows that it is very difficult to change the organisation and mechanism of health systems once established. In terms of Australia, it is unlikely that changes to the tiers of government will be made any sooner, rendering health system reform problematic. Lessons from other countries demonstrate a need for **bipartisan agreement** across different governments (state and national) and with opposition parties, so that more joined-up approaches to the design, development and implementation of health system reform can be undertaken.

Future directions and challenges for health care systems

Globally health systems face similar issues and challenges – including changing demographics with an ageing population that has more chronic and complex health needs, a rise in technological advances that are costly to implement, a rise in the resistance to antibiotics, and the spread of infectious diseases. These challenges are complex, requiring responses that involve a number of different stakeholder groups who often have very different values and cultures and different interests and perspectives.

Ageing and non-communicable diseases (NCDs)

The increasing prevalence of chronic conditions is placing unprecedented demand on health care systems globally and is a priority for action (Sum et al. 2018). How we manage chronic disease has seen a push to provide services outside of the hospital settings and out into primary care, the focus being a better understanding of health determinants, risk factors and multiple morbidities combined with a reorientation of current health funding and delivering services through better design. For example, derived from the Chronic Care Model, the concept of patients having a Medical Home to manage their primary health care needs has been widely supported across the United States through the **Patient Centered Medical Home (PCMH)** model (Peikes et al. 2012). Australia's **Health Care Home (HCH)** model has been adapted from the PCMH to address the complex health care needs of people living with chronic conditions within a different fiscal environment (Department of Health 2016). The concept of medical homes links to the principles of patient-centred, comprehensive and coordinated care through integrated services. Its prime focus is to reduce spending whilst simultaneously improving quality as there is strong evidence internationally that integrated health systems with a strong focus on primary care will produce more efficient outcomes than fragmented systems. Such integration can be difficult given the power of hospitals and the different professional groups in the health system.

Role of the consumer and technology

The success of providing patient-centred, integrated and coordinated care is reliant on developing technology and the role of the consumer. We have seen a paradigm shift in how people access health care and the role of social media, social networks and digital communities (see Chapter 16). There has been an upsurge in digital health with consumers progressively taking control of their health information and being involved in managing their own health care. In many countries consumers now have access to their personally controlled **electronic health record (EHR)** and new opportunities exist as a result of wearable apps and interactive systems enabling health service delivery to be managed in their own homes. This is vital to achieving the health reform many systems desire, but here in Australia there continue to be major trust issues between consumers and governments on who should have access to this data or how this data should be used. This then results in a fragmentation of the use of personally controlled EHRs, particularly in an Australian health care context, in spite of the evidence that suggests improvements in both patient engagement and health care outcomes (Milani & Franklin 2017).

Moving from volume to value

Many health care systems around the globe have a dominant fee-for-service model and this incentivises over-provision of services, which contributes nothing to improving health (Case study 4.1). We are seeing a shift in focus from rewarding activity and volume to models that reward value and effective patient outcomes. The work by Porter and Lee (2013) and West et al. (2014) suggests that if the focus and goals of health systems are to provide high-quality care, and if this is realised, then this will lead to efficiency savings. This suggests that, in Australia, consideration needs to be given to how to

Case Study 4.1

Comparing health care systems

The OECD uses a series of indicators to compare the health care systems of different countries. Table 4.3 presents the most commonly cited indicators for Australia, the USA and the UK. Public views expressed through the media often claim that more money needs to be spent on health care to improve population health outcomes; however, this is not necessarily the case, as demonstrated in Table 4.3. Consider the information presented in the table and answer the questions below.

Case study questions

1. Given the quantitative data shown in the table, does increasing financial expenditure equal improved health outcomes? If not, what are the reasons for this?

2. Does assessing purely quantitative data in relation to health care systems illustrate the effectiveness? If not, what more could be assessed?

3. Reflecting on the above, revisit the WHO building blocks earlier in the chapter, then go to the Commonwealth Fund web page https://www.commonwealthfund.org/publications/fund-reports/2017/jul/mirror-mirror-2017-international-comparison-reflects-flaws-and and compare/contrast the top 10 high-income countries' health care systems. What are the main differences between the top five countries, and why?

4. Examine the health risk factors, what strikes you about these data? With these two indicators related to chronic disease, what impact do you think this has on overall health care systems spending?

incorporate incentives to reward outcomes that focus on value and quality (Norman & Robinson 2015). This will require a shift in thinking by many health care systems that will need to continue to reduce waste and unnecessary variation, changing health care delivery models using data more effectively to drive the change and engaging with all stakeholders to transform health care systems to providing economically sustainable quality care (Katz & Baum 2017).

Governance and stewardship leadership

Although effective policy is important to system reform, it is cultures and behaviours that shape the system, and as such they will have considerable impact on the development and implementation of health policy. Shifting mindsets and changing culture is a major challenge for system integration, especially in systems like Australia that have privileged silo-based working (Brown et al. 2013). Reform of this nature will require effective leadership that can navigate the complex system and the different organisations and powerful professions. West et al. (2014) note the importance of taking a collective leadership approach, rather than traditional command and control structures; they suggest that the former will 'provide the optimum basis for caring cultures'.

TABLE 4.3 THE MOST COMMONLY CITED INDICATORS FOR COMPARING THE HEALTH CARE SYSTEMS OF AUSTRALIA, USA AND UK

	Australia	USA	UK
Total population	25,000,000	326,000,000	66,000,000
Gross national income per capita (PPP International $)	$45.10	$52.10	$38.50
Life expectancy at birth (years)	Male 81 Female 85	Male 76 Female 81	Male 77 Female 81
Probability of dying under five (per 1000 live births)	6	8	5
Total expenditure on health per capita (International $ 2012)	$4357	$9403	$3495
Total expenditure on health as % of GDP (2017)	9.6	17.8	9.7
Health risk factors prevalence of obesity BMI >30	28	38	26
Health risk factors prevalence of self-reported smoking	13	19	13

GDP=gross domestic product; PPP=purchasing power parity.

Source: Data from OECD Health Statistics (2018) https://www.oecd.org/els/health-systems/health-data.htm

PAUSE
for
REFLECTION
...

- What are the dominant and powerful professions in health care systems? Give reasons for your answers.
- Who are the dominant stakeholder groups in health care systems? And why?
- Are there any differences in these groups between the UK, the USA and Australia? If so, what are they and what could be the reasons for this?
- What are the three biggest challenges, in your view, facing the Australian health care system now and into the future, and why?

Summary

In this chapter we focus on the different systems of health care found worldwide.

- This included a brief description of what we mean by a health system, including the goals, elements and characteristics of international health systems.
- Health system development is based on a number of factors, including a society's views, values and cultures; we have also seen that future policy reforms are often influenced by past choices.
- The chapter explored the performance of systems and compared two very different health system models – that of a predominantly market-based model (US) and a predominantly public-based model (UK).
- International lessons for Australia include that, although systems strive for efficiency, policies that reward activity can actually have a negative impact on efficiency, and we are seeing a number of systems moving from a focus on volume to one on value and patient experience.
- International policy directions are shifting to more integrated systems of care that focus on the whole patient experience – this involves breaking down the traditional silos and power structures.
- It is early days in terms of this policy direction; however, early evidence suggests that system integration will require policies that incentivise this type of approach and have access to data that can measure performance and governance. It will also require effective leadership, throughout the system, that can motivate and drive change.
- Finally, Australia has much to learn from other countries while also having much to offer – policy-makers need to look to international evidence and consider how this evidence translates to their own health system setting.

Review Questions

1 Is it possible to have a health service that is free for all? Give reasons for why or why not in your answer.
2 Discuss whether health care is a *right* or a *commodity*. Should health care be treated like a commodity and traded in the marketplace? Give reasons for your answers.
3 What characteristics would you say the perfect health care system should have? Explain each characteristic.
4 Do you think the population in general needs more education about the health care system? Talk about the reasons why this may be important.
5 Identify the key aspects of the US health care system.
6 Identify the key aspects of the UK health care system.
7 Reflect on how the US and UK systems have changed over the past 20 years. Why have they changed?

References

Ackoff, R.L., Rovin, S., 2003. Redesigning society. Standford Business, Standford, CA.

Australian Institute of Health and Welfare, 2018. Australia's health 2018. Australia's health series no. 16. AUS221. Canberra: AIHW. Available from: https://www.aihw.gov.au/getmedia/7c42913d-295f-4bc9-9c2 4-4e44eff4a04a/aihw-aus-221.pdf.aspx?inline=true.

Brown, L., Katterl, R., Baywoood, P., et al., 2013. Medicare Locals: a model for primary healthcare integration? PHCIRS Policy Issue Review. Primary Healthcare Research and Information Service, Adelaide.

Collins, C., Green, A., Hunter, D., 1999. Health sector reform and the interpretation of policy context. Health Policy (New York) 47 (1), 69–83.

Department of Health, 2016. Primary Health Care Advisory Group final report: better outcomes for people with chronic and complex health conditions. Department of Health, Canberra. http://www.health .gov.au/internet/main/publishing.nsf/Content/76B2BDC12AE54540CA257F72001102B9/$File/Primary -Health-Care-Advisory-Group_Final-Report.pdf.

Frenk, J., 2010. The global health system: strengthening national health systems as the next step for global progress. PLoS Med. 7, e1000089.

Gilson, L., 2012. Health Policy and Systems Research: A Methodology Reader. Alliance for Health Policy and Systems Research. World Health Organization, Geneva.

Katz, I., Baum, F., 2017. National strategic framework for Aboriginal and Torres Strait Islander Peoples' mental health and social and emotional wellbeing 2017–2023. Australian Government, Health Minister's Advisory Council, Canberra.

Kulesher, R.R., Forrestal, E.E., 2014. International models of health systems financing. J. Hosp. Admin. 3 (4), 127.

Lameire, N., Joffe, P., Wiedemann, M., 1999. Healthcare system – an international review: an overview. Nephrol. Dial. Transplant. 14 (Suppl. 6), 3–9.

Milani, R.V., Franklin, N.C., 2017. The role of technology in health living medicine. Prog. Cardiovasc. Dis. 59 (5), 487–491.

Norman, R., Robinson, S., 2015. Lessons from Albion: can Australia learn from England's approach to primary healthcare funding? J. Health Organ. Manag. 29 (7), 925–932.

O'Reilly, J., Busse, R., Hakkinen, U., et al., 2012. Paying for hospital care: the experience with implementing activity based funding in five European countries. Health Econ. Policy Law 7, 73–101.

Organization of Economic Coorperation and Development OECD, 2018. Health statistics 2018. http:// www.oecd.org/els/health-systems/health-data.htm.

Peikes, D., Zutshi, A., Genevro, J.L., et al., 2012. Early evaluations of the medical home: building on a promising start. Am. J. Manag. Care 18, 105–116.

Porter, M.E., Lee, T.H., 2013. The strategy that will fix health care. Available from: https://www.hbs.edu/ faculty/Pages/item.aspx?num=45614.

Quadagno, J., 2010. Institutions, interest groups, and ideology: an agenda for the sociology of health care reform. J. Health Soc. Behav. 51 (2), 125–136.

Schneider, E.C., Sarnak, D.O., Squires, D., et al., 2017. Mirror, mirror 2017: international comparison reflects flaws and opportunities for better U.S. health care (Don Mills). https://www.commonwealthfund.org/publications/fund-reports/2017/jul/mirror-mirror-2017-international-comparison-reflects-flaws-and.

Smith, R.D., Hanson, K., 2012. Health Systems in Low- and Middle-income Countries: An Economic and Policy Perspective. OUP, Oxford.

Stevens, F., Van der Zee, J., 2007. Healthcare delivery systems. Blackwell Encyclopedia Sociol. 37, 312–324.

Sum, G., Hone, T., Atun, R., et al., 2018. Multimorbidity and out-of-pocket expenditure on medicines: a systematic review. BMJ Glob. Health 3 (1), e000505.

Trompenaars, F., Hampden-Turner, C., 1998. Riding the Waves of Culture: Understanding Diversity in Global Business. McGraw-Hill, New York.

Tuohy, C., 1999a. Accidental Logics: The Dynamics of Change in Healthcare Arena in United States, Britain and Canada. OUP, New York.

Tuohy, C.H., 1999b. Dynamics of a changing health sphere: the United States, Britain, and Canada. Health Aff. 18 (3), 114–134.

United States Congress, 2009–10. H.R.3590 - Patient Protection and Affordable Care Act. https://www.congress.gov/bill/111th-congress/house-bill/3590/.

Van Olmen, J., Criel, B., Van Damme, W., et al., 2012. Analysing Health System Dynamics: A Framework. ITG Press, Antwerp.

van Rensburg, H., 2012. Health and Health Care in South Africa. Van Schaik, Pretoria.

West, M., Steward, K., Eckert, R., et al., 2014. Developing Collective Leadership for Healthcare. Kings Fund, London, pp. 7–8.

World Heath Organization (WHO), 1946. Preamble to the constitution of the World Health Organization (WHO) as adopted by the International Health Conference, New York 19–22 June 1946. WHO, Geneva.

World Health Organization (WHO), 2000. The world health report 2000: health systems: improving performance. WHO, Geneva.

World Health Organization (WHO), 2007. 'Everybody's business', strengthening health systems to improve health outcomes: WHO's framework for action. WHO, Geneva.

World Health Organization (WHO), 2010. The world health report: health systems financing: the path to universal coverage. WHO, Geneva. http://www.who.int/whr/2010/en/.

World Health Organization (WHO), 2013. The determinants of health. WHO, Geneva. http://www.who.int/hia/evidence/doh/en/.

World Health Organization (WHO), 2018. Health topics: health systems. WHO, Geneva. http://www.who.int/topics/health_systems/en/.

Wranik, D., 2012. Healthcare policy tools as determinants of health system efficiency: evidence from the OECD. Health Econ. Policy Law 7, 197–226.

Further Reading

Braithwaite, J., Hibbert, P., Blakely, B., et al., 2017. Health system frameworks and performance indicators in eight countries: a comparative international analysis. SAGE Open Med. 5, 1–10.

Gonzalo, J.D., Haidet, P., Papp, K.K., et al., 2017. Educating for the 21st-century health care system. Acad. Med. 92, 35–39.

Mossialos, E., Wenzl, M., Osborn, R., et al., 2017. International Profiles of Health Care Systems. Commonwealth Fund, New York.

Pappagiani, M., Tziomalos, K., 2018. Health care reform in China: challenges and opportunities. Curr. Med. Res. Opin. 34, 821–823.

Pawson, R., Greenhalgh, J., Brennan, C., et al., 2014. Do reviews of healthcare interventions teach us how to improve healthcare systems? Soc. Sci. Med. 114, 129–137.

Tichenor, M., Shirdar, D., 2017. Universal health coverage, health systems strengthening, and the World Bank. BMJ 358, j3347.

World Health Organization (WHO), 2008. Closing the Gap in a generation – health equity through action and the social determinants of health. WHO, Geneva.

Online Resources

Australian Institute of Health and Welfare (AIHW) and the Australian Bureau of Statistics (ABS) – both the AIHW and ABS has a range of resources and publications illustrating the health of the Australian population: https://www.aihw.gov.au and http://www.abs.gov.au/AUSSTATS/.

Organisation for Economic Co-operation and Development (OECD) – the OECD brings together the governments of countries committed to democracy and the market economy from around the world. The OECD analyses the financial sustainability, efficiency and quality of health and long-term care systems in member countries: http://www.oecd.org/

World Health Organization (WHO) – the WHO website provides many resources for comparing health care systems in other countries: http://www.who.int/en/

CHAPTER 5

Public health in Australia

Helen Keleher

Key learning outcomes

When you finish this chapter you should be able to:

- ◆ understand public health and population health
- ◆ explain the aims of population health approaches to health
- ◆ describe the pathways into public health careers
- ◆ describe the public health system in Australia and the responsibilities of different levels of government for public health
- ◆ provide an overview of how major public health issues are handled
- ◆ consider the politics of public health.

Key terms and abbreviations

acquired immune deficiency syndrome (AIDS)

Council of Academic Public Health Institutions of Australia (CAPHIA)

environmental health officer (EHO)

health equity

health gap

human immunodeficiency virus (HIV)

Master of Public Health (MPH)

new public health

old public health

population strategy

prevention paradox

public health outcome funding agreements (PHOFAs)

social determinants of health (SDH)

Introduction

Public health is a broad field that involves all of us, on a daily basis, whether as health professionals or as citizens. Public health is a field of practice, research and advocacy designed to protect and improve the health of individuals, families, communities and populations, locally and globally (Association of Schools and Programs of Public Health (ASPPH) 2018) (Box 5.1). This chapter will explain public health, discuss pathways into public health careers, the connections between public

---

Public health is your health

On a global scale, public health improves the conditions of living that affect the health of all of us. Public health is at the forefront of containing deadly contagious diseases such as ebola, measles, malaria and HIV/AIDS. Public health seeks to reduce the incidence of preventable diseases, minimise the consequences of catastrophic events, provide the basics of sanitation, safe food and safe water, and promote healthier lifestyles.

You are only as healthy as the world you live in

Your health is determined not only by your own genetics and personal choices, but also by the environment around you. Public health investigates the ecology of health – from social networks and economic circumstances to our environment – and then minimises health risks.

Public health is moral and smart

Public health efforts allow us to save lives – your life, the lives of your family and friends, and the lives of people around the world. If we can save lives, we should. We'll not only make people healthier, but we'll also address soaring health care costs by preventing unnecessary death and disease.

Source: Association of Schools and Program of Public Health (2018). https://www.aspph.org

---

health and the social determinants of health, and how public health is organised and delivered in Australia, including the public health responsibilities of the three levels of government.

The classic definition of public health, from Winslow (1920), is that public health is the art and science of preventing disease and injury, prolonging life and promoting health through the organised efforts of society.

Public health is described by the Public Health Association of Australia (2015, p. 7) as:

◆ the distribution, determinants and significance of health, sickness and disabilities in communities
◆ the social, behavioural and biological sciences in relation to health and disease
◆ the impact of the physical and social environment on health, and the prevention and control of disease
◆ the economic, social and personal resources required for the optimum health of individuals
◆ the health problems and needs of the community, and the distribution and utilisation of health resources
◆ the structure and organisation and function, planning and management of health services and health information systems, and
◆ the causes and likely remedies for a reduction of social and economic inequities in health status, especially the inequities between Indigenous and non-Indigenous populations.

'Old' and 'new' public health

'**Old public health**' in the 19th and early 20th centuries focused on hygiene, sanitation, control of infectious diseases and the provision of clean water. '**New public health**' developed in the latter part of the 20th century as the emphasis moved towards a focus on the broad determinants of health and the conditions of life where people live, work and play. Public health became increasingly understood in terms of how to achieve healthy populations and the quality of people's lives and well-being without losing the foundations provided by old public health measures. New public health has become a movement that has learnt from the political and practical experience of past successes and failures in public health, and aims to achieve higher standards of health for populations, particularly those who have the least resources and experience disadvantages of various types (Keleher & MacDougall 2015).

The drivers for public health are both philosophical and economic. Philosophically, the values for public health are based on notions of health for all, social justice and equity (Commission on the Social Determinants of Health 2008; Nuffield Council on Bioethics 2007). The economic drivers for public health are about reducing the costs of illness and treatment through preventing ill-health and promoting and protecting the public's health, and the maintenance of a healthy workforce (Swedish National Institute of Public Health 2011). In Tuohy's terms (Tuohy 1999), public health is maintained by strong networks, which is characteristic of public health delivery systems. No single organisation can effectively deliver a public health service. While public health is primarily a public-sector government activity, delivery of some activities is reliant on sound relationships between governments at all levels, universities and research institutes, as well as with the private sector such as general practice, cancer screening services, road safety organisations, the alcohol and drug sector, water utilities and so on. All societies need public health, provided in the most efficient and effective ways.

Pathways into public health

Public health practitioners come from a wide range of disciplines including medicine, nursing, epidemiology, biostatistics, economics, social sciences, political science, psychology, allied health, environmental health and health promotion. Public health can be studied as a discipline at undergraduate and postgraduate levels.

- The different types of undergraduate program include Public Health, Health Sciences, Health Promotion and the profession of environmental health officers.
- At postgraduate level, the **Master of Public Health (MPH)** program is the main route into public health for graduates of other disciplines. It is popular with clinicians who wish to broaden their understanding and fields of practice.

The peak body for academic schools of public health is the **Council of Academic Public Health Institutions Australia (CAPHIA**; www.caphia.com.au). This is an organisation of schools of public health that work together to advance public health education, research and workforce development.

The public health workforce

Public health systems rely on an infrastructure based on good education and experience that is particularly reliant on its workforce. The public health workforce is necessarily multidisciplinary, stemming from occupational groups that include those of medicine, epidemiology, biostatistics, social sciences, environmental health, nursing, health promotion, health communication, the various allied health groups, public policy, health service management and health economics (Gebbie et al. 2003). People with these disciplinary backgrounds have often studied public health at postgraduate level and find a wide range of careers in government and non-government sectors and in academia. For example, a social science graduate from a Master of Public Health course may discover a strong affinity with epidemiology and biostatistics, while a graduate from health promotion may study a Master of Public Policy course and find a career in government, working on policy issues associated with health promotion or health inequalities.

Any single public health issue requires a multidisciplinary response. Many major public health programs represent 'investments in large-scale, longer term public health programs over 30–50 years that utilise a breadth of strategies and methods to achieve reductions in harm' (Keleher 2017, p. 2). Public health programs seek improved population health outcomes from significant, and often socially entrenched, problems, analysing what is needed to improve health outcomes from those problems from the evidence, and often building the evidence over time. For example, road safety efforts to reduce deaths from vehicle and bike accidents have required legislative, institutional, policy and program responses that have aimed to 'change the story' behind the problems, which are complex and therefore cannot be solved by simplistic solutions.

Public health efforts are coordinated and evidence based, backed by clear legislative and policy frameworks that inform road safety campaigns. The legislation is complemented by national strategies that provide clear roles and responsibilities across levels of government within agreed national goals, objectives and priorities. However, the acceptance of legislation has been dependent on law enforcement backed by concerted public education programs.

To inform public education, researchers in biostatistics and epidemiology interpret the trends in the incidence and prevalence of road deaths and injuries, engineers and police advise on the causes of road traffic accidents, and program managers develop the overall program plans, budgets and the various components of the whole program. The campaign materials have often included graphic footage that involves all of the people associated with film- or documentary-making, while the health communication experts work on shaping the key messages, designing them to influence people's behaviour on roads.

Public health professionals are distinguished by their preparedness to advocate for neglected public health issues and to stand up for what might be politically unpopular solutions to public health problems. Examples are sex education in schools that includes comprehensive information about sexually transmitted infections and how to prevent them, access to health services through bulk-billing, and a functional welfare state to support the health of disadvantaged or vulnerable groups.

PAUSE
for
REFLECTION
...

What social conditions and settings have had the greatest impact on your life? How might they reflect public health issues?

Population health

Population health can be narrowly defined in terms of risks and associated health outcomes, but also more broadly to encompass the multiple determinants of health. The Public Health Agency of Canada (2011) argues for an even broader conceptualisation of population health, saying that it should expect outcomes that go far beyond just health improvement for populations. The benefits of a population health approach should extend to include integrated health systems that work in sustainable partnerships across sectors, increase economic growth and productivity, and strengthen social cohesion and citizen engagement.

Geoffrey Rose (1981, 1992, 2001), now regarded as a classic thinker and researcher about public and population health, posed a key question for public health: 'Why are some people healthy and others not?' To answer that question, Rose said (1992, p. 62):

> In order to grasp the principles of public health, one must understand that society is not merely a collection of individuals but is also a collectivity, and the behavior and health of its individual members are profoundly influenced by its collective characteristics and social norms. Given time, these collective and societal characteristics can be changed either by the behavior of individuals, such as opinion formers and health educators, or by the mass effects of changes in the economy, the environment, or technical developments. The efforts of individuals are only likely to be effective when they are working with the societal trends.

Population health is an approach used within public health systems – it is a framework for thinking about why some populations are healthier than others, as well as the policy development, research and resource allocation that flow from this (Van Wave et al. 2010; Young 1998). The aims of population health are twofold: to improve the health of the whole population, and to decrease the inequities in health status between different social groups.

A narrow view of population health is that 'population health rests largely on shaping the distribution of risk in a population so that fewer people are exposed to risky situations' (Berkman & Melchior 2006, p. 55). A broader view of population health is that it seeks to influence the health outcomes of whole populations, or sub-populations, and the distribution of outcomes across those various populations (e.g. youth, children, refugees, older people) (Kindig 2007).

Population health is a growing field of practice that encompasses the generation of data, data mining and data analysis, which are the foundation of population health research. As the availability of data grows, there is increasing demand for professionals with skills in these fields:

> People who study the health of populations are focused on understanding the distribution of health and disease patterns and determining why they occur, as well as defining the characteristics of population subgroups that do not enjoy the same level of health as the general population. These are called priority population groups. Disciplines that take a population health approach to their work include social epidemiology, health promotion and planning. These disciplines see their work through the lens of populations rather than individuals.   *(Keleher 2015, p. 65)*

Both high-risk and population strategies have been developed to influence the distribution of illness across the population. A **high-risk strategy** is one that targets the right patient at high risk of developing a more serious condition, such as pregnant women or overweight men who are smokers. A **population strategy** is one that attempts to control the determinants of incidence, and thus to shift the distribution of exposure across the whole population. This gives rise to the **prevention paradox**, which is that a large number of people at low risk may give rise to more cases than the small number who are at high risk – that is, 'a preventive measure that brings large benefits to the community offers little to each participating individual' (Rose 1992, p. 38). In other words, many people must take precautions such as immunisation in order to prevent illness in only a few.

Equity

How we can decrease health and social inequities is a key concern of population health work. Health inequities are caused by avoidable circumstances and unfair socio-economic conditions. Differences in access to health care also contribute to health inequities, which are those inequalities in health deemed to be unfair or stemming from some form of injustice (Keleher & MacDougall 2015).

Health equity explains the rights of people to have equitable access to services on the basis of need, and the resources, capacities and power they need to act upon the circumstances of their lives that determine their health. Health inequality is an observable, often measurable, difference in health status between individuals, groups or populations, whatever the cause. In Australia, the '**health gap**' describes the inequities between population groups that may be described by culture, socio-economic status, or place (i.e. where they live).

Social determinants of health

The **social determinants of health (SDH)** are the social conditions in which people live and work, and they represent a significant shift in thinking about how to resolve issues of health inequity and disadvantage (Commission on the Social Determinants of Health 2008). Collectively, the SDH are recognised as the best predictors of health – the causal pathways for both individuals and populations. The evidence that has been systematically collected and analysed demonstrates how pathways through societal, political, environmental and economic determinants translate into illness and disease. The social conditions and settings in which people live their lives not only influence how people behave, but also have a direct impact on the health of individuals, families, communities and populations.

Public health is increasingly concerned with the evidence about how to address the determinants of health. The world-views of the social science disciplines involved in public health are influenced by contemporary social–ecology/equity debates, and since the early 21st century 'new public health' has increasingly been influenced by the evidence emerging about the social, economic, political and environmental determinants of health (Baum 2016). The new public health is a socio-political movement that argues for the need for social and political action to control disease and improve the health of populations while simultaneously addressing inequities. Its proponents see the need for action on social and economic environments to improve the public's health and to reduce health inequalities where these are avoidable, and especially where they are unjust or unfair (Commission on the Social Determinants of Health 2008). These determinants include access to health care and public health interventions; socio-economic environments including income, education, employment, social support, gender and culture; physical environments including urban design, clean air and water; genetics or biology; and individual and group behaviour including social norms for particular groups (Kindig 2007).

In theory, population health work should take account of the patterns of health determinants, and the policies and interventions that link outcomes with determinants. But in reality only a narrow range of determinants is considered in population health work by governments focusing on relationships between patterns of illness and disease in relation to socio-economic factors and, to a lesser extent, racial and ethnic group differences. Good population health requires **intersectoral collaboration** and approaches to programs, as well as a focus on the needs of those with disadvantaged health status, with the aim of reducing health and social inequities. Typically, both public health and population health strategies are more 'upstream' than medical treatment services, which are classified primarily as 'downstream'. Upstream strategies are focused on social and environmental change and on health-promoting policies and practices.

Universal and targeted public health approaches

Universal approaches to public health are those available to everyone at no cost or very little cost. **Targeted public health** approaches are those focused on particular population groups – those at higher risk for contracting a communicable disease, for example (Case study 5.1).

Public health places emphasis on high-quality, universal programs such as immunisation, maternal and infant health, and cancer screening programs that are available to the whole population.

Case Study 5.1

HIV / AIDS Prevention
• •

In the field of HIV prevention and control, the rapid and coordinated mobilisation of governments and community has enabled significant activity through community education and awareness-building and behaviour change, both in the most at-risk groups from contracting HIV and in the general community. The response to HIV / AIDS has achieved progress towards its targets in a shorter timeframe compared with other public health issues. It has done so despite raising controversial social questions about sexuality and human rights that had not previously been openly discussed, and despite requiring difficult conversations at the individual and also policy level. Government and civil society organisations worked closely together to ensure efforts to change attitudes and behaviours were well targeted and involved mobilisation of opinion and action within key groups. This enabled introduction of policies and regulations that may otherwise have become points of resistance. However, while the achievements in this health area are remarkable, there is some concern that Australia is becoming complacent about HIV / AIDS prevention, and winding back strategies rather than embedding them (Keleher 2017, p. 3).

Sources: Keleher, H. (2017). Review of prevention and public health strategies to inform the primary prevention of family violence and violence against women. Report commissioned to VicHealth by the Department of Premier and Cabinet. VicHealth and Victorian State Government, Melbourne; Kindig, D. (2007). Understanding population health terminology. Milbank Quarterly 85(1),139–161.

Funding of public health

Public health funding in Australia is estimated on an annual basis via a protocol developed to inform the National Public Health Expenditure Project, which measures expenditure against nine types of population-level activities undertaken or funded by state and territory health departments that address issues related to populations rather than individuals (Australian Institute of Health and Welfare (AIHW) 2018). These activities are communicable disease control; selected health promotion; organised vaccination; environmental health; food standards and hygiene; breast, cervical and cancer screening programs; prevention of hazardous and harmful drug use; public health research; and administration of funding for public health. Until 2009, this was managed through **Public Health Outcome Funding Agreements (PHOFAs)** with the states and territories. Overall, public health receives about 2% of the total recurrent Commonwealth allocation from the health budget (AIHW 2018, p. 59).

Arguably, the low ceiling on public health expenditure can be attributed to debates about the role of governments in the lives of the public and, therefore, their role in public health. Conservative public management has seen a trend in the role of government in health care to minimise government engagement to that of a contract manager seeking accountability for outputs, as well as greater involvement of markets and competitive forces to 'reform' health care, including public health, as governments look to reduce expenditure and increase end-user costs. We have seen the privatisation of housing, water and transport, food, food safety, hospitals and medical care – all of which have public health impacts, especially on the health of the poorest. When the interests of private industry dominate, public health interests can be suppressed.

Public health – which seeks prevention and capacity-building for the long term with social objectives that include access and equity – is vulnerable to cut-backs as health is increasingly considered to be a market-place commodity, or the demands of hospital waiting lists become politically embarrassing for governments. One of the tensions for public health is the extent to which governments are prepared to allow the allocation of public expenditure for public health to the private sector.

Responsibilities for public and population health

Different levels of government carry diverse and distinct levels of responsibility for the work involved in public health. Australia has three levels of government: the federal government, the governments of the six states and two territories, and local governments in all states and territories, all with their own jurisdictions. All levels of government have responsibilities for public health policy, planning and implementation.

Federal responsibilities

The main federal bureaucracy with public health responsibilities is the Department of Health. Apart from Medicare (see Chapter 2), the Pharmaceutical Benefits Scheme (see Chapter 7) and aged care (see Chapter 8), the Department of Health is responsible for the funding of family planning services, the supply of blood products (mainly through the Red Cross), and food safety such as applications for genetic modification of foods and the labelling of products. It is also responsible for some funding for specific health promotion programs, such as harm reduction from drugs and anti-violence programs. The Commonwealth has been guided by a process of identifying National Health Priority Areas for which strategies were then developed but responsibility for them has shifted to the National Health and Medical Research Council (https://www.nhmrc.gov.au/about-us/publications/nhmrc-corporate-plan-2018-2019), whose job it is to fund research rather than develop national strategies. This means that increasingly state/territory governments will develop and fund their own strategies, making them relevant to local services and responsive to local issues and communities. Funding for service delivery is allocated on the basis of this planning.

State and territory government responsibilities

The responsibilities for population health activities are steered and often directed by public health departments in state/territory governments, each of which is headed by the Chief Health Officer, or Manager of Public Health, who has statutory responsibility to the Minister for Health for the health of the population. Public health units in government departments are responsible for population-based programs (such as immunisation and vaccination), to ensure that the whole population is protected from preventable communicable (or infectious) diseases, and for managing disease outbreaks (such as *Salmonella* poisoning from contaminated food or influenza outbreaks).

State and territory governments have public health responsibilities for disease control and health protection, which covers communicable diseases such as legionellosis, tuberculosis, HIV/AIDS, SARS and avian influenza. These governments are required by federal law to manage effective epidemiological surveillance systems for the identification of public health issues, for the development and implementation of interventions to raise awareness and provide education to the population, and for the monitoring of the outcomes of those interventions. State and territory governments are also responsible for the administration of many public health issues, including dangerous drugs and poisons, emergency responses (e.g. floods, fires, bioterrorism), health promotion, immunisation, maternal and child health (funded by states/territories and administered by local governments), school health and dental health. State governments are also responsible for health promotion such as healthy nutrition, physical activity, mental health promotion, promoting safe environments, sexual and reproductive health, and reducing tobacco-related harm.

Every jurisdiction in Australia has a *Public Health Act* that sets out the requirements for individuals, organisations and governments and their agencies for the control of infectious diseases, the control of a range of risks to public health, and measures that must be taken to promote and protect health. Some of these measures are enacted at federal level and others at state or local level. Policy for public health frequently combines diverse but complementary approaches to creating better health, including legislation, fiscal measures, taxation, and organisational and behavioural change. Public health policy is highly influential on the actions that can be taken by public health professionals. When governments develop strong evidence-based policy platforms for the regulation and management of public health issues, the practice of public health is made stronger and is more effective.

Local government responsibilities

Specific local government public health responsibilities include:

- ◆ legislative responsibility for the administration of the Commonwealth *Food Act 1984* (Victoria State Government 1984)
- ◆ food premises, food production, food selling
- ◆ the built and social environment, including cultural, community and recreational development
- ◆ environmental hazards, including waste disposal
- ◆ the provision of community services: youth and aged care (e.g. home and community care such as meals on wheels, home maintenance and personal home care services)
- ◆ land use planning
- ◆ roads, drains and footpaths.

Local government is a key player in public health. Indeed, one could argue that almost every local government program is about the promotion of health and well-being and the health of local populations. For example, local governments are involved in the promotion of healthy environments through local amenities such as footpaths, walkways and bicycle paths linked to active transport strategies, reduction of harm from illicit drugs and alcohol abuse, and community renewal programs for disadvantaged neighbourhoods. Community renewal may be linked to state / territory-government-funded programs for early childhood or learning networks that promote lifelong learning opportunities at local levels.

PAUSE
for
REFLECTION
...

There has been continued resistance from industry so as to undermine and oppose public health efforts to control tobacco use, at every level. The resistance is well funded and coordinated, targeting governments, industry and community. 'As the sophistication of tobacco reduction efforts has increased over time, so too have the resistance efforts' (Keleher 2017, p 3).

Consider how legislation, taxation, organisational change and behavioural change have been used in public health efforts aimed at tobacco control. How successful have they been?

How are public health issues handled?

There is no single way in which any issue is handled, but generally federal, state, territory and local governments will have officers who have responsibility for particular issues. Frequently, governments work across jurisdictions to develop responses to specific issues. Environmental health officers (EHOs) in local government have statutory responsibilities – that is, they are responsible for the development, regulation, enforcement and monitoring of laws and regulations governing public health, building and environmental management. As an example, if there was an outbreak of gastroenteritis affecting a larger than usual number of people, the treating doctors, whether in clinics or a hospital, would be required to notify the local health authorities of the outbreak. This would be classified as a significant incident. Case study 5.2 describes some aspects of an EHO's work.

Case Study 5.2

Environmental health officers
. . . .

Environmental health officers (EHOs) investigate possible sources of food contamination, taking samples to send to laboratories. They interview people and gather as much information as possible, sending information to the state / territory Chief Health Officer, whose Department of Health would have oversight of the outbreak and its control. If a food outlet is found to have sold or provided contaminated food, it is closed down until the premises are declared safe, and the owners may be prosecuted. In these ways, the relevant local government would work closely with the state / territory Department of Health.

EHOs also have responsibility for the *prevention* of such outbreaks, so their work has an educational role. For example, they inspect premises to ensure that food is hygienically prepared, stored and served in places such as shops, cafés, food-processing factories and dairies, and collect food samples for chemical and microbiological analysis. They conduct food hygiene education seminars and other community health education programs for food handlers in such places as school canteens, market stalls and fund-raising barbecues.

For the prevention and management of diseases and conditions that feature highly in the burden of disease data, federal, state and territory governments engage in strategic planning. These planning processes can be quite extensive and result in documents that set out the government's approach to the issue; where responsibilities lie for action on the issue; how prevention, health protection and health promotion should be addressed; and how action will be monitored. Indicators may be used to track and measure progress to monitor the effectiveness of the strategy. For example, the Department of Health has a National HIV / AIDS Strategy (Department of Health 2014), which was first developed in 1989 and has been reviewed and renewed approximately every few years. It sets out requirements for epidemiology and surveillance so that the incidence and prevalence of new infections are carefully monitored. It also sets out expectations for treatment and support of people living with HIV / AIDS (see Case study 5.1).

Public health: libertarian to egalitarian

Tensions between narrow and broad approaches to public health will continue as individual versus broad approaches, based on the determinants of health, are debated by governments, bureaucrats, advocates, academics and practitioners. Just as previous chapters have discussed the role of the public and private sectors in health insurance (see Chapters 1, 2 and 3), public health must be debated on the spectrum from libertarian to egalitarian:

- Libertarian positions represent choice and personal responsibility for health needs.
- Egalitarian positions represent a rights-based universality with equal access for equal need.

Neither health care for individuals nor public health for populations is a typical commodity. It might be, some argue, that the private sector is more efficient, but in Australia the reverse is true in the provision of public health: the public sector is not only more efficient but also carries more of the risks and handles emergencies and the seriously complex issues that the private sector would find unprofitable, such as policy development and issues such as disease prevention that rely on complex solutions.

Public health suffers from lack of funding, but additional funding will make a real difference only if there are more concerted intersectoral efforts to tackle the causes of problems such as poverty, low levels of education and literacy, and degraded environments, rather than 'soft' targets such as physical activity and obesity. The failure of public health systems is more likely to occur if public health maintains a narrow focus, rather than a broad focus through intersectoralism. Health is not necessarily created within the health sector, so intersectoral activity is essential for public health success.

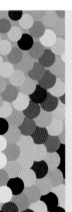

Summary

In this chapter, the following have been addressed:

- an explanation of the breadth of public and population health
- the importance of public health infrastructure within the public sector
- approaches to public health, including upstream–downstream approaches
- a brief overview of the public health workforce
- an introduction to how public health issues are handled
- the responsibilities of different levels of government for public health
- public health futures and what is required to promote and protect the health of the public.

An accompanying video exploring the themes of this chapter is hosted on Evolve: http://evolve.elsevier.com/AU/Willis/understanding/.

Review Questions

1 What are three key characteristics of the population health approach?
2 What are the implications for policy and programs of a narrow approach to population health that is focused on diseases?
3 Critically reflect on how well Australia's public health efforts are doing in increasing health equity and reducing inequities among the population.
4 Whose business in the health sector is not related to public health?

References

Association of Schools and Programs of Public Health, 2018. https://www.aspph.org.

Australian Institute of Health and Welfare (AIHW), 2018. Australia's health 2018, AIHW, Canberra. Cat. no. AUS 221. https://www.aihw.gov.au/reports/australias-health/australias-health-2018/contents/table-of-contents.

Baum, F., 2016. The New Public Health, fourth ed. OUP, South Melbourne.

Berkman, L.F., Melchior, M., 2006. The shape of things to come. How social policy impacts social integration and family structure to produce population health. In: Siegrist, J., Marmot, M. (Eds.), Social Inequalities in Health. OUP, Oxford, pp. 55–72.

Commission on the Social Determinants of Health, 2008. Closing the Gap in a Generation: Health Equity Through Action on the Social Determinants of Health. World Health Organization, Geneva.

Department of Health, 2014. Seventh National HIV Strategy 2014–2017. DOH, Canberra. http://www.ilo.org/wcmsp5/groups/public/—ed_protect/—protrav/—ilo_aids/documents/legaldocument/wcms_302435.pdf.

Gebbie, K., Rosenstock, L., Hernandez, L.M. (Eds.), 2003. Who Will Keep the Public Healthy? Educating Public Health Professionals for the 21st Century. National Academies Press, Washington, DC.

Keleher, H., 2015. Population health. In: Keleher, H., MacDougall, C. (Eds.), Understanding Health, fourth ed. OUP, Melbourne, (Chapter 6).

Keleher, H., 2017. Review of prevention and public health strategies to inform the primary prevention of family violence and violence against women. Report commissioned to VicHealth by the Department of Premier and Cabinet. VicHealth and Victorian State Government, Melbourne.

Keleher, H., MacDougall, C. (Eds.), 2015. Glossary. Understanding Health, fourth ed. OUP, Melbourne.

Kindig, D., 2007. Understanding population health terminology. Milbank Q. 85 (1), 139–161.

Nuffield Council on Bioethics, 2007. Public Health Ethical Issues. Nuffield Council on Bioethics, London.

Public Health Agency of Canada (PHAC), 2011. What is the Population Health Approach? PHAC, Ottawa. https://www.hse.ie/eng/about/who/population-health/population-health-approach/.

Public Health Association of Australia (PHAA), 2015. Public Health Association of Australia constitution and rules. https://www.phaa.net.au/documents/item/29.

Rose, G., 1981. Strategy of prevention: lessons from cardiovascular disease. BMJ 282, 1847–1851.

Rose, G., 1992. The Strategy for Preventative Medicine. OUP, New York.

Rose, G., 2001. Sick individuals and sick populations. Bull. World Health Organ. 79 (10), 960–966.

Swedish National Institute of Public Health (SNIPH), 2011. Public Health Priorities in Sweden. SNIPH, Stockholm.

Tuohy, C., 1999. Accidental Logics: The Dynamics of Change in the Health Care Arena in United States, Britain and Canada. OUP, New York.

Van Wave, T.W., Scutchfield, F.D., Honoré, P.A., 2010. Recent advances in public health systems research in the United States. Annu. Rev. Public Health 31, 283–295.

Victoria State Government, 1984. The Food Act 1984. https://www2.health.vic.gov.au/public-health/food-safety/food-safety-laws-local-government-and-auditors/food-safety-laws-and-regulations/food-act-1984.

Winslow, C.E.A., 1920. The untilled fields of public health. Science 51(1306), 23–33.

Young, T., 1998. Population Health Concepts and Methods. OUP, New York.

Further Reading

Keleher, H., 2015. Population health. In: Keleher, H., MacDougall, C. (Eds.), Understanding Health, fourth ed. OUP, Melbourne.

UCL Institute of Health Equity, 2010. Fair Society, Healthy Lives: the Marmot Review, UCL Institute of Health Equity, London.

Online Resources

Association of Schools and Programs of Public Health. This resource-rich site is for students of public health, and has been established to assist them to prepare for careers in education, advocacy, research and practice. Available from: https://www.aspph.org.

UCL Institute of Health Equity – provides a wealth of resources on the social determinants of health and public health. Available from: www.instituteofhealthequity.org.

CHAPTER 6

Primary health care in Australia

Helen Keleher

Key learning outcomes

When you finish this chapter you should be able to:

- describe the primary health care system in Australia
- explain how primary health care contributes to health equity
- explain the continuum from selective to comprehensive primary health care
- identify the multidisciplinary professionals who work in community-based health settings
- discuss health reformist agendas for primary health care.

Key terms and abbreviations

Aboriginal Community Controlled Health Organisation (ACCHO)

Aboriginal Community Controlled Health Services (ACCHSs)

Australian Health Ministers Advisory Council (AHMAC)

Australian Institute of Health and Welfare (AIHW)

commissioning

Community Health Program (CHP)

community health services (CHSs)

comprehensive needs assessments (CNAs)

comprehensive primary health care (CPHC)

Commission on the Social Determinants of Health (CSDH)

general practitioner (GP)

health system

Indigenous Australians' Health Programme (IAHP)

National Aboriginal Community Controlled Health Organisation (NACCHO)

neoliberal

prevention

primary care

primary care organisations (PCOs)

primary health care (PHC)

Primary Health Care Access Program (PHCAP)

Primary Health Networks (PHNs)

selective primary health care (SPHC)

social determinants of health (SDH)

social gradient

social model of health

universalism

'welfarism'

World Health Organization (WHO)

Introduction

All health professional groups covered in this book will work in or with the primary **health system** in some way. For most Australians, contact with the health system involves a visit to a **general practitioner (GP)** or pharmacist, or perhaps a physiotherapist, whose services are part of a much broader and complex primary health network. Although many health professionals will work in hospitals, understanding of the primary health system is essential for effective care because no part of the health system works in isolation from other components of the system.

At this point it is worth defining what is meant by a system and how we frame both the problems within systems and the values we use to decide the directions of change. A system is a group of elements or components that make up the parts of that system. Those parts are interrelated, interdependent and interact. Together they form a complex whole which develops patterns over time. Those patterns can be changed but change is often slow and not as dynamic as we might want. Systems also have boundaries from where boundary judgements are made. Those judgements are often based on values which define what is included and excluded in how we think about that system. Following Bacchi (2012), boundary judgements frame a problem and the approaches we take to problem-solving in a system, and this in turn affects the success of different types of solutions.

Australia's health system is dominated by hospitals and the provision of acute care, but since about 2010 the primary health care sector has attracted much overdue attention. That year saw the release of the first National Primary Health Care Strategy (Department of Health and Ageing 2010), which recognised that community-based primary health care is the front line of health care for most Australians. Since then, the **Australian Institute of Health and Welfare (AIHW)** has produced a series of data driven reports that document the performance of the health system against key indicators (Australian Institute of Health and Welfare (AIHW) 2016).

In 2014–15, (AU)$56 billion was spent on primary health care. This is almost as much as the $62 billion that was spent on hospitals in 2014–15 (AIHW 2016); this is a level of expenditure that indicates the need for the same level of policy attention to primary health care as has been traditionally given to hospitals.

This chapter explains the concepts of primary health care and primary care and how that translates into Australia's systems for primary health care. The **social model of health** is explained both as the foundation of community-based services and as a strategy to address health inequities. Concepts of 'welfarism' and **universalism** will be explored in this context. In addition, the framing of Bacchi's 'What's the problem represented to be?' will underpin the 'Pause for Reflections' throughout this chapter.

Primary health care

Primary health care (PHC) is a model of community-based health service delivery and a philosophy about equity and fairness in terms of access to affordable, accessible and appropriate health care. Primary health care is as relevant to Australia as it is to any low- or middle-income country. In Australia, PHC operates through a wide range of services such as **community health services** (CHSs), Aboriginal health services, women's health services, mental health services and youth health services.

These services are primarily publicly funded and operate on a **social model of health** emphasising equity of access and affordability.

The concept of PHC was articulated and documented at the first International Conference on Primary Health Care in 1978, held in the city of Alma-Ata, Kazakhstan, which was a state of the former USSR. The *Declaration of Alma-Ata* has become a landmark document that still guides primary health care today (World Health Organization (WHO) and UNICEF 1978). It documents the principles of the social model of health in the following terms:

◆ Health is a fundamental human right, and the attainment of the highest possible level of health is a most important worldwide social goal whose realisation requires the action of many other social and economic sectors in addition to the health sector.

◆ The existing gross inequality in the health status of people, particularly between developed and developing countries as well as within countries, is politically, socially and economically unacceptable and is, therefore, of common concern to all countries.

◆ The people have a right and duty to participate individually and collectively in the planning and implementation of their health care.

◆ Primary health care is essential health care based on practical, scientifically sound and socially acceptable methods and technology made universally accessible to individuals and families in the community through their full participation and at a cost that the community and country can afford to maintain at every stage of their development in the spirit of self-reliance and self-determination. It forms an integral part both of the country's health system, of which it is the central function and main focus, and of the overall social and economic development of the community. It is the first level of contact of individuals, the family and community with the national health system, bringing health care as close as possible to where people live and work, and constitutes the first elements of a continuing health care process (World Health Organization and UNICEF 1978).

Three salient principles of primary health care from the *Declaration of Alma-Ata* stand out:

1 a commitment to shift health resources from urban hospitals to community-based settings

2 a reduced reliance on highly specialised doctors and nurses and greater mobilisation of community-based health care

3 an explicit link between health and social development, and the social and environmental determinants of health. Primary health care work is conceived not as an isolated and short-lived intervention but as part of a process of health-creating environments (WHO 2005).

In Australia, primary health care services range from universally provided services such as maternal and child health, for which all new parents are eligible, to services for very marginalised groups such as programs for the homeless or drug-using groups. Comprehensive approaches to the rehabilitation of people living with mental illness might include treatment and medication management, counselling, employment support and education in basic living skills to enable independent living.

Primary health care is necessarily part of the publicly funded health system, provided at little or no cost to those who access services, and is regarded as a 'not-for-profit' model of service delivery. Universal services like this are resisted by the conservative, **neoliberal** push for the privatisation of health services. Both primary health care policy and service delivery are driven by those core values mentioned above (social justice, human rights and equity), which are connected to the concepts of both '**universalism**' and '**welfarism**'. The connection operates through a shared concern with the health and welfare of all people, but especially vulnerable groups: those with disadvantaged health and those living in poor circumstances or marginalised socially who cannot afford to use privatised health services that require co-payments at the point of service. Primary health care is necessarily provided in a multidisciplinary environment where there is commitment to the social model of health.

Primary care

Primary care services are provided by a whole range of public and private providers, such as GPs, community nurses, allied health practitioners, mental health professionals, youth workers and Aboriginal and Torres Strait Islander health practitioners who work from a range of different settings.

Primary care and primary health care form a continuum of care from treatment and disease management through to social determinants of health and disease, as outlined in Fig. 6.1, which shows that primary care is a more defined occasion of care than the services provided by a primary health care team. That said, it is still considered best practice for integrated primary care centres to provide a suite of services that may include GPs, dentists nurses, allied health practitioners, pre- and

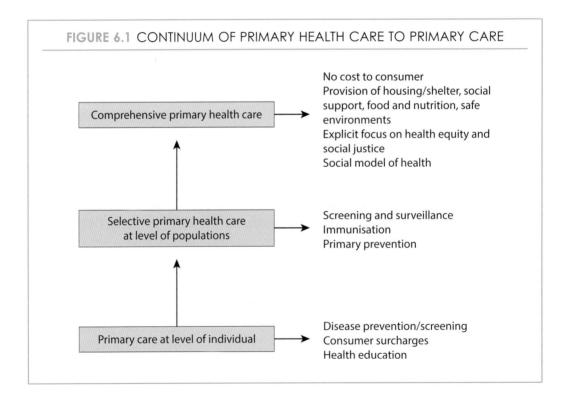

FIGURE 6.1 CONTINUUM OF PRIMARY HEALTH CARE TO PRIMARY CARE

Comprehensive primary health care → No cost to consumer / Provision of housing/shelter, social support, food and nutrition, safe environments / Explicit focus on health equity and social justice / Social model of health

Selective primary health care at level of populations → Screening and surveillance / Immunisation / Primary prevention

Primary care at level of individual → Disease prevention/screening / Consumer surcharges / Health education

post-hospital care, screening, education and other preventive health services (Doggett 2007), which is how many community health centres operate across Australia.

Sometimes primary care is a person's first point of contact with the health system for a particular condition, although there has been an alarming trend towards hospital emergency departments being used for that purpose. Reforms to the system through Primary Health Networks are one measure intended to curb this trend.

Australia has a strong primary care sector based on general practice, which is dominated by self-employed practitioners in private practice. The bulk of income for general practice is derived from patient payments, subsidised by Medicare or other insurers such as Veterans Affairs, Transport Accident or Workcover. The size of the general practice subsidies is reviewed regularly by governments, and frequently becomes a political issue.

PAUSE
for
REFLECTION
...

In Chapter 1 we noted that in the 2014 Budget, the Australian Government announced plans to charge a $7 co-payment for visiting a general practitioner. Days later (then) Health Minister Peter Dutton claimed the charge was necessary to make Medicare sustainable. The proposed charge was later watered down to $5 but was scrapped amid a fierce backlash from the Australian Medical Association and patients.

What was the problem that the government was trying to solve? What additional problems would it have created?

Primary care organisations (PCOs)

Primary Health Networks (PHNs), 30 in total across Australia, were developed in 2015 to replace an earlier model of PCOs called Medicare Locals, which ran from 2013 to 2015. These in turn, were a reform of the Divisions of General Practice, which had operated since 1992 until 2013. Divisions were GP membership organisations to support general practices, but Medicare Locals and now PHNs were given a much broader brief and objectives.

Medicare Locals were tasked with the responsibility for:

- improving the patient journey through developing integrated and coordinated services
- providing support to clinicians and service providers to improve patient care
- identifying the health needs of local areas and developing locally focused and responsive services
- facilitating the implementation and successful performance of primary health care initiatives and programs.

In reality, the 61 Medicare Locals across Australia were not given sufficient time or funding to fulfil these objectives before they were reconfigured into PHNs, which were established with just two key objectives:

1 to increase the efficiency and effectiveness of medical services for patients, particularly those at risk of poor health outcomes, and

2 to improve coordination of care to ensure patients receive the right care in the right place at the right time.

PHNs aim to help improve primary health outcomes across the region through health systems improvement and the **commissioning** of efficient and effective primary health services (Department of Health 2018). Key to both Medicare Locals and PHNs is that their task is specifically to be system enablers rather than service providers. We are beginning to see a stronger emphasis in PHNs on improving health access and equity through advocacy and action.

All PHNs conduct **comprehensive needs assessments (CNAs)** to identify population health priorities for each local area but health promotion and prevention programs are not funded. Generally, the CNAs conducted by PHNs are much more comprehensive than the population health work of Divisions of General Practice and we should expect that PHNs will continue to strengthen population health data and analysis to inform decision-making.

PHNs are using commissioning as a mechanism for purchasing services, which involves processes of planning, purchasing and monitoring services for a geographically defined population or sub-population that also takes account of the needs of individual clients with conditions requiring specific services (Harris et al. 2015). Theoretically, commissioning is based on robust priority-setting through population health needs assessment, but in practice this has been difficult to achieve because of limited budgets for the commissioning of services.

The drivers for reform

Australia has concentrated its spending on providing **selective primary health care (SPHC)** through general practice, with a focus on providing primary care interventions in treatment and disease management in the private sector (Table 6.1). We all need general practice services from time to time, and we all like to be sure that they will be available and accessible when we need them. General practice is, however, not able to provide the wide range of health programs and social services that people may need, and has limited capacity to address health inequities.

Moreover, the cost of seeing a doctor in Australia is increasing. A 2018 report (AIHW) showed that half of all patients in 2016–17 – 10.9 million people – had out-of-pocket costs for non-hospital Medicare services. There is huge variation across PHN areas in the out-of-pocket costs which people pay. Furthermore, 7% of people aged 15 years and over, or an estimated 1.3 million people, said the cost of services was the reason that they delayed or did not seek specialist, GP, imaging or pathology services when they needed them. The report shines a spotlight on how much patients pay out-of-pocket for specialist, GP, diagnostic imaging and obstetric services (otherwise known as the 'gap'). It also looks at where patients have reported delaying or not using health services because of cost.

The people who are least likely to have reasonable access to affordable health services are those marginalised by poverty, culture, race, disability, addiction, chronic illness, social stereotyping and difference. These are determinants that magnify the experience of illness, diminish people's ability to participate socially and economically to their fullest capacity, and reduce opportunities for them to lead healthy and productive lives. Moreover, when people are not able to access needed

TABLE 6.1 THE CONTRAST BETWEEN SELECTIVE AND COMPREHENSIVE PRIMARY HEALTH CARE

Characteristic	Selective	Comprehensive
Main aim	Reduction/elimination of specific disease	Improvement in overall health of the community and individuals
Strategies	Focus on curative strategies, with some attention to prevention and promotion	Comprehensive strategy with curative, rehabilitative, preventive and health promotion aspects that seeks to remove the root cause of ill-health
Planning and strategy development	External, often 'global', programs with little tailoring to local circumstances	Local and reflecting community priorities – professionals 'on tap, not on top'
Participation	Limited engagement on the terms of outside experts and tending to be sporadic	Engaged participation that starts with community strengths and their assessment of health issues, ongoing and aiming for community control
Engagement with politics	Professional and claims to be apolitical	Acknowledges that primary health care is inevitably political and engages with local political structures such as consumer advocate groups or other 'civil' society activist groups
Forms of evidence	Limited to assessment of disease prevention strategy based on traditional epidemiological methods usually conducted out of context and extrapolated to the situation	Complex, multiple methods, involving a range of research methods including epidemiology and qualitative and participatory methodology

Source: Baum, F. (2013). Community Health Services in Australia. In: Germov, J. (Ed.) Second Opinion: An Introduction to Health Sociology, fifth ed., OUP, Melbourne, pp. 484–502.

care their conditions can easily deteriorate, leading to the requirement for more complex tertiary level care.

In the last few years, significant Australian- and state-level reports and research have been published which are influencing the directions for strategy and actions for improved effectiveness in the care of people with chronic conditions. The Australian Government has published a National Strategic Framework for Chronic Conditions (Australian Health Ministers' Advisory Council (AHMAC) 2017), which highlights the continuing need to strengthen primary health care, particularly to better manage the large numbers of patients with multiple chronic conditions, and identifies outcomes and indicators for measurement of progress and change. The Grattan Institute reports (Duckett et al. 2017; Swerrissen et al. 2016) have highlighted the following key issues:

- Avoidable hospital admissions cost the health system more than $320 million each year. Providing better care for people with diabetes, asthma, heart disease and other chronic conditions could save a significant proportion of this, as well as improve the working and social lives of the people affected.
- Despite the government spending more than $1 billion each year on planning, coordinating and reviewing chronic disease management, many people with chronic conditions do not receive the best care.
- The demand for hospital services can be reduced by better coordinating the care of people with complex and chronic and management of these conditions in primary care.

Two major changes are recommended by the authors:

1 The first step should be to gather more information about what happens in general practice. We know, roughly, how long a general practice visit is, but we have no idea why the patient went to the doctor or what was decided. Without data, there is no sound basis for system reform. A new payment should be made to general practices to gather and supply the necessary data.

2 The second change required is to build on the development of local primary care systems. PHNs need to be strengthened and given explicit responsibility for creating more effective and efficient primary care systems in their local areas. In particular, they need to be held accountable for making improvements that will reduce unnecessary hospital admissions – those which could have been prevented with better primary care.

PAUSE
for
REFLECTION
...

Potentially preventable hospitalisations accounted for nearly 2.7 million bed days nationally in 2015–16 – equivalent to 9% of all public and private hospital bed days. An avoidable or potentially preventable hospitalisation is one that may have been prevented by timely and appropriate provision of primary or community-based health care. Five conditions contribute most to the number of days spent in hospital for potentially preventable hospitalisations nationally. Those conditions are chronic obstructive pulmonary disease, diabetes complications, congestive heart failure, cellulitis, and kidney and urinary tract infections.

What is the problem? Is it that people are not using GPs and primary health providers to stay well, or is it that they cannot afford to pay for primary health services? Or is the problem one of inequities? Once the problem is defined, what do you see are the solutions?

From the social model of health to the determinants of health

The **social determinants of health (SDH)** are understood as the social conditions in which people live and work – the social characteristics of living and working environments. Broad thinking about the SDH has been recognised and asserted by the **World Health Organization** since the *Declaration of Alma-Ata* (WHO and UNICEF 1978), and again in the goals and targets set to achieve the vision of *Health for all by the year 2000* (WHO 1981) and then the re-launch of primary health care in the WHO report *Primary health care: now more than ever* (WHO 2008).

From 2005 to 2008, the WHO held a **Commission on the Social Determinants of Health (CSDH)** to concentrate attention on those social determinants of health that are amenable to change. The CSDH was set up to 'mobilize emerging knowledge on social determinants in a form that could be turned swiftly into policy action ... where needs are greatest' (Commission on the Social Determinants of Health 2007, p. 6). The SDH that are of greatest interest to the WHO are income, employment, the **social gradient**, early childhood, access to health care, education, secure and affordable food sources, social support, gender, culture and social exclusion.

The CSDH reports point to the specific features of those social contexts that create or mitigate health, and the pathways by which social conditions translate into health impacts. The SDH can, of course, have both positive and negative effects. They are interrelated and frequently require government action to address them. For example, poverty and maldistribution of wealth, psychosocial deprivation, powerlessness, low literacy and low levels of health service use are all causes of poor health, but these complex issues cannot be resolved by the health sector unless it works in partnership with other relevant government sectors.

One of the key policy directions of the CSDH (2007) is the role of the health system as a determinant of health, particularly in reducing health inequities. The association between a strong primary health care sector and reduced health inequities has long been identified. The CSDH made the case that primary care services such as general practice can address health inequities by improving access to quality care. As illustrated in Case study 6.1, the integration of primary care with multilevel community-based strategies that use outreach and seek to address the social and economic determinants of health are likely to be effective in addressing health inequities because of the range of multidisciplinary and integrated models of care within the services that run those services.

Health systems can determine health outcomes via the types of interventions developed, for example through health care to reduce the unequal consequences of disease or ill-health. The health system determines health by the way in which it provides access to health care services, but also by putting in place public health programs and by involving other policy bodies to improve health, particularly for disadvantaged groups and communities. Conceptually, the health system plays a role as a social determinant of health at three levels:

1 at the macro level: through public policy and equitable resource allocation processes to enable affordable, appropriate and timely access to needed care

2   at the meso (community) level: through decentralised policy and participatory decision-making that includes soundings from communities about their access to care, gaps and needs

3   at the micro level: through factors related to the organisation of the health care system.

PAUSE
for
REFLECTION
...

Which types of client that are seen by members of your profession are likely to gain benefit from a multidisciplinary, integrated primary health service? In what ways do the services provided by those in your profession work to increase health equity?

Case Study 6.1

The Mt Spencer Community Health Service

The Mt Spencer Community Health Service was formed in the 1970s when local doctors saw a need for a community health service (CHS) that incorporated a social worker, community nurses and a physiotherapist to assist elderly people living in the area. The services were funded jointly by the Commonwealth and the state governments, through the Community Health Program. As demand increased, the services that were provided grew to include community health nursing, physiotherapy, social work services, a family planning clinic, which later became the women's health clinic, volunteer services, occupational therapy and dietetics. The CHS focused on people experiencing social disadvantage or economic hardship, who are more susceptible to higher rates of disease and ill-health.

Today, Mt Spencer delivers primary health care services across four sites. These services span allied health, dental, drug and alcohol, mental health, casework/counselling, family violence, health promotion, community development and sexual and reproductive health services. The CHS believes strongly in the value of health promotion to help reduce inequities, using a social model of health and community development approaches for outreach programs to local communities. Two GPs visit the CHS to conduct clinics. One clinic is for people with mental illness who need GP care. A practice nurse visits one of the local homeless services to encourage clients to use the clinic when required. The other clinic is for people with diabetes. Both clinics are fully bulk-billed, and are guided by the General Practitioners in Community Health Services Strategy (Department of Human Services 2005). They both enable access for clients with higher levels of complex and chronic conditions who are unable to access affordable services and who might otherwise present to hospital emergency departments. All other services are provided at little or no cost to people with a health care, pension or student card. Waiting-list times vary, but the CHS is proud to have established four dental chairs and special clinics for people with conditions such as HIV/AIDS who would otherwise find it difficult to get dental treatment.

Mt Spencer CHS staff work in partnership with other organisations and their local community to create supportive environments for health, develop policy, advocate for change and develop people's ability to improve their own health in ways that matter to them.

Community health and community-based services

As indicated in Case study 6.1, in the early 1970s the Whitlam Federal Labor Government established the **Community Health Program (CHP)**. This program established a service sector for the delivery of primary health care across Australia through locally managed community health centres that provided 'integrated primary health care'. Based on a social model of health and with a strong focus on equity and participation, the centres comprised multidisciplinary teams that provided medical and nursing services as well as community development and advocacy / social action on social and environmental problems of concern to the community (Baum 2013). Many provided low-cost financial counselling and support referrals to housing services. Boosted by the WHO's commitment to primary health care under its inspirational leader Dr Halfdan Mahler, the community health movement gathered strength to form the Australian Community Health Association. By 1981, the Fraser Liberal Government had ended its involvement in the CHP and the program effectively ceased to exist.

In 1983, the Hawke Labor Government restored 1975 levels of community support, but in the absence of any overarching policy for primary health care the program was vulnerable. Funding community health had become the responsibility of the states and territories. Victoria and South Australia led the way, continuing to establish community health centres in areas of social and economic deprivation and pioneering new models of service delivery.

The original service profiles of the CHS were designed to meet the needs of local communities and were established to promote the social model of health. Services included community (or district) nursing, allied health, women's health, drug and alcohol services, child, youth and family services, community mental health and sexual health services. In recent years, drug and alcohol services have largely been moved to specialist services. In Victoria, public dental health services are being integrated into community health services and programs – a trend which is likely to increase as chronic disease and early intervention programs are strengthened across all states and territories. Chronic disease programs increasingly focus on early intervention and education and support for self-management, with an emphasis on effective strategies to facilitate access to early CHS interventions and disease management for people living in disadvantaged circumstances.

Today, across the states and territories, CHSs vary in their governance arrangements, how they employ staff, and the types of programs they fund. Community health services are now funded through a mix of block grants from the Commonwealth and from state and territory funding. Victoria is the only state to have CHSs report directly to boards of management. Staff members of CHSs in Western Australia, Queensland, South Australia and Tasmania are employees of their respective state departments of health, and report directly to district managers. Queensland also funds non-government organisations to provide CHS. The CHSs in Western Australia and New South Wales are part of population health units in state-run, area-based health services.

Most jurisdictions now fund health promotion, community development and capacity-building, although some of this funding may be limited to a focus on **prevention** and early intervention for chronic disease, such as diabetes. Community development in health has not been well supported, with governments preferring to fund primary care through clinical streaming, and chronic disease programs focused on self-management gaining momentum in all states. Programs funded for disease management strive to maintain a primary health focus by organising work through multidisciplinary teams, working from a social model of health as much as possible, and developing collaborations and partnerships with other service providers and sectors in order to improve health outcomes.

Supporters of community health models continue to advocate for services that address the lack of equity in the distribution and delivery of primary care services, and the need to strengthen primary health care approaches in order to address social inequity. A strong emphasis is placed on multidisciplinary teams and partnerships with, for example, schools, workplaces, migrant services and welfare and social services.

Dedicated women's health services have also been established in each state and territory, supported through Australia's National Policy on Women's Health. Founded solidly on the social model of health, participation and local management, this network of women's health services has a particular focus on the development of information and resources (e.g. on violence against women and on reproductive health), education and training, health promotion and community development.

Indigenous primary health care

In Australia, Indigenous communities have led the way in the design and implementation of **comprehensive primary health care (CPHC)**, especially through the **Aboriginal Community Controlled Health Organisation (ACCHO)**, and **Primary Health Care Access Program (PHCAP)**. There are more than 150 **Aboriginal Community Controlled Health Services (ACCHSs)** across Australia, delivering primary health care services. Their national peak body is the **National Aboriginal Community Controlled Health Organisation (NACCHO)**. ACCHOs are initiated and operated by local Aboriginal communities expressly to deliver holistic, comprehensive, and culturally appropriate health care to the community that controls it, through a locally elected board of management (National Aboriginal Community Controlled Health Organisation 2014).

The National Aboriginal and Torres Strait Islander Health Plan 2013–2023 (Department of Health 2013) is the policy framework that will guide policies and programs to improve Aboriginal and Torres Strait Islander health until 2023. This Plan has a much stronger approach to strengthening the social and cultural determinants of Indigenous health. Following the release of the Plan, in 2014, the Australian Government established the **Indigenous Australians' Health Programme (IAHP)** consolidating four existing funding streams: primary health care, child and maternal health programs, Stronger Futures in the Northern Territory (Health) and programs covered by the Aboriginal and Torres Strait Islander Chronic Disease Fund.

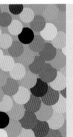

Summary

In summary, primary health care is a broad model of care that incorporates primary care in community-based services that are delivered by a range of practitioners. These services are guided by Australia's health system policy frameworks as well as by service delivery models, characterised by the type of care provided, the settings in which that care is provided, the people providing the care and the specific activities or goals involved or the models' underlying values (Doggett 2007).

We should not be under the illusion that, in a relatively rich country like Australia, there is no need for improved primary health care systems and programs. The need for primary health care in Australia has never been greater than now. System improvements require goals to first increase efficiency and effectiveness of the vast number of health providers across Australia. Second, system goals must also seek to increase access to affordable health services, which is likely to impact on a reduction in health inequalities in Australia as the social divide expands.

In this chapter, we have explored the concepts of primary health care, primary care and community-based service delivery in the context of the Australian health care system. Key points include:

- the global context for primary health care and its history
- different models of primary care / primary health care in the context of their capacity to address health inequities
- the importance of maintaining comprehensive primary health care services as a strategy to address health inequities
- the role of Primary Health Networks as enablers of system reform.

Review Questions

1   What are the differences and synergies between primary care and primary health care? How do you expect these to affect your work as a health care practitioner in the future?
2   From your reading of this chapter, how would you define the underpinning values of comprehensive primary health care, and how does it differ from selective primary health care?
3   For what reasons, and for which groups of people, might Australia need to develop a stronger primary health care service delivery system?
4   How does primary health care conform to the principles of a social model of health?
5   What groups in the Australian population might be best serviced by a primary health care model of service?

References

Australian Health Ministers' Advisory Council (AHMAC), 2017. National Strategic Framework for Chronic Conditions. Australian Government, Canberra.

Australian Institute of Health and Welfare (AIHW), 2016. My healthy communities. Australian Government, Canberra. https://www.myhealthycommunities.gov.au.

Australian Institute of Health and Welfare (AIHW), 2018. Australia's health 2018. Australia's health series no. 16. AUS221. AIHW, Canberra. https://www.aihw.gov.au/getmedia/7c42913d-295f-4bc9-9c24 -4e44eff4a04a/aihw-aus-221.pdf.aspx?inline=true.

Bacchi, C., 2012. Introducing the 'What's the problem represented to be?' approach. In: Bletsas, A., Beasley, C. (Eds.), Engaging With Carol Bacchi: Strategic Interventions and Exchanges. University of Adelaide Press, Adelaide. https://www.adelaide.edu.au/carst/docs/wpr/wpr-summary.pdf.

Baum, F., 2013. Community heath services in Australia. In: Germov, J. (Ed.), Second Opinion: An Introduction to Health Sociology, fifth ed. OUP, Melbourne, pp. 484–502.

Commission on the Social Determinants of Health, 2007. A conceptual framework for action on the social determinants of health: a draft discussion paper, WHO, Geneva.

Commission on the Social Determiannts of Health, 2008. Closing the Gap in a generation: health equity through action on the social determinants of health, WHO, Geneva.

Department of Health, 2013. National Aboriginal and Torres Strait Islander Health Plan 2013–2023. Australian Government, Canberra. http://www.health.gov.au/natsihp.

Department of Health, 2018. Primary Health Networks (PHNs). Australian Government, Canberra. http://www.health.gov.au/internet/main/publishing.nsf/Content/PHN-Home.

Department of Health and Ageing, 2010. Building a 21st century primary health care system. Australia's First National Primary Health Care Strategy. Publication no. 6594. Australian Government, Canberra.

Department of Human Services, 2005. General practitioners in community health services strategy. Victorian Government Department of Human Services, Melbourne.

Doggett, J., 2007. A new approach to primary care for Australia. Centre for Policy Development, occasional paper no. 1. Centre for Policy Development, Sydney.

Duckett, S., Swerissen, H., Moran, G., 2017. Building better foundations for primary care. Grattan Institute, Melbourne. https://grattan.edu.au/wp-content/uploads/2017/04/Building-better-foundations-for-primary-care.pdf.

Harris, M., Gardner, K., Powell Davies, G., et al., 2015. Commissioning primary health care: an evidence base for best practice investment in chronic disease at the primary-acute interface: an Evidence Check rapid review brokered by the Sax Institute (www.saxinstitute.org.au) for NSW Health, Sydney.

National Aboriginal Community Controlled Health Organisation (NACCHO), 2014. Definitions. NACCHO, Canberra. http://www.naccho.org.au/about/aboriginal-health/definitions/.

Swerissen, H., Duckett, S., Wright, J., 2016. Chronic failure in primary medical care. Grattan Institute, Melbourne. https://grattan.edu.au/wp-content/uploads/2016/03/936-chronic-failure-in-primary-care.pdf.

World Health Organization (WHO), 1981. Global strategy for health for all by the year 2000 (Health For All Series 3). WHO, Geneva.

World Health Organization (WHO), 2005. The Bangkok Charter for health promotion in a globalized world. 6th Global Conference on Health Promotion. WHO, Geneva.

World Health Organization (WHO), 2008. Primary health care: now more than ever. WHO, Geneva.

World Health Organization (WHO) and UNICEF, 1978. Declaration of Alma-Ata, International Conference on Primary Health Care, Alma-Ata, USSR. WHO, Geneva.

Further Reading

Commission on the Social Determinants of Health, 2007. A conceptual framework for action on the social determinants of health: a draft discussion paper, WHO, Geneva.

Online Resources

Australian Primary Health Care Research Institute (APHCRI) – funded by the Australian government for research to drive policy development for primary health care. The site provides a wealth of reports and other resources: http://aphcri.anu.edu.au.

Primary Health Care Research and Information System (PHCRIS) – an Australian site for the exchange of information about primary health care, particularly for the purposes of policy and research. The site is rich with resources for practice, as well as conference reports, a research round-up and journal-watch: www.phcris.org.au.

World Health Organization (WHO) – WHO site for primary health care. It includes speeches by the Director-General and links to primary health care in WHO regions, as well as the World Health Report 2008, Primary health care: now more than ever: www.who.int/topics/primary_health_care/en/.

CHAPTER 7

The Pharmaceutical Benefits Scheme

Erica Sainsbury

Key learning outcomes

When you finish this chapter you should be able to:

- explain the purpose of the Pharmaceutical Benefits Scheme (PBS) and its relationship to government health and medicines policy
- describe the key elements of the PBS including authorised prescribers, authorised suppliers of medicines, types of benefits, the Schedule of Benefits, eligibility requirements, co-payments, the Safety Net scheme, generic substitution, Closing the Gap
- explain why the cost of the Pharmaceutical Benefits Scheme is high
- describe a number of key reforms to the PBS which have been undertaken to contain cost increases
- identify a number of key challenges to the sustainability of the PBS in the future.

Key terms and abbreviations

authority-required benefit	Pharmaceutical Benefits Advisory Committee (PBAC)
bioequivalence	Pharmaceutical Benefits Scheme (PBS)
brand equivalence	private prescriptions
brand premium	quality-adjusted life-year (QALY)
Closing the Gap (CTG)	quality of life (QOL)
concession card holders	quality use of medicine (QUM)
Consumer Price Index (CPI)	reciprocal health care agreement (RHCA)
co-payment	reference pricing
general patients	repatriation beneficiaries
generic brand	repeats
generic substitution	restricted benefit
mandatory price disclosure	Safety Net scheme
National Medicines Policy (NMP)	Schedule of Pharmaceutical Benefits
originator brand	Therapeutic Goods Administration (TGA)
patent	weighted average disclosed price (WADP)

Introduction

Although a scheme to provide free medicines to war veterans (the Repatriation Pharmaceutical Benefits Scheme) was in place in Australia from 1919, moves towards a more general **Pharmaceutical Benefits Scheme** (PBS) initially arose as a result of political decisions made during the last years of World War II. Following the devastation of the war, the Australian Labor government led by John Curtin aspired to create a better, fairer and more efficient Australia, and one of the most significant aspects to be reformed was the health system. In 1944, all Australian residents became entitled to obtain specified medicines free of charge when they presented a doctor's prescription to a pharmacist. There was considerable opposition to the scheme, however, particularly by doctors, who succeeded in having the legislation declared unconstitutional. Nonetheless, successive governments persevered, and in the 1950s a small number of expensive but life-saving and disease-preventing medicines were made available free of charge to pensioners, widows and returned servicemen and women. By 1960, the list (Schedule) of medicines had expanded significantly, and the general public was also able to benefit from cheaper medicines. Pensioners and veterans still received free medicines, and members of the public paid 5 shillings (equivalent to (AU)\$7.27 in 2017) (Goddard 2014; GSK & ViiV Healthcare 2018; Vitry et al. 2015). The PBS operating today is the direct result of ongoing changes and reforms to this 1960 Scheme.

Purpose and philosophy of the PBS

The PBS sits underneath the **National Medicines Policy** (NMP), the objective of which is to provide for:

1 timely access to the medicines that Australians need, at a cost individuals and the community can afford
2 medicines meeting appropriate standards of quality, safety and efficacy
3 **quality use of medicines (QUM)**, and
4 maintaining a responsible and viable medicines industry.

(Department of Health and Ageing 1999, p. 1)

The PBS contributes to delivering the first outcome, particularly the affordability of medicines needed by Australians. Three key elements of this approach are important:

1 medicines must be affordable to the individual who needs them
2 the overall cost of medicines must be affordable by society, as they are subsidised by taxation, and
3 because the subsidies are paid from taxation, the benefits are available to Australian citizens and residents (with minor exceptions).

How the PBS operates

In Australia, there are two ways of pricing prescribed medicines:

1 pharmaceutical benefits – a list of specific medicines approved by the **Pharmaceutical Benefits Advisory Committee (PBAC)** for subsidisation by the government. These

medicines have a fixed price, maximum quantity and maximum number of **repeats**, and are listed in the **Schedule of Pharmaceutical Benefits** (the 'Schedule').

2 **private prescriptions** – all medicines other than pharmaceutical benefits. Their price is determined by market forces including competition between pharmacies.

If more than the maximum PBS quantity of a medicine is prescribed, that prescription becomes private and is not eligible for government subsidisation. Additionally, some medicines are listed as benefits only for certain medical conditions and not others; if a medicine is prescribed for a non-approved condition, that prescription is also private.

The PBS covers two broad categories of patients: **general patients** and **concession card holders**. Concession card holders include individuals and families who are eligible for welfare or social security, including the old age pension, disability support and unemployment or low-income support (Department of Human Services 2018), together with **repatriation beneficiaries** (eligible war veterans, former members of the Australian Defence Force and their widows/widowers and dependents) (Department of Veterans' Affairs 2018). General patients are all other eligible patients. The two groups differ in the amount they pay for their subsidised medicines.

General patients pay a fixed or 'agreed' price for a particular medicine, but only up to a certain limit, and if the agreed price is greater than that limit then the government subsidises the difference. Concession card holders pay much less for their medicines, with the government subsidising the rest. In 2019, the two limits, or '**co-payments**', were $40.30 and $6.50 respectively. Fig. 7.1 illustrates this.

PAUSE *for* **REFLECTION** ...

If the aim of the PBS is to help make medicines more affordable for Australians, why not cover the costs of all medicines completely? What might be the reason for having co-payments, and a restricted Schedule of medicines?

The Safety Net scheme

Even with partial government subsidies, the cost of medicines for many families can still be very high, particularly when patients have several medical conditions and are on multiple medicines. To help keep medicines affordable for these patients, the PBS includes a **Safety Net scheme**, introduced in 1986 (Department of Health 2018a). Under this scheme, the PBS defines a 'family unit', which may be an individual patient, a couple or a family with dependent children; couples may be married or de facto, and of the opposite or same sex. When payments for PBS medicines for a family unit reach a threshold amount in a calendar year, they become eligible for an additional Safety Net benefit. For the rest of the year, general patients pay the concession card holder co-payment for their medicines, while concession card holders pay nothing for their PBS medicines. On 1 January of the following year, the Safety Net benefit ends, and patients pay the 'normal' amount until they reach the Safety

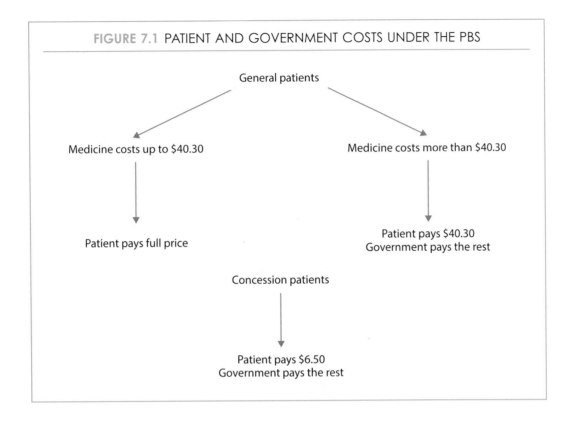

FIGURE 7.1 PATIENT AND GOVERNMENT COSTS UNDER THE PBS

Net threshold for the new year. In 2019, the Safety Net threshold for general patients was $1550.70 and for concession card holders was $390.00.

The co-payment amounts and Safety Net thresholds increase annually on 1 January according to the **Consumer Price Index (CPI)**. Table 7.1 (overleaf) shows increases in these payments over the past 5 years.

Closing the Gap (CTG)

In 2008, state, territory and federal governments in Australia made a commitment to working together to remove the health disparities experienced by Indigenous Australians in comparison with non-Indigenous Australians. Several strategies were adopted to achieve this 'Closing the Gap', and seven specific targets were set in health, education and employment.

In relation to health, the cost of medicines needed by Indigenous Australians with chronic diseases was identified as a barrier to improving health outcomes, and in 2010 the **Closing the Gap (CTG) co-payment program** was established to reduce the cost of medicines for eligible Aboriginal and Torres Strait Islander people. This program allows individuals who would otherwise pay the general co-payment to receive their medicines for the concessional charge. Individuals who would

TABLE 7.1 CO-PAYMENTS AND SAFETY NET THRESHOLDS 2015–19

Year	Co-payment concession	Co-payment general	Safety Net threshold concession	Safety Net threshold general
2015	$6.10	$37.70	$366.00	$1453.90
2016	$6.20	$38.30	$372.00	$1475.70
2017	$6.30	$38.80	$378.00	$1494.90
2018	$6.40	$39.50	$384.00	$1521.80
2019	$6.50	$40.30	$390.00	$1550.70

Source: Department of Health (2019). Fees, patient contributions and safety net thresholds, http://www.pbs.gov.au/info/healthpro/explanatory-notes/front/fee

normally pay the concessional charge receive their PBS medicines for free (Department of Health 2018b). In the first 7 years of its operation, more than 23 million medicines have been supplied under the program (Fig. 7.2).

Restricted benefits and authorities

As indicated above, some PBS medicines can be prescribed only for specific conditions. These medicines may be classified as either a **restricted benefit** or an **authority-required benefit**. Authority-required benefits must have a specific code included on the prescription before a pharmacist can dispense the medicine under the PBS. The code indicates that the patient has a particular medical condition and / or has met certain required criteria. If the code is absent, the pharmacist can still dispense the medicine but at the private price. A restricted benefit may have similar criteria, but no code is required on the prescription.

Table 7.2 on p. 106 includes examples of restricted and authority-required benefit criteria. These examples illustrate the level of detail that may be required.

Patents, originator brands and generic substitution

For a new medicine to become available to Australian patients, it must be approved by the **Therapeutic Goods Administration (TGA)**, an Australian Government agency which requires evidence of the quality, safety and effectiveness of the medicine (Vitry et al. 2015). This requires a large investment of money and time by the pharmaceutical company which develops the medicine, and these costs must be recouped from sales. The company has a 20-year **patent** for this medicine (Duckett et al. 2013), which prevents other companies from developing their own version while the patent lasts. If the medicine is listed in the PBS, the agreed price is intended to help compensate the company for development costs, and is often higher than the actual manufacturing cost. The medicine is marketed

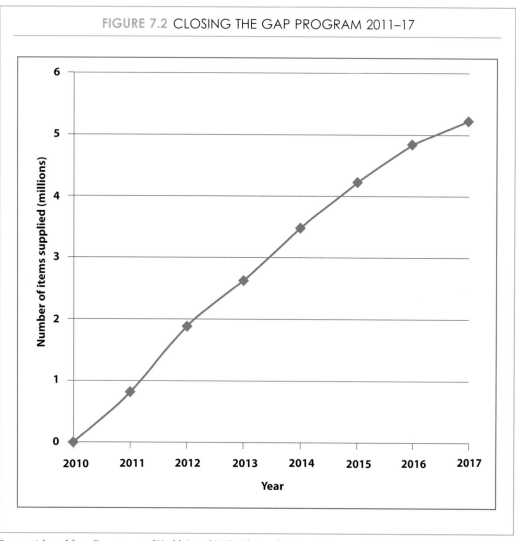

FIGURE 7.2 CLOSING THE GAP PROGRAM 2011–17

Sources: Adapted from Department of Health (2018b). The Closing the Gap – PBS co-payment measure, http://www.pbs.gov.
au/info/publication/factsheets/closing-the-gap-pbs-co-payment-measure; Department of Prime Minister and Cabinet (2018)

with a particular brand name, known as the **originator brand**. For example, the originator brand
of atorvastatin for the treatment of high cholesterol was Lipitor®.

Once the patent expires, other companies are free to develop and market their own brand of
the medicine. Because they do not have to provide safety and effectiveness evidence, the costs of
producing this new **generic brand** are much lower than the agreed price for the originator brand.
For prescribers, pharmacists and patients the introduction of generic brands means the same medicine
is available as two or more brands. **Generic substitution** is the replacement of one brand, usually
the originator, with a generic brand of the same medicine. For example, generic brands of atorvastatin

TABLE 7.2 EXAMPLES OF RESTRICTED AND AUTHORITY-REQUIRED BENEFIT CRITERIA

Type of benefit and medicine	Medical condition	Other criteria
Restricted benefit – alendronate	Established osteoporosis	Clinical criteria: Patient must have fracture due to minimal trauma, AND Patient must not receive concomitant treatment with any other PBS-subsidised anti-resorptive agent for this condition.
Authority-required benefit – glatiramer	Multiple sclerosis treatment phase: continuing treatment	Clinical criteria: The condition must be diagnosed as clinically definite relapsing-remitting multiple sclerosis, AND Patient must have previously received PBS-subsidised treatment with this drug for this condition, AND Patient must not show continuing progression of disability while on treatment with this drug, AND Patient must have demonstrated compliance with, and an ability to tolerate this therapy.

Source: www.pbs.gov.au

include Lorstat®, and Trovas®. Generic substitution may be suggested by the prescriber or pharmacist, or requested by the patient; however, it must never occur without the patient's agreement.

Generic substitution is also restricted by **brand equivalence**. This means that a generic manufacturer must demonstrate that its brand behaves similarly to the originator brand in the human body. All brands which can demonstrate equivalence may be used interchangeably. Some brands have been shown not to be equivalent, and so cannot be substituted, for example the Coumarin® and Marevan® brands of warfarin, a blood-thinning medicine. The introduction of generic medicines has led to a reduction in the price of medicines for patients; however, there have also been a number of significant additional consequences.

Eligibility for the PBS

All Australian residents with a valid Medicare card are eligible to receive medicines under the PBS. In addition, visitors from a small number of overseas countries are able to receive subsidised medicines while they are in Australia. These countries have **reciprocal health care agreements** (RHCAs) with Australia, meaning that Australians also have access to some health benefits when visiting these countries. Currently Australia has RHCAs with the United Kingdom, Ireland, New Zealand, Malta, Italy, Sweden, the Netherlands, Finland, Norway, Belgium and Slovenia (Department of Health 2018c).

Prescribing PBS medicines

Several different categories of health professional are authorised to prescribe medicines under the PBS, namely doctors, dentists, optometrists, midwives and nurse practitioners. Doctors are permitted to prescribe any PBS medicine, whereas the other professions can prescribe from specific lists of medicines relevant to their practice (Department of Health 2018d). Optometrists, midwives and nurse practitioners must also hold special qualifications, called endorsements, in order to prescribe.

Supplying PBS medicines

Most PBS medicines are supplied by pharmacists when a patient presents a valid prescription from an authorised prescriber. The pharmacists must be working in a pharmacy which is approved by the Department of Human Services. Some PBS medicines are supplied through hospitals, and doctors working in remote areas can also be approved to supply PBS medicines (Department of Health 2018e).

PAUSE
for
REFLECTION
...

Earlier chapters introduced the idea that health care systems can be described using three models – the *public-integrated*, the *public-contract* and the *private-insurance* models. How would you describe the PBS in terms of these models?

How are medicines listed in the PBS?

Historically, once a medicine was approved for use in Australia by the TGA, the manufacturer could apply to the PBAC for listing in the Schedule. Since 2011, however, parallel processes for application to the TGA and PBAC have been introduced to reduce delays (Vitry et al. 2015). The PBAC evaluates each application and, if satisfied that the medicine meets specific criteria for safety, effectiveness and cost-effectiveness compared with other currently available medicines, it can recommend that the medicine be listed in the Schedule. The PBAC also recommends the maximum allowable quantity and number of repeats, and whether the medicine should be a restricted or an authority-required benefit (Department of Health 2018f). Medicines can be recommended for listing on the basis of either cost minimisation or cost-effectiveness. If a new medicine is considered to have similar safety and efficacy to an already listed medicine, it is added at a similar price. If a new medicine is considered to be more cost-effective than current therapy, it can be added at a higher price. Cost-effectiveness is more difficult to estimate than safety and efficacy, but a commonly used value is the cost per **quality-adjusted life-year (QALY)** (Vitry et al. 2015).

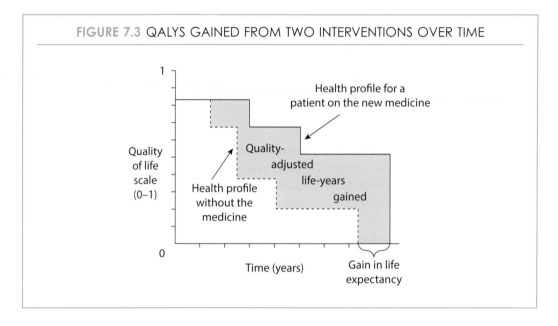

FIGURE 7.3 QALYS GAINED FROM TWO INTERVENTIONS OVER TIME

The QALY takes into account both quality and quantity of life and is a measure of the benefit to a patient resulting from the new medicine. **Quality of life (QOL)** is estimated on a scale from 0 to 1, where 0 represents death and 1 represents perfect health. For each year the QOL is estimated both with and without the medicine until the end of life. These values are graphed against each other and the area between the lines is a measure of the QALYs added as a result of the medicine (Fig. 7.3).

There is no single agreed threshold for the cost of QALY, although a figure of $50,000 is commonly quoted (Neumann et al. 2014; Vallejo-Torres et al. 2016). A study by George et al. (2001) revealed that from 1992 to 1996 the PBAC approved new medicines with costs of up to $42,000/QALY and rejected medicines with costs greater than $76,000/QALY. Between these values, some medicines were approved and others were not.

Societal affordability

As described earlier, the PBS is critical to implementation of the first arm of the National Medicines Policy (NMP) – timely access to the medicines that Australians need, at a cost individuals and the community can afford. Co-payments and the Safety Net are designed to assist with individual afford-ability and access, but these individual needs must be balanced with the overall cost to the Australian community. The second half of this chapter outlines ways that governments have attempted to create and maintain this balance, but it is important first to understand the scale of the issue.

The real costs of medicines

Table 7.3 lists agreed prices for a number of medicines, and the patient and government contributions for each. Even from this small sample, it is clear that costs differ dramatically. For atorvastatin and

TABLE 7.3 GOVERNMENT AND PATIENT CONTRIBUTIONS TO COSTS (AU$) OF MEDICINES (1 FEBRUARY 2019)

Condition / medicine	Actual cost of medicine	General patients		Concession card holders	
		Cost to patient	Gov't subsidy	Cost to patient	Gov't subsidy
High cholesterol / atorvastatin	15.87	21.63	0	6.50	9.37
Gastric reflux / esomeprazole	22.05	27.81	0	6.50	15.55
Asthma / fluticasone + salmeterol inhaler	61.63	40.30	21.33	6.50	55.13
Heart disease / dabigatran	88.62	40.30	48.32	6.50	82.12
Prostate cancer / goserelin	899.89	40.30	859.59	6.50	893.39
Leukaemia / Imatinib	1839.51	40.30	1799.21	6.50	1833.01
Multiple sclerosis / fingolimod	2209.33	40.30	2169.03	6.50	2202.83
Cervical cancer / Bevacizumab	3851.64	40.30	3811.34	6.50	3845.14

Source: www.pbs.gov.au

esomeprazole, only concession patients receive the subsidy, because the general price is below the co-payment. For conditions which are more debilitating or life-threatening, particularly cancers, the medicines are extremely expensive, and the cost of unsubsidised treatment is much higher than the ability of most people to pay. As a society, providing affordable treatments which can improve quality of life and extend patients' lifespan is generally considered compassionate and appropriate. However, society must be able to pay for this as part of its overall goal of providing services to its members. It is therefore important to look at the bigger picture of overall PBS costs.

Expenditure on the PBS is a significant fraction of health spending, and costs generally increase each year. Fig. 7.4 shows expenditure on PBS medicines over the past five decades, with the lower bar representing government costs and the upper bar patient contributions. From 2007 to 2017, total expenditure rose from $6.62 billion to over $10 billion, with government expenditure rising from $5.47 billion to $8.71 billion and patient contributions rising from $1.15 billion to $1.34 billion.

Because the government contribution is sourced from taxation and the government is accountable to taxpayers for the ways their taxes are spent, it is important to understand the reasons underlying the high costs, and which medicines are the most expensive as a whole. There are two main reasons why a particular medicine may be high cost; either the medicine itself is expensive, or it is prescribed for many people. Table 7.4 illustrates how this works.

FIGURE 7.4 GOVERNMENT AND PATIENT EXPENDITURE ON PBS MEDICINES 1967–2017

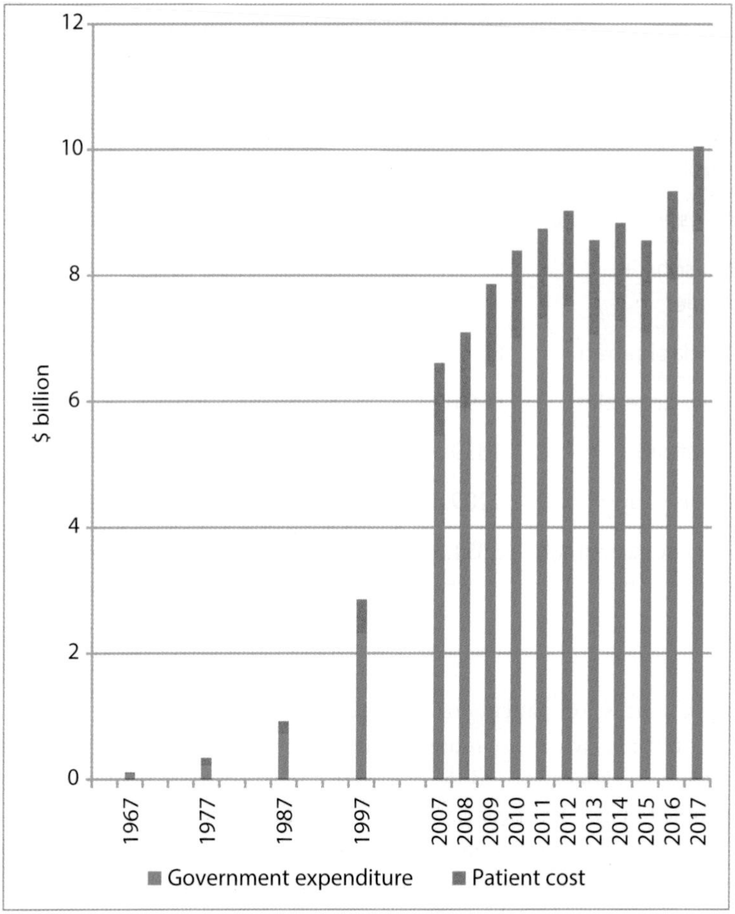

Source: Department of Health (2017). Expenditure and prescriptions twelve months to 30 June 2017, http://www.pbs.gov.au/info/statistics/expenditure-prescriptions-twelve-months-to-30-june-2017

TABLE 7.4 ACTUAL COST (AU$) OF PBS MEDICINES: YEAR ENDING 30 JUNE 2017

Medicine	Total number of prescriptions (million)	Average cost in 2016/17	Total cost ($ million)
atorvastatin	7.126	14.12	64.7
esomeprazole	6.283	27.33	140.0
fluticasone + salmeterol inhaler	2.767	64.04	132.4
fingolimod	0.065	2287.71	146.2

Source: Adapted from Department of Health (2017). Expenditure and prescriptions twelve months to 30 June 2017, http://www.pbs.gov.au/info/statistics/expenditure-prescriptions-twelve-months-to-30-june-2017

Although the government cost was small for each atorvastatin prescription, the large number of prescriptions resulted in an overall cost of almost $65 million. Fingolimod was prescribed relatively infrequently, but was responsible for contributing more than twice as much as atorvastatin to overall cost.

PAUSE
for
REFLECTION
...

In 2017, nine of the ten most highly prescribed medicines were for the treatment of high cholesterol, high blood pressure, gastric reflux, asthma and diabetes. The life expectancy of Australians is rising, with boys born in 2016 expected to reach an average of 80.4 years, and girls an average of 84.6 years (Australian Institute of Health and Welfare 2018). What implications can you see for the PBS in the light of these two observations?

Pharmaceutical Benefits Scheme reforms

Governments have been concerned about the increasing cost of PBS medicines for several decades, and several measures have been progressively trialled to attempt cost containment. This section outlines some key policy and process changes used.

Patient contributions

Patient contributions have been a feature of the PBS since 1960, when general patients paid a small amount for each prescription, nominally equivalent to $0.50. This amount remained constant until 1971, when it became $1.00, with additional increases every few years until 1990, when the co-payment reached $15.00. Since then, the co-payment has increased each year according to the CPI.

Initially, pensioners and repatriation beneficiaries received free medicines, but other concession card holders paid the same as general patients. In 1983, a reduced co-payment for concession card holders was introduced, and in 1990 pensioners became liable for the same co-payment as other concession card holders. The concession co-payment was extended to repatriation beneficiaries in 1992, with the result that all patients were charged a co-payment (Department of Health 2018a). While co-payments contribute to the total cost of medicines, Fig. 7.4 shows that government costs are increasing more rapidly than patient costs; therefore patient contributions have not by themselves been able to contain overall costs.

Closing loopholes – Medicare cards and Safety Net early supply

As previously described, PBS medicines are intended only for individuals with a valid Medicare card. However, until 2002 patients were not required to show their card when having a PBS prescription filled, and it was difficult for pharmacists to establish the eligibility of a particular patient. Since 2002 pharmacists have been required to check Medicare numbers before providing PBS medicines.

A second loophole is related to the Safety Net scheme and the dispensing of repeats. Repeats are allowed for many PBS medicines to save the patient from unnecessary doctor's visits; commonly 1 month's supply is prescribed with five repeats, meaning the patient sees the doctor every 6 months. Before 2006, patients could have their repeats dispensed whenever they chose. This meant a patient could obtain a month's supply one day, and the following day receive another month's worth from the next repeat. This is problematic for several reasons. Firstly, it is inconsistent with QUM, because it may lead to patient confusion if the doctor decides to stop the medicine or change the dosage while the patient still has a stockpile. The patient may accidentally keep taking the medicine, and may suffer harm as a result.

A second problem is that of wastage, because dispensed medicines cannot legally be supplied to anyone else. This is cost inefficient because both the patient and the government have paid for medicines that are never used. The Safety Net allows patients with high medicine costs to access concessional benefits once they reach a threshold each year. This creates an incentive to maximise savings by having as many prescriptions as possible dispensed before the concession ends on December 31, and this trend was increasingly seen in the early years of the 21st century. Pharmacists were frequently pressured to dispense the original and five repeats of a medicine on six consecutive days towards the end of December, meaning the patient received 6 months' worth of medicine effectively at once. In 2006, a requirement to wait either 4 or 20 days (depending on the medicine) between repeat dispensing at the concessional price was introduced. If the prescription was dispensed earlier, the patient had to pay the full price (as if they did not have the concession). If the patient was trying to reach the threshold by having prescriptions filled early, those prescriptions did not count towards the threshold. This significantly reduced the incentive to have prescriptions filled earlier than needed and resulted in significant savings in government expenditure (Department of Health and Ageing and Medicines Australia 2013). Both measures have been reasonably effective in managing the loopholes; however, as with patient contributions, they have not been able to constrain increasing costs overall.

To what extent do you think health professionals such as doctors and pharmacists should be expected to police the appropriate use of the PBS?

Price controls – reference pricing, generic substitution and mandatory price disclosure

The major strategies to contain PBS costs have involved generic medicine policies. As described previously, generic brands are generally cheaper than originator brands; however, before 1990 the use of generic brands in Australia was relatively low. In an effort to increase the generic share of the market, the Minimum Pricing Policy was introduced in 1990, which set the benchmark for government subsidy of a medicine on the basis of the cheapest brand. If different brands had different prices, the government subsidy would cover only the cheapest, or 'reference', brand. This resulted in **'brand premiums'**, where a patient who received the generic brand would pay only the co-payment, but a patient who received the originator brand would pay more than the co-payment (Box 7.1). This policy was applicable only where the brands were considered therapeutically equivalent (McManus et al. 2001).

Under this policy, generic substitution was permitted only if the prescribing doctor suggested or approved it. Four years after introducing the policy, 83% of prescriptions were still being dispensed with the brand premium, and only 17% at the cheaper benchmark rate (McManus et al. 2001). In 1994, the government widened generic substitution by permitting pharmacists to substitute brands at the point of dispensing provided that the:

1 brands were therapeutically equivalent and therefore could be interchanged
2 patient agreed to the substitution
3 prescriber had not prohibited substitution.

This third condition was an important change because the prescriber no longer needed to be consulted if a box on the prescription was not ticked and the other two conditions were met. Substitution was therefore permitted unless the prescriber specifically forbade it. McManus et al. (2001)

BOX 7.1   HOW THE BRAND PREMIUM WORKS

Sulfasalazine tablets (for rheumatoid arthritis) come as Salazopyrin-EN® ($4.00 brand premium), and the generic Pyralin EN® (no brand premium). General patients pay $40.30 for Pyralin EN® and $44.30 for Salazopyrin-EN®, while concession patients pay $6.50 for Pyralin EN® and $10.50 for Salazopyrin-EN®. The government subsidy is identical for both.

showed a significant change in dispensing patterns 5 years later, when only 55% of prescriptions were being dispensed with the brand premium, and 45% at the cheaper rate.

Initially, **reference pricing** was effective in keeping prices relatively low. Research comparing the prices of 150 PBS medicines against seven comparable countries in 2000 showed that Australian prices were much lower than those in Canada, Sweden, the UK and the USA, and similar to those in France, New Zealand and Spain. Although the differences could not be explained completely, the report concluded that reference pricing was likely to have played an important role (Australian Productivity Commission 2001).

Subsequently, however, Australian prices rose in comparison to other countries. By 2011, Australian prices were higher than those in France, New Zealand, Spain, Sweden and the UK. Costs had also risen in comparison with Austria, Belgium, Finland, Germany, Italy and the Netherlands, although USA prices remained significantly higher than in Australia (Duckett et al. 2013).

Cost differences were particularly noticeable for generic medicines. Although from 2005 the government reduced the price of a medicine by 12.5% (16% from 2011; Roughead et al. 2018) when the first generic brand was PBS listed, this resulted in relatively limited government savings. It was expected that, as more manufacturers introduced generic brands, increased competition would continue to reduce prices to the government; what actually happened was that manufacturers offered competitive discounts to pharmacists, resulting in the government reimbursing pharmacists at prices often considerably higher than the pharmacists had paid (Vitry et al. 2015).

To counter this, major PBS reforms were introduced in 2007 and 2010 to align the price paid by the government for generic medicines to the price paid by pharmacists to purchase them. The reforms included three strategic components (Vitry et al. 2015):

1 dividing PBS medicines into two lists or 'formularies', F1 and F2
2 regular mandatory price reductions
3 **mandatory price disclosure**.

All PBS medicines became classified as either F1 or F2. Medicines with only a single brand were classified as F1; medicines with multiple brands were classified as F2. F1 medicines are re-classified as F2 when the first generic brand is PBS listed. A series of fixed price reductions was initially applied to the F2 list to bring prices down in stages, following which the calculation of price has been based on price disclosure.

The price disclosure policy requires manufacturers to report (disclose) the actual prices charged to pharmacists for each generic medicine, including any discounts. A weighted average is calculated for each item across all manufacturers (**weighted average disclosed price** or WADP), which is used to set the government price (Roughead et al. 2018; Vitry et al. 2015). Government savings as a result of these reforms were estimated at over $1 billion from 2010/11 to 2012/13, and 160 medicines were reduced in price by an average of 42% (range 10%–98%) between 2012 and 2014 (Vitry et al. 2015). Fig. 7.5 shows the impact on the average cost to the government of three highly prescribed medicines for the years ending 30 June from 2010 to 2017 (Department of Health 2017). Atorvastatin and simvastatin are F2 medicines, while esomeprazole is F1. Dramatic reductions in the cost of the statins reflect the introduction of generic brands; esomeprazole costs have fallen more slowly because only the originator brand is currently available.

FIGURE 7.5 CHANGES TO AVERAGE COST FOR ATORVASTATIN, SIMVASTATIN AND ESOMEPRAZOLE

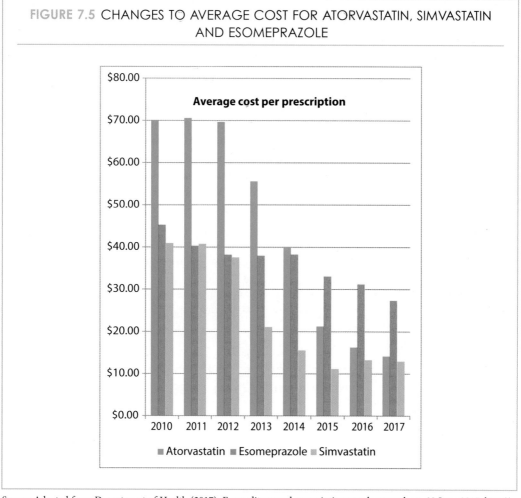

Source: Adapted from Department of Health (2017). Expenditure and prescriptions twelve months to 30 June 2017, http://www.pbs.gov.au/info/statistics/expenditure-prescriptions-twelve-months-to-30-june-2017

Are generics the same?

While the increasing use of generics has resulted in significant cost savings, other concerns have been raised about them. A common perception is that because the generic brand is cheaper it must be inferior. This is not true. All originator and generic brands must meet the same, very high, TGA standards of safety, quality and efficacy. In addition, to be listed as interchangeable, generic brands must demonstrate **bioequivalence**. Bioequivalence requires that the patient should expect the same response whether taking the generic or originator brand, and is measured experimentally. Volunteers take the medicine at a particular time, and at defined times afterwards give blood samples in which the concentration of the medicine is measured. Graphs of blood concentration against time are drawn (Fig. 7.6) and bioequivalence is determined by the closeness of the concentration–time curves, specifically the maximum concentration that is achieved (C_{max}) and the area under the curve (AUC). Statistical analysis is used to decide whether the values are sufficiently close (McLachlan et al. 2007) and if they are the brands are considered bioequivalent.

Even when bioequivalence has been established, however, a significant issue remains that patients may become confused when they receive different brands of the same medicine at different times. Common medicines may have a large number of different brands (atorvastatin has 14). Most pharmacies do not stock all brands of every medicine, but may only have two or three different ones. If patients visit different pharmacies, there is a strong chance they will be given different brands, and if they do not realise that two packets with different names contain the same medicine they may accidentally take both simultaneously and thus receive an overdose (McLachlan et al. 2007).

PAUSE

for

REFLECTION

...

How could the problem of confusion for patients taking different brands of the same medicine be minimised?

FIGURE 7.6 CONCENTRATION TIME CURVES FOR TWO BRANDS OF A MEDICINE AFTER A SINGLE ORAL DOSE

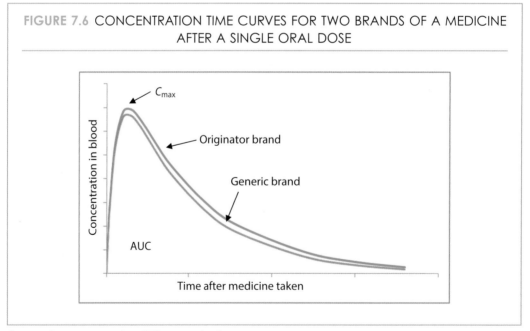

C_{max}=maximum concentration; AUC=area under the curve.

Looking to the future

Although it is impossible to predict the future precisely, Australia's population and life expectancies will clearly continue growing. The *2015 intergenerational report* (Commonwealth of Australia 2015) estimated that in 2054/55 the population would reach nearly 40 million, and average life expectancies would be 3–4 years longer. Importantly, the proportions of Australians over 65 and over 85 are expected to increase substantially, and the proportion in the traditional working age group will decline. These changes have significant implications for the costs of medicines. Not only will individuals live longer, but they will also remain active and healthy for longer as new and improved treatments are discovered. Many of these treatments will be medicines, many of these medicines will be expensive and individuals will take medicines for longer. These factors will combine to put pressure on the PBS and its funding as part of the significant challenges that the health care system will face overall. Australian society will need a clear vision of its values and priorities, and wise leadership from its governments, as it seeks to navigate and meet these challenges effectively and efficiently.

Summary

The PBS is a key arm of the National Medicines Policy, which seeks to provide timely and affordable access to the medicines that Australians need at a cost that society can sustain. A specific list (Schedule) contains medicines which have demonstrated safety, effectiveness and cost-effectiveness, and for which government subsidy of costs is available. Medicine prices are capped for individuals and families with and without concession cards, and a special scheme provides additional support for Indigenous Australians.

Eligibility for subsidised medicines is possession of a valid Medicare card, or being a visitor from specific overseas countries. Doctors, dentists, optometrists, nurses and midwives can prescribe PBS medicines, and most prescriptions are dispensed by pharmacists.

The costs to pharmaceutical companies of developing new medicines are very high, and some of these costs are recouped through the PBS while the medicine's patent remains in place. As a consequence, the introduction of a new medicine may result in significant cost to the government particularly if the medicine is used by many patients. Once the patent expires, other manufacturers can develop generic brands, which are much cheaper because they do not have the development costs associated with the originator brand. Government policies over the past decade have focused on reducing total costs of a medicine by requiring compulsory price reductions once generic brands are available. These reforms have slowed the growth in PBS expenditure, but have not reversed it. Some concerns have also been expressed about the quality and safety of generics, with the major risk being the chance of patients becoming confused and taking two brands of the same medicine simultaneously.

Future challenges to the PBS include population growth, particularly in older age groups as life expectancies increase, and the continual development of new and expensive medicines. Cost pressures on the PBS will need to be managed by effective and ongoing government policies and reforms if these medical and medicinal advances are to benefit Australians in ways that both individuals and society can continue to afford.

Review Questions

1   What is the major purpose of the Pharmaceutical Benefits Scheme and how does it relate to the National Medicines Policy?

2   Why is access to the Pharmaceutical Benefits Scheme restricted to Australian citizens and permanent residents?

3   How does the Safety Net scheme operate to assist families who need a large number of medicines?

4   Who benefits from the Closing the Gap co-payment scheme, and how do they benefit?

5   How would you explain to a patient the similarities and differences between the originator and generic brands of a medicine?

6   Why is it important that generic substitution be permitted only when the brands are bioequivalent?

7   What is the meaning of the term 'quality-adjusted life-year', and how is it used to determine which medicines are listed on the Schedule of Pharmaceutical Benefits?

8   How did the introduction of mandatory price disclosure affect the price of medicines in Australia, and why?

9   What are the critical challenges that must be addressed to ensure that the Pharmaceutical Benefits Scheme continues to achieve its purpose into the future?

10   In Chapter 1, it was stated that 'Efficiency, effectiveness and equity are core drivers for health system performance'. How important a role has each of these drivers played in shaping the Pharmaceutical Benefits Scheme to its current structure?

References

Australian Institute of Health and Welfare, 2018. Australia's health 2018: in brief. Cat. no. AUS 222. AIHW, Canberra. https://www.aihw.gov.au/getmedia/fe037cf1-0cd0-4663-a8c0-67cd09b1f30c/aihw-aus-222 .pdf.aspx?inline=true.

Australian Productivity Commission, 2001. International pharmaceutical price differences. http:// www.pc.gov.au/inquiries/completed/pharmaceutical-prices/report/pbsprices.pdf.

Commonwealth of Australia, 2015. 2015 intergenerational report: Australia in 2055. https:// static.treasury.gov.au/uploads/sites/1/2017/06/2015_IGR.pdf.

Department of Health, 2017. Expenditure and prescriptions twelve months to 30 June 2017. http:// www.pbs.gov.au/info/statistics/expenditure-prescriptions-twelve-months-to-30-june-2017.

Department of Health, 2018a. Fees, patient contributions and Safety Net thresholds. http:// www.pbs.gov.au/info/healthpro/explanatory-notes/front/fee#_1.

Department of Health, 2018b. The Closing the Gap – PBS co-payment measure. http://www.pbs.gov.au/ info/publication/factsheets/closing-the-gap-pbs-co-payment-measure.

Department of Health, 2018c. About the PBS. http://www.pbs.gov.au/info/about-the-pbs#Who_is _eligible_for_the_PBS.

Department of Health, 2018d. Prescribing medicines – information for PBS prescribers. http://www.pbs .gov.au/info/healthpro/explanatory-notes/section1/Section_1_2_Explanatory_Notes#PBS-prescribers.

Department of Health, 2018e. Supplying medicines – what pharmacists need to know. http:// www.pbs.gov.au/info/healthpro/explanatory-notes/section1/Section_1_3_Explanatory_Notes.

Department of Health, 2018f. Procedure guidance for listing medicines on the Pharmaceutical Benefits Scheme. www.pbs.gov.au/industry/listing/procedure-guidance/files/procedure-guidance-listin g-medicines-on-the-pbs.docx.

Department of Health, 2019. Fees, patient contributions and Safety Net thresholds. http://www.pbs .gov.au/info/healthpro/explanatory-notes/front/fee.

Department of Health and Ageing, 1999. National Medicines Policy. http://www.health.gov.au/internet/ main/publishing.nsf/Content/B2FFBF72029EEAC8CA257BF0001BAF3F/$File/NMP2000.pdf.

Department of Health and Ageing and Medicines Australia, 2013. Trends in and drivers of Pharmaceutical Benefits Scheme expenditure. http://www.pbs.gov.au/publication/reports/trends-in-and-drivers-of -pbs-expenditure.pdf.

Department of Human Services, 2018. Health Care card: who can get a card. https:// www.humanservices.gov.au/individuals/services/centrelink/health-care-card/eligibility#a4.

Department of Prime Minister and Cabinet, 2018. Closing the Gap: Prime Minister's report 2018. https:// pmc.gov.au/resource-centre/indigenous-affairs/closing-gap-prime-ministers-report-2018.

Department of Veterans' Affairs, 2018. Veterans' health cards. https://www.dva.gov.au/ health-and-wellbeing/veterans-health-cards.

Duckett, S., Breadon, P., Ginnivan, L., et al., 2013. Australia's bad drug deal: high pharmaceutical prices. https://grattan.edu.au/wp-content/uploads/2014/04/Australias_Bad_Drug_Deal_FINAL.pdf.

George, B., Harris, A., Mitchell, A., 2001. Cost-effectiveness analysis and the consistency of decision making: evidence from pharmaceutical reimbursement in Australia (1991 to 1996). Pharmacoeconomics 19, 1103–1109.

Goddard, M., 2014. How the Pharmaceutical Benefits Scheme began. Med. J. Aust. 201(1 Suppl.), S23–S25.

GSK & ViiV Healthcare, 2018. The Pharmaceutical Benefits Scheme in Australia: an explainer on system components. https://au.gsk.com/media/421635/gsk-viiv-the-pbs-in-australia-feb-2018.pdf.

McLachlan, A., Ramzan, I., Milne, R., 2007. Frequently asked questions about generic medicines. Aust. Prescr. 30 (2), 41–43.

McManus, P., Birkett, D., Dudley, J., et al., 2001. Impact of the minimum pricing policy and introduction of brand (generic) substitution into the Pharmaceutical Benefits Scheme in Australia. Pharmacoepidemiol. Drug Saf. 10 (4), 295–300.

Neumann, P., Cohen, J., Weinstein, M., 2014. Updating cost-effectiveness: the curious resilience of the $50,000-per-QALY threshold. N. Engl. J. Med. 371 (9), 796–797.

Roughead, E., Kim, D.S., Ong, B., et al., 2018. Pricing policies for generic medicines in Australia, New Zealand, the Republic of Korea and Singapore: patent expiry and influence on atorvastatin price. WHO S. E. Asia J. Public Health 7 (2), 99–106.

Vallejo-Torres, L., García-Lorenzo, B., Castilla, I., et al., 2016. On the estimation of the cost-effectiveness threshold: why, what, how? Value Health 19, 558–566.

Vitry, A., Thai, L., Roughead, E., 2015. Pharmaceutical pricing policies in Australia. In: Babar, Z. (Ed.), Pharmaceutical Prices in the 21st Century. Springer International, Switzerland.

Further Reading

Babar, Z. (Ed.), 2015. Pharmaceutical Prices in the 21st Century. Springer International, Switzerland (in particular Chapter 1: Vitry, A., Thai, L., Roughead, E., Pharmaceutical pricing policies in Australia).

Commonwealth of Australia, 2015. 2015 intergenerational report: Australia in 2055. https://static.treasury.gov.au/uploads/sites/1/2017/06/2015_IGR.pdf.

Goddard, M., 2014. How the Pharmaceutical Benefits Scheme began. Med. J. Aust. 201 (1 Suppl.), S23–S25.

Grove, A., 2016. The Pharmaceutical Benefits Scheme: a quick guide. http://parlinfo.aph.gov.au/parlInfo/download/library/prspub/4482670/upload_binary/4482670.pdf;fileType=application/pdf.

GSK & ViiV Healthcare, 2018. The Pharmaceutical Benefits Scheme in Australia: an explainer on system components. https://au.gsk.com/media/421635/gsk-viiv-the-pbs-in-australia-feb-2018.pdf.

McLachlan, A., Ramzan, I., Milne, R., 2007. Frequently asked questions about generic medicines. Aust. Prescr. 30 (2), 41–43.

Online Resources

Department of Health – The Pharmaceutical Benefits Scheme: http://www.pbs.gov.au/pbs/home.

CHAPTER 8

The aged care sector: residential and community care

Suzanne Hodgkin and Anne-Marie Mahoney[a]

Key learning outcomes

When you finish this chapter you should be able to:

◆ understand the implications of an ageing population for health and social care systems

◆ describe recent aged-care reforms that have impacted on policy and funding

◆ critically assess the impact of government policy on aged-care service delivery

◆ understand community care for older people.

Key terms and abbreviations

active ageing	formal services
Aged Care Assessment Service (ACAS)	health gap
Aged Care Funding Instrument (ACFI)	healthy ageing
ageing in place	Home Care Packages (HCP)
assessment	iatrogenic
'Baby Boom' generation	life expectancy
chronic obstructive pulmonary disease (COPD)	medical model
chronological age	refundable accommodation deposit (RAD)
Commonwealth Home Support Program (CHSP)	residential aged-care facility (RACF)
consumer-directed care (CDC)	residential services
coronary heart disease	retirement
dementia	workforce shortfalls
diversity	

[a]We acknowledge the contribution by Jeni Warburton to the chapter in the 3rd edition of this book.

Introduction

As the population ages in Australia, it becomes crucial to maintain good population health. The population profile has significantly changed over the last decade, with the older generation (those aged 65 and over) continuing to grow and it is projected that by 2057 this cohort will double. On 30 June 2017, 3.8 million Australians were aged 65 years and over (Australian Institute of Health and Welfare (AIHW), 2017). By contrast, the proportion of older Indigenous Australians aged 65 and over is very low. An Indigenous Australian is considered to be 'older' when aged 50 and over, which reflects the **life expectancy** gap. The Australian Institute of Health and Welfare considers that this demographic change will create both pressure and opportunities for Australia's health and welfare systems. The Australian federal government has implemented policies associated with **healthy ageing**, ageing well and increased choice for consumers of health care services. Australians have one of the highest life expectancies in the world, although many older Australians are living with one or more chronic illnesses.

In the health domain, concerns about the economics of ageing have required refocused policy towards practices, services and behaviours directed at keeping growing numbers of older people well and out of costly care settings such as hospital and residential care. This is reflected in the current aged-care reform agenda, where health and aged-care services are increasingly provided in the home and in the community. This approach is supported through a model of interprofessional practice (see Chapter 1) aimed at improving health and maintaining the independence of Australia's older people. Over a quarter of a million people (259,000) were using residential care (permanent or respite), home care or transition care services in Australia on 30 June 2017. In addition, in 2016–17 almost 723,000 people were assisted in their home under the Commonwealth Home Support Program (AIHW 2017).

Older Australians are not a homogeneous group, with many of them living independent, active and highly productive lives. The diversity of older Australians has a significant influence on the ageing process and the need to access health and welfare services. The proportion of older people participating in exercise, social and cultural activities has increased since 2012 (Australian Bureau of Statistics (ABS), 2016). Of Australia's older population, 75% report their health as good, very good or excellent (AIHW, 2017). The proportion of older people continuing in the labour force has doubled since 2000. The profile of older Australians is also changing; in 2016, 57% of the older population were aged 65–74, 30% were aged 74–84 and 13% were aged 85 and over (AIHW, 2017). Interestingly, the predictions for 2046 are that 1 in 5 Australians will be aged 85 and over.

At the other end of the age spectrum, there are a growing number of much older people, including centenarians. According to the latest census data, in 2017 there were almost 4000 centenarians living in Australia. Longevity can be a health challenge: as people become older, they are more likely to face complex health issues (AIHW, 2018). If we look at burden of disease data from *Australia's health 2018* (AIHW, 2018), we see the burden from **coronary heart disease** was highest among older people aged 75–84, with **dementia** the second leading cause of burden, followed by **chronic obstructive pulmonary disease** (COPD), stroke and lung cancer. The leading causes of burden among the very old (aged 95 and over) include chronic conditions (dementia, coronary heart disease and stroke).

Chronological age is becoming less of an indicator of health status, with an emphasis on maintaining good health for longer.

Diversity is key here, with older people varying enormously in terms of their health and well-being. Older people in Australia, as elsewhere, have highly diverse life circumstances, which affect their capacity to age well. These include their economic circumstances, their social and family situation, where they live, their cultural background and so on, which contribute to their health and well-being as they age. Such factors can also lead to serious inequities in terms of health outcomes, particularly for Indigenous Australians, who generally have the worst health outcomes characterised by a heavier burden of disease and shorter lifespans than non-Indigenous Australians. Currently, Indigenous Australians can expect to live 10 years less than their non-Indigenous counterparts (AIHW, 2018). Although there have been some improvements in overall health and well-being of this group, there continue to be large disparities, which are referred to as the **health gap.** Social determinants of health have a significant impact on this gap (see Chapters 5 and 6). The Council of Australian Governments continues to work on improving the health and well-being of Indigenous Australians.

A less well-known example is provided by rural older people. In Australia, demographic ageing is more prominent in rural Australia and rural older people experience poorer health outcomes related to increased mortality (Hodgkin et al. 2018). Many of these health challenges are affected by the service environment, as a result of the difficulties of delivering services efficiently and effectively across rural locations. This chapter will explore some of these issues and the health and aged-care context of an ageing Australia, starting with a brief outline of the ageing context (see Chapter 9 for more details on rural health).

Population ageing

Australia's population, like that of most developed countries, is ageing as a result of increasing **life expectancy**, which, in turn, has been achieved by sustained low fertility, low infant mortality and social progress in the spheres of public health, biomedicine, education, nutrition, housing and workplace safety. These are some of the social determinants of health. A growth in the number of older Australians can be attributed to the increasing life expectancy. On average, Australian women aged 65 and over can expect to live to around 87, and men to 84 (AIHW, 2017). As mentioned earlier, there is a significant difference for Indigenous Australians, who are generally affected by aged-related conditions at a younger age and have a lower comparative life expectancy. An Indigenous female born between 2010 and 2012 has a life expectancy of 73.7 years and a male 69.1 years (AIHW, 2017).

PAUSE
for
REFLECTION
…

Life expectancy in Australia has improved dramatically in the past century. Consider the variation between the life expectancies of Indigenous and non-Indigenous Australians. What do you think contributes to this variation? Consider this question in the light of related disadvantage, such as income, education, location and housing options for this population.

While very old age, particularly beyond 80 years, is a significant accomplishment for both the individual and society, there is also no doubt that this group places critical demands on the health and aged-care systems. While most people live at home in the community, some require significant health interventions and live in residential aged-care facilities. However, it needs to be remembered that this is not the norm; indeed, at any one time only 7.5% of the population aged over 70 years lives permanently in residential aged care. In 2016, 5.2% of those aged 65 and older were living in care accommodation, such as residential aged care (AIHW, 2017). However, although the population in residential care at any one time is small, as people live longer the risk of moving into residential care increases. This will have a significant impact on service provision.

Of particular concern here is the growing prevalence of **dementia**, the most common of which is Alzheimer disease. Dementia was added to the Australian National Health Priorities in 2013, recognising the significant health burden this disease presents to the individual and to the community (AIHW, 2012). The number of people with dementia is expected to increase over time, reflecting Australia's ageing population. The number of cases increased by 40% in a decade – from an estimated 252,000 in 2006 to 354,000 in 2016. In 2018, an estimated 376,000 people had dementia in Australia and this figure is expected to grow to 550,000 by 2030 (AIHW 2018). In 2018, 61% of people with dementia were women, and 43% were aged 85 and over. An estimated 8.7% of people aged 65 and over in Australia had dementia in 2018.

The question of how to provide dignified care for those with dementia is a profound one, particularly as they frequently reside side by side with non-demented residents in facilities that have not been designed to cater for the specific needs arising from memory loss, confusion and disorientation.

PAUSE *for* REFLECTION ... Older people, particularly those over age 85, are more likely to experience chronic diseases. They are also at increased risk of dementia and mental health challenges. Consider some of the areas of professional practice that are needed to maximise these people's capacity to live a good life even in very old age. What are some of the factors that might impede their access to interprofessional support? Chapter 1 provides some useful insights about this as you reflect on this question (see also Chapters 20 and 23 for more on the problem of aged care).

A brief history of aged care in Australia

The growth of the older population that has occurred over the past century has had a significant impact on Australia's welfare system and social policy (Warburton, 2014). Support for a continuing government role in the provision of services to older people and in the payment of pensions remains strong (Hodgkin, 2014). This is despite recent political discourse highlighting tensions between generations, and presenting older people as a drain on government spending (Dow et al. 2016).

These tensions are played out in the policy arena; with who should pay, and who should provide, at the forefront in approaches to aged care. Issues such as this, as well as other changes to the arrangements for the care of older people, have been shaped by a set of evolving socio-economic, demographic, political and cultural circumstances In the early colonial days, there were few older people and those who were sick or destitute were housed in poor-houses run by church-based benevolent societies. Pensions were introduced in 1908; although meagre, these at least indicated some recognition of the importance of supporting the aged. Yet most people were cared for within the family. As the welfare state developed in the post-war period, the federal government began to take responsibility for providing support for vulnerable older people. The *Aged Persons Homes Act 1954* provided federal grants to the voluntary sector to provide nursing homes. This marked the beginning of governmental control over aged-care homes and, for the next two decades, policy developments were oriented towards **residential services** based on a **medical model** of health (Gibson, 1994, pp. 157–158). During the resulting period of unrestrained growth between 1963 and 1972, the number of nursing-home beds approved under the legislation doubled to 51,286. A federal funding program led to the establishment of many smaller nursing homes across Australia, as well as the provision of hostel beds, day centres and day hospitals. As a result of rapid social and cultural change over this period, advances in biomedicine and technology prompted institutional change across all spheres of life. Hospital care became reorganised, medical specialisation flourished and the focus on ageing changed to become understood as both a social and a medical problem.

Although the financial incentives of this period significantly boosted the number of nursing-home and hostel beds, community care initiatives lagged behind. Thus, many frail elderly Australians had little choice but to leave their homes when they reached the point of being unable to care for themselves. The problem of lost rights loomed large by the 1980s; the media reported many instances of neglect and abuse of frail elders in institutional settings, and government reviews signalled an urgent need for closer scrutiny and tighter regulations (see Chapter 20 for a case study). In October 2018, similar media reports precipitated the announcement of a Royal Commission into Aged Care Quality and Safety to commence in 2019 – this in addition to the establishment of a new Aged Care Quality and Safety Commission (Department of Health 2018a).

Recent government policies have espoused the value of keeping older adults living in the community for as long as possible, with this emphasis strongly endorsed by older adults (Wiles et al. 2012). These initiatives have significantly changed the way that residential and community care programs are funded and delivered. Terms contained in recent policy documents such as 'rebalanced care' signal an overt shift in funding from residential to community care.

PAUSE *for* REFLECTION ... Recent aged-care reform has a focus on enabling older Australians to remain in their own homes for as long as possible. The primary goal of these reforms is to support individuals to remain in their community. There are particular challenges facing older people who are reliant on health and welfare services to remain as independent as possible. What are some of the foreseeable issues with this approach to maintaining older people's independence?

Ageing, illness and dependency

Ageing is inevitably accompanied by physical decline; bodily 'wear and tear' and the effects of age-related conditions reduce stamina, function and independence. Older people commonly have conditions such as those identified within the National Health Priorities initiative. This initiative identifies priority areas for focus on expenditure and improving health outcomes (Parliament of Australia 2017).

Common conditions such as arthritis, cardiovascular disease, diabetes and sensory loss are chronic. When acute health 'events' such as stroke or heart attack occur, an individual's capacity for self-care and participation in social life may be significantly compromised. As a result, older people are highly represented in acute settings such as hospitals: 3% of reported hospital admissions for those aged 65 and over resulted from injury due to a fall (AIHW 2018). For many older people, the risk of falling and the fall episode influence decision-making about access to community supports or transition to residential aged care.

Mental deterioration, too, affects self-care abilities. The effects of dementia, for example, are profound. Over time, often more than 10 years, individuals with dementia become increasingly impaired as they lose specific mental capacities such as memory, comprehension and reasoning; physical functions are also affected, for example bladder and bowel control. People with dementia may also use a mix of health and aged-care services. In 2017, 89,500 people with dementia were living in permanent residential aged care (AIHW 2018).

It should be noted that, although the rates of poor health and disability increase with age, they are not uniformly distributed across the older population; the burden of ill-health and disability is disproportionately higher for some groups, including those from rural and remote areas and Indigenous people (AIHW 2018). Those in rural and remote areas tend to have poorer health outcomes. These outcomes may be correlated to a combination of access to services, lifestyle risk factors and regional / remote environment compared with major urban environments (AIHW 2017). It is very important to remember that the majority of older people live independently in their own homes, requiring minimal (if any) intervention or support. The need for, and use of, health services is dependent on local structural factors such as access to services, the availability of family and community support and the cultural significance of taking up **formal services.** Rural and remote areas have fewer residential aged-care places available, with 38% of facilities in remote areas and 72% in very remote areas having fewer than 20 places. Older Australians in remote or very remote areas account for only 0.7% of people aged 65 and over in permanent residential care (AIHW 2015).

Ageing and wellness

The experience of ageing affects all aspects of life, from housing and income to health, family relationships and social participation. A major aim of the health care system is to positively influence our health behaviours to prevent disease and reduce ill-health (AIHW 2018, p. 374). In 2015 the World Health Organization (WHO) moved from **active ageing** to **healthy ageing. Healthy ageing** is about creating the environments and opportunities that enable people to be and do what they value in their lives, defined as 'the process of developing and maintaining the functional ability that enables well-being in older age' (WHO 2015, p. 28). Functional ability includes a person's ability:

◆ to meet their basic needs
◆ to learn, grow and make decisions
◆ to be mobile
◆ to build and maintain relationships, and
◆ to contribute to society.

Healthy ageing is the focus of WHO's work on ageing between 2015 and 2030 (WHO, 2015), emphasising the need for action across multiple sectors and enabling older people to remain a resource to their families, communities and economies.

Following the lead taken by the World Health Organization, the Australian Government has recognised that health care systems need to be transformed so that they can ensure affordable access to evidence-based medical interventions that respond to the diverse needs of older people. Cities and communities around the world are working towards being more aged-friendly. An aged-friendly world enables people of all ages to participate in community activities and treats everyone with respect regardless of their age.

The importance of the social aspect in maintaining good health in later life is now well accepted. Older people may have quite different ageing trajectories as they grow older. Public policy should not be based upon an erroneously homogeneous group or a 'one-size-fits-all' approach. Burns et al. (2017) support the view that individuals who get into or are in good shape before age 65 have the best chances of ageing well.

Retirement is traditionally regarded as the onset of 'old age' and, by representing withdrawal from active life, can actually promote ill-health and lead to the early onset of health problems (Harvey & Thurnwald 2009). Retirement can lead to deterioration of mental health as older people lose social connections and move away from workforce engagement (Lucas et al. 2017). This is a major concern, as Australia's **'Baby Boom' generation** now represents a significant proportion of retirees, and hence there is a growing need to ensure that they maintain social and productive involvement in society. Certainly, concerns about a shrinking workforce have led the Australian government to implement new policies aimed at extending the working lives of people and keeping them in paid work longer.

PAUSE *for* REFLECTION ...   The series of government intergenerational reports highlights the costs of health as people age, raising concerns about generating enough tax revenue to support the growing older population. At the same time, the age of access to the pension is rising. Thus, overall, there is a growing expectation that older people need to work longer. Is this equitable, and should there be exceptions? What are some of the health implications of working longer?

Service provision, use and dependency

In Australia, government-funded aged care is principally a Commonwealth Government function. Current expenditure on aged-care services across all Australian states and territories in 2016–17 was $17.5 billion per annum with approximately 69% of this on residential aged care; by 2055, aged-care spending is projected to nearly double as a proportion of GDP (Australian Government Aged Care Financing Authority 2017). Growth in spending can be attributed to societal changes such as increasing age, increased prevalence of chronic disease, and risk factors.

In recent decades, arrangements for the delivery of aged-care services have changed dramatically. In the latter half of the last century, governments around the world, regardless of their political persuasions, refocused their health and human service policies through the lens of neoliberal, free-market philosophies. As a consequence, Australian aged-care services operate in a competitive financial environment, with a combination of approved non-profit and for-profit providers. In 2014, some aged-care providers were listed on the stock exchange for the first time. The following section provides an outline of residential care and community care, and considers the impact of recent reform.

Residential care

Residential care programs include long-term and respite care. The shift away from residential services towards those provided within the community is evident in changes to the future proposed allocation of residential places and community care packages. To highlight this, the Australian Government currently allocates places based upon population ratios and is aiming to reduce residential aged-care places down from 84.5 per thousand people aged over 70 in 2012, to 78 per thousand people aged over 70 in 2022 (Australian Government Aged Care Financing Authority 2017). In contrast, it is set to increase community care places, from 18 per thousand people aged 70 and over in 2102 to 45 per thousand people aged over 70 in 2022. Despite these changes, funding for residential care will, by necessity, increase owing to projected increases in the ratio of numbers of older people per population. This is set to substantially increase, the Productivity Commission (2011) projecting the need for an additional 105,000 residential beds by 2025.

The increasing marketisation of aged-care services has been found to have reduced applicability in rural and remote settings (Baldwin et al. 2015). While the for-profit sector has increased its ownership of residential care beds to 30%, the majority of these are metropolitan based (Baldwin et al. 2015). An analysis of trends in residential care by Baldwin et al. (2015) found that, in metropolitan areas, the trend has been in the development of fewer yet larger services and an increase in for-profit providers. In contrast, smaller and often government-owned services were the norm in outer regional and remote locations. At a structural level, this led Baldwin et al. (2015) to predict a two-tiered system of residential care in Australia, characterised by a metropolitan / rural divide.

The *Living Longer, Living Better Act* (Australian Government 2013) introduced a number of key reforms. Entry to all Commonwealth funded services is through the Commonwealth 'gateway' *My Aged Care,* which acts primarily as a first-level **assessment** service. For residential and packaged community care services, a formal assessment is required through the **Aged Care Assessment Service (ACAS)**.

Since 2014, these reforms have also increased the contribution that older people make towards their care. All older people entering residential care are means tested on a combination of both assets and income to determine this contribution and eligibility for a Commonwealth subsidy paid to their provider. A daily payment (or service fee) is paid by all residents, currently set at a maximum of 85% of the single aged pension. In addition, residents pay a 'rent' fee in the form of a **refundable accommodation deposit (RAD)** paid as a deposit and / or or a daily equivalent payment. The total contribution that older Australians made to their care in 2015 was $4.2 billion, exclusive of the RAD fees (Australian Government Aged Care Financing Authority 2017).

Since the removal of the distinction between 'high care' and 'low care' in 2014, all residents entering residential care, including those with higher care needs, are required to make a contribution towards their accommodation. Both levels of care are now legally referred to as **residential aged-care facilities (RACFs)** and all permanent aged-care residents are assessed by the **Aged Care Funding Instrument (ACFI)**.

This combination of sector reforms has resulted in an increase in the average age of entry into residential care, now at 84.6 years, with the median length of stay reduced to 3 years (Australian Government Aged Care Financing Authority 2017). Residents often have complex conditions (Andrews-Hall et al. 2007; King et al. 2013) including cardiovascular diseases, diabetes mellitus, dementing illnesses and psychological disorders. With the majority of residents remaining in residential care until they die, there is a growing need for intensive palliative care services (Phillips & Currow 2017). The Productivity Commission Report (2011) highlighted the need for all care staff to be skilled in providing palliative care.

Community care

The Home and Community Care (HACC) program, first introduced in the 1980s, was a jointly funded and managed program by the Commonwealth and States and Territories. Since 2017, services provided to people aged 65 and over under the old HACC program have transitioned to Commonwealth funding and control. In July 2015, the **Commonwealth Home Support Program (CHSP)** consolidated the following into one program: the HACC Program, planned respite from the National Respite for Carers Program, the Day Therapy Centres Program and the Assistance with Care and Housing for the Aged Program. The CHSP program is designed to provide a modest amount of single service care. Older people with complex needs are supported through the **Home Care Packages (HCP)** program, which provides a range of services to support older people to remain at home (Department of Health 2018b). The packages are subsidised by the Commonwealth Government, although if an individual has capacity they may be asked to make a financial contribution to the cost of their care.

Older people with complex needs can find it extremely difficult to access care. In 2017, the Australian Government established a national prioritisation queue to better understand unmet need. As of 31 December 2017, around 45% of all people waiting for a package had been allocated a lower-level package and only 5% were assigned at the assessed level (Australian Government Aged Care Financing Authority 2017). Despite the Australian Government announcing additional packages in the 2017 and 2018 budgets, a cap remains on the number of home care packages, thus creating a mismatch between community expectation and access to services (Jorgensen & Haddock 2018).

Consumer-directed care

A significant focus of recent aged-care reform has been **consumer-directed care (CDC)**. The intention behind CDC is to give older people more choice and control in the type of service they receive; thus in 2017 all new and existing home care packages were assigned to consumers, rather than aged-care providers. This has introduced competition among home care providers, who must now market their services and broker services from other providers. In rural and remote areas this is problematic for a number of reasons. Lack of markets and problems around service delivery are compounded by the reduced availability of and proximity to primary health care services.

As CDC is relatively new in Australia, research into its effectiveness is scant. One systematic review found older people reported varying preferences for CDC (Ottmann et al. 2013), while other studies have highlighted significant implementation issues (Douglas et al. 2017; Gill & Cameron 2015; Laragy & Allen 2015).

Workforce challenges

Over several decades, policy-makers, peak bodies, unions, providers and researchers have nominated widespread **workforce shortfalls** as a continuing and pressing threat to the aged-care industry. Conservative estimates call for a tripling of the current direct care workforce by 2050 to meet projected care needs. The concerns about meeting projected consumer demands and care standards are endorsed in the recently Government commissioned report from the Aged Care Workforce Strategy Taskforce (2018).

Workforce estimates indicate a worsening of the current situation due to the ageing and imminent retirement of a large number of aged-care workers. Industry and policy demands for high-quality and cost-effective care into the future are threatened by skill shortfalls as well as by reported dissatisfaction with current training courses. Regional and rural communities are particularly impacted by both workforce and skill shortages. Across the sector, shortages are more prevalent outside the major cities and vacancies are harder to fill. Equally, factors such as distance from services and training organisations, smaller workforce pools, the diverse service mix and the relatively poor health status of rural aged consumers will impact on care delivery capacity and costs. The complexity of regional and rural workforce issues is well described in a recent study of community aged-care managers' experiences (Savy et al. 2017).

Comparatively low pay, lack of career potential, **de-skilling** of professional nurses, heavy workloads and little control over workload are the reasons cited for the current workforce issues (Cheek et al. 2003; Hodgkin et al. 2017; Nay et al. 2014). As a result, the profile of aged-care workers has changed over the past few decades, with fewer registered nurses in the field and more Vocational Education and Training (VET)-prepared workers with a Certificate III or IV in Aged Care Work (Productivity Commission 2011). The issue of who will care and what kind of skill-mix will achieve best practice is of at least the same magnitude as concerns about the future growth in the numbers of long-term care residents.

PAUSE
for
REFLECTION
...

Although there are services that provide some element of care for older people, much is left to family carers in looking after their ageing family members. Reflect on some of the dilemmas this places on families, particularly in an era of **'ageing in place'**, where older people are increasingly expected to remain in their homes even when they become old and frail.

The care is packaged to meet the care requirements of each individual. Information is made available to consumers on the My Aged Care website https://www.myagedcare.gov.au.

Case study 8.1 explores issues in aged care.

Case Study 8.1

Issues in aged care

With the support of her family and a home care package, Laine lived independently with her cat (Mr Darcy). Laine was beginning to become very forgetful, and was also becoming less trusting of her care team. She began to experience visual hallucinations, imagining that she was in danger. This led to a distrust of the care team and, as a consequence, she was refusing to let them into her home.

Laine developed a sacral pressure area and was being seen by the district nurse. It was February, and a period of very hot days meant that Laine was not drinking enough to maintain adequate hydration. She became increasingly confused and lethargic. The district nurse contacted one of Laine's daughters and suggested that Laine should go to hospital.

Laine's daughter took her to the local emergency department after much persuasion and coercion. Her triage category meant a very long wait before being seen by a doctor. This increased Laine's agitation and confusion as well as her dehydration. The emergency department was busy, noisy and a frightening place for Laine, who just wanted to go home.

Laine was given some intravenous fluids and a CT brain was performed. She was agitated and disorientated as to time and place, although knew her daughter and begged to be taken home. In the early hours of the following morning she was admitted to a general medical ward for aged-care assessment and review. It was determined that for her safety she would be required to move into a residential-care facility.

Laine remained on the medical ward for 2 weeks, becoming increasingly confused and scared. She was diagnosed with vascular dementia. The medical team commenced her on risperidone 1.5 mg daily to 'manage' her hallucinations and confusion. The medication made her unsteady on her feet and drowsy. Laine was admitted to a residential-care facility's locked dementia unit, where she lived until she died some 3 years later.

Case study questions

What issues does this case study raise about:

1   The **iatrogenic** effects of acute hospital stay on older patients?
2   The need for improved pathways between services and transition services for older people?
3   Psychosocial support for consumers and carers of older people?

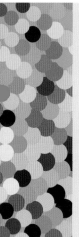

Summary

Overall, and in light of our discussion in this chapter, the complexity of the residential and community care is perhaps best expressed in terms of balance:

- between residential and community care, and how formal services can be developed and delivered that support the needs of all older people, whatever their health and social status
- between illness and wellness approaches, which represent the diversity of needs and service approaches.

Health care policies are moving towards a multidisciplinary approach, which supports the principle of healthy ageing across the diversity of older people. The advent of consumer-directed care, based on need and consumer choice, is touted as another positive move towards more universal change, acknowledging that older people have capabilities, rights and value within our societies.

Review Questions

1   Consider what impact the changing population profile in Australia is likely to have on care arrangements in the future. What will be the major challenges faced by our health and social care systems?
2   What are the issues associated with developing an appropriately trained and skilled health workforce in aged care?
3   Consider the question of who speaks for older people. What are the constraints on consumer involvement by older people in health care?
4   Discuss the issue of balance in relation to the delivery of appropriate, cost-effective health care to all older Australians.

References

Aged Care Workforce Strategy Taskforce 2018 Department of Health, Canberra. https://consultations.health.gov.au/aged-care-policy-and-regulation/aged-care-workforce-strategy/.

Andrews-Hall, S., Howe, A., Robinson, A., 2007. The dynamics of residential aged care in Australia: 8-year trends in admission, separations and dependency. Aust. Health Rev. 31 (4), 611–622.

Australian Bureau of Statistics, 2016. 4430.0 – Disability, ageing and carers, Australia: summary of findings, 2015. https://www.abs.gov.au/ausstats/abs@.nsf/0/C258C88A7AA5A87ECA2568A9001393E8 ?Opendocument.

Australian Government, 2013. Living Longer, Living Better Act. Australian Government, Canberra. https:// www.legislation.gov.au/Details/C2016C00170.

Australian Government Aged Care Financing Authority, 2017. Fifth report on the funding and financing of the aged care sector, July. Australian Government, Canberra. https://agedcare.health.gov.au/sites/ default/files/documents/08_2017/design_version_2017_acfa_annual_report.pdf.

Australian Institute of Health and Welfare (AIHW), 2012. Risk factors contributing to chronic disease. AIHW cat. no. PHE 157. AIHW, Canberra.

Australian Institute of Health and Welfare (AIHW), 2015. Residential aged care and home care 2014–2015. https://www.gen-agedcaredata.gov.au/Resources/Access-data/2015/December/Residential-aged -care-and-Home-Care-2014-15-suppo.

Australian Institute of Health and Welfare (AIHW), 2017. Older Australia at a glance. https://www.aihw.gov .au/reports/older-people/older-australia-at-a-glance/contents/demographics-of-older-australians/ australia-s-changing-age-and-gender-profile.

Australian Institute of Health and Welfare (AIHW), 2018. Australia's health 2018. Australia's health series no. 16. AUS 221. Canberra: AIHW. https://www.aihw.gov.au/getmedia/7c42913d-295f-4bc9-9c2 4-4e44eff4a04a/aihw-aus-221.pdf.aspx?inline=true.

Baldwin, R., Chenoweth, L., Dela Rama, M., et al., 2015. Quality failures in residential aged care in Australia: the relationship between structural factors and regulation imposed sanctions. Australas. J. Ageing 34 (4), E7–E12. doi:10.1111/ajag.12165.

Burns, R.A., Browning, C., Kendig, H.L., 2017. Living well with chronic disease for those older adults living in the community. Int. Psychogeriatr. 29 (5), 835–843. doi:10.1017/S1041610216002398.

Cheek, J., Ballantyne, A., Jones, J., et al., 2003. Ensuring excellence: an investigation of the issues that impact on registered nursing providing residential care to older Australians. Int. J. Nurs. Pract. 9 (2), 103–111.

Department of Health, 2018a Aged Care Quality and Safety Commission. Department of Health, Canberra.

Department of Health, 2018b Ageing and aged care. Home care packages program. https:// agedcare.health.gov.au/programs/home-care-packages-program.

Douglas, H.E., Georgiou, A., Tariq, A., et al., 2017. Implementing information and communication technology to support community aged care service integration: lessons from an Australian aged care provider. Int. J. Integr. Care 17 (1), 9. doi:10.5334/ijic.2437.

Dow, B., Joosten, M., Kimberly, H., et al., 2016. Age encounters: exploring age and intergenerational identity. J. Intergener. Relatsh. 14 (2), 104–118. doi:10.1080/15350770.2016.1160731.

Gibson, D., 1994. Reforming aged care in Australia: change and consequence. J. Soc. Policy 25 (2), 157–179.

Gill, L., Cameron, D., 2015. Innovation and consumer directed care: identifying the challenges. Australas. J. Ageing 34 (4), 265–268. doi:10.1111/ajag.12222.

Harvey, P.W., Thurnwald, I., 2009. Ageing well, ageing productively: the essential contribution of Australia's ageing population to the social and economic prosperity of the nation. Health Sociol. Rev. 18 (4), 379–386.

Hodgkin, S., 2014. Intergenerational solidarity at the state and family level: an investigation of Australian attitudes. Health Sociol. Rev. 23 (1), 53–56.

Hodgkin, S., Warburton, J., Hancock, S., 2018. Predicting wellness among rural older Australians: a cross-sectional study. Rural Remote Health 18 (3), 4547. doi:10.22605/RRH4547.

Hodgkin, S., Warburton, J., Savy, P., et al., 2017. Workforce crisis in residential aged care: insights from rural, older workers. Aust. J. Public Admin. 76 (1), 93–105.

Jorgensen, M., Haddock, R. 2018. The impact of the home care reforms on the older person, the aged care workforce and the wider health system. (Deeble Institute issues brief; no. 27). Australian Healthcare and Hospitals Association, Deakin West, ACT. https://ahha.asn.au/publication/health-policy-issue -briefs/deeble-issues-brief-no-27-impact-home-care-reforms-older.

King, D., Wei, Z., Howe, A., 2013. Work satisfaction and intention to leave among direct care workers in community and residential aged care in Australia. J. Aging Soc. Policy 25 (4), 301–319. doi:10.1080/ 08959420.2013.816166.

Laragy, C., Allen, J., 2015. Community aged care case managers transitioning to consumer directed care: more than procedural change required. Aust. Social Work 68 (2), 212–227.

Lucas, A.R., Daniel, F., Guadalupe, S., et al., 2017. Time spent in retirement, health and well-being. European Psychiatry 41, S339–S340. doi:10.1016/j.eurpsy.2017.02.298.

Nay, R., Garratt, S., Fetherstonhaugh, D., 2014. Older People: Issues and Innovations in Care, fourth ed. Elsevier, London.

Ottmann, G., Allen, J., Feldman, P., 2013. A systematic narrative review of consumer-directed care for older people: implications for model development. Health Soc. Care Community 21 (6), 563–581. doi: 10.1111/j.1742-6723.2009.01168.x.

Parliament of Australia, 2017. The National Health Priority Areas Initiative. https://www.aph.gov.au/ About_Parliament/Parliamentary_Departments/Parliamentary_Library/Publications_Archive/CIB/ cib9900/2000CIB18.

Phillips, J.L., Currow, D.C., 2017. Would reframing aged care facilities as a 'hospice' instead of a 'home' enable older people to get the care they need? Collegian 24 (1), 1–2.

Productivity Commission, 2011. Caring for older Australians, Commonwealth of Australia, Canberra. www.pc.gov.au/inquiries/completed/aged-care/report/aged-care-volume1.pdf.

Savy, P., Warburton, J., Hodgkin, S., 2017. Challenges to the provision of community aged care services across rural Australia: perceptions of service managers. Rural Remote Health 17 (2), 4059. doi:10.22605/RRH4059.

Warburton, J., 2014. Ageing and social policy in Australia. In: Harper, S., Hamblin, K. (Eds.), International Handbook of Ageing and Public Policy. Edward Elgar, Cheltenham, pp. 301–317.

Wiles, J.L., Leibing, A., Guberman, N., et al., 2012. The meaning of "aging in place" to older people. Gerontologist 52 (3), 357–366. doi:10.1093/geront/gnr098.

World Health Organization (WHO), 2015. World report on ageing and health. WHO, Geneva.

Further Reading

Warburton, J., 2014. Ageing and social policy in Australia. In: Harper, Sarah, Hamblin, Kate (Eds.), International Handbook of Ageing and Public Policy. Edward Elgar, Cheltenham, pp. 301–317.

Online Resources

Myagedcare website: www.myagedcare.gov.au.

CHAPTER 9

Rural health systems: spotlight on equity and access

Bernadette Ward and Rachel Tham

Key learning outcomes

When you finish this chapter you should be able to:

- consider how rural health is defined from a range of perspectives
- understand the nuances between the health status of rural and urban populations and links with the social determinants of health
- explain the importance of equity and access in improving population health
- discuss the challenges of implementing equity and access interventions
- consider the role of primary health care in improving the health status of rural populations
- be aware of the challenges in recruiting and retaining the rural health workforce.

Key terms and abbreviations

Aboriginal Community Controlled Health Organisations (ACCHOs)
Aboriginal health workers (AHWs)
acceptability
access
Access Relative to Need (ARN) index
Accessibility/Remoteness Index of Australia (ARIA)
affordability
approachability
appropriateness
Australian Health Practitioner Regulation Agency (AHPRA)
Australian Standard Geographic Classification – Remoteness Areas (ASGC-RA)
availability and accommodation
big data

general practitioner (GP)
geographical classification systems
horizontal equity
Index of Relative Socio-economic Advantage and Disadvantage (IRSAD)
Modified Monash Model (MMM)
National Disability Insurance Scheme (NDIS)
nurse practitioner (NP)
primary health care (PHC)
Rural, Remote and Metropolitan Areas (RRMA) classification
rural workforce incentive programs
telehealth
Urgent Care Centre (UCC)
utilisation
vertical equity

Introduction

Australia is a vast and geographically diverse continent with a population of approximately 25 million people. The majority of the population (71%) lives in major cities while the remainder is typically sparsely spread across rural and remote communities within an area of 7.5 million square kilometres.

Addressing the relatively poor health status of rural populations is a national priority in many countries and, in Australia, the health of rural communities is frequently highlighted in the media. However, there is little discussion on what we actually mean by 'rural health'. People living in rural (or metropolitan) areas are not homogeneous populations. That is, within these populations there are vast differences in health status and access to care. In such a high-income country as Australia these inequities are objectionable – so in this chapter we explore what rural health is and how it is influenced by geography; the social determinants of health; the health system, workforce and funding; health policy; and rural communities.

What is rural health?

Definitions and classifications are important because they assist policy-makers and health service planners to allocate financial and human resources to the health system within and across locations, service models and disciplinary groups in order to meet health needs. Internationally, policy-makers struggle to reach consensus on the definition of rural health, resulting in no consistent definition of this term. Definitions range between geographical, demographical, sociological and cultural perspectives (Wilson et al. 2009) owing to diverse settings and health needs.

What do we mean by rural health in Australia?

In Australia, health is considered from physical, mental and social perspectives in addition to the organisational, social and cultural systems that produce health outcomes. In general, 'rural health' usually refers to the health status of individuals and communities in 'regional' and 'remote' areas. Classifications of 'rural' have underpinned the evolving definition of rural health.

How are rural, regional and remote areas defined and classified in Australia?

In Australia, several **geographical classification systems** have evolved in the attempt to differentiate rural locality and remoteness from urban (metropolitan) areas. Initially, the **RRMA (rural, remote and metropolitan areas)** and **ARIA (Accessibility / Remoteness Index of Australia)** classifications were based on population size and road distance to service centres (Australian Institute of Health and Welfare (AIHW) 2004). It was soon recognised that more-accurate measures were needed. The **ASGC-RA (Australian Standard Geographical Classification – Remoteness Areas)** classification was based on a refinement of enhanced ARIA (Department of Health 2013). It differentiates between levels of accessibility and location as follows: (RA 1) major cities, (RA 2) inner regional, (RA 3) outer regional, (RA 4) remote and (RA 5) very remote. ASGC-RA differentiates between cities that are

TABLE 9.1 COMPARISON OF MODIFIED MONASH MODEL AND ASGC-RA GEOGRAPHICAL CLASSIFICATION SYSTEMS

MMM	Population size	ASGC-RA	Example locations
1	All	RA 1	Most capital cities, Newcastle, Geelong, Gold Coast
2	>50,000	RA 2 & 3	Bendigo, Launceston, Cairns, Darwin
3	15,000–50,000	RA 2 & 3	Coffs Harbour, Mt Gambier, Shepparton, Broken Hill, Kalgoorlie
4	5000–15,000	RA 2 & 3	Ararat, Port Augusta, Moree, Warwick
5	0–5000	RA 2 & 3	Gundagai, Naracoorte, Bega, Margaret River
6	0–5000	RA 4	Bourke, Kununurra, Charleville, Queenstown
7	0–5000	RA 5	Derby, Tennant Creek, Nhulunbuy, Weipa

Source: Modified from Department of Health – Rural and Regional Australia (2017). General Practice Rural Incentives Programme (GPRIP) program guidelines, http://www.health.gov.au/internet/main/publishing.nsf/content/general_practice_rural_incentives_programme-programme-guidelines

major (e.g. capital cities such as Sydney (RA 1)) or outer regional cities (e.g. Darwin (RA 2)), and it defines remote areas more tightly than ARIA (AIHW 2004).

The **Modified Monash Model (MMM)** has recently been developed from the ASGC-RA to create a new seven-level geographical classification system that distinguishes different town sizes in inner and outer regional Australia (Table 9.1) in order to overcome distributional inequities, particularly in relation to recruitment and retention incentives for the health workforce (**general practitioners (GPs)** in particular). This system takes six sentinel indicators of rural health workforce recruitment and retention into account: hours worked, work in a public hospital, working after-hours, ability to have time off, employment opportunities for a partner and choice of schools available locally (Humphreys et al. 2012).

Although there is no perfect geographical classification system, the MMM addresses some deficiencies of previous systems. The MMM was adopted by the Australian Department of Health in 2015 and is now the classification system of choice for funding a range of health activities including the National Disability Insurance Scheme (NDIS), aged-care services and workforce incentive and training programs (Aged Care 2019; Allied Health Professional Australia (AHPA) 2019; Department of Health 2019; Department of Human Services 2018).

The use of geographical classifications systems alone for developing appropriate policy, allocating financial and human resources and developing innovative models of service delivery can be problematic, as they do not account for socio-demographic indicators such as health status, population density, environmental factors, community resources, availability of communication and transport systems and health literacy (McGrail & Humphreys 2009a, 2009b; Levesque et al., 2013).

PAUSE
for
REFLECTION
...

Take time to review the key components of ASGC-RA and MMM. What are the key differences between them?

You can get a better understanding of the differences by looking at the classification of the following locations using the ASGC-RA tool on the Department of Health website: (http://www.doctorconnect.gov.au/internet/otd/publishing.nsf/content/home): Charters Towers; Townsville; Port Fairy; Ballarat; Gundagai; Hobart; Sale; Mildura.

Find out their population size and regroup them using the MMM criteria in Table 9.1. Which ones are grouped together under ASGC-RA but grouped differently under MMM?

Rural health status and the rural–urban differential

On a population basis, Australians living in rural and remote areas generally experience poorer health outcomes than their metropolitan counterparts. Health status is typically measured in terms of both morbidity and mortality. For example, there are higher rates of asthma, lung disease, arthritis, injury, harmful alcohol drinking levels, being overweight or obese and poorer oral health amongst people living in rural and remote areas. Similarly, life expectancy decreases with increasing remoteness (AIHW 2008, 2010). Although a relatively higher proportion of Indigenous Australians live in MMM5–7 locations compared with non-Indigenous Australians, this does not entirely account for the generally lower health status reported by people living in these remote areas. With the advent of **'big data'** we can identify differences within rural settings. This gives a more nuanced understanding of the health status of rural sub-populations and provides the opportunity to develop more targeted approaches to addressing inequitable health outcomes.

PAUSE
for
REFLECTION
...

Go to the Rural and Remote Health Report on the AIHW website: https://www.aihw.gov.au/reports/rural-health/rural-remote-health/contents/rural-health.

This report highlights that Australians living in inner / outer regional and remote areas have poorer health status and lower life expectancy than their counterparts in major cities. It appears that mortality rates increase with remoteness.

Now go to 'My Healthy Communities': https://www.myhealthycommunities.gov.au.

If you look at health status and outcomes by local area comparisons you will find the rural–metropolitan differential in health status is not so clear. That is, indicators of incidence of some diseases and risk factors are higher in major cities than in some outer regional and remote areas.

These data highlight health differences both across and within populations.

Links with the social determinants of health

As you have seen, the Australian population is diverse and experiences varying levels of health and well-being. If we are trying to understand these differences, it is useful to look at some of the social determinants of health and how they are distributed across Australia.

Socio-economic factors are important determinants of your potential to live a life of advantage or relative poverty, thereby your wellbeing. One way of measuring this is the **Index of Relative Socio-economic Advantage and Disadvantage (IRSAD)**. IRSAD is based on Australian Bureau of Statistics census data and combines income, occupation, education and housing information to measure of people's access to material and social resources and ability to participate in society.

PAUSE
for
REFLECTION
...

Go to the IRSAD interactive map and type in the postcode or name of any rural town or metropolitan suburb to identify geographically advantaged and disadvantaged areas: (http://www.abs.gov.au/ausstats/abs@.nsf/Lookup/by%20Subject/2033.0.55.001~2016~Main%20Features~IRSAD%20Interactive%20Map~16).

You will find varying levels of advantage across rural and metropolitan Australia. Overall, Australians living in rural and remote areas experience higher levels of disadvantage compared with their metropolitan counterparts.

In a country like Australia, these inequalities are unacceptable but to address them we need to understand equity and access.

Equity

Health care is a fundamental human right, and so the need to improve equity of access to health services and reduce health status inequities are commonly cited objectives for governments and policy-makers alike (Starfield 2011). The terms '**health inequality**' and '**health inequity**' are sometimes used interchangeably, but they are not the same. We will now examine the difference between these two, and how equity is addressed in the delivery of rural health services.

Inequality refers to the uneven distribution of health outcomes that can be attributed to biological variations (e.g. cystic fibrosis, a medical condition that is inherited) or predetermined factors (e.g. age). In the case of **inequity**, the difference is not only due to inequality, but it is also avoidable. Put simply, it looks like Fig. 9.1.

One measure of an equitable health service is whether, at an aggregated level, people in rural and remote areas can access health services and achieve similar health outcomes to their metropolitan counterparts. This is called **horizontal equity**.

FIGURE 9.1 VISUALISING THE DIFFERENCE BETWEEN EQUALITY AND EQUITY

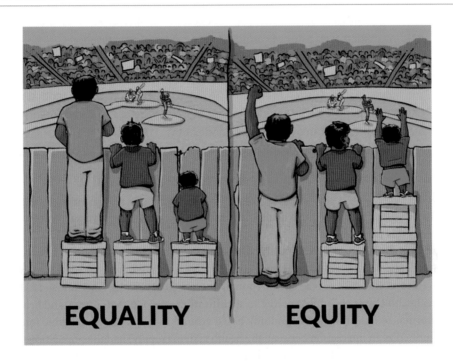

Source: Interaction Institute for Social Change / artist: Angus Maguire. www.interactioninstitute.org and www.madewithangus.com

When considering how equity can be measured, we need to think about equity of 'what' and for 'whom'. The 'what' can be understood in terms of equitable inputs (resources to ensure that everyone has adequate access to services), outputs (ensuring that all groups achieve similar health outcomes such as life expectancy or morbidity) or both (Starfield 2011). The 'whom' refers to which marginalised group is the focus of interventions aimed at improving equity. This is called **vertical equity**. Invariably this means that the concept of equity is values based and thus there is a need to include the voices of marginalised populations to reflect the values of these groups in any health decision-making.

One of the challenges in addressing health inequities is the inextricable link to the social determinants of health and the absence of clearly defined measures of health equity. The National Health Performance Framework has a strong focus on health equity and includes health system performance measures of access (see Online Resources section), but there is still much to be achieved in this area.

PAUSE

for

REFLECTION

...

Across Australia there are differences in the rates of potentially avoidable hospitalisations. For example, reduced availability of services is associated with increased rates of cardiovascular-related hospitalisations.

Look at where you live: https://www.heartfoundation.org.au/for -professionals/heart-maps/australian-heart-maps.

Similarly, the *Australian Atlas of Health Care Variation* (2018) highlights the differences in potentially avoidable hospitalisations across 18 clinical items: http://acsqhc.maps.arcgis.com/home/index.html.

These differences in health outcomes are inequitable as they can be remedied.

Access

In Australia, we subscribe to having a health care system where there is universal (equitable) access. But what does this mean?

Access to health care is central to health care systems around the world but, as a concept, access is difficult to define. Access is defined as the degree of 'fit' between the characteristics of providers and health services and the ability of the clients (potential access) (Penchansky & Thomas 1981). The act of accessing health care is generally referred to as **utilisation** (also *realised* access), and health system equity performance indicators are commonly based around this input. This dynamic interplay can also be described as an interaction between the health system (supply) and the population (demand).

Levesque et al. (2013) extends this further and describes the *dimensions* of access as follows:

- *Approachability*: identifying that a service exists, that it can be used and can change a client's health status.
- *Acceptability*: social and cultural factors that influence a client's preference for a service.
- *Availability and accommodation*: the existence and geographical location of a service and appropriately skilled personnel that can potentially be reached by clients.
- *Affordability*: financial and time costs related to using the service.
- *Appropriateness*: the fit between a client's health care needs and the timeliness and care spent trying to provide the correct treatment and care.

As outlined in Fig. 9.2, these dimensions interact with the ability of the client to perceive their needs, seek health care, reach and pay for the service, and ultimately utilise the service. Not surprisingly, these characteristics are, in turn, linked to many social determinants of health.

PAUSE

for

REFLECTION

...

Think about a health service that you know of and consider each dimension of access and how it might apply to that service. How accessible do you think the service is? Could you 'rate' the service on each dimension of access? Would your access rating differ if you were from another population group? How would you rate the accessibility of the service for vulnerable populations?

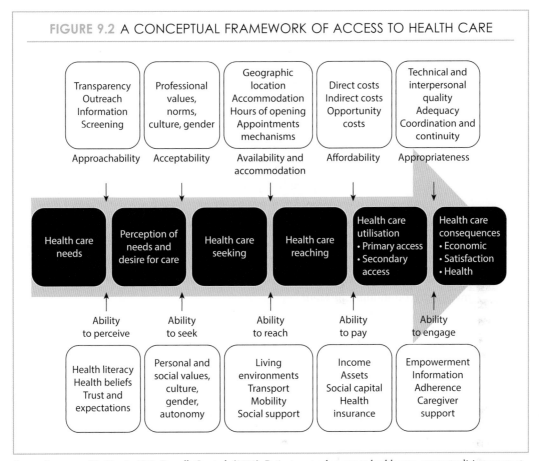

FIGURE 9.2 A CONCEPTUAL FRAMEWORK OF ACCESS TO HEALTH CARE

Source: Levesque, J.F., Harris, M.F., Russell, G., et al. (2013). Patient-centred access to health care: conceptualising access at the interface of health systems and populations. Int. J. Equity Health 12, 18

The dimensions of access are not independent of each other. For example, in rural Australia the use of bulk-billing (when a health service provider bills Medicare directly for the rebate fee only) may improve the affordability of a service. However, this could inadvertently affect the viability, and resultant availability, of some health services as the Medicare rebate may not cover the true cost of delivering a service. Similarly, increasing acceptability (e.g. reconfiguring the gender and cultural mix of staff) for one group in the population may compromise acceptability for another group and/or reduce service availability (Li et al. 2014).

Improving access

In 2018, the Australian Government announced the Stronger Rural Health Strategy (Department of Health 2018). The strategy primarily focuses on improving access to medical practitioners. Although this is important; access comprises more than this. There is much to be done to improve access before utilisation (and ultimately health outcomes) can be improved. Reliable measurement of some dimensions can be difficult and, to further complicate matters, consumers often make 'trade-offs' between dimensions. Across Australia there are numerous schemes aimed at improving access to health care for rural residents. There are travel schemes that provide financial assistance to access health care, but these generally apply only to attending the nearest service provider. Some residents may pay additional travel and accommodation costs to see their preferred provider (Ward et al. 2015).

PAUSE
for
REFLECTION
...

There is information online about the availability of health services.

Go to Healthmap and look at the availability of key health services by MMM category. https://healthmap.com.au/.

Although these demonstrate availability, there is scarce detail about other dimensions of access and the ability of clients to utilise those services.

Explore 'My Healthy Communities' to see how a rural community you know of is performing in terms of experiences and utilisation of health services – there are indicators that align with the dimensions of access outlined above: http://www.myhealthycommunities.gov.au/.

Can you identify differences in health service utilisation and experiences across geographical areas?

Improving access in rural and remote Australia has generally focused on health system characteristics. This has included altered models of care and workforce initiatives, such as fly-in, fly-out women's health practitioners, which have improved availability and acceptability of services for some communities (Kildea et al. 2010). Similarly, the presence of **Aboriginal Community Controlled Health Organisations (ACCHOs)** has improved approachability in many communities (Jongen et al. 2014). However, the approaches and underlying evidence have been *ad hoc* (World Health Organization (WHO) 2006).

One of the difficulties for policy-makers charged with improving access is **equity** – systematically determining which health services should be accessible in rural and remote areas. In response, Thomas et al. (2014) have identified 'core' primary health care (PHC) services that rural and remote Australians can expect to access, and the AIHW has developed a geospatial **Access Relative to Need (ARN) index**. This index uses GP workforce, census, hospital, morbidity and mortality data to report on people's access to GPs relative to their predicted need for PHC across Australia (AIHW 2014). The ARN index shows health outcomes improving more when consumers have improved access to GPs in geographical areas of high health need than they do when there is improved access to GPs in areas of low health need. This is very important, because it demonstrates that the need for PHC services is not only about where you live; it is also about your health status. As per Fig. 9.3, the ARN index demonstrates that when you take health status into account, the predicted need for PHC services in rural and remote areas is very different for Indigenous and non-Indigenous populations. For Indigenous Australians the need for PHC services is very high throughout these areas, but for

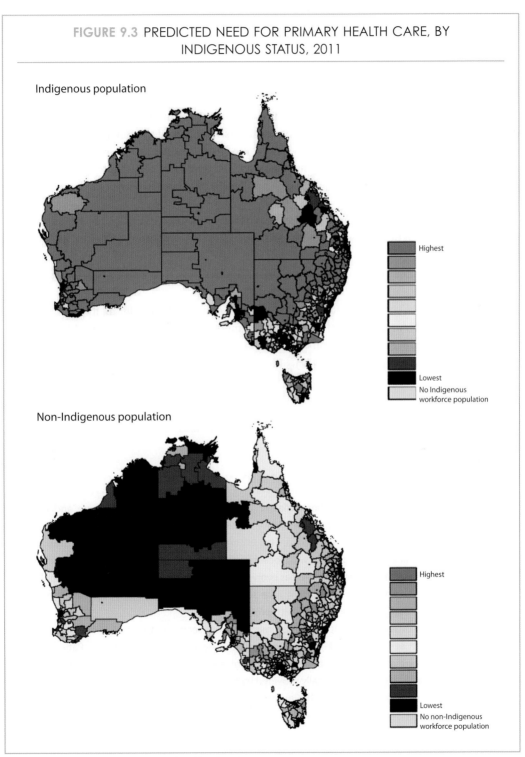

FIGURE 9.3 PREDICTED NEED FOR PRIMARY HEALTH CARE, BY INDIGENOUS STATUS, 2011

Source: Australian Institute of Health and Welfare (2014)

non-Indigenous Australians the need is very low. So, to address inequitable health outcomes, both health need and socio-demographic factors (e.g. the ARN index) need to be considered when planning PHC services.

Rural health service models

Due to the extensive geographical distances that separate rural communities, no single health service model can meet the diverse health needs of rural Australians while maintaining economic and operational efficiency. Hence, a variety of service models are needed to ensure equitable health outcomes. Research has shown that a comprehensive PHC approach (see Chapter 6), characterised by interdisciplinary team approaches, yields the best health outcomes in situations characterised by limited resources (Starfield 1998).

Many rural health services have developed innovative service models to meet communities' needs in diverse geographical and cultural settings. These have evolved to be 'fit for purpose', such as:

- ◆ transitioning to integrated and comprehensive PHC services such as ACCHOs (Jongen et al. 2014)
- ◆ outreach services such as the Royal Flying Doctor Service and other fly-in, fly-out health services (O'Sullivan et al. 2017), and networked models for allied health, mental health and community health services (Dyson et al. 2012)
- ◆ GP-based and nurse practitioner (NP)-supported hospitals (see Case study 9.1)
- ◆ virtual outreach services using digital technology (Bradford et al. 2016).

Case Study 9.1

Innovative approaches to rural health workforce challenges

Heathcote is a small town located approximately 110 kilometres north of Melbourne and 46 km south-east of Bendigo, with a population of 2793. In socio-economic terms, Heathcote is one of the most disadvantaged communities in Victoria. This is compounded by insufficient public transport, poor health literacy and disengagement with local health services.

Heathcote Hospital, established in 1894, has evolved into Heathcote Health, which provides publicly funded acute, aged, community and urgent care services. The service employs approximately 80 full-time equivalent staff, of which 57 are health professionals.

The Heathcote Urgent Care Centre (UCC) is similar to those seen in many small rural communities, whereby the health service is 'block-funded' to provide time-sensitive medical care. Patients may receive definitive care at the UCC or be referred to regional/metropolitan hospitals in Bendigo or Melbourne. UCC medical care is traditionally provided by private GPs who are remunerated via Medicare bulk-billing. Over the last few decades, the number of GPs in Heathcote decreased and it has been challenging to engage GPs to provide after-hours urgent care services, and to integrate care between Heathcote Health, the GPs and the regional/metropolitan hospitals.

In response to GP workforce shortages, Heathcote Health developed an NP model of care. The model aimed to identify those who are disadvantaged, do not access health care, or conversely are frequent attenders of UCC or acute hospital care. NP case management services were intended to reduce avoidable hospitalisations, increase health literacy and improve integration of care for consumers with complex health needs.

In 2016, Heathcote Health conducted a 6-month NP pilot project. A NP provided extended scope of practice for patients in the UCC (e.g. suturing, some pathology ordering and medication prescribing, mental health referrals). Active case management enabled hospital and district nurses, and GPs, to refer consumers to receive care in their homes. Heathcote Health funds the NP service, which is, in part, supported by access to Medicare NP items.

Evaluation of the NP project found a reduction in avoidable hospitalisations, avoidable UCC and GP service presentations and increased integration of acute, community, GP and regional/metropolitan hospital services for consumers. Feedback from the broader community, patients and health staff is very positive. Heathcote Health has subsequently extended the model and now also provides NP palliative care, midwifery and aged-care services. The service is currently supporting the training of additional NPs and has been called upon by other small rural health services to share the model. While similar models of care have been the 'norm' in other parts of rural Australia, via the advanced practice remote area nurse program, for communities that are relatively close to regional and metropolitan centres, this is a relatively new and innovative approach to tackling workforce challenges.

Workforce

There is inequitable distribution of health workers between metropolitan and rural and remote areas. Except for Aboriginal and Torres Strait Islander health practitioners, commonly known as **Aboriginal health workers (AHWs)**, more than 75% of health practitioners registered with the **Australian Health Practitioner Regulation Agency (AHPRA)** (see Chapter 1) are located in MMM 1 (major cities). The geographical spread of the health workforce does not reflect the distribution of the population and highlights the reduced access to health practitioners in rural and remote areas. While the majority of registered AHWs are located in rural and remote areas, AHWs often take on numerous roles, many are unregistered, and shortages remain in remote areas (Community Affairs References Committee 2012).

Health professionals face substantial barriers to entering and staying in rural and remote locations, including accessing professional development, excessive workload and limited opportunities for partners and children (Li et al. 2014; McGrail et al. 2017). A study of medical graduates has found those who spent at least 1 year studying in rural hospital/PHC settings were more likely to be practising in a rural location 9 years post-graduation (O'Sullivan et al. 2018). It is unknown whether this applies to other health professions.

To date, many **rural workforce incentive programs** have been aimed at medical students and practitioners and have not taken interdisciplinary practice (see Chapter 1), the role of AHWs (Mason 2013) and role substitution between health practitioners (Laurant et al. 2018) into account. For example, in some locations practitioners have extended scopes of practice that enable them to provide clinical services that, in metropolitan areas, would be provided by another discipline, for example nurse practitioners (see Case study 9.1). In locations with housing shortages, incentive programs for non-AHWs often include housing. Such resources are not always available to AHWs (Community Affairs References Committee 2012). The adoption of the MMM geographical classification system means that professional workload and social factors that are critical to retaining health practitioners will now be considered in workforce incentive schemes (Humphreys et al. 2012). Although the MMM is based on research with rural GPs, there are opportunities to apply similar principles to AHWs, nursing, community and allied health workforce incentive programs.

PAUSE
for
REFLECTION
...

There is a plethora of workforce interventions aimed at addressing the inequity of access in rural and remote areas that have included: expanding and/or changing the scope of practice for existing providers (Maier & Aiken 2016); role substitution (Laurant et al. 2018), developing new health disciplines (Kurti et al. 2011), establishing university Departments of Rural Health and Rural Clinical Training Schools, increasing student intakes, recruiting rural medical/dental students and international medical/dental graduates,; and providing incentive/support programs (Community Affairs References Committee 2012).

Visit the Health Workforce site: http://www.health.gov.au/internet/main/publishing.nsf/Content/work-co-rur and explore the range of programs aimed at addressing the maldistribution of the Australian health workforce.

What do you think makes a difference to *recruiting* and *retaining* health professionals? Why is it an ongoing concern?

Financing rural health services

There is substantial evidence that PHC is a cost-effective approach to health care in rural and remote areas (Zhao et al. 2014). Building on the health-financing information provided in Chapters 2 and 3, the inequitable access to good-quality health services in rural and remote areas highlights the need for more equitable resourcing mechanisms for those with the greatest health needs. Funding of rural and remote services is typically based on geographical classification systems, population–health service provider ratios and/or estimates of population need. The reduced availability of doctors means that many rural health services have been unable to access additional Medicare funding because the doctors are not present to generate fees. Programs such as the Medical Specialist Outreach Assistance Program and the Medical Outreach Indigenous Chronic Disease Program use salaried or Medicare-billing doctors in an effort to address these inequities but, to date, funding policies have failed to adequately take the burden of disease into account for rural and remote health service delivery. There is evidence that the funding of ACCHO services addresses some social determinants of health by providing economic benefits to local communities (Alford 2014) and there are currently trials under way to determine whether new general practice funding models can improve quality of patient care, but there is still much to be done in these areas.

More-sophisticated funding approaches that address the inequities in health outcomes are needed. The ARN Index (AIHW 2014) is a promising policy tool for health service policy-makers and planners allocating limited resources. Similarly, the Index of Access developed by McGrail et al. (2016) is underpinned by measures of service availability, proximity to services and population health needs. Currently, these models focus only on GPs and remote area nurses. However, in time they may be applied to other health care providers.

It's not all bad news

We should, however, be cautious about jumping to the conclusion that rural health is an inherently problematic environment to work in. The pleasures and fulfilment of rural living and working, such as satisfaction with life and work, work variety and community connectedness, are well documented (Bourke et al. 2010; McGrail et al. 2010). In addition, rural communities are important incubators of innovation and change agents (Tham et al. 2014) that can drive improvements in the social determinants of their health along with advocating and driving health service models to be designed and delivered in ways that respond to their community needs.

Where to from here?

The rural health system needs to match the dynamic needs of rural communities while becoming sustainable, responsive and strengthening rural community development. There is an identified need to continually assess the impact of rural health policy and reorientate the policy in line with changing needs, improve health equity, involve rural health service users in planning and strengthen a people-centric approach to rural health systems (Box 9.1).

BOX 9.1   T E L E H E A L T H

Improving access to health care is multidimensional. In recent years, the Medicare **telehealth** items have led to innovative service models and an exponential increase in the availability of e-health across medical, nursing and allied health services.

Several systematic reviews have reported that there is clear evidence that rural telehealth consultations can lead to equivalent health outcomes to those obtained via face-to-face care (Flodgren et al. 2015). A recent systematic review (Bradford et al. 2016) identified key factors to consider when implementing and sustaining telehealth interventions in rural and remote areas:

Continued

BOX 9.1   TELEHEALTH—cont'd

- Vision: clear realistic vision of the purpose of the service.
- Ownership: deliberate and consultative service development with all stakeholders; supportive management; clinicians who champion the service by actively engaging and participating in service delivery.
- Adaptability: trial and modify the service model according to needs of patients and health service; remain responsive to requirements of all stakeholders.
- Economics: deliver cost savings or facilitate prioritisation of services for health services; provide value for patients; achieve comparable care with clinical benefits.
- Efficiency: have defined, efficient processes for managing activity; quantity not necessarily the marker of success – high levels of activity are not required to be sustainable.
- Equipment: careful consideration of the equipment used and the technical requirements for support.

For rural outpatient and PHC consultations, cost outcomes largely depend on the distances between sites and the frequency of telehealth utilisation (Wade et al. 2010). While there is improved access, timeliness of care and savings from a patient perspective, these may offset the additional staffing and infrastructure costs borne by the health service (Rietdijk et al. 2012; Rubin et al. 2013).

Summary

- Increasingly, geographical classification systems are commonly used to define rural health and are becoming more sensitive to geographical maldistribution of health practitioners.
- Residents of rural Australia tend to have poorer health status than their metropolitan counterparts, but this is not always the case.
- Health status is closely linked to the social determinants of health so some 'answers' to improving health outcomes may lie outside the health system.
- Equity is not the same as equality.
- Embedding measures of equity and access into the health care system means making value judgements about what resources are allocated to rural and remote health services.
- The concept of access is multidimensional and invariably involves trade-offs linked to measures of equity.
- Access to appropriate health service models is important when addressing inequity and improving health outcomes.
- Innovative solutions are needed to address workforce maldistribution and develop models of care that meet the needs of rural communities.

Review Questions

1 Why are geographical classifications of 'rural' important in addressing the health status inequities experienced by many residents of rural areas?

2 How can we enhance the 'accessibility' of health care? How might we measure and compare access?

3 How can health policy decision-makers work with rural communities to develop models of health care and workforce programs that address the needs of the population?

4 How can workforce incentives be equitably distributed to recruit and retain rural health professionals?

References

Aged Care, 2019. Modified Monash Model Suburb and Locality Classification – Home Care Subsidy. https://agedcare.health.gov.au/funding/aged-care-fees-and-charges/modified-monash-model-suburb-and-locality-classification-home-care-subsidy.

Allied Health Professional Australia (AHPA), 2019. NDIS pricing guide update. https://ahpa.com.au/news-events/1129-2/.

Australian Institute of Health and Welfare (AIHW), 2004. Rural, regional and remote health – a guide to remoteness classifications. Cat. no. PHE 53. AIHW, Canberra.

Australian Institute of Health and Welfare (AIHW), 2008. Australia's health 2008. Cat. no. AUS 99. AIHW, Canberra.

Australian Institute of Health and Welfare (AIHW), 2010. Whose health? How population groups vary. Australia's health 2010. AIHW, Canberra, pp. 227–280.

Australian Institute of Health and Welfare (AIHW), 2014. Access to primary health care relative to need for Indigenous Australians. Cat. no. IHW 128. AIHW, Canberra.

Alford, K., 2014. Economic value of Aboriginal community controlled health services. NACCHO, Canberra. http://apo.org.au/node/39333.

Australian Atlas of Health Care Variation 2018. http://acsqhc.maps.arcgis.com/home/index.html.

Bourke, L., Humphreys, J.S., Wakerman, J., et al., 2010. From 'problem-describing' to 'problem-solving': challenging the 'deficit' view of remote and rural health. Aust. J. Rural Health 18 (5), 205–209.

Bradford, N., Caffery, L., Smith, A., 2016. Telehealth services in rural and remote Australia: a systematic review of models of care and factors influencing success and sustainability. Rural Remote Health 16, 3808.

Community Affairs References Committee, 2012. The factors affecting the supply of health services and medical professionals in rural areas. Senate Enquiry. Parliament House, Commonwealth of Australia, Canberra.

Department of Health – Rural and Regional Australia, 2017. General Practice Rural Incentives Programme (GPRIP) program guidelines. http://www.health.gov.au/internet/main/publishing.nsf/content/general_practice_rural_incentives_programme-programme-guidelines.

Department of Health, 2013. Reform of the ASGC-RA rural classification system. http://www.health.gov.au/internet/publications/publishing.nsf/Content/work-review-australian-government-health-workforce-programs-toc~chapter-4-addressing-health-workforce-shortages-regional-rural-remote-australia~chapter-4-reform-asgc-ra-rural-classification-system.

Department of Health, 2018. Stronger Rural Health Strategy – factsheets. http://www.health.gov.au/internet/main/publishing.nsf/Content/stronger-rural-health-strategy-factsheets.

Department of Health, 2019. Modified Monash Model. http://www.health.gov.au/internet/main/publishing.nsf/Content/modified-monash-model.

Department of Human Services, 2018. Rural Health Workforce Strategy (RHWS) incentive programs. https://www.humanservices.gov.au/organisations/health-professionals/services/medicare/general-practice-rural-incentives-program.

Dyson, K., Kruger, E., Tennant, M., 2012. Networked remote area dental services: a viable, sustainable approach to oral health care in challenging environments. Aust. J. Rural Health 20 (6), 334–338.

Flodgren, G., Rachas, A., Farmer, A., et al., 2015. Interactive telemedicine: effects on professional practice and health care outcomes. Cochrane Database Syst. Rev. (9), CD002098, doi:10.1002/14651858. CD002098.pub2.

Humphreys, J., McGrail, M., Joyce, C.M., et al., 2012. Who should receive recruitment and retention incentives? Improved targeting of rural doctors using medical workforce data. Aust. J. Rural Health 20, 3–10.

Jongen, C., McCalman, J., Bainbridge, R., et al., 2014. Aboriginal and Torres Strait Islander maternal and child health and wellbeing: a systematic search of programs and services in Australian primary health care settings. BMC Pregnancy Childbirth 14 (251), 1471–2393.

Kildea, S., Kruske, S., Barclay, L., et al., 2010. 'Closing the Gap': how maternity services can contribute to reducing poor maternal infant health outcomes for Aboriginal and Torres Strait Islander women. Rural Remote Health 10 (3), 6.

Kurti, L., Rudland, S., Wilkinson, R., et al., 2011. Physician's assistants: a workforce solution for Australia? Aust. J. Prim. Health 17 (1), 23–28.

Laurant, M., van der Biezen, M., Wijers, N., et al., 2018. Nurses as substitutes for doctors in primary care. Cochrane Database Syst. Rev. (7), CD001271, https://www.cochrane.org/CD001271/EPOC_nurses-substitutes-doctors-primary-care.

Levesque, J.F., Harris, M.F., Russell, G., 2013. Patient-centred access to health care: conceptualising access at the interface of health systems and populations. Int. J. Equity Health 12, 18. doi:10.1186/1475-9276-12-18.

Li, J., Scott, A., McGrail, M., et al., 2014. Retaining rural doctors: Doctors' preferences for rural medical workforce incentives. Soc. Sci. Med. 121, 56–64.

Maier, C.B., Aiken, L.H., 2016. Task shifting from physicians to nurses in primary care in 39 countries: a cross-country comparative study. Eur. J. Public Health 26 (6), 927–934.

Mason, J., 2013. Review of Australian Government health workforce programs. http://www.health.gov.au/internet/main/publishing.nsf/Content/work-health-workforce-program-review.

McGrail, M.R., Russell, J., Humphreys, J.S., 2016. Index of Access: a new innovative and dynamic tool for rural health service and workforce planning. Aust. Health Rev. 41, 492–498.

McGrail, M.R., Humphreys, J.S., 2009a. Geographical classifications to guide rural health policy in Australia. Aust. N. Z. Health Policy 6, 28. doi:10.1186/1743-8462-6-28.

McGrail, M.R., Humphreys, J.S., 2009b. The index of rural access: an innovative integrated approach for measuring primary care access. BMC Health Serv. Res. 9, 124. doi:10.1186/1472-6963-9-124.

McGrail, M.R., Wingrove, P.M., Petterson, S.M., et al., 2017. Measuring the attractiveness of rural communities in accounting for differences of rural primary care workforce supply. Rural Remote Health 17 (2), 3925.

McGrail, M., Humphreys, J.S., Scott, A., et al., 2010. Professional satisfaction in general practice: does it vary by size of community? Medical Journal of Australia 193 (2), 94–98.

O'Sullivan, B., McGrail, M., Russell, D., et al., 2018. Duration and setting of rural immersion during the medical degree relates to rural work outcomes. Med. Educ. 52 (8), 803–815.

O'Sullivan, B.G., McGrail, M.R., Stoelwinder, J.U., 2017. Reasons why specialist doctors undertake rural outreach services: an Australian cross-sectional study. Hum. Resour. Health 15 (1), 3. doi:10.1186/s12960-016-0174-z.

Penchansky, R., Thomas, J.W., 1981. The concept of access: definition and relationship to consumer satisfaction. Med. Care 19 (2), 127–140.

Rietdijk, R., Togher, L., Power, E., 2012. Supporting family members of people with traumatic brain injury using telehealth: a systematic review. J. Rehabil. Med. 44 (11), 913–921.

Rubin, M.N., Wellik, K.E., Channer, D.D., et al., 2013. Systematic review of telestroke for post-stroke care and rehabilitation. Curr. Atheroscler. Rep. 15 (8), 343. doi:10.1007/s11883-013-0343-7.

Starfield, B., 1998. Primary Care: balancing health needs, services and technology. OUP, Oxford.

Starfield, B., 2011. The hidden inequity in health care. Int. J. Equity Health 10 (1), 15.

Tham, R., Buykx, P., Kinsman, L., et al., 2014. Staff perceptions of primary healthcare service change: influences on staff satisfaction. Aust. Health Rev. 38 (5), 580–583.

Thomas, S.L., Wakerman, J., Humphreys, J.S., 2014. What core primary health care services should be available to Australians living in rural and remote communities? BMC Fam. Pract. 15, 143. doi:10.1186/1471-2296-15-143.

Wade, V.A., Karnon, J., Elshaug, A.G., et al., 2010. A systematic review of economic analyses of telehealth services using real time video communication. BMC Health Serv. Res. 10, 233. doi:10.1186/1472-6963-10-233.

Ward, B., Humphreys, J., McGrail, M., et al., 2015. Which dimensions of access are most important when rural residents decide to visit a general practitioner for non-emergency care? Aust. Health Rev. 39 (2), 121–126.

Wilson, N.W., Couper, I.D., De Vries, E., et al., 2009. A critical review of interventions to redress the inequitable distribution of healthcare professionals to rural and remote areas. Rural Remote Health 9 (2), 12–29.

World Health Organization (WHO), 2006. Health workforce 2030: a global strategy on human resources for health. WHO, Geneva.

Zhao, Y., Thomas, S., Guthridge, S.L., et al., 2014. Better health outcomes at lower costs: the benefits of primary care utilisation for chronic disease management in remote Indigenous communities in Australia's Northern Territory. BMC Health Serv. Res. 14 (1), 463.

Further Reading

Bradford, N., Caffery, L., Smith, A., 2016. Telehealth services in rural and remote Australia: a systematic review of models of care and factors influencing success and sustainability. Rural Remote Health 16, 3808. www.rrh.org.au/journal/article/3808.

McGrail, M.R., Russell, D.J., Humphreys, J.S., 2016. Index of Access: a new innovative and dynamic tool for rural health service and workforce planning. Aust. Health Rev. 41, 492–498.

Thomas, S.L., Wakerman, J., Humphreys, J.S., 2015. Ensuring equity of access to primary health care in rural and remote Australia – what core services should be locally available? Int. J. Equity Health 14 (1), 111. https://doi.org/10.1186/s12939-015-0228-1.

Thomas, S.L., Zhao, Y., Guthridge, S.L., et al., 2014. The cost-effectiveness of primary care for Indigenous Australians with diabetes living in remote Northern Territory communities. Med. J. Aust. 200 (11), 658–662. doi:10.5694/mja13.11316.

Online Resources

National Aboriginal Community Controlled Health Organisation (NACCHO): https://www.naccho.org.au/.

National Health Performance Framework: http://meteor.aihw.gov.au/content/index.phtml/itemId/392569.

National Rural Health Alliance: www.ruralhealth.org.au.

Primary Health Care Access Program: http://www.atns.net.au/agreement.asp?EntityID=4384.

CHAPTER 10

Indigenous health systems and services

Colleen Hayes and Kerry Taylor[a]

Key learning outcomes

When you finish this chapter you should be able to:

- identify the key elements of Indigenous health systems and services in Australia, including both traditional and contemporary models
- understand the factors that make Indigenous-controlled health systems and services still relevant and necessary
- identify specific features of an Indigenous health service
- critique current funding and policy priorities for Indigenous health services
- reflect on what practitioners and organisations can do to sustain and collaborate successfully with Indigenous health systems and services.

Key terms and abbreviations

Aboriginal-controlled Medical Service (AMS)

Anangu

Australian Human Rights Commission (AHRC)

Central Australian Aboriginal Congress (CAAC)

Close the Gap

Closing the Gap

community control

cultural awareness

cultural competence

cultural safety

First Peoples

knowledges

mainstream

National Aboriginal Community Controlled Health Organisation (NACCHO)

Ngaanyatjarra, Pitjantjatjara, Yankunytjatjara Women's Council (NPYWC)

Ngangkari

non-government organisations (NGOs)

1967 Referendum

self-determination

social capital

[a]Revised and updated from John Reid, Kerry Taylor and Colleen Hayes, 2016.

Introduction

If asked to identify where the first Indigenous[b] health services started in Australia, many people might think about somewhere like the Aboriginal-controlled Medical Service (AMS) in Redfern that was established in the 1970s. However, Indigenous health systems and 'services' have been in place for thousands of years prior to the arrival of Western health care.

In this chapter we will look at the contemporary contexts of Indigenous health, but begin with an overview of the pre-existing and continuing systems and services that Indigenous people relied on prior to and since colonisation. We will discuss the interface between what is sometimes labelled 'traditional' and 'Western, non-Indigenous or **mainstream**' systems, and consider the key elements of Indigenous health services and why they remain relevant and necessary.

The oldest health care systems and services in the world

It may surprise some readers to know that the health care systems and services that extend back tens of thousands of years still have relevance today in some regions. When terms such as 'traditional' are used, this can imply practices of a past era, but in fact Indigenous traditional health care and services are ongoing and adaptive.

A brief look at health statistics today highlights major disparities between Indigenous and other Australians. Indigenous Australians die younger, live with higher rates of acute and chronic illness, are more prone to accidents and injuries and suffer higher rates of mental health problems. Many would know the history that has led to this state and we will not go over it in this chapter. The experience of colonisation for Indigenous peoples around the world has often resulted in similarly poorer health outcomes (Baba et al. 2014; Taylor & Guerin 2014). For additional information on the current health state of Indigenous Australians, see the Further Reading section.

Health care systems and services were in place long before the colonising events that forever changed the health and well-being of Indigenous Australians. Evidence suggests that Indigenous people enjoyed a level of health that was once envied by the British (Gammage 2011). Indigenous health care drew upon **knowledges** and skills developed over thousands of years. Within a relatively short period of contact with non-Indigenous people, however, health and well-being deteriorated owing to introduced diseases, decimation of populations through conflict, dispossession and dislocation and profound and rapid changes in lifestyle that continue to have impacts today (see Fig. 10.2).

While Indigenous healers might now be contacted by phone, the principles underlying their practice remain consistent and tied to the unique but diverse world-views of Indigenous peoples. Indigenous healers or traditional healers are generally identified by other healers and then educated

---

[b]A brief note on terminology: the term 'Indigenous' is not routinely accepted by all groups throughout Australia. We use this term advisedly. Chapter author Colleen Hayes, for example, identifies as Arrernte-Kaytetye rather than as Indigenous. Across Australia there are hundreds of different names for the **First Peoples** that reflect their specific homelands and language groups. The best advice is to simply ask locally about the preferred terminology for any location or individual. In this text for national distribution, we use Indigenous to imply Aboriginal and Torres Strait Islander peoples. Where appropriate we may use other relevant terms.

in the practice, which focuses largely on maintaining holistic well-being. Physical, psychological and social well-being are integrated in Indigenous conceptualisations of health and this traditional model still operates today throughout some parts of Australia.

In central Australia, for example, traditional healers are currently employed within some Aboriginal-controlled health services. Even where they are not formally employed, many of these healers retain ongoing relationships with patients within mainstream health services. Aboriginal Liaison Officers and/or family members can assist patients to access the services of traditional healers when requested. One organisation that employs traditional healers is the Ngaanyatjarra, Pitjantjatjara, Yankunytjatjara Women's Council (NPYWC). The Ngaanyatjarra, Pitjantjatjara, Yankunytjatjara (NPY) are the major language groups associated with the tri-state regions of the top of South Australia, Western Australia and the Northern Territory. According to the NPYWC:

> **Ngangkari** are **Anangu** traditional healers, who have received special tools and training from their grandparents. Anangu have a culturally based view of causation and recovery from physical and mental illness and attribute many illness and emotional states to harmful elements in the Anangu spiritual world. *(Ngaanyatjarra, Pitjantjatjara, Yankunytjatjara Women's Council Ngangkari Program 2013).*

Ngangkari is the NPY word for traditional healer; Anangu is the NPY term for people, and has come to imply Aboriginal people. Box 10.1 outlines the aims of the NPYWC's Ngangkari Program.

BOX 10.1 THE NGANGKARI PROGRAM

The Ngangkari (traditional healers) Project of the Ngaanyatjarra, Pitjantjatjara, Yankunytjatjara (NPY) Women's Council aims to:

- provide Anangu and Yarnangu (people) from the NPY region in central Australia with ngangkari traditional healing to promote the work and skills of ngangkari, as a means of ensuring that their work is highly valued and respected within the broader mainstream mental health and public health system
- educate health and mental health workers about the role and work of ngangkari
- provide direction for the development of culturally appropriate mental health services in the region.

The ngangkari believe that collaboration and mutual respect between Western health and human services and ngangkari lead to the best outcomes for Anangu and Yarnangu. They say Western and Anangu and Yarnangu practitioners have different but equally valuable skills and knowledge and both are needed to address the significant problems Anangu and Yarnangu face …

The effectiveness of their work in Indigenous mental health was acknowledged in 2009 with a prestigious award from the Royal Australian and New Zealand College of Psychiatrists, and also with the Dr Margaret Tobin Award for excellence in mental health service delivery.

(Reproduced with permission from Ngaanyatjarra, Pitjantjatjara, Yankunytjatjara Women's Council Ngangkari Program 2018)

For further reading about the work of Ngangka<u>r</u>i today, we recommend the award-winning publication *Traditional Healers of Central Australia: Ngangkari*, by Ngaanyatjarra, Pitjantjatjara, Yankunytjatjara Women's Council, available through the NPYWC's online store (see Further Reading section) or some bookstores. There is also a DVD about their work, called Ngangka<u>r</u>i, available through Ronin Films (see Online Resources).

Traditional healers in other parts of Australia will have other names and practices. What is important for non-Indigenous practitioners to acknowledge is that they may meet clients or patients who bring their own explanations of illness and well-being to their encounter with Western medical systems and services. In addition to accessing traditional healers, Indigenous Australians may also draw upon an extensive pharmacopoeia of traditional medicines. (For further information, see Low's book *Bush Medicine: A Pharmacopoeia of Natural Remedies*, listed in Further Reading.)

It should also be recognised that people often engage in health-promoting practices that are determined by their own cultural values and beliefs. Rather than asking people to choose, optimum health outcomes may be achieved by facilitating collaborative responses, as in Case study 10.1.

Case Study 10.1

Best of both worlds

As an Aboriginal person, my definition of health was and still is about traditional healing and the beliefs and values that come with that; but today for me, I can't go one without the other. Western health care is also needed to deal with the things that my cultural healing practices did not have to deal with before colonisation. As an example from my own experience of caring for a very sick child, I wanted to try to draw on every option available to him. I did not close one door to the other. I did not think any less of the treatments – both were a priority and of value. When my son was only little, I found him one day, feverish, hot and unsettled … the usual things we would do for a hot child did not seem to help as he became sicker throughout the day. I had taken him to the Aboriginal Congress (in Alice Springs) but this was a new illness for me to understand … so we went to hospital for treatment where they told me he had meningitis.

While we were waiting with him, my mother, who was also a trained health worker in Western health care, said, 'You have to go and pick up that old man … grandfather.' My grandfather was a healer and I had stopped thinking about what other treatment my son might need because I was only thinking about what the hospital could do for him, which was good, but he was still very sick. My grandfather knew that his grandson was sick before I even told him … his own healer's messages had already told him and he was waiting for me to pick him up from out bush. When he came to hospital we had prepared the room, telling the nurses what he was going to do, and asked them to respect us, be quiet and stand back. Even though I felt it was a Western sickness, I still needed my grandfather's healing hands to make sure that my son would get fully better.

He strengthened him by rubbing his hands over his body, and especially his head to help him fight the sickness. This happened around 6 p.m. and by 9 p.m. he was sitting up in bed playing.

While we have trust and value Western medicine for dealing with certain health problems, it would not have been enough for our son to recover. For us, we needed to have access to the depth of knowledge, skills and healing practices that would heal not only his body but his whole being. I felt so much better knowing that my grandfather was coming to do this. And he not only healed my son, but he strengthened my son who has grown into a very healthy and strong young man today. Some people might say this is about faith and the power of belief. How is that any different to Western health practice? People believe antibiotics work and they would say they have a lot of scientific evidence to prove this. Well, Aboriginal people believe in their practices that have thousands of years of evidence as proof as well. The two systems don't have to compete with each other. They can work together for the best outcome for the patient and that is the most important thing.

(Colleen Hayes, personal communication, 2015)

Why do we have Indigenous-controlled health systems and services today?

There is no question that the overall health of Indigenous Australians today is worse on all standard indicators compared with other Australians (Durey & Thompson 2012). The requirement for additional resources and different approaches to address the needs of this specific population should be obvious. However, not all Australians would understand the requirement for separate services for Indigenous people. It is therefore necessary to look at what prompted the development of these services and why they remain relevant today.

The first of the contemporary Aboriginal Community Controlled Health Services (ACCHSs) was established in Redfern, Sydney in 1971 'by community activists in response to ongoing discrimination against Aboriginal people within mainstream health services; to address the poor health and premature deaths of Aboriginal people; and to provide a culturally appropriate system of health care' (Aboriginal Medical Service 2015).

General practitioners, other medical specialists, religious groups, Aboriginal community leaders and other **non-government organisations (NGOs)** were concerned about the state of health of the Aboriginal people who were living in the city of Sydney at the time. Many of these Aboriginal people had migrated from rural and regional parts of the state of New South Wales looking for better employment and lifestyle opportunities after the **1967 Referendum**, when rights to freedom of movement for Aboriginal people became more flexible. Places like Redfern, which historically had always had an Aboriginal presence, both before and since colonisation, was the gathering place of many of who had voluntarily moved or were forced to move because of economic, cultural or political (policy) factors that impacted on their lives.

At this time, access to mainstream health care for Indigenous Australians was hampered by barriers that were both systemic and individual. Racism, discrimination, mistrust, miscommunication and a lack of **cultural awareness** meant that access, even where possible, did not translate into positive health care experiences for many Indigenous Australians. For some, access was hampered by remoteness. Services were simply unavailable or required extensive separation from families and communities in order to access them. A lack of transport and finances also affected people's uptake of services. Overall, however, the major gap for Indigenous Australians was the lack of access to a comprehensive primary health care service. Whereas the majority of Australians today enjoy the benefits of a First World health care system, Indigenous Australians were and are still experiencing health outcomes that are more commonly associated with Third World conditions. This disparity suggests that something was / is wrong with the system.

PAUSE
for
REFLECTION
...

According to John Reid,

This was not just Redfern of the early 1970s. This was Alice Springs, this was Port Augusta, the same scenario described about the initial establishment of the first AMS [Aboriginal Medical Service] in Australia in Sydney, is reflected or had been replicated right across the country at that period of time. All of which can be analysed through the prism of post-colonisation to give meaning and inspiration to the freedom fighters from yesteryear who fought and struggled, including begging, borrowing and donating to set up such essential services for their mob.

The model of health care in the ACCHSs aligned most closely with primary health care (PHC), which had emerged internationally as the approach with the greatest potential to address disparities in health for vulnerable and marginalised populations including Indigenous Australians. PHC aimed to make health care *accessible*, by providing services close to where people lived, and *affordable*, by focusing on low-technology and preventive and health-promoting services; and, importantly, to make services *culturally appropriate* to ensure the uptake and efficacy of care.

The establishment of the ACCHSs was a political movement based on the premise of the principle of **self-determination** – proving to the mainstream community that Aboriginal people could organise and raise funds to set up health care centres and systems that could cater for the culturally diverse needs of their constituency. Redfern, the **Central Australian Aboriginal Congress (CAAC)** in Alice Springs and others that followed also represented the political voice of the Aboriginal community, who were fighting for human rights in health, education and employment: important factors in enhancing a person's **social capital** and maintaining their subjective and communal wellbeing. The early ACCHSs were a staunch statement about the importance of self-determination (see Box 10.2).

BOX 10.2 PERSPECTIVES FROM SOME OF THE PIONEERING ACCHSS

Redfern Aboriginal Medical Service, Sydney, New South Wales

The Aboriginal Medical Service (AMS) has pioneered the concept of Aboriginal community-controlled health care services as the only successful way of improving the health of Aboriginal communities.

> Our experience in Redfern has proved that Aboriginal people are capable of solving their own problems: if we are given control of the resources and facilities and allowed to do it our way.
> *(Aboriginal Medical Service 2018)*

Central Australian Aboriginal Congress (CAAC), Alice Springs, Northern Territory

> [The CAAC's] first service was a 'Tent Program', providing shelter to Aboriginal people in town. As time went by, other Aboriginal organisations grew up to take care of issues like housing, education, and land. But health remained a great concern for Aboriginal people, and in 1975, Congress started a Medical Service in a house in Hartley Street. A doctor was employed and transport and welfare services set up.
> *(Central Australian Aboriginal Congress 2018)*

Pika Wiya Health Service, Port Augusta, South Australia

> The Pika Wiya Health Service Aboriginal Corporation provides services to Aboriginal and Torres Strait Islanders of Port Augusta and Davenport, with outreach services to the Northern Flinders Ranges community: Copley, Leigh Creek, Nepabunna and communities isolated in this area as well as Roxby Downs, Andamooka and surrounding areas … Pika (meaning 'sickness') Wiya (meaning 'no') is derived from the Pitjantjatjara language, which is one of the many Aboriginal languages spoken in the area covered by the health service. The Pika Wiya Health Service Aboriginal Corporation was established by the determination of three local Aboriginal women.
>
> Early in the 1970s, a group of Aboriginal women met in Port Augusta. One of them was a nurse. At the meeting they were told that a sick man was lying in the sand hills just out of town. The women went out and gave what assistance they could and called an ambulance. As a result of the sharing of this and other stories, the women decided that Port Augusta needed a medical service for Aboriginal people. But at the time, neither state nor federal government were interested in providing money, so the women wrote to the World Council of Churches in Geneva, Switzerland and outlined their plight. The World Council of Churches gave them a grant and with this money the Aboriginal Medical Service, Port Augusta was formed.

Continued

BOX 10.2 PERSPECTIVES FROM SOME OF THE
PIONEERING ACCHSS — cont'd

The Aboriginal Medical Service in Redfern, although struggling themselves, loaned them a doctor, who came over regularly. There were no funds for accommodation so the doctor had to sleep on the floor of the clinic, and bandages had to be washed and re-used. The Aboriginal Medical Service evolved into the Pika Wiya Health Service Inc. in 1984.

Since then, Pika Wiya has gone through a number of transformations. The Service has grown and has evolved into one of the largest leading Aboriginal Medical Services in South Australia.

(Deadly Vibe 2015)

Kambu Health, Southeast Queensland

Kambu Health was founded by a group of local residents – Ken Dalton, Cecil Fisher, Roberta Thompson, Faye Carr, Bill Robinson and Doreen Thompson – to address the growing health needs of the local Aboriginal and Torres Strait Islander community. Originally there was a meeting called by the people of the community to get a housing co-operative to be incorporated with Southern Suburbs Football Team. The health service was run from a room in the home of Doreen Thompson. It provided culturally appropriate health care by doctors who travelled up from Aboriginal and Islander Community Health Service Brisbane for one day a week.

In 1975–6, a house was purchased by the housing co-op, and the medical staff moved into one of the rooms there. It was from there the doctor and [nursing] sister would go to Wacol Hostel and conduct an outside clinic … The growth of the co-op and the medical centre was such that there was soon a need to expand, so a new medical centre was built beside the old nursing house at 27 Roderick Street, Ipswich. The staff now consisted of a doctor, nursing sister, bookkeeper, CEO and medical receptionist.

In 1988 the medical centre became incorporated in its own right and was named the Aboriginal and Islander Community Health Service Ipswich. By 1994 the staff had increased again to a CEO, finance officer, doctor, two health workers, a trainee health worker, a driver, nutrition field officer, trainee receptionist and trainee admin assistant, all managed by a community-elected Board of Directors.

Today, Kambu Aboriginal and Torres Strait Islander Corporation for Health employs over 60 staff (not including visiting specialists), and provides comprehensive medical and specialist services to Ipswich and the surrounding areas. Clinics are now located in Ipswich, Goodna and Laidley.

(Kambu Aboriginal and Torres Strait Islander Corporation for Health 2015)

Most ACCHSs have good information on their web pages about their histories, services and systems of care. It is obvious from the examples provided that a common theme has been the persistence of a few individuals in striving to improve health outcomes for their communities. It would be worth checking your local region for information relevant to your interests. We have provided some web addresses in the Online Resources section of this chapter.

The ACCHSs differ in their structure, policy implementation, service focus and workforces, reflecting the diversity of Indigenous Australia. The **National Aboriginal Community Controlled Health Organisation (NACCHO)** is Australia's peak national representative body for Indigenous health, representing over 150 ACCHSs (National Aboriginal Community Controlled Health Organisation (NACCHO) 2019).

Adhering to many of the principles of a primary health care model, Aboriginal-controlled services are, by necessity, initiated by the community and located within Aboriginal communities and, importantly, have governance structures that ensure **community control**. Being incorporated ensures a legal accountability. Common to all ACCHSs are the principles shown in Fig. 10.1.

Indigeneity is not a cause of ill-health, so how do people explain the health burden on Aboriginal and Torres Strait Islander people today? No one would suggest that Indigenous Australians did not suffer illness or injury prior to colonisation. However, cultural practices and protocols were largely protective, as evidenced by surviving tens of thousands of years on this continent. The links between colonisation and the complex state of Indigenous health today are both explicit and implicit.

The consequences of dislocation, dispossession and radical changes in living conditions over several generations has had a profound physiological and psychological effect on Indigenous peoples, manifesting in many diverse and complex ways: heart disease, high blood pressure and other forms of chronic disease, mental health issues, including suicide, alcohol abuse, elevated levels of smoking and family violence.

Look at the increased incidence of diabetes as an illustrative example. The diet of Indigenous Australians prior to colonisation was believed to be well balanced and nutritionally sound. Considerable physical energy was required to obtain food. With the loss of lands came a loss of access to traditional diets. Instead, successive governments and other groups provided Indigenous Australians with inferior and potentially harmful food through the periods of missions and reserves and even in lieu of wages in some employment settings such as the cattle industries. The staples of these diets were most often flour, sugar, tea, low-quality fatty meat and tobacco. The pathways to chronic diseases were established.

Fig. 10.2 examines just some of the overt links between colonisation and health today.

Funding for ACCHSs

Funding is possibly the greatest threat to the successful achievement of the original goals of Aboriginal Community Controlled Health Services. What is common to almost all ACCHSs is the way in which they have had to develop with relatively little financial support in their early days. While health care services are often taken for granted for most Australians, Indigenous Australians have had to fight to secure funding and, even now, to maintain adequate funding. According to Alford (2014, p. 7):

FIGURE 10.1 KEY FEATURES OF ABORIGINAL COMMUNITY-CONTROLLED HEALTH SERVICES

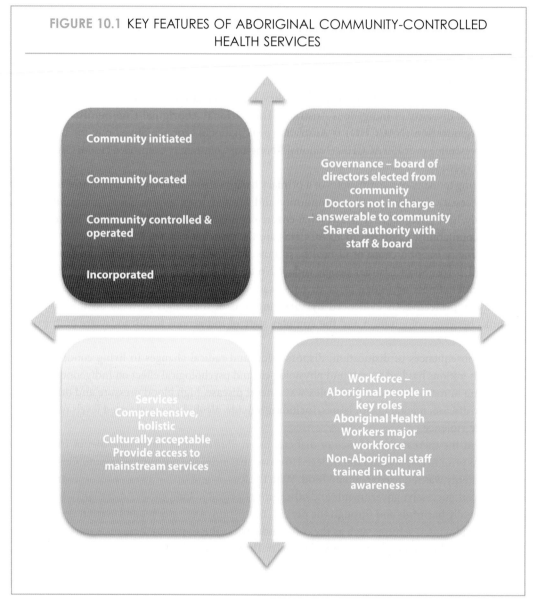

Sources: Adapted from http://www.ntgpe.org/workingwell/working_well1_1.htm; Miller & Speare (in Willis et al. 2012)

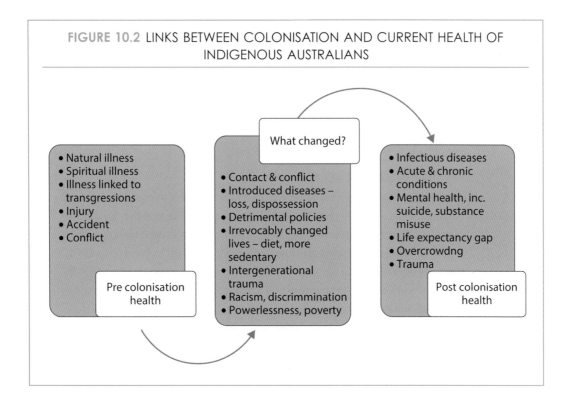

FIGURE 10.2 LINKS BETWEEN COLONISATION AND CURRENT HEALTH OF INDIGENOUS AUSTRALIANS

Unlike government funding for mainstream health services which has risen and continues to rise, Australian government funding for Indigenous health was substantially reduced in 2012–13 and was projected to fall further behind Aboriginal and Torres Strait Islander population growth and overall health expenditure in the three years 2013–14.

Some positive news was welcomed by NACCHO in 2018 with the following communiqué from NACCHO chair John Singer:

> The National Aboriginal Community Controlled Health Organisation (NACCHO) welcomed the Budget announcement of a new needs based funding formula model for the Indigenous Australians' Health Program (IAHP) … This new model for our 144 Aboriginal Community Controlled Health Service (ACCHS) provides funding for our primary health care services … NACCHO Chair Mr John Singer believes 'that funding certainty is critical to ACCHSs achieving good health outcomes. It is important to strengthen and expand ACCHS role as primary care providers in our communities as there will be 1 million Aboriginal people by 2030,' …
>
> NACCHO welcomes the 5-year funding agreements and grandfathering arrangements under this new model. NACCHO welcomes the new money for preventing and treating complex chronic health conditions such as eye disease ($34.3 million) hearing loss ($30.0 million) and crusted scabies

($4.8 million). Acknowledges the new investment in remote renal services and infrastructure with a **MBS** item for dialysis. Also, the $105.7 over four years to deliver additional residential aged care places and home care packages in remote Indigenous communities ... Aboriginal controlled health services provide about three million episodes of care each year for about 350,000 people and employ about 6000 staff. *(https://www.naccho.org.au/wp-content/uploads/Government -announces-new-funding-model-for-ACCHS.pdf)*

PAUSE
for
REFLECTION
...

A consumer's view of ACCHSs

I am happy to go to the hospital when I need to but for most things I will always go to Congress – the Aboriginal Congress in Alice Springs. I like that they are already familiar with my cultural views, they understand my ways – I don't have to explain certain things, like my kinship structure and why I might want to bring other family into the consultation. That is not seen as a problem or a disruption and it's common. There is a lot more flexibility because they understand that some people might live out of town and even though we have appointments like in mainstream services, there is more flexibility of the walk-in appointments at times because if people travel in from remote areas they may not always know exactly when they will arrive.

There are more Aboriginal staff employed there and the non-Aboriginal staff undergo some cultural training and have to work in alignment with the way Aboriginal people are comfortable. The doctors seemed to have good training in cultural awareness and are open to options that fitted with my lifestyle, like knowing that I might be out bush and can't always come back each day or on a specific day. They are in touch with what goes on for Aboriginal people in terms of our mobility and obligations and things like that. They also offer transport for those who don't have it, which is a lot of our people and they give advice about social and emotional issues. It's a comprehensive service with things like alcohol support, quit smoking and other services that are in house, so you don't have to go to a lot of different places.

(Colleen Hayes, personal communication, 2018)

Despite strong evidence for the efficacy and value of ACCHSs, there is an ongoing need to fight for their place in Australian health care (Baba et al. 2014; Rollins 2014). Successive governments have found it difficult to separate their responsibility for funding from trying to assert control.

The benefits of ACCHSs are considered substantial and to have positive impacts on more than health (Case study 10.2). The report *Economic value of Aboriginal community controlled health services* found that, in addition to their effectiveness in improving health care, Indigenous-operated health organisations deliver significant economic benefits to the communities they serve, providing

Case Study 10.2

An example of the principles that define ACCHSs: The Purple House (Western Desert Dialysis) – Alice Springs

The Purple House is the name of a health care service that has arisen from the tenacity and persistence of a small group of people for whom today's impressive renal and holistic services have come too late. Purple House is a shorthand term, based on the original centre in Alice Springs, which is actually a house painted purple! This house is the operational base for a network of services that seeks to provide an ongoing connection to family and country for those people affected by renal failure. The organisation's full name, Western Desert Nganampa Walytja Palyantjaku Tjutaku, means 'making all our families well'.

With the knowledge that what they were setting out to achieve would not benefit them directly, the group's thoughts were for the future and their countrymen and women who would experience the almost inevitable trajectory towards renal failure, which is at epidemic proportions throughout many Aboriginal populations. The Purple House story is well worth hearing. When Pintupi people from the Western Desert found themselves faced with the need to leave their homes in order to access renal services, the genesis for this unique and innovative health service emerged. After being repeatedly told by governments that dialysis services in remote homelands was unviable, this group took matters into their own hands and, using the growing regard for contemporary Indigenous art, sold two major works at auction raising over a million dollars.

For Pintupi, receiving dialysis treatment meant little if the person's spirit was sick. Health is more than physical well-being and this holistic view of health is reflected in the service's core values of compassion, caring for family and connection to country. A major goal of the Purple House and the satellite centres now established is to ensure this ongoing connection for people.

Far from living on the machines, away from family and culture, the original Purple House is a vibrant environment for patients, where the CEO, along with any other staff member, can be found making cups of tea for families, who are working in the yard preparing bush medicines or cooking kangaroo in a fire pit. As the model demonstrated its success and sustainability, other remote populations sought to partner with Western Desert Dialysis and there are now mobile and permanent dialysis services in some eight remote communities. For more information, see Western Desert Nganampa Walytja Palyantjaku Tjutaku Corporation (2018).

---

well-paid jobs for 3200 Aboriginal people, boosting education with on-site training and offering valuable career paths' (Rollins 2014, p. 11).

Recently there have been moves to re-accredit and re-register services under the Office of the Registrar of Indigenous Corporations (ORIC), placing AHCCSs under the Office of Prime Minister, as are all Indigenous matters. Governance has admittedly been challenging for some services, but the erosion of the key principle of community control may undo the many benefits and gains achieved to date.

Indigenous Australia is a culturally diverse population and the models of health systems and services are by necessity reflective of this diversity (Baba et al. 2014). What works in one region may not work in another. As you might have noticed with each of the examples of ACCHSs in Box 10.2, the common impetus for development was a lack of access or acceptable services. ACCHSs filled a service delivery gap; all commenced as initiatives of the local communities that they serve, and are controlled by them.

While there remains a gap in health outcomes between Indigenous and non-Indigenous Australians, there also remains a need for such services. This of course does not mean that mainstream services cannot do much to improve the effectiveness and experience of health care they provide to Indigenous Australians. Increased employment of Indigenous people across all sectors of mainstream health services, better cultural safety education, policy and accountability, and greater partnering with Indigenous organisations will all go a long way to improving outcomes for Indigenous clients.

Where to from here?

Fig. 10.2 showed a basic connection between colonisation and contemporary health problems. However, health is not determined by health care alone. Health is widely accepted as determined by social circumstances of individuals and groups. Over the last decade, the disparities between Indigenous and non-Indigenous Australians have highlighted more than ever the need for Indigenous control over and participation in health services. Two campaigns aimed at addressing inequalities in outcomes have been rolled out since 2008 – **Close the Gap** and **Closing the Gap**.

Close the Gap is a public awareness campaign focused on closing the health gap. It's run by numerous NGOs, Indigenous health bodies and human rights organisations, including the **Australian Human Rights Commission (AHRC)**.

Closing the Gap is the Government's program with six key targets:

◆ To close the life-expectancy gap within a generation
◆ To halve the gap in mortality rates for Indigenous children under five within a decade
◆ To ensure access to early childhood education for all Indigenous four-year-olds in remote communities within five years
◆ To halve the gap in reading, writing and numeracy achievements for children within a decade
◆ To halve the gap in Indigenous Year 12 achievement by 2020
◆ To halve the gap in employment outcomes between Indigenous and non-Indigenous Australians within a decade.

(Davidson H, 2014 https://www.theguardian.com/world/blog/2014/feb/12/
close-the-gap-and-closing-the-gap-whats-the-difference)

Unfortunately in 2018 the report card for Closing the Gap has not been well scored in the majority target areas. Far from being less necessary since their inception in the 1970s, ACCHSs remain essential to reduce disparities in health outcomes.

Sustainability for ACCHSs may require strategic partnerships with mainstream services to achieve the best outcomes for Indigenous consumers (Lloyd & Wise 2011). We know that, irrespective of financial support, Indigenous Australians will continue to hold their own health beliefs and conduct their own health care practices at the individual and community levels. However, there are undoubtedly health care challenges today that are beyond even successive governments' resources to manage and it will only be through sustained and collaborative efforts that improvements in the health of Indigenous Australians will be made. Taylor and Thompson (2011, p. 302) suggest that:

> … partnerships with Aboriginal services offer a powerful mechanism for helping build mainstream providers' sociocultural awareness and overcoming 'paternalistic' care where mainstream health providers see themselves as the experts and the Aboriginal patient as naïve recipients. In this way, partnerships can honour the knowledge of Aboriginal people. Importantly, as more Aboriginal health professionals become involved in the health system, institutional racism (that is, normative and codified differential access in health structures) should be broken down.

Racism is still a major barrier to health for Indigenous Australians. While some improvements have resulted from the uptake of key philosophical frameworks such as **cultural safety** and **cultural competence** within mainstream services, Baba et al. (2014, p. 1) suggest that the:

> … pervasive influence of racism' that results in reduced healthcare-seeking behaviour, unhealthy lifestyles and mental health issues means that AMSs or ACCHSs remain 'crucial in addressing the negative impacts of continued discrimination on Indigenous health by providing comprehensive, culturally appropriate, community empowering health services.

Inadequate funding and resources, along with efforts to control the autonomy of organisations, may be hampering the original goals of putting Indigenous health into Indigenous hands. Indigenous health services and systems have proven their worth in ensuring better outcomes for Indigenous Australians. Both traditional and contemporary models of Indigenous health services remain relevant and active today. Working together with mainstream services offers the greatest potential for improving the health and well-being of Indigenous Australians today.

Summary

Indigenous health systems and services existed well before the introduction of Western medical services and remain relevant and necessary across Australia today.

Aboriginal-controlled services arose from the paradigm of self-determination for Aboriginal people and a failure of mainstream services to adequately provide for Indigenous people. There are fundamental differences in the way Indigenous services are structured that reflect Indigenous ways of thinking, feeling and valuing.

Some positive examples of Indigenous health care systems and services are found in the case studies.

Changes to funding and governance may be impacting on the original aims of Aboriginal- controlled health services. Positive and respectful partnerships are necessary.

Review Questions

1   How relevant are the traditional health care systems and services in contemporary Australia? Can you provide examples of how these might impact on health today?

2   What are some of the current challenges to the sustainability of ACCHSs today?

3   How can mainstream services improve the experience of health care for Indigenous Australians?

4   From your reading of this chapter and reviewing information on their web site, what are the key features that make the Purple House an example of an ACCHS?

5   There is a tension between mainstream health systems and Indigenous health systems. What are the advantages and disadvantages of Australia having multiple health systems, e.g. Indigenous, private, complementary?

References

Aboriginal Medical Service, 2015. Our history. https://amsredfern.org.au/.

Aboriginal Medical Service, 2018. redfernoralhistory.org/Organisations/AboriginalMedicalService/tabid/208/Default.aspx.

Alford, L., 2014. Investing in Aboriginal Community Control Makes Economic Sense. National Aboriginal Community Controlled Organisation, Canberra.

Baba, J., Brolan, C., Hill, P., 2014. Aboriginal medical services cure more than illness: a qualitative study of how Indigenous services address the health impacts of discrimination in Brisbane communities. Int. J. Equity Health 13, 56. http://www.equityhealthj.com/content/13/1/56.

Central Australian Aboriginal Congress (CAAC), 2018. Past, present, future, Alice Springs, CAAC. www.caac.org.au/about-congress/past-present-future.

Davidson, H., 2014. Close the Gap and Closing the Gap – what's the difference? The Guardian https://www.theguardian.com/world/blog/2014/feb/12/close-the-gap-and-closing-the-gap-whats-the-difference. 12 Feb.

Deadly Vibe, 2015. Pika Wiya means 'no sickness'. Deadly Vibe Group. www.deadlyvibe.com.au/2013/08/pika-wiya-means-no-sickness-2.

Durey, A., Thompson, S., 2012. Reducing the health disparities of Aboriginal Australians: a time to shift focus. BMC Health Serv. Res. 12, 151.

Gammage, B., 2011. The Biggest Estate on Earth: How Aborigines Made Australia. Allen & Unwin, Sydney.

Kambu Aboriginal and Torres Strait Islander Corporation for Health, 2015. Ipswich and West Moreton Areas. kambuhealth.com.au/ipswich-and-west-moreton-areas.php.

Lloyd, J., Wise, M., 2011. Improving Aboriginal health: how might the health sector do things differently? Aust. Rev. Public Affairs 2.

Miller, A., Speare, R., 2012. Health care for Indigenous Australians. In: Willis, E., Reynolds, L., Keleher, H. (Eds.), Understanding the Australian Health Care System, second ed. Elsevier, Australia.

National Aboriginal Community Controlled Health Organisation (NACCHO), 2018. Government announces new funding model for ACCHS. https://www.naccho.org.au/wp-content/uploads/Government-announces-new-funding-model-for-ACCHS.pdf.

National Aboriginal Community Controlled Health Organisation (NACCHO), 2019. About us. https://www.naccho.org.au/about/.

Ngaanyatjarra, Pitjantjatjara, Yankunytjatjara Women's Council, 2018. Ngangkari program. https://www.npywc.org.au/ngangkari/.

Rollins, A., 2014. End funding uncertainty in Aboriginal controlled health care. Med. J. Aust. 26 (7), 11. https://ama.com.au/ausmed/end-funding-uncertainty-aboriginal-controlled-health-care-ama.

Taylor, K., Guerin, P., 2014. Health Care and Indigenous Australians: Cultural Safety in Practice. Palgrave MacMillan, Melbourne.

Taylor, K., Thompson, S., 2011. Closing the (service) gap: exploring partnerships between Aboriginal and mainstream health services. Aust. Health Rev. 35, 297–308.

Western Desert Nganampa Walytja Palyantjaku Tjutaku Corporation, 2018. Purple House. https://www.purplehouse.org.au.

Further Reading

Funding of ACCHSs – Aboriginal Community Controlled Health Service funding: report to the sector 2011. https://www.lowitja.org.au/sites/default/files/docs/Overburden_Funding-Report-to-ACCHS-2011.pdf.

Hayman, N., Armstrong, R., 2014. Health services for Aboriginal and Torres Strait Islander people: handle with care. Med. J. Aust. 200 (11), 613.

Larkin, S.L., Geia, L.K., Panaretto, K.S., 2006. Consultations in general practice and at an Aboriginal community controlled health service: do they differ? Rural Remote Health 6, 560. http://www.rrh.org.au/articles/subviewnew.asp?ArticleID=560.

Low, T., 1990. Bush Medicine: A Pharmacopoeia of Natural Remedies. Angus & Robertson, Sydney.

Morgan, G., 2006. Unsettled Places: Aboriginal People and Urbanisation in New South Wales. Wakefield Press, Adelaide.

Ngaanyatjarra, Pitjantjatjara, Yankunytjatjara Women's Council, 2013. Traditional Healers of Central Australia; Ngangkari, by the Ngaanyatjarra, Pitjantjatjara, Yankunytjatjara.

Online Resources

For a history of the various ACCHSs or Aboriginal Medical Services (AMSs) the following websites are useful.

Central Australian Aboriginal Congress: www.caac.org.au.

Information about traditional healers – watch the film Ngangkari (National Indigenous Documentary Fund Series 5), Dir. Erica Glynn. www.roninfilms.com.au/feature/778.html.

Kambu Health in Southeast Queensland. http://kambuhealth.com.au/our-history.php.

Ngaanyatjarra, Pitjantjatjara, Yankunytjatjara Women's Council. www.npywc.org.au/.

Northern Territory General Practice Education online resources: https://www.ntgpe.org/workingwell/working_well1_1.htm.

Overview of Australian Indigenous health – Australian Indigenous HealthInfoNet, 2019. Overview of Aboriginal and Torres Strait Islander health status. www.healthinfonet.ecu.edu.au/health-facts/overviews.

Redfern AMS: redfernoralhistory.org/Organisations/AboriginalMedicalService/tabid/208/Default.aspx and http://redfernoralhistory.org/Organisations/AboriginalMedicalService/tabid/208/Default.aspx.

The Indigenous Health and Cultural Competency (IH&CC) education resources for emergency department staff: https://acem.org.au/Content-Sources/Advancing-Emergency-Medicine/Cultural-competency/Indigenous-Health-and-Cultural-Competency-Resource/Indigenous-Health-and-Cultural-Competency.

Women's Council Aboriginal Corporation: http://www.npywc.org.au/shop/.

CHAPTER 11

Organising care for the mentally ill in Australia

Julie Henderson and Louise Roberts

Key learning outcomes

When you finish this chapter you should be able to:

- briefly describe the features of the mental health care system in Australia
- outline changes in the delivery of mental health care in Australia arising from the National Mental Health Strategy
- identify the health professionals who provide care to the mentally ill
- describe a recovery approach to mental health care.

Key terms and abbreviations

Australian Health Ministers' Advisory Council (AHMAC)
Better Outcomes in Mental Health Care (BOiMHC)
capacity
carer
case management
chronic mental illness
community mental health services (CMHS)
consumer
de-institutionalisation
emergency departments (EDs)
federalism
feminisation of care
general practitioners (GPs)
institutionalisation

integrated care
involuntary care
National Community Mental Health Care Database (NCMHCD)
National Disability Insurance Scheme (NDIS)
non-government organisation (NGO)
primary care
primary carers
Primary Health Networks (PHNs)
primary mental health care
recovery
social inclusion
stepped care
stigma
treatment orders
World Health Organization (WHO)

Introduction

This chapter provides an overview of the delivery of mental health care in Australia. In Chapter 1, you read about the impact of 'new public management' and neoliberalism on the delivery of health care. Among the changes identified was the introduction of practices from the private market to increase the efficacy and productivity of health care, such as the outsourcing of service delivery and competitive tendering by private companies to provide services. This has involved the use of a greater range of service providers to deliver mental health care and increased opportunities for interprofessional practice. This chapter picks up on some of those themes, arguing that mental health care delivery in Australia from the 1990s has adopted features of a market model. Some of the changes identified in this chapter are the reduction of the role of the state in providing mental health care; privatising care through use of **non-government organisations** (NGOs), **private, for-profit primary care** and private hospital services; and greater consumer and carer involvement in the control and management of mental health services. The chapter will identify the role of these services in delivering mental health care.

Mental health, as defined by the **World Health Organization (WHO)** Mental Health Action Plan 2013–20, is 'a state of well-being in which the individual realizes his or her own abilities, can cope with the normal stresses of life, can work productively and fruitfully, and is able to make a contribution to his or her community' (World Health Organization (WHO) 2013, p. 6). Mental illness is a widespread health problem. The WHO estimates that 400 million people worldwide experience depression, with a further 81 million experiencing low-prevalence disorders such as bipolar affective disorder (60 million) and schizophrenia (21 million) (WHO 2014). Based on 2016 population estimates approximately 8.5 million Australians aged 16 to 85 have experience of a mental health disorder in their lifetime, with 1 in 5 or 3.8 million estimated to experience mental illness in each year (Australian Institute of Health and Welfare (AIHW) 2017a). Rates are higher within Aboriginal and Torres Strait Islander communities, with 29% of people self-reporting mental health issues in the 2014–15 National Aboriginal and Torres Strait Islander Social Survey (ABS 2016). The most common disorders are depression and anxiety, with approximately 14.4% of Australian adults experiencing an anxiety disorder in the last 12 months and 6.2% an affective disorder. Approximately 3% of the Australian population experience severe mental health disorders such as schizophrenia and bipolar affective disorder (AIHW 2017a; National Mental Health Commission 2012).

The past 60 years have witnessed a global change from institutional to community mental health care. This change has been driven, in part, by a greater focus on the human rights of people with mental illness and reduction of **stigma**. The United Nations (UN) *Principles for the protection of people with mental illness and for the improvement of mental health care* (1991) call for the end of discrimination and the full participation in society of people with mental illness. People with mental illnesses are entitled to the right to live in the community and to have care delivered in 'the least restrictive environment and with the least restrictive or intrusive treatment appropriate to the patient's health needs' (United Nations General Assembly 1991, p. 4). Australia became a signatory to this resolution, committing Australia to its goals.

Mental health care in Australia

Mental health care in Australia was traditionally provided by the state in stand-alone psychiatric hospitals. From 1955 there has been movement towards **de-institutionalisation** of psychiatric patients based on a belief that mental illness can be prevented by early intervention and that long-term **institutionalisation** leads to poor mental health outcomes. The first wave of de-institutionalisation involved the establishment of community services such as day hospitals, community housing, community mental health centres and outpatient care for the newly diagnosed and the acutely ill. Older people, people with drug and alcohol problems and the intellectually disabled were moved into separate services. People with severe or **chronic mental illness** were excluded from the first wave of de-institutionalisation.

De-institutionalisation accelerated from the late 1980s, with a focus on de-institutionalising the chronically mentally ill and establishing community services for them to live outside of psychiatric hospitals. De-institutionalisation at this time involved the movement of inpatient facilities from psychiatric hospitals to psychiatric wards in general hospitals supported by the National Mental Health Strategy, agreed by state, territory and federal health ministers in 1992.

National Mental Health Strategy (1992–)

The National Mental Health Strategy originally consisted of three documents: the *National Mental Health Strategy* and the first *National Mental Health Plan* released in 1992, and the *Mental health statement of rights and responsibilities*, initially released in 1991 (Australian Health Ministers 1991) and re-released in 2012 (Commonwealth of Australia 2012). Subsequent 5-year *National Mental Health Plans* were released in 1998 and in 2003. These were followed in 2009 by the *National Mental Health Policy 2008* (Department of Health and Ageing 2009a) and the *Fourth National Mental Health Plan 2008* (Department of Health and Ageing 2009b), and in 2017 by the *Fifth National Mental Health and Suicide Prevention Plan* (Council of Australian Governments (COAG) 2017).

The goals of the original National Mental Health Strategy were to (1) move service delivery and funding for mental health services from psychiatric hospitals to general hospitals and the community, (2) create better links between government support services and NGOs, and (3) foster uniform mental health legislation across the country (Australian Health Ministers 1992). As a result, the number of psychiatric hospitals fell from 59 in 1989 to 20 in 2005 and to 17 in 2015–16 (AIHW 2018). Fig. 11.1 outlines all specialist mental health services available in 2015–16.

Of note is that, by 2015–16, only 24% of public psychiatric beds were offered in psychiatric hospitals. Also of note is the extent of private service provision through private hospitals' beds and residential services operated by non-government services.

Closure of psychiatric beds was accompanied by the development of community mental health services. Services ranged from community mental health teams, which assessed, monitored and maintained people in the community, to residential services such as supported accommodation, and services that provided social and employment activity. Recent estimates from the AIHW indicate that approximately 9.4 million community mental health care service contacts were provided to approximately 410,000 patients in 2015–16, a significant shift in service provision from hospital care (AIHW 2018).

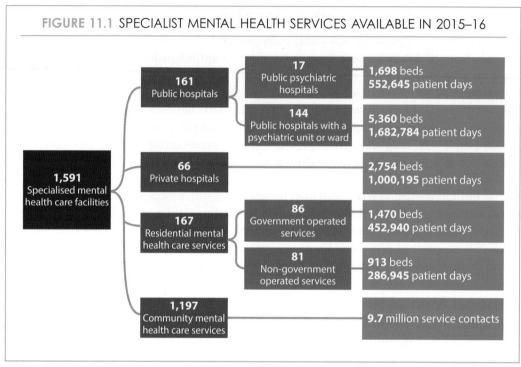

FIGURE 11.1 SPECIALIST MENTAL HEALTH SERVICES AVAILABLE IN 2015–16

Source: Australian Institute of Health and Welfare (2018) National mental health establishments database, Tables FAC.1, FAC.4, FAC.20 and FAC.24. https://www.aihw.gov.au/getmedia/e3d29485-4296-4bf2-afe3-816ba08de75b/Specialised-mental-health-care-facilities-15-16.xlsx.aspx

The second and third *National Mental Health Plans* focused on prevention and early intervention, development of service partnerships, development of mechanisms for **consumer** and **carer** participation, and research and service evaluation (Australian Health Ministers 1998, 2003). There was growing recognition at this point that specialist mental health services only supported people with chronic mental illness, leading to gaps in service delivery for people with depression and anxiety disorders and for younger people first experiencing mental health symptoms (McGorry 2007). This was addressed through Medicare funding changes, which promoted the role of primary care (**general practitioners, GPs**) in providing mental health care, and through targeted programs for younger people such as Headspace. Consumer and carer participation in mental health services increased through monitoring the level of their involvement in management boards of both government and non-government services.

The *National Mental Health Policy 2008* and the *Fourth National Mental Health Plan* shifted the focus to **recovery**-based services and **social inclusion** through promoting access to housing, education and employment opportunities for people with mental illness. There was also a greater focus on integrated community care, with Medicare Locals providing leadership for integration at a regional level. The *Fifth National Mental Health and Suicide Prevention Plan* also focuses upon regional planning for primary mental health care (COAG 2017). The Coalition Government amalgamated Medicare Locals into **Primary Health Networks** (PHNs) in 2015 and transferred responsibility for federally funded programs such as Headspace and access to psychological services to the PHNs (Henderson et al. 2018). The central role of PHNs in primary mental health is to plan and tender for **stepped care** services. Stepped care is defined as 'an evidence-based, staged system comprising a hierarchy of interventions, from the least to the most intensive, matched to the individual's needs' (Department of Health 2016, p. 2). Stepped care makes efficient use of existing resources through reserving more-intensive treatments such as seeing a psychologist for people with greatest need and providing cost-effective options such as online programs for people with lesser need (Bower & Gilbody 2005). More information about primary care can be found in Chapter 6. In addition to regional planning, the *Fifth National Mental Health and Suicide Prevention Plan* also focuses upon suicide prevention, Aboriginal and Torres Strait Islander (Chapter 10) mental health and clinical services for people with severe and complex illness.

PAUSE
for
REFLECTION
...
Consider the policy shift from institutional care of those with mental illness to community- and primary-based mental health care. How does this shift reflect the ideas of 'new public management' and a welfare model of care delivery?

Privatisation and integration

Underpinning many of the changes associated with the National Mental Health Strategy has been a movement from a reliance on government services to the use of private, for-profit services. This shift towards a market model of care is underpinned by a view of people with mental illness as consumers who can exercise control over their care through deciding between services. Privatisation has resulted in the use of more service providers and greater complexity in service delivery. To overcome complexity, mental health policy has promoted integration between services. Banfield et al. (2012) argue that service and interprofessional partnerships have been on the policy agenda from the first *National Mental Health Plan*, but have become a priority area from the fourth plan. **Integrated care** is seen as a means of managing the demands on the health care budget while improving access to and the quality of services and addressing gaps in service delivery (Petrich et al. 2013).

In practice, service integration has had mixed results. Petrich et al. (2013) argue that services are currently fragmented owing to the dispersion of the population, to **federalism** resulting in two layers of government and blurred lines of accountability between the federal and state governments, and to differences in approach to private services between the major political parties. The dispersion of the population leads to poorer access to services for rural and remote people. An evaluation of rural and remote mental health services in 2011 found that people had difficulty in accessing specialist mental health services, and that the gap between access and demand was growing (Department of Health and Ageing 2011). In 2015, there were 13 full time psychiatrists per 100,000 people in major cities compared with 4 per 100,000 in outer regional areas, 5 per 100,000 in remote areas and 2 per 100,000 in very remote areas (National Rural Health Alliance 2017). (See Chapter 9 for more insights into rural health.)

Federalism results in the state governments providing specialist mental health services and the federal government funding the **National Disability Insurance Scheme (NDIS)** (Chapter 12) and primary care, leading to difficulties in coordinating services (Petrich et al. 2013). Creating partnerships between public and private services has been identified as difficult. McDonald et al. (2011) argue that ways of working may not be compatible between public and private services. Private-service providers such as GPs seek results for specific patients, whereas government services focus on populations. Furthermore, GPs and other private-service providers may have difficulty in negotiating bureaucratic systems (McDonald et al. 2011). This is significant as, in 2015–16, GPs provided the most Medicare-subsidised mental health-specific services (30.6%) (AIHW, 2017a).

Delivering community mental health care

In the discussion that follows, we outline some of the people involved in service delivery for people with mental health disorders. For some groups (e.g. GPs, NGOs), this involvement has been prompted by policy; for other groups (e.g. paramedics and emergency services), it has come about as a result of de-institutionalisation.

Community mental health provision

Community mental health care is provided in the community and hospital based outpatient settings. The **National Community Mental Health Care Database (NCMHCD)** is used to collate and describe the care provided by these services (AIHW 2018). **Community mental health services (CMHS)** provided 9.4 million service contacts nationally during 2015–16. These episodes of care were provided to 414,176 clients, an average of 23 service contacts per client (AIHW, 2017a). Fig. 11.2 provides information about diagnosis and contact with community mental health services. This figure demonstrates that people with schizophrenia receive community mental health services most commonly, followed by people experiencing depression.

Mental health care in the community is delivered through **case management** by multidisciplinary teams consisting of psychiatrists, mental health nurses, social workers, occupational therapists and psychologists, among others. For mental health professionals, core skills include the ability to identify mental disorders and assess and manage risk, a basic knowledge of psychotropic medications and their side-effects, use of educational strategies with patients and carers, and skills in improving engagement. Advanced skills usually require specific training, such as cognitive behavioural therapy (CBT) and specific counselling expertise. Meadows et al. (2012) provide more information about the roles and skills of community mental health teams.

Primary care

A second source of support for mental health is primary care promoted by strategies to increase collaboration between primary care and specialist mental health services. **Better Outcomes in Mental**

FIGURE 11.2 COMMUNITY MENTAL HEALTH CONTACTS VIA DIAGNOSIS

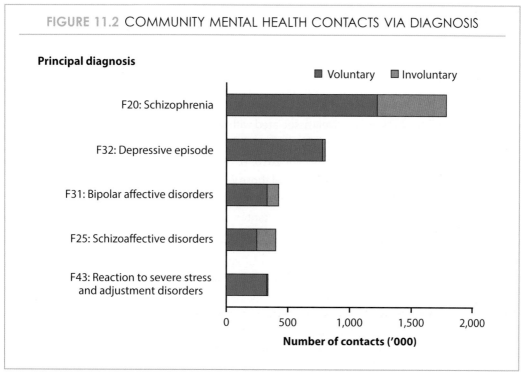

Source: Australian Institute of Health and Welfare (2018) National community mental health care database (state and territory community mental health care), Table CMHC.25

Health Care (BOiMHC) was launched in July 2001 to improve access to **primary mental health care** (Fletcher et al. 2009). The first cycle of reforms allowed GPs to claim through Medicare for psychological interventions and referrals to psychologists and social workers for people with depression and anxiety disorders (Hickie & Groom 2002; Fletcher et al. 2009, Medicare 2010). This was extended in November 2006 through the Better Access program, which allowed psychologists, and some social workers and occupational therapists, to claim services under the Medicare Benefits Scheme upon referral by a GP (Fletcher et al. 2009). The 2011 Budget lowered the number of consultations available through the Better Access program and reduced Medicare rebates for GP mental health care planning, opting instead to target resources through Medicare Locals and NGOs (Henderson & Fuller 2011) and later through PHNs.

GPs have become a major source of care, because they are viewed as the first point of contact for someone with a mental health disorder. According to the BEACH data, 12.4% of all GP encounters were mental health related, with depression being the most common at approximately one-third, or 32.1%, during 2015–16 (AIHW, 2017a). Funding has also been targeted towards the provision of multidisciplinary primary care to people aged 12–25 years. One initiative is the establishment by the federal government of Headspace, Australia's National Youth Mental Health Foundation, for people with mental health and substance abuse problems (Hickie & McGorry 2007).

PAUSE
for
REFLECTION
...

The Mental Health Council of Australia has expressed concern that community care will be exclusively associated with primary care when 'not all community-based or "non-hospital" mental health services provide primary care' (Mental Health Council of Australia 2010, p. 3). Community mental health services traditionally service the needs of those with serious and disabling mental illness. A focus on primary care is viewed as a threat to the specialist focus of community mental health services. How important is the role of primary care in delivering mental health services? Where should the focus of care delivery be?

Non-government organisations

A third source of care has been the use of non-government services to provide support services for people with mental illness. The National Mental Health Strategy (Australian Health Ministers 1992) argued for the use of a combination of government and NGO service providers to meet the needs of the mentally ill. NGOs competed for government funding through tendering to provide services. Funding occurred on 'a contractual basis dependent upon the NGOs' definition of objectives and priorities for service delivery', tying the services provided by NGOs to government priorities (Australian Health Ministers' Advisory Council (AHMAC) 1989, p. 44).

Recent changes have resulted in the NDIS organising support services for people with mental illness. The NDIS provides individualised care through a market model in which people are assessed and given a budget to purchase the services that they require. Consumer advocates question the role of the NDIS in meeting the needs of people with mental illness as the NDIS provides services to those with ongoing disability and mental illness is often episodic (NMHC 2017). Further, many people are falling through gaps in the system, leading to a need for alternative funding (COAG 2017; NMHC 2017).

Paramedics and emergency services

As the care of those with mental illness shifted from institutions to community-based and primary care, mental illness and suicidal behaviour (e.g. self-injury, overdose, suicidal ideation and suicide attempts) became a major public health issue. The increase in need led to services such as the mental health triage service and instigation of mental health liaison teams within hospital **emergency departments (EDs)**. Emergency services such as paramedics (Chapter 25), the police and front-line services have taken an increasing role in the provision of services to those with mental illness (Parsons et al. 2011; Roberts & Henderson 2009; Shaban 2005). As a result, EDs have become a second entry point for mental health care alongside GPs. In 2016–17, there were an estimated 276,954 ED presentations with a mental health-related principal diagnosis in Australia. The rate of mental health-related ED presentations was 113.6 per 10,000 population (AIHW, 2016, 2017b). The majority of the mental health-related ED presentations in 2016–17 were classified as either urgent or semi-urgent (79.2%). Over forty-four percent (44.8%) of mental health-related ED presentations arrived via ambulance, air ambulance or helicopter rescue service (AIHW 2017b). Paramedics, as the primary prehospital emergency medical care providers, have been forced to consider role changes with their increasing responsibility in the care of those with mental illness.

Legislation has supported extended powers for paramedics and other accredited health practitioners. Under the *Mental Health Acts* (e.g. South Australia (2009; s. 56), Victoria (2014; s. 350) and New South Wales (2007; s. 19, 20 and 23)), paramedics and accredited health professionals are authorised to restrain and transport those experiencing suspected mental illness to a designated mental health facility or a health care facility where appropriate assessment and further care can be arranged (e.g. an ED). The *Mental Health Acts* provide for the use of 'reasonable force', physical and mechanical restraint and sedation, by those trained to provide it, for the individual under their care. As these roles and responsibilities expanded, the aim was to reduce the role of the police as de-facto community mental health providers and allow their role to return to managing behaviour and providing support as requested.

Informal carers

Families and friends of the mentally ill also provide a major source of care. The original *National Mental Health Strategy* document stated that 'many people with mental disorders are cared for in the community by "unpaid" carers' (Australian Health Ministers 1992, p. 26), where a carer was defined as 'a person whose life is affected by virtue of his or her having a close relationship with a consumer, or who has a chosen and contracted caring role with a consumer' (Australian Health Ministers 1991, p. 23). In representing the families of the mentally ill as carers they are viewed as a having the **capacity** but also a responsibility to provide care to mentally ill family members. There are currently few data on the number of people caring for people with mental health disorders, although earlier estimates suggest that 2.6 million Australians are caring for someone with a disability of some sort (AIHW 2009). Of these people, one-third are **primary carers**. Responsibility for providing day-to-day care falls disproportionately on women (two-thirds of primary carers). This is sometimes referred to as the **feminisation of care**. Adoption of a carer role has been associated with poorer mental and physical health. Pirkis et al. (2010) found that the carers of people with mental illness were more likely to be women, to be aged between 55 and 64 years old, and to experience significant levels of depression and distress. Despite this, governments presume that carers are not only willing but able to provide care to families and friends with mental illness, and that people with mental illness want to be cared for by their families. To address this problem, the National Mental Health Commission is working with state and territory bodies to establish a Lived Experience Steering Group to engage and co-design with service providers and policy groups' policy, practice and research priorities (National Mental Health Commission, 2017)

What are the implications of service change, including bed closure and the privatisation of mental health care and the construction of family members as carers on the families and friends of the mentally ill? What support do families need to provide care? Is there enough support for families?

The consumer

The following discussion focuses on the consumer of mental health services. We outline a recovery approach to mental illness and explore the roles of consumer rights and the manner in which these are reflected in legislation.

Recovery

Mental health policy and legislation in Australia is underpinned by a recovery approach to mental illness. Recovery is not about curing a mental illness, but instead about finding a satisfying way of living with the illness (Anthony 1993). A recovery approach is consumer focused and based on mental health services working in partnership with mental health consumers to meet their own goals (Farkas et al. 2005). This assumes an advocacy role on the part of the service providers, and the participation of consumers and carers in the development of care plans (Case study 11.1).

Case Study 11.1

Primary mental health care

This case study relates the experience of a young man presenting with symptoms of early psychosis complicated by his cannabis use. It demonstrates the use of primary mental health care services to deliver mental health care in a de-institutionalised setting.

Tim is a 21-year-old university student in his second year of studying commerce. He presents to the student health and counselling services as his study performance is slipping from credit-plus grades to resubmissions and uncompleted assessments. A close friend has also noticed that Tim's income has dropped as Tim, who usually gets shifts as a shelf-packer, has not accepted shifts or gone to work for almost 2 months. The friend tries to ask Tim if he is alright, but Tim gets agitated and states that he is fine. On a recent visit with his parents, they have an argument around Tim asking for some money to hold him over and their disappointment with his poor university performance. They are concerned that something is occurring, but are not aware of his cannabis use and hearing of voices. They suggest he should maybe move back home if he is finding it hard to study and meet demands, but Tim insists that he will work it out and he wants to remain independent.

The health and counselling services provide GP services and allied health support through government-funded shared-care agreements. When Tim sees the nurse practitioner he is evasive, and attributes his poor grades to his increased cannabis use. He knows it is affecting his concentration and short-term memory; he is not putting in the study time and has less energy. After several sessions to discuss his cannabis use and how the service can best assist him, Tim reluctantly discloses that he is very fearful that he is 'going mad' because he has had the experience of auditory hallucinations. Tim is reluctant to disclose this to the nurse practitioner because he doesn't want to be labelled a 'psycho'. The cannabis stops the experience of the auditory hallucinations and Tim feels relaxed when stoned.

Tim agrees to reduce his drug use. He is able to make the connection for himself between his reasons for using the drugs to dull the auditory hallucinations and the unwanted effects on his performance overall. He is still concerned about how the voices are going to affect him if he stops the cannabis use. The counsellor and Tim work on a plan to stop his cannabis use by identifying a quit date and learning mindfulness as an alternative relaxation strategy. Tim utilises the services of the drug information and telephone support line, which is available 24/7, many times over the first few months when he feels the need for help to stay on track.

Tim consents to his counsellor discussing his situation with the other team members within the service, but not with his parents. With Tim's involvement, a management plan based on the early psychosis prevention and intervention centre guidelines is agreed.

Case study questions

1 What could Tim's treatment plan include?

2 Who within the service or outside the service might be involved in Tim's care?

3 Would specialist mental health services be required in Tim's care? What might prevent their involvement?

4 Should Tim's parents be informed of and involved in his care?

5 Consider other carers or people that Tim may require for support, and how this would be incorporated into any management plan.

6 What effect would Tim's behaviour and cannabis use have had on friends and family and his relationships with them?

Consumer rights

One aspect of recovery is a greater focus upon consumer rights. Consumer rights came to the fore with the release of *Human rights and mental illness: report of the national inquiry into human rights of people with mental illness* (Human Rights and Equal Opportunity Commission 1993), more commonly known as the Burdekin Report, which identified abuses of human rights occurring in both hospital and community mental health settings. The National Mental Health Strategy has been associated with the development of the *Mental health statement of rights and responsibilities* (Australian Health Ministers 1991; Commonwealth of Australia 2012) and National standards for mental health services (Department of Health 2010), which established principles for protecting the rights of the mentally ill and their carers. Following from the UN's *Principles*, the *Mental health statement of rights and responsibilities* views mental health consumers as having the right to social inclusion and participation on an equal basis with others without discrimination of any kind. Mental health consumers have the right to:

1 respect for their individual human dignity and worth at all ages and stages of life

2 respect for their privacy and confidentiality (Commonwealth of Australia 2012).

In 2008, Australia also endorsed the UN *Convention on the Rights of Persons with Disabilities*. This convention is based on a social model of disability that shifts the focus from a person having a disability to society and the barriers to the full participation of people with disabilities, including mental illness, in that society (Kämpf 2008). The convention focuses on social inclusion through the attainment of social, political and economic rights, along with non-discrimination on the basis of disability (Weller 2010). This is a departure from previous views of rights for people with mental illness, which focus on limiting government interference with the freedom of people with mental health problems.

Despite an increasing focus upon rights, the *National report on mental health and suicide prevention* (Mental Health Commission 2017) found that there is concern that consumer engagement with services is often tokenistic, standards are not rigorously applied, payment for participation is inconsistent and human rights and a recovery-orientated approach are not reflected well in policy.

The focus on human rights and protecting the rights of those living with mental illness has been an important driver of current state and territory mental health legislation. Australia's *Mental Health Acts* focus on the provision of comprehensive mental health care to support recovery; maintenance of people's freedoms, rights and dignity in conjunction with their protection, protection of others and provision of services; and the limited conferral of powers to facilitate the care of those who may not have the insight to make those decisions for themselves.

The guiding principle of Australia's *Mental Health Acts* is the provision of the best therapeutic outcomes for individuals in the least restrictive way possible and in the least restrictive environment (e.g. voluntary treatment). Treatment should also be provided as close as practicable to the individual's family, carers, support networks and place of residence, and should be designed in consultation with the individual, family and / or carers or significant others. As part of the principle of collaboration, most *Mental Health Acts* provide guidance that information sharing is essential and should be done to benefit the individual, family / carers and those who care for them across interprofessional boundaries. Each individual's age, needs and cultural background should be considered when providing care, and review of care should be consistent and offer the opportunity for appeal.

The *Mental Health Acts* also provide a framework for assessment and safeguarding when **involuntary care**, such as **treatment orders** provided in the community setting, inpatient care or emergency crisis care, is required. Risk of serious harm is a criterion for involuntary care, and occurs when an individual's mental health is viewed as deteriorating to a point where the risk is high. Despite legislation, once someone gets to the stage of being a high risk to themselves or others, the likelihood of the police being involved increases (Bradbury et al. 2014).

A major challenge for involuntary care under current *Mental Health Acts* is the notion of capacity. Lack of capacity to make decisions regarding one's own health care is used alongside risk as a measure for the need for involuntary care. The difficulty with the concept of capacity is that someone may be able to make decisions in some areas but not in others, and it is dependent on the environment and circumstances. This creates difficulties with assessment in community or acute settings, as the time and past history required to ascertain the capacity or needs of an individual are often not readily available and may lead to early decisions that involuntary care is required (Ryan 2011; Bradbury et al. 2014). It also raises questions regarding the resources and training required to equip those in the acute setting to assess for capacity.

Ryan (2011) argues that the person, person's family, GP, carer(s) or mental health practitioner can pre-plan and have mechanisms in place for when a person's capacity diminishes that clearly outline treatment pathways that have been generated by agreement and collaboration (e.g. advance care directives). These mechanisms assist in maintaining the individual's rights to choice of treatment, where and how, and in the early identification of deterioration, which would enable early interventions that are consistent with the principles of human rights.

PAUSE
for
REFLECTION
…

Consider the term 'risk' and the challenges to providing care 'in the least restrictive way possible' for health professionals when caring for those with mental illness. How could a person's ability to problem-solve be affected by mental illness?

Summary

This chapter has described the delivery of mental health care in Australia, and makes the following key points.

- There has been a global trend towards community care in the past 60 years. This movement has been driven by concern about the human rights of people with mental illness.
- Mental health care in Australia was provided in institutions until 1955. A first wave of de-institutionalisation led to community services for people with acute mental health problems. A second wave of de-institutionalisation from the 1980s focused on the community services for people with chronic mental illness.
- The National Mental Health Strategy was launched in 1992. The main goals of the strategy were to move service delivery from psychiatric hospitals to general hospitals and the community, to create better links between government support services and NGOs and to foster uniform mental health legislation across the country.

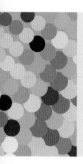

- Mainstreaming has resulted in the closure of psychiatric hospitals and fewer beds for the mentally ill in public hospitals. Community-based services have been and are continuing to be developed.
- The National Mental Health Strategy has resulted in greater use of non-governmental services, emergency services, GPs and family and friends of the mentally ill to provide care.
- The rights of the mentally ill and their carers have been addressed through changes in mental health legislation, development of policies to identify these rights and more recently by the *Convention of Rights of People with Disabilities*.

An accompanying video exploring the themes of this chapter is hosted on Evolve: http://evolve.elsevier.com/AU/Willis/understanding/.

Review Questions

1   Identify two factors that have assisted and two factors that have prevented change in mental health service delivery in the past 20 years.

2   List at least four social determinants of mental health. What strategies could be developed to improve social inclusion in these areas?

3   Rosen et al. (1993) provide the following definition of case management:

   'The role of drawing together into one coherent system all services necessary to meet the needs of the service user, whether in the community or the hospital. This includes meeting the needs for psychiatric or physical treatment, family and social relationships; basic survival needs like food, safe accommodation, employment, leisure, cultural and spiritual needs.'

   Consider whether you think this is ambitious, or representative of what clients have a right to expect.

4   What are the positive and negative effects of privatising mental health care delivery in Australia?

5   How much evidence is there of consumer participation in the design and delivery of mental health services? Is the reform and policy direction of increased consumer participation reflected in the real experience of consumers?

References

Anthony, W., 1993. Recovery from mental illness: the guiding vision of the mental health service system in the 1990s. Psychosoc. Rehabil. J. 16 (4), 11–23.

Australian Bureau of Statistics (ABS), 2016. Aboriginal and Torres Strait Islander people with a mental health condition. http://www.abs.gov.au/ausstats/abs@.nsf/Lookup/by%20 Subject/4714.0~2014-15~Feature%20Article~Aboriginal%20and%20Torres%20Strait%20Islander%20 people%20with%20a%20mental%20health%20condition%20(Feature%20Article)~10.

Australian Health Ministers, 1991. Mental health statement of rights and responsibilities, AGPS, Canberra.

Australian Health Ministers, 1992. National Mental Health Strategy. AGPS, Canberra.

Australian Health Ministers, 1998. Second national mental health plan. Mental Health Branch, Commonwealth Department of Health and Family Services, Canberra.

Australian Health Ministers, 2003. National mental health plan 2003–2008. Australian Government, Canberra.

Australian Health Ministers' Advisory Council (AHMAC), 1989. Mental health discussion paper: a paper presented to Australian Health Minister Advisory Council in Oct 1989. AGPS, Canberra.

Australian Institute of Health and Welfare (AIHW), 2009. Carers National Data Repository scoping study: final report. AIHW, Canberra.

Australian Institute of Health and Welfare (AIHW), 2016. Emergency department care 2015–16: Australian hospital statistics. Health services series no. 72. Cat. no. HSE 182. AIHW, Canberra.

Australian Institute of Health and Welfare (AIHW), 2017a. Mental health services – in brief 2017. Cat. no. HSE 192. AIHW, Canberra. https://www.aihw.gov.au/reports/mental-health-services/mental-healt h-services-in-brief-2017/contents/table-of-contents.

Australian Institute of Health and Welfare (AIHW), 2017b. Emergency department care 2016–17: Australian hospital statistics. Health services series no. 80. Cat. no. HSE 194. AIHW, Canberra.

Australian Institute of Health and Welfare (AIHW), 2018. Mental health services in Australia. AIHW, Canberra. https://www.aihw.gov.au/reports/mental-health-services/mental-health-services-i n-australia/report-contents/specialised-mental-health-care-facilities.

Banfield, M., Gardner, K., Yen, L., et al., 2012. Co-ordination of care in Australian mental health policy. Aust. Health Rev. 36, 153–157.

Bower, P., Gilbody, S., 2005. Stepped care in psychological therapies: access, effectiveness and efficiency: narrative literature review. Br. J. Psychiatry 186, 11–17.

Bradbury, J., Ireland, M., Stasa, H., 2014. Mental health emergency transport: the pot-holed road to care. Med. J. Aust. 200 (6), 348–351.

Commonwealth of Australia, 2012. Mental health statement of rights and responsibilities, Commonwealth of Australia, Canberra. http://www.health.gov.au/internet/main/publishing.nsf/Content/ E39137B3C170F93ECA257CBC007CFC8C/$File/rights2.pdf.

Council of Australian Governments (COAG), 2017. Fifth national mental health and suicide prevention plan. Commonwealth of Australia, Canberra.

Department of Health, 2010. National standards for mental health services. Commonwealth of Australia, Canberra. http://www.health.gov.au/internet/main/publishing.nsf/Content/mental-pubs-n-servst10.

Department of Health, 2016. PHN Primary mental health care flexible funding pool implementation guidelines: stepped care. Commonwealth of Australia, Canberra. http://www.health.gov.au/internet/ main/publishing.nsf/Content/2126B045A8DA90FDCA257F6500018260/$File/1PHN%20Guidance%20 -%20Stepped%20Care.pdf.

Department of Health and Ageing, 2009a. National mental health policy 2008. Commonwealth of Australia, Canberra.

Department of Health and Ageing, 2009b. Fourth national mental health plan – an agenda for collaborative government action in mental health 2009–2014. Commonwealth of Australia, Canberra.

Department of Health and Ageing, 2011. Mental health service in rural and remote areas program evaluation, January 2011 version 1.3, final evaluation report. Commonwealth of Australia, Canberra. http://www.health.gov.au/internet/main/publishing.nsf/Content/mental-pubs-m-mhsrraev.

Farkas, M., Gagne, C., Anthony, W., et al., 2005. Implementing recovery orientated evidence based programs: identifying the critical dimensions. Community Ment. Health J. 41 (2), 141–158.

Fletcher, J., Pirkis, J., Kohn, F., et al., 2009. Australian primary mental health care: improving access and outcomes. Aust. J. Prim. Health 15, 244–253.

Henderson, J., Fuller, J., 2011. "Problematising" Australian policy representations in responses to the physical health of people with mental health disorders. Aust. J. Soc. Issues 46 (2), 183–203.

Henderson, J., Javanparast, S., McKean, T., et al., 2018. Commissioning and equity in primary care in Australia: views from Primary Health Networks. Health Soc. Care Community 26 (1), 80–89.

Hickie, I., Groom, G., 2002. Primary care-led mental health service reform: an outline of the *Better Outcomes in Mental Health Care* initiative. Australas. Psychiatry 10 (4), 376–382.

Hickie, I., McGorry, P., 2007. Increased access to evidence-based primary mental health care: will the implementation match the rhetoric? Med. J. Aust. 187 (2), 100–103.

Human Rights and Equal Opportunity Commission, 1993. Human rights and mental illness: report of the national inquiry into human rights of people with mental illness, AGPS, Canberra.

Kämpf, A., 2008. The Disabilities Convention and its consequences for mental health laws in Australia. Law Context 26 (2), 10–36.

Meadows, G., Fafhall, J., Fossey, E., et al., 2012. Mental Health in Australia: Collaborative Community Practice, third ed. OUP, Melbourne.

Mental Health Commission, 2017. National report on mental health and suicide prevention. http://mentalhealthcommission.gov.au/media/202298/NMHC17-3367_National_Report_ACC2.pdf.

McDonald, J., Davies, G., Jayasuriya, R., et al., 2011. Collaboration across private and public sector primary health care services: benefits, costs and policy implications. J. Interprof. Care 25, 258–264.

McGorry, P., 2007. The specialist youth mental health model: strengthening the weakest link in the public mental health system. Med. J. Aust. 187 (7), S53–S56.

Medicare Australia, 2010. National Health and Hospital Network – mental health – flexible care packages for patients with severe mental illnesses. http://www.medicareaustralia.gov.au/provider/budget-2010/mental-health.jsp.

Mental Health Council of Australia (MHCA), 2010. Community mental health and primary mental health care background paper. https://mhaustralia.org/sites/default/files/imported/component/rsfiles/publications/Community_Mental_Health_and_Primary_Mental_Health_Care_Background_Paper_July_2010.pdf.

National Mental Health Commission (NMHC), 2012. A contributing life, the 2012 national report card on mental health and suicide prevention. NMHC, Sydney.

National Mental Health Commission (NHMC), 2017. The 2017 report on mental health and suicide prevention. NMHC, Sydney.

National Rural Health Alliance, 2017. Mental health in rural and remote Australia: Fact sheet. http://
ruralhealth.org.au/sites/default/files/publications/nrha-mental-health-factsheet-dec-2017.pdf.

Parsons, V., O'Brian, L., O'Meara, P., 2011. Mental health legislation: an era of change in paramedic clinical
practice and responsibility. Int. Paramed. Pract. 1 (2), 9–16.

Petrich, M., Ramamurthy, V.L., Hendrie, D., et al., 2013. Challenges and opportunities for integration in
health systems: an Australian perspective. J. Integr. Care 21 (6), 347–359.

Pirkis, J., Burgess, P., Hardy, J., et al., 2010. Who cares? A profile of people who care for relatives with
mental disorder. Aust. N. Z. J. Psychiatry 44, 929–937.

Roberts, L., Henderson, J., 2009. Paramedic perceptions of their role, education, training and working
relationships when attending cases of mental illness. JEPHC. 7 (3), doi:10.33151/ajp.7.3.175.

Rosen, A., Miller, V., Parker, G., 1993. AIMHS (Area Integrated Mental Health Services) Standard Manual.
NSW Department of Health, Royal North Shore Hospital and Community Mental Health Services,
Sydney.

Ryan, C., 2011. Capacity as a determinant of non-consensual treatment of the mentally ill in Australia.
Psychiatr. Psychol. Law 18 (2), 248–262.

Shaban, R., 2005. Accounting for assessments of mental illness in paramedic practice: a new theoretical
framework. JEPHC. 3 (3), 10–21.

United Nations (UN) General Assembly, 1991. Principles for the protection of people with mental illness
and for the improvement of mental health care, United Nations, New York. http://un-documents.net/
pppmi.htm.

United Nations (UN), 2008. Convention on the Rights of Persons with Disabilities. UN, New York. https://
www.un.org/development/desa/disabilities/convention-on-the-rights-of-persons-with-disabilities
.html.

Weller, P., 2010. The right to health: the Convention on the Rights of Persons with Disabilities. Altern. Law
J. 35 (2), 66–71.

World Health Organization (WHO), 2013. Mental health action plan 2013–2020. WHO, Geneva. https://
apps.who.int/iris/bitstream/handle/10665/89966/9789241506021_eng.pdf;jsessionid=C1886122289D4
EFC12307AFBB2879A63?sequence=1.

World Health Organization (WHO), 2014. Mental disorders: Fact sheet 396. http://www.who.int/
mediacentre/factsheets/fs369/en/.

Further Reading

Australian Health Ministers, 1992. National Mental Health Strategy. Australian Government, Canberra.

Australian Institute of Health and Welfare (AIHW), 2017. Mental health services – in brief 2017. Cat. no.
HSE 192. AIHW, Canberra.

National Mental Health Commission (NMHC), 2017. The 2017 report on mental health and suicide
prevention. NMHC, Sydney.

Meadows, G., Fafhall, J., Fossey, E., et al., 2012. Mental Health in Australia: Collaborative Community
Practice, third ed. OUP, Melbourne.

Online Resources

Australian government mental health and well-being publications: http://www.health.gov.au/internet/main/publishing.nsf/Content/mental-pubs.

Australian Institute of Health and Welfare: www.aihw.gov.au.

BeyondBlue: www.beyondblue.org.au.

Black Dog Institute: www.blackdoginstitute.org.au.

Headspace: www.headspace.org.au.

Mental Health Australia: http://mhaustralia.org/.

Mental Health Carers ARAFMI Australia: www.arafmiaustralia.asn.au.

Mental Illness Fellowship of Australia Inc: www.mifa.org.au.

National Mental Health Consumer and Carer Forum: www.nmhccf.org.au.

Orygen (National Centre of Excellence in Youth Mental Health): orygen.org.au.

Reach Out: au.reachout.com.

SANE Australia: www.sane.org.

World Health Organization, Mental health page: www.who.int/mental_health/en/.

CHAPTER 12

People living with disability: navigating support and health systems

Caroline Ellison[a]

Key learning outcomes

When you finish this chapter you should be able to:

- ◆ identify some key factors and barriers impacting on health and development of quality life for a diverse range of Australians living with disability
- ◆ understand the importance of a holistic approach and challenges faced in providing overall health care for people living with disability
- ◆ describe the concepts of **self-management** and **individualised funding models,** quality and safeguarding including the **National Disability Insurance Scheme (NDIS)** and their interface with the Australian health system
- ◆ briefly outline roles undertaken by disability professionals in Australian health care and human services systems
- ◆ outline some areas in which **developmental educators (DEs)** and other disability professionals engage with the Australian disability support and health systems in assisting individuals living with disability to achieve quality of life.

Key terms and abbreviations

ableist	individualised funding
activities of daily living (ADLs)	medical model
block-funded	National Disability Insurance Agency (NDIA)
developmental educators (DEs)	National Disability Insurance Scheme (NDIS)
Developmental Educators Australia Incorporated (DEAI)	National Health Priority Areas (NHPAs)
	person-centred approach
disability	self-determination
general practitioner (GP)	social model
human rights model	Technical and Further Education (TAFE)
impairment	transdisciplinary

[a]We acknowledge the contribution by Kerrie Lante to the chapter in the 3rd edition of this book.

Introduction

Approximately 4.3 million Australians live with **disability** (Australian Bureau of Statistics (ABS) 2015) and, globally, this numbers more than a billion, according to the World Health Organization (WHO 2014). While most individuals living with disability in Australia are not sick, a higher proportion will experience or self-report more complex general health issues (Australian Institute of Health and Welfare (AIHW) 2014; Carey et al. 2017; Foubert et al. 2014). Carey et al. (2017) report that individuals with long-term disability require supports to engage in **activities of daily living (ADLs)** or to interact with and navigate complex support and health systems. Disability is described as a limitation, restriction or **impairment** lasting, or likely to last, for at least 6 months and restricting everyday activities. There are many various disabilities, usually resulting from accidents, illness or genetic disorders. Disability may affect a person's mobility, communication or learning. It can also affect their employability, income and participation in education and social activities.

People living with disability are at greater risk of experiencing mental health difficulties (Chapter 11) having negative physical outcomes associated with ageing sooner than the general population (AIHW 2010), and are often less able to engage with support systems to achieve positive outcomes (AIHW, 2017; Keane 1996; Williamson et al. 2017). The Australian Institute of Health and Welfare (AIHW 2018) reports that 41% of people living with significant impairment and/or disability experience poor to fair health, compared with 6.5% for those living without disability. They note that people living with significant impairments were more likely to have acquired a long-term health condition related to the **National Health Priority Areas (NHPAs)** at a younger age than people without disability. For example the AIHW (2010, p. 2) showed that:

> Among people aged 15–64 years with a specific long-term health condition of NHPAs, the comparisons between people with severe or profound disability and those without disability showed that:
> - ◆ the proportion who had diabetes or a high sugar level before age 25 was 23% versus 7%
> - ◆ the proportion who acquired arthritis before age 25 was 14% versus 6%
> - ◆ the proportion who first experienced osteoporosis before age 45 was 43% versus 31%.

This has implications for disability support and health professionals in understanding how an individual's impairment can interplay with and impact on their health, community participation, independence and need for disability support. For example, the Survey of Disability, Ageing and Carers reported that nearly 700,000 Australians live with intellectual disability (ABS 2015), many of whom frequently experience communication difficulties and psychiatric disability (AIHW 2008), are misunderstood or are misinterpreted by service providers in health and disability support service systems. Research has established that adults living with intellectual disability are more susceptible to sedentary lifestyle diseases owing to low levels of physical activity (McKeon et al. 2013; Stanish et al. 2006). Emerson (2005) found that 25–34-year-old adults living with intellectual disability have an activity level equivalent to that of a 75-year-old. With such high levels of sedentary behaviour an increasing demand is placed on health systems (Lante et al. 2014).

Case study 12.1 helps illustrate how an individual's impairment can interplay with and impact on their health and the need for effective communication in the health care setting. The questions following the case study ask you to consider how changes from the allied health professionals and the support worker could impact on Nancy's health care management.

Case Study 12.1

Nancy, a 25-year-old female living with intellectual disability and mental health needs, presents to a rheumatologist at the local hospital. The rheumatologist notices Nancy's file indicates that 4 years ago she presented to hospital, at that time with her mother who was listed as her carer. No diagnosis was made; however, potential lupus was recorded. Today Nancy has a support worker, Lucy, accompanying her. During the consultation the rheumatologist asks questions including 'What are your symptoms?' and 'When did they start?' Nancy replies, 'My body aches' and then continues to ask what is wrong and why this is happening. To assist, Lucy asks Nancy 'Did your body ache before or after Christmas' to which the reply was 'Before, it was just before we went away.' From this information Lucy could inform the rheumatologist that this had started 2 weeks ago, adding that she had heard Nancy complain of body aches on and off over the past year. Lucy then asked Nancy, waiting for a response, between each question, if she could tell the rheumatologist 'What part of your body aches?', 'Can you walk around when your body aches?' and 'When your body aches do you get tired?'

A blood test and 24-hour urine test were ordered. Nancy had to wait some time at pathology for the blood test and became extremely anxious. Lucy reassured Nancy while waiting and tried to explain the process. Nancy was called to have the blood test and said she wanted Lucy to accompany her. The nurse would not allow this, indicating 'It's against the rules, I'll get in trouble from my boss.' Following the test Nancy appeared with some containers and said 'We can go now.' Lucy asked what the containers were for and was told 'For the other test, the nurse told me what to do.' Upon discussion when Lucy dropped Nancy back home it was obvious that Nancy did not understand why or how she had to do the 24-hour urine test. As Lucy was not present when this was explained to Nancy, she could not explain this to Nancy herself. Nancy did not complete the test, however, but indicated to everyone that she had and that she took the sample back to the hospital the next day. The rheumatologist presumed that something went wrong at pathology's end.

After further tests and upon the return visit to the rheumatologist, Nancy was informed that she had connective tissue disorder and was prescribed medication. Nancy replied 'Ok' and carried on the conversation. She was given a piece of paper and told 'This is about a similar disorder but most of it applies to you, if you want to know more you can Google it.' She was also told that it was important that if she ever had a temperature she must go straight to hospital.

Continued

Case study questions

1 Given the above, do you believe Nancy understands her condition? What, if any, follow-up steps do you believe are needed and why?

2 What could the a) rheumatologist, b) nurse and c) Lucy have done differently to help Nancy to successfully complete the urine test and understand her newly diagnosed condition?

3 What further information could have been provided to Nancy around the medication she was prescribed? Is Nancy likely to take the medication? Why/why not? What could occur between health and disability professionals to assist Nancy to take and manage her medication? What might the interactions be between the National Disability Insurance Scheme and the health system?

The Productivity Commission (2011) report on disability care and support identified problems with the current disability policy (Bacchi 2016) and acknowledged an inadequate, fragmented support system for individuals living with disability in Australia. Addressing these concerns, in 2013 the Commission's proposed National Disability Insurance Scheme was launched and in 2019 the roll-out continues, giving groups of people living with disability access to individualised packages of resources to support daily living and have a life of their choice.

The *National Disability Insurance Scheme (NDIS) Act* (C'mwlth 2013), based on the United Nations *Convention on the Rights of People* and ratified by the Australian Government in 2008, was first proposed in the Productivity Commission (2011) report. The *NDIS Act* (2013 C'mwlth *s4*) has 17 general principles guiding action; principle one states that 'People with disability have the same right as other members of Australian society to realise their potential for physical, social, emotional and intellectual development' (p. 6). Other principles outline their right to participate in economic and social life in line with their ability to receive support across their life-span, to be supported to exercise choice in the pursuit of their goals, to be respected, to have dignity and to ensure control over their own life is maximised. Despite this, accessing timely and effective health care for people living with disabilities is often restricted owing to physical and organisational (i.e. health care staff attitudes) barriers (Victorian Health Promotion Foundation (Vic Health) 2012). International systematic literature reviews concur with these findings and add that barriers to accessing health care stem from factors such as a lack of formal training for health care around understanding disability, lack of communication and advocacy skills between individuals living with disability and health care providers and often complex transport, finance and other access barriers (Ervin et al. 2014; Williamson et al. 2017).

The NDIS is based on a Medicare-type model and is currently funded by directing funds from consolidated revenue, although it is proposed there may be a tax levy imposed in the future. As of August 2018, full roll-out of the NDIS continues in all states including Western Australia, as well as various reviews and evaluations to ensure that the scheme meets its aims and objectives. Cost estimates have increased to $22 billion annually (Productivity Commission 2017).

Four guiding principles govern the NDIS:

♦ actuarial estimate of long-term costs – to ensure financial sustainability

♦ long-term view of funding requirements – unlike previous models the NDIS takes a life-long view of an individual's need for support

♦ investment in research, innovation and outcome analysis – to facilitate capacity-building

♦ investment in community participation and building social capital – to further access to and use of mainstream services and increased social and economic participation by people living with disability (**National Disability Insurance Agency (NDIA)** 2014).

According to Bonyhady (2014) the concept of an insurance scheme to support individuals is not necessarily new; however, broadening a scheme to include people living with diverse needs and moving away from a diagnostic approach to a **person-centred approach** means that the NDIS is developing and being refined as it is being rolled out.

The introduction of the NDIS and subsequent funding changes between the Commonwealth and state governments built on a number of existing individualised Australian funding models, particularly in Victoria and Western Australia. However, 5 years since the initial pilot sites and an ongoing national roll-out, tensions exist between the NDIA, costings and high compliance costs linked to audits and other processes which are not funded making long-term sustainability uncertain for smaller organisations. This is likely to impact on long-term choice and control for individuals, who may find they have a limited number of options to support them. This could undermine the concept of choice and control.

Individualised funding is conceptually and philosophically about maximising independence, choice and control over supports and services, and allowing a person living with disability to have a valued role within their community (Carey et al. 2017; Government of Western Australia 2013). At the forefront of this notion is the individual being at the centre of and involved in decisions affecting their life. However, there is a pricing structure for health, therapeutic and daily living supports provided, and the NDIS is working with service providers to assist them to transition from current funding models to compliance with the new scheme.

The NDIS already has powerful implications for how disability, health and therapeutic professionals provide services to people living with disability. Developing a collaborative interprofessional model within the health sector focusing on the **medical model**, the **social model** and the **human rights model** of disability (focus on removal of environmental and attitudinal barriers and access to the same human rights as other citizens) (Mallett & Runswick-Cole 2014) needs to be at the forefront of service development in these sectors (Bonyhady 2014). For example, in an article discussing the benefits of reliable, regular, persistent and assertive support, the following case study of Peter, who lives with psychosocial support needs, highlights the importance of his understanding about his diabetes and mental health needs. This was achieved through a holistic support plan that included Peter, his parents, a home visiting nursing support service, a local general practitioner (GP) and disability supports. It highlights the need for supports that do not restrict a person but overcome barriers and create opportunities via health and disability staff working collaboratively for **self-determination** (Springgay & Sutton 2014).

PAUSE
for
REFLECTION
...

Check out

Access *newparadigm*, the *Australian Journal on Psychosocial Rehabilitation*, at: http://dro.deakin.edu.au/eserv/DU:30061988/wilson-consumerchoices-2014 .pdf.

Go to Publications and Resources and access *newparadigm*.

Turn to past editions and access the summer 2014 edition.

Go to the article on p. 16 – 'Psychosocial disability: the urgent need for reform in assessment and care' by Springgay & Sutton (2014).

Read the full case study of Peter on p. 19. It is under the heading 'Benefits of reliable, regular, and persistent and assertive support'.

Now consider the following:

- What is the importance of the role for each person in Peter's support plan?
- What were the identified barriers for Peter and how were these identified? Reflect on the outcome for Peter and his family if these barriers were not identified.
- Once an ideal placement is found for Peter, what adjustments need to be made to his support plan, who should initiate this, who should be involved and what steps will need to take place for this to occur?
- What would the potential health outcomes have been for Peter if a collaborative, interprofessional approach had not been not taken?

Concepts of disability, health and support

As stated by Keane (1996), the concept of health can be a difficult construct for some people living with disability to define. In research conducted by Ellison et al. (2011), participants living with disability most often described health as being free from negative impacts of illness or disease. In addition, participants' comments reflected the perception that having health was linked to being mobile, able to engage in activities of daily living to their satisfaction, having activities to keep busy, and having the opportunity and ability to form and maintain relationships.

Unchanged since 1948, the World Health Organization (WHO 1946) defines health as 'a state of complete physical, mental and social well-being and not merely the absence of disease and infirmity'. On this basis, no person who identifies as living with disability could attain the status of having health. This raises numerous questions including:

1 Is this an ableist perspective?

2 What are the implications of this for people living with disability and their interactions with Australia's disability support and health system?

3   What are the issues for health professionals educated around this definition and their potential view of the capacity for individuals living with disability to live a quality life and be actively involved in health related decisions?

In a paper discussing 'Why people are so messed up about dis/ability' Goodley (2014, pp. 117–136) states that we live in an **ableist** culture that provokes responses to individuals living with disability that can be described as fascination, anxiety, projection and devaluation. These are also often the responses of the health and support system professionals. Therefore there is a need for support professionals to understand a person's differing perception of health, especially when communicating with them. What has been problematic is health professionals who view individuals living with disability as not having the capacity for positive health and participation in decision-making around their health, within the context of their disability (Bacchi, 2016; Douglas et al. 2015; Stuifbergen et al. 1990). The challenge for professionals is to ensure information is provided so that the person living with disability understands and comprehends, so as to make and take informed choices and actions. Information may need to be provided in alternate formats to what currently exists.

PAUSE *for* **REFLECTION** ...   Considering the balance between duty of care and an individual's right to make decisions, how can you professionally ensure people living with disability are involved in decision-making around their health care? In addressing this question, consider people living with various needs, including their cultural background, cognitive impairments, communication difficulties and intellectual disabilities.

What supports and services are needed to facilitate capacity building for decision-making in individuals living with disability and awareness and understanding of the need to build capacity in health and support providers? Do these supports and services exist?

The NDIS is not the panacea to overcome all challenges and there is a risk it could be seen as a vehicle for resource 'handballing' or 'buck-passing'. The 2013 *NDIS Act* is clear that people living with disability can be supported by the NDIS in a coordinated manner to access generic and mainstream supports available outside of the NDIS. The purpose of the NDIS is not to replace or provide services that are available to the rest of society and for the cost of such services to be transferred to the NDIS. For example, state governments are still obliged to provide accessible and affordable public transport and not defer transport to the responsibility of the NDIS.

Skills and knowledge linked to collaborative health and disability supports

Like the rest of our community, people living with disability are not a homogeneous group. People may have lifelong conditions with which they are born, their disability may be invisible or visible, the effects of their disability may be constant or episodic, and levels of care and support required may range from occasional to 24 hours per day. However, there is specific knowledge about living with the interaction between disability and health that can be useful for support professionals to consider. The *NDIS Act* indicates a strong need for individuals to be at the centre of decision-making around planning for support, and the scheme is seeking outcomes that reflect this. So disability, therapy and health professionals need to work collaboratively with each other, the individual and their family and supports.

Professionals working with people living with disability, their families and supports to achieve the individual's expressed goals and choices need to listen and discuss with the individual and those who support the person:

1 health care issues which may impact on support, management and education of the person
2 the impact of impairments on some bodily systems and how this impacts on daily living and community participation for the person
3 specific personal care, communication issues and the link to a person-centred approach to managing health implications of some impairments and syndromes on the person
4 specific health care issues relevant to some people living with disability, which can include the use of medication, epilepsy, incontinence, impact of ageing and increased risk of psychological and mental health issues
5 lifestyle issues, which may affect or be affected by the person's physical and emotional well-being, including nutrition, housing and accommodation, relationships, sexuality, grief and loss and vulnerability to abusive relationships
6 the interaction between the disability and health professionals' duty of care and a person's freedom to choose and the right to 'dignity of risk'
7 provision of opportunities for capacity-building and experience around decision-making that allows for experience, learning, skill development and growth in the ability to make decisions.

To ensure these discussions can occur in a way that is accessible and understandable to all, allied health professionals, disability professionals and **developmental educators (DEs)** need to work collaboratively to ensure the person living with disability can make informed decisions.

PAUSE *for* REFLECTION ··· Search for health education material and general information on informed consent and consider how you can (a) provide accessible and understandable information to people living with intellectual disability and (b) ensure they have the capacity to give informed consent for a routine medical procedure.

Disability professionals in Australia

Disability professionals constitute a relatively new stream in Australia and in most states and territories there is lobbying for recognition as an allied health profession. One of the first associations to lobby for a discrete group of disability professionals, Developmental Educators Australia Incorporated (DEAI), was established in South Australia where DEs were recognised in the allied health professional stream in 2012, alongside and equivalent to speech pathologists, psychologists, occupational therapists and other allied health disciplines. The DEAI is pursuing national recognition and registration with Allied Health Professions Australia (AHPA).

DEs are part of the human service system, educated to understand the myriad functions and roles of health and support professionals in lives of people living with disability (Bottroff et al. 2000). DEs and other disability professionals use this understanding to enhance the health, self-determination and control of people living with disability and their supports through promoting a **person-centred approach** to support and advocacy and assisting individuals to navigate access to relevant support and health services (Bottroff et al. 2000). Person-centred approaches put the individual at the centre of decision-making processes and both take and create opportunities to inform and empower individuals to be actively involved in the management of their health (Nankervis 2006).

The roles of disability professionals are complex, with a need for varied but specific skills and knowledge. DEs are multi-skilled professionals who can work within a **transdisciplinary** and interprofessional framework with other professionals, such as speech pathologists, occupational therapists, physiotherapists, psychologists and social workers. Rather than *replace* these professions, the DE *facilitates* a holistic, coherent response to supports for people living with disability, primarily in their local community as opposed to a particular 'centre-based' responses.

Prior to the mid 1990s, relatively untrained personnel were often in the position of providing core services and support to people living with a disability. This often led to suboptimal outcomes and a lack of opportunity for self-determination and control over their lives for individuals and their families. Encouragingly, government policy has now moved to ensure that personnel working in the sector have at least Certificate III level training in disability and related areas. Increasingly, this has resulted in university-trained professionals providing planning, coordination and guidance around the individual and their family being in control of supports. DEs often pursue further qualifications in areas such as counselling, special education, occupational therapy, speech pathology, rehabilitation counselling, community development and/or management to meet the needs of engaging in such diverse environments.

PAUSE *for* REFLECTION ... Much work done by DEs and other disability professionals may appear similar to that of other allied health professionals such as speech pathologists, psychologists, physiotherapists and occupational therapists. Can you foresee any potential difficulties emerging due to these professional similarities? How might these issues be resolved?

The changing face of the disability profession

The work of disability professionals may range from one-to-one services and localised group supports to policy development and involvement in disability campaigns. With regard to interactions between community-based allied health and disability professionals, there is a need for disability professionals to be employed in primary health care, not just within disability support systems that deal with education, employment, community participation and daily living. The acute health care system has a clear need for community disability professionals to be involved in clinical care pathways to assist individuals with disabilities who are re-entering the community from acute or community-based health care settings.

The disability profession has to date been publicly funded at no cost to service consumers or their families. However, there have been some minimal private disability support services with costs generally covered by the individual living with disability or his/her family. The broader availability of individualised funding under the NDIS should increase opportunities for individual services and practices to emerge, giving individuals living with disability and families increased choice (Bigby 2014). There is also an opportunity under the NDIS for individuals and families to choose who provides support and assists in the achievement of goals and development of a chosen life and lifestyle. This can include support from service providers who may not have specific disability training and skills but are valued by the individual and/or their family. Although this may seem a move away from quality, it is not necessarily so. The NDIS is about ensuring that people living with disability have maximum choice and control over their lives and is likely to see the need for building capacity of such supports.

Currently, few disability professionals in Australia work in their own private practice; however, under the NDIS there are increased opportunities for DEs and disability professionals to establish private practices, with individuals living with disability and family no longer restricted to trying to access supports from already '**block-funded**' state services and having the case manager, coordinator or support worker allocated. The NDIS provides resources to the individual and/or family so they can purchase the services and supports of choice. Disability professionals can also be found working as consultants in a broad range of non-disability-specific settings including research, education, family support and sexuality and with other disadvantaged individuals such as those from refugee backgrounds. Their work is often varied and can include advocacy, individual counselling, group education, public presentations and the production of written materials such as audits, resources, articles and reports, and individual lifestyle, behaviour and skills development programs. Areas of employment for disability professionals include:

- disability-specific non-government organisations
- generic human service non-government organisations
- government and health departments
- educational organisations, such as universities and **Technical and Further Education (TAFE)** campuses, where DEs are involved in professional training and research
- local government.

Case study 12.2 outlines an example of the work of DEs and other disability professionals. The questions at the end of the case study ask you to consider how DEs and other disability and allied

Case Study 12.2

Frank is a 71-year-old individual living with intellectual disability in supported accommodation in a community setting. He has reducing vision, slightly elevated blood pressure and cholesterol levels and type II diabetes. The deterioration of his eyesight is not linked to his diabetes. For the past 40 years, Frank has walked independently and unaided approximately 5 km each way, daily, into a local shopping and tourist area where he talks to shop owners, has coffee and sells The Big Issue, a fundraising magazine. Recently, it was reported that while crossing a busy road, Frank was hit by a tram (without injury to himself or anyone on the tram). There are other reports that Frank is becoming agitated when walking on the footpath, as he is bumping into people due to his limited vision. Frank has also been seen by staff on 'days off' eating foods that are considered not in keeping with his prescribed diabetes eating plan. The disability professionals supporting Frank have attempted to reduce his walks into town but this has seen an increase in aggressive verbal outbursts at home. Frank has also refused support staff offers to drive or accompany him into town, resulting in a decision by the staff to call a case meeting involving the accommodation manager, case manager (DE), doctor, dietitian, Frank's brother (his family contact) and several staff providing day-to-day support.

Case study questions

Using your knowledge from previous chapters on models of health such as health promotion, primary care and primary health care, reflect on what constitutes an effective person-centred approach to supporting Frank to be involved in the management of his health care.

1 Who are the key stakeholders in these decisions? Should Frank be at the meeting? Should the meeting have been called with Frank's consent?

2 What are the issues and concerns that need to be discussed and considered? Whose perspective should be given priority?

3 What assumptions about Frank's ability to participate, make decisions and the impact of his disability on his health status are potentially being made by the disability and health professionals?

4 How might disability and allied health professionals work together to create a person-centred approach to assisting Frank to remain active and involved in the community with minimal negative impact on his health?

5 Discuss the potential risk in cases like Frank's that disability and health professionals can use 'duty of care' as a new form of 'institutionalising' people living with disability in the community.

health professionals might best work towards assisting people living with disability to access the daily activity support and health care they need to live a productive, valued and healthy life.

Responsibility for disability health care – specialised or generic services, segregated or community?

There is ongoing debate as to whether people living with disability should have specialised segregated health care services or whether they should access mainstream generic community-based services. The 2013 *NDIS Act* and current government policy is a move away from specialised disability services and for people living with disability and their supports to access mainstream services with access to resources via an individualised package.

PAUSE *for* REFLECTION ...

Should people living with disability access disability-specific health services or generic health services?

What added pressure does accessing generic health services put on allied health professionals? How may they need to adjust their practice to accommodate people living with disability accessing their services?

Decisions about health and lifestyle are impacted on by economic, social and systems issues combining to affect the well-being of people living with disability. The cost of healthy foods, medications, therapies and support to be active are difficult to afford on a disability support pension. Although risk factors for a range of health conditions are higher than in typical community members, individuals living with disability are often not targeted in primary health campaigns on healthy lifestyle (Keane 1996). In addition, individuals living with disability often have to receive support from a myriad of allied health professionals all with discipline-specific jargon and strategies, and not always aware of strategies, equipment or advice being suggested by another and how this advice can contradict or compete for limited time and fiscal resources. This, along with the dominant paradigms apparent in the Australian health system around curing illness and the promotion of lifestyle changes with emphasis on the individual being responsible for their own health, can be challenging to individuals living with disability who have limited economic and social resources. Also to be considered is the impact on health of carers and significant others supporting individuals living with disability. As both health and disability support resources become stretched, the negative impacts on the health of the non-paid supports in an individual's life are emerging rapidly (AIHW 2004).

Disability professionals have much to contribute to provision of quality health services. Concepts such as consumer self-determination, person-centred approaches and consumer contribution to planning have been part of disability research and practice for over 25 years. A further shift from multidisciplinary approaches to better-developed collaboration, interprofessional practice and a transdisciplinary approach is needed. In a transdisciplinary approach, allied health professionals move beyond traditional disciplinary boundaries to share skills and knowledge with individuals, caregivers and other team members as facilitators of services, acting as consultants providing indirect services rather than just delivering therapies (Cloninger 2004). This approach has proven effective and it supports the philosophy of person-centred approaches to services. However, the principles and practice of interprofessional and transdisciplinary approaches need to continue to spread through disability support and health care systems.

The NDIS Quality and Safeguards Commission is an independent agency established to improve the quality and safety of NDIS supports and services and it will have implications for practice for all health and disability supports. The Commission aims to regulate the NDIS market, provide national consistency, promote safety and quality services, resolve problems and identify areas for improvement. It brings together, under a nationally consistent approach that applies across Australia regulations, education opportunities, safeguarding functions and regulatory powers around the use of restrictive practices which can include medication, behaviour support strategies, restricting movement and locking doors. Details of the codes or conduct, policies, legislation and rules can be found at https://www.ndiscommission.gov.au/about/legislation-rules-policies. It is critical that all health and human services professionals are aware of and are familiar with these rules and regulations.

Summary

In this chapter, we have outlined key information about supporting people living with disability to navigate disability support in the context of the Australian health care system.

The complexities around people living with disability accessing health care and their daily support needs have been briefly described. In a health and human service environment with limited funding and resources, competition for resources among interest groups representing both the dominant medically oriented clinical services and the broader public health groups continues to be an issue of the health system. The complexities of the relationship between disability and the health care system, especially considering the changing environment with the NDIS, will necessitate the consideration of how disability and health care services manage the care of people living with disability (Department of the Prime Minister and Cabinet 2014).

The roles of disability professionals have been defined within the health care system. These roles are diverse and are undertaken in various settings in the health care system from clinical treatment of patients to primary health care and health promotion advocacy work.

The status of the disability profession in Australia has been described, and although the disability profession is still under-recognised it has growing influence within allied health and human service sectors.

Review Questions

1 What is the NDIS and why is it significant for the health care of people living with disability?

2 Identify health and human services organisations in your local area that employ professionals with an understanding of disability.

3 List the diversity of roles that are undertaken, or could be undertaken, by DEs and disability professionals in those organisations.

4 Outline what structural changes would need to be introduced into Medicare to allow DEs and other disability professionals to work with GPs and other allied health professionals in providing multidisciplinary primary care.

5 Describe your approach to working under the 2013 *NDIS Act* in supporting a person living with disability around an emergency, short-term or long-term chronic health care situation. What do you need to understand in order to approach this in a person-centred way? Who and or what information and resources might assist? What do you understand your responsibilities are under the NDIS Quality and Safeguarding Commission legislation and rules?

References

Australian Bureau of Statistics (ABS), 2015. Disability, ageing and carers, Australia: summary of findings, 2015. Cat. no. 4430.0. ABS, Canberra.

Australian Institute of Health and Welfare (AIHW), 2004. Carers in Australia: assisting frail older people and people with a disability. Cat. no. AGE 41 (Aged Care Series). AIHW, Canberra.

Australian Institute of Health and Welfare (AIHW), 2008. Disability in Australia: intellectual disability. AIHW bulletin no. 67. Cat. no. AUS 110. AIHW, Canberra.

Australian Institute of Health and Welfare (AIHW), 2010. Health of Australians with disability: health status and risk factors. AIHW bulletin no. 83. Cat. no. AUS 132. AIHW, Canberra.

Australian Institute of Health and Welfare (AIHW), 2017. Life expectancy and disability in Australia: expected years living with and without disability. Cat. no. DIS 66. AIHW, Canberra.

Australian Institute of Health and Welfare (AIHW), 2018. Australia's health 2018. Cat. no. AUS 221. AIHW, Canberra. https://www.aihw.gov.au/reports/australias-health/australias-health-2018/contents/table-of-contents.

Bacchi, C., 2016. Problematizations in health policy: questioning how "problems" are constituted in policies. SAGE Open 6(2), 2158244016653986.

Bigby, C., 2014. The NDIS – a quantum leap towards realising social rights for people with intellectual disability. In: Rice, S., Day, A. (Eds.), Social Work in the Shadow of the Law. Federation Press, Alexandria, NSW, pp. 305–321.

Bonyhady, B., 2014. Tides of change: the NDIS and its journey to transform disability support. Australian Journal of Psychosocial Rehabilitation Summer, 7–9.

Bottroff, V., Grantley, J., Brown, R., I, 2000. Tertiary education for professionals in the field of disability studies: roads of progress and crossroads. Int. J. Pract. Approaches Disabil. 24(1), 18–24.

Carey, G., Malbon, E., Reeders, D., et al., 2017. Redressing or entrenching social and health inequities through policy implementation? Examining personalised budgets through the Australian National Disability Insurance Scheme. Int. J. Equity Health 16, 192. doi:10.1186/s12939-017-0682-z.

Cloninger, C.J., 2004. Designing collaborative educational services. In: Orelove, F.P., Sobsey, P.D., Silberman, R.K. (Eds.), Educating Children With Multiple Disabilities: A Collaborative Approach, fourth ed. Paul H Brookes, Baltimore, pp. 1–29.

Department of the Prime Minister and Cabinet, 2014. Reform of the Federation White Paper, roles and responsibilities in health. Issue paper 3, December. https://federation.dpmc.gov.au/sites/default/files/issues-paper/Health_Issues_Paper.pdf.

Douglas, J., Bigby, C., Knox, L., et al., 2015. Factors that underpin the delivery of effective decision-making support for people with cognitive disability. Res. Pract. Intellect. Dev. Disabil. 2, 37–44.

Ellison, C.J., White, A.L., Chapman, L., 2011. Avoiding institutional outcomes for older adults living with disability: the use of community-based aged care supports. J. Intellect. Dev. Disabil. 36 (3), 175–183.

Emerson, E., 2005. Underweight, obesity and exercise among adults with intellectual disabilities in supported accommodation in Northern England. J. Intellect. Disabil. Res. 49, 134–143.

Ervin, D.A., Hennen, B., Merrick, J., et al., 2014. Healthcare for persons with intellectual and developmental disability in the community. Front. Public Health 2 (Jul), art–no. 83.

Foubert, J., Levecque, K., Van Rossem, R., et al., 2014. Do welfare regimes influence the association between disability and self-perceived health? A multilevel analysis of 57 countries. Soc. Sci. Med. 117, 10–17.

Goodley, D., 2014. Dis/ability Studies. Theorising Disablism and Ableism. Routledge, New York.

Government of Western Australia, 2013. Disability Services Commission, individualised funding policy. http://www.disability.wa.gov.au/Global/Publications/Reform/Procurement%20reform/Individualised%20Funding%20Policy.pdf.

Keane, S., 1996. Health medication and consent to intervention. In: Annison, J., Jenkinson, J., Sparrow, W., et al. (Eds.), Disability a Guide for Health Professionals. Nelson, Melbourne, pp. 307–335.

Lante, K., Stancliffe, R.J., Bauman, A., et al., 2014. Embedding sustainable physical activities into the everyday lives of adults with intellectual disabilities: a randomized controlled trial. BMC Public Health 14, 1038.

Mallett, R., Runswick-Cole, K., 2014. Approaching Disability. Critical Issues and Perspectives. Routledge, New York.

McKeon, M., Slevin, E., Taggart, L., 2013. A pilot survey of physical activity in men with an intellectual disability. J. Intellect. Disabil. 17 (12), 157–167.

Nankervis, K., 2006. Planning for support. In: Dempsey, I., Nankervis, K. (Eds.), Community Disability Services: An Evidence-Based Approach to Practice. UNSW Press, Sydney, pp. 110–144.

National Disability Insurance Agency, 2014. 2013–2014 Annual Report. NDIA, Canberra. https://www.ndis.gov.au/search?keywords=2013–2014+annual+report.+.

National Disability Insurance Scheme Act 2013 (Cwlth). http://www.comlaw.gov.au/Details/C2013A00020.

Productivity Commission, 2011. Disability Care and Support. Productivity Commission, Canberra. Productivity Commission Inquiry Report no. 54.

Productivity Commission, 2017. National Disability Insurance (NDIS) Costs, Study Report. Productivity Commission, Canberra.

Springgay, M., Sutton, P., 2014. Psychosocial disability: the urgent need for reform in assessment and care. Australian Journal of Psychosocial Rehabilitation Summer, 16–19.

Stanish, H.I., Temple, V.A., Frey, G.C., 2006. Health-promoting physical activity of adults with mental retardation. Ment. Retard. Dev. Disabil. Res. Rev. 12, 13–21.

Stuifbergen, A.K., Becker, H.A., Ingalsbe, K., et al., 1990. Perception of health among adults with disabilities. Health Values 14 (2), 18–26.

Williamson, H.J., Contreras, G.M., Rodriguez, E.S., et al., 2017. Health care access for adults with intellectual and developmental disabilities: a scoping review. OTJR (Thorofare N J) 37 (4), 227–236.

World Health Organization (WHO), 1946. Preamble to the Constitution of the World Health Organization (WHO) as adopted by the International Health Conference, New York, 19–22 June, 1946; signed on 22 July 1946 by the representatives of 61 States (Official Records of the World Health Organization, no. 2, p. 100) and entered into force on 7 April 1948. WHO, Geneva. https://www.who.int/about/who-we-are/constitution.

World Health Organization (WHO), 2014. Disability and health. Factsheet no. 352. http://www.who.int/mediacentre/factsheets/fs352/en/.

Further Reading

Australian Government, 2018. National Disability Insurance Scheme (Quality Indicators) Guidelines 2018. Australian Government, Canberra. https://www.legislation.gov.au/Details/F2018N00041.

Bigby, C., 2003. Ageing With a Lifelong Disability. A Guide to Practice, Program and Policy Issues for Human Services Professionals. Jessica Kingsley, London.

Brown, I., Percy, M., 2007. A Comprehensive Guide to Intellectual and Developmental Disabilities. Paul H. Brookes, Baltimore, MD.

Browning, M., Bigby, C., Douglas, J., 2014. Supported decision making: understanding how its conceptual link to legal capacity is influencing the development of practice. Res. Pract. Intellect. Dev. Disabil. 1 (1), 34–45.

Crozier, M., Muenchberger, H., Colley, J., et al., 2013. The disability self-direction movement: considering the benefits and challenges for an Australian response. Aust. J. Soc. Issues 48, 455–472.

O'Brien, E., Rosenbloom, L. (Eds.), 2009. Developmental Disability and Ageing. Mac Keith Press, Cambridge.

Queensland Government, 2017. Queensland health guide to informed decision-making in healthcare, second ed. http://www.health.qld.gov.au/consent/documents/ic-guide.pdf.

VicHealth, 2012. Disability and Health Inequalities in Australia Research Summary: Addressing the Social and Economic Determinants of Mental and Physical Health. VicHealth, Victoria. Publication no. P-053-HI.

Online Resources

Developmental Educators Australia Inc. (DEAI): provides information on DEs and promoting the profession to the general public: http://www.deai.com.au.

Department of Social Services: has produced a series of short videos explaining the National Disability Advocacy Program. These videos can be viewed at: https://www.youtube.com/playlist?list=PLrjsEoziQ mWSJbkTp28wys7MWLBvBcVXH.

NDIS: provides updated information on the NDIS and its roll-out, inclusive of set prices for supports; information is available for not only for people currently involved in the scheme but also for other people living with disability, family and carers, providers and the community: http://www.ndis.gov.au/.

National Disability Services (NDS): provides information, representation and policy advice; promotes and advances services which support people with all forms of disability to participate in all domains of life: http://www.nds.org.au.

People with Disability: provides useful information and links around disability and human rights, the social model, advocacy, legislation and disability-specific organisations: http://www.pwd.org.au.

Reports on services provided under the National Disability Agreement: information about people who used disability support services and the agencies and outlets that provided services. Key trends in service provision are examined: http://www.aihw.gov.au/publication-detail/?id=60129547855.

CHAPTER 13

Australian workers' compensation systems

Alex Collie and Tyler Lane

Key learning outcomes

When you finish this chapter you should be able to:

- describe the Australian system of compensation for work-related injury and illness
- understand the interaction between Australia's workers' compensation systems and the health care system
- describe the positive and negative impacts that involvement in compensation processes can have on health and well-being
- understand the impact that work and the employment relationship has on recovery and return to work following work-related injury and illness.

Key terms and abbreviations

benefits
claim
claims management organisation
claims manager
general practitioner (GP)
iatrogenic nature
independent medical assessments (IMAs)
insurance
occupational rehabilitation
regulator
return to work (RTW)
social contract
social determinants of health (SDH)
work disability
work disability duration

Introduction to work and health

Work injury and illness are substantial public health issues. Workers' compensation systems are the primary means by which Australian governments have chosen to address the recovery and **occupational rehabilitation** of injured and ill workers. Although Australia has a complex federated system of workers' compensation systems, these systems share some common underlying principles and approaches. There is substantial interaction between workers' compensation and public and private health care systems.

There is a growing body of evidence that employment and safe work are determinants of health (Marmot 2005; Waddell & Burton 2006). There is also a growing body of evidence that **return to work (RTW)** after injury or illness can promote recovery (Rueda et al. 2012). Despite this, disability due to work injury remains a significant economic and health burden both in Australia and internationally. Prevention of **work disability**, promotion of RTW and effective management of workplace injury are central mandates of Australia's workers' compensation systems.

Estimates of the burden of workplace injury and illness in Australia demonstrate the significance of the problem, both in health and in economic terms. In 2013–14, there were nearly one-quarter of a million work-related injury claims for absence from work that were accepted by the nation's workers' compensation jurisdictions (Collie et al. 2016). The direct and indirect costs of work-related injury and illness for 2012–13 were estimated to be in excess of (AU)$60 billion (Safe Work Australia (SWA) 2016).

Societal factors play a major role in determining the recovery and RTW outcomes of injured workers. For example, the strength and quality of an injured worker's relationship with their employer has been shown to be a major determinant of RTW following work-related injury or illness.

Australian workers' compensation systems

Australia has a complex and fragmented system of workers' compensation (Case study 13.1). In total there are 11 main workers' compensation systems in operation across the nation (Table 13.1). Each of the eight Australian states and territories has developed its own workers' compensation system, and there are also three Commonwealth systems. Each of these systems has adopted policy settings and practices that attempt to maximise RTW and the recovery of those injured, while also ensuring their ongoing financial sustainability. These systems operate under an '**insurance** model', with premiums collected from employers based on the risk of work injury occurring at any given employer/workplace. Some higher-risk industries attract higher premiums (e.g. forestry, mining), whereas lower-risk industries generally attract lower premiums (e.g. the community and public sectors). The systems rely on substantial investments that seek to cover the current and future costs of compensation (i.e. the outstanding liabilities) with the objective of achieving full funding (for their investments and assets to be sufficient to pay for all future costs of the compensation system). The systems thus operate within relatively tight financial constraints.

Each of the main systems is established under state, territory or Commonwealth legislation. There is substantial variability between the systems with respect to their structure, coverage, benefits

Case Study 13.1

Introduction of Workers' Compensation in Australia

Workers' compensation legislation preceded many of the national health care reforms by decades. The first formal workers' compensation system to be enacted was in South Australia in 1900, followed by Western Australia (1902), Queensland (1905) and Tasmania (1910). These statutes were based on similar approaches in the UK and New Zealand. These early compensation systems prescribed the amounts of compensation that employers had to pay if an employee suffered 'personal injury by accident arising out of and in the course of' their employment. They did not remove the right of employees to sue their employers (as modern workers' compensation legislation does except under specific circumstances), although an employee could not both recover damages from a court and receive workers' compensation. The introduction of these systems reflects an underlying, and at that time unstated, proposition that work and working circumstances are an important social determinant of health. The legislation was specifically designed to ensure that, in the event of a worker being harmed in the course of work, the employer should provide compensation. Since the late 20th century it has been increasingly recognised that work, and being in work, is positively associated with health status. The **social determinants of health (SDH)** remind us that work and employment facilitate improved health in many ways, for instance by providing supportive social networks and income to pay for life's necessities, health care and other needs. Modern workers' compensation systems seek to minimise the dislocation from the workplace (period of time off work) and maximise the health status of the injured person. This is both to ensure that the optimal health state is achieved and to reduce the costs of health care provision to injured workers.

provided, claims management practices and, in some cases, interactions with health care and legal and financial systems. The legislation defines the limits of each system.

These financial and legal structures within the workers' compensation systems mean that, as well as having important public health objectives, Australia's workers' compensation systems can equally be considered from a financial or a legal systems perspective.

Workers' compensation is a good example of a **social contract**. Before the implementation of workers' compensation arrangements, an injured worker's only means of receiving compensation was to sue their employer for negligence at common law. With the onset of workers' compensation, injured workers have foregone the right to sue their employers in return for the provision of health care, wage replacement and other benefits provided by the compensation systems.

In addition to workers' compensation, Australia maintains a variety of other systems of income support for people with health conditions that affect their ability to work. These include life insurance, motor vehicle accident compensation and social security. The most recent estimates demonstrate that more than 750,000 Australians of working age with health-related work disability will receive income support from one of these systems annually, and the total direct cost of income replacement alone is estimated at $37.2 billion (Collie et al. 2018). Workers' compensation represents a substantial component of this overall 'systems of systems'.

TABLE 13.1 WORKERS' COMPENSATION REGULATORS IN AUSTRALIA, COVERAGE OF EMPLOYED WORKFORCE (2015–16) AND NUMBER OF SERIOUS CLAIMS WITH 1 WEEK OR MORE INCAPACITY (2014–15)

Jurisdiction	Authority/ regulator	Employees covered by workers' compensation	Employees covered by self-insurance	Claims ≥1 week incapacity
New South Wales	State Insurance Regulatory Authority (SIRA)	3,055,800	790,000 (approx.)	33,800
Victoria	WorkSafe Vic	2,607,300	147,000 (approx.)	21,970
Queensland	WorkCover Qld	1,979,580	163,165	24,710
Western Australia	WorkCover WA	1,243,900	104,637	11,640
South Australia	ReturnToWork SA	500,000 (approx.)	Data not collected	7950
Tasmania	WorkCover Tas	207,200	10,488 (FTE)	2480
Northern Territory	NT WorkSafe	120,000	4999	1080
Australian Capital Territory	WorkSafe ACT	136,000 (private sector approx.)	3000 (approx.)	1720
Commonwealth	Comcare/ Seacare/DVA	375,954	167,726	1900

FTE=full-time equivalent.

Source: Data drawn from the Australian workers' compensation statistics published by Safe Work Australia (SWA 2017, 2018)

System structure and operation

Each workers' compensation system is regulated by a government authority. The **regulator** is responsible for ensuring that the system operates within the boundaries of the relevant legislation, and ultimately for achieving the objectives of the workers' compensation legislation. Employers and workers are often considered the 'clients' of workers' compensation systems, as they are the parties involved in, and responsible for, the RTW and rehabilitation process. Management of compensation **claims** is a core function of the systems, but is achieved in different ways in different jurisdictions. Some systems have 'in-house' claims management functions whereby the regulatory authority also conducts the claims management, whereas other systems outsource the claims management function to private insurers or other claims management providers.

The systems share many common features. They generally provide coverage for employees of working age within the relevant jurisdiction. Many common work-related physical conditions are eligible for compensation, including acute traumatic injuries and chronic or gradual-onset conditions (e.g. chronic lower-back pain). Musculoskeletal conditions are the most common condition dealt with in Australian workers' compensation systems. Some diseases are also compensable, and each jurisdiction maintains a list of occupational diseases for which workers' compensation may be paid. Most jurisdictions also accept 'psychological injury' or mental health claims, mainly due to workplace stress. However, there are substantial variations between jurisdictions in this area, and the process for demonstrating eligibility for a stress or psychological injury claim is qualitatively different (and usually more difficult to meet) than those for more apparent physical injuries. A summary of the regulators in each Australian jurisdiction, the number of employees covered, and number of 'serious' workers' compensation claims (exceeding 1 week of work incapacity) is provided in Table 13.1.

Benefits or payments

Benefits are provided to eligible workers with a work-related injury or illness, regardless of fault. Benefits or payments provided by workers' compensation systems typically include health care expenses (medical and hospital costs, fees of allied health practitioners) and income replacement payments to injured workers for the period of time they are away from work. In many cases, systems will also pay the costs associated with occupational or vocational rehabilitation and retraining. Some injured workers with a permanent injury or disability may also be eligible to receive lump-sum payments.

Health care and other medical expenses are typically provided on the basis that they are 'reasonable and necessary' as determined by the claims management organisation. Income replacement payments are usually capped at a percentage of the worker's pre-injury earnings. Some jurisdictions have time limits on the duration for which benefits will be provided (e.g. 130 weeks in Victoria), whereas others have no such time limit (e.g. Comcare).

Changes to benefit levels or to the maximum allowable duration of benefits are relatively common. For example, a maximum benefit time limit of 5 years was introduced in the New South Wales workers' compensation scheme in 2012, whereas the South Australian workers' compensation system restricted benefits to a maximum of 2 years in 2014.

PAUSE *for* REFLECTION …

The Australian government provides an annual overview of the performance of the nation's work health and safety and workers' compensation systems. This includes analysis of injury rates, work disability duration and costs of compensation in the major workers' compensation jurisdictions. The annual *Comparative performance monitoring* report is available at the Safe Work Australia website (www.safework.gov.au).

Compare the return to work rates between different jurisdictions. Examine the differences in outcomes.

Process

All jurisdictions now place substantial emphasis on **returning to work** as a primary goal of rehabilitation. Most require employers to develop RTW plans for injured workers, and require injured workers to meet certain obligations such as participation in RTW planning and attending assessments, and to make reasonable efforts to return to work.

The process of making a workers' compensation claim is largely consistent between jurisdictions. Workers who have incurred an injury at work and are intending to make a workers' compensation claim must provide their employer, and in some cases their insurer, with information about their injury. This information is captured on a 'claim form', which is usually paper based, and must usually be accompanied by a medical certificate from a general practitioner (GP) or other qualified medical practitioner. The employer must then notify the claims management organisation of the claim within a specified time, and that organisation usually has a period of time to determine whether the claim is eligible for workers' compensation benefits under the legislation, and to accept or deny the claim.

If the claim is accepted, the injured person becomes eligible for the benefits described earlier; however, these are usually provided on an as-needs basis, with the claims management organisation having policies and work practices in place to determine the need for certain benefits.

In many cases, an RTW plan is developed that involves the employer, the worker and the claims management organisation, and usually health care professionals. The requirements for RTW planning vary somewhat between jurisdictions, and different approaches may be taken depending on the severity of the worker's injury and / or the duration for which they have been away from work (**work disability duration**). RTW plans usually include a list of actions to be taken to enable a return to work, and the person responsible for each action. They may include:

♦ suitable duties being offered, including alternative duties or changes in duties
♦ health care and rehabilitation requirements during the period away from work and while returning to work
♦ modifications to the working environment, including hours of work, changes to work tasks and changes to the physical work environment
♦ timeframes for returning to work, often including a graduated re-entry to the workplace
♦ an approach to monitoring and evaluating progress.

In most jurisdictions, employers have legal obligations with respect to the return to work. These include obligations to:

♦ consult with the worker and other involved parties, such as medical or rehabilitation practitioners
♦ develop or be involved in the development of an RTW plan
♦ provide suitable duties for injured workers who have some work capacity.

Interaction with the health care system

Workers' compensation systems purchase health care services on behalf of their clients (injured workers and employers) from the public and private health care systems. They do so within certain policy settings and using processes and procedures intended to ensure that workers receive appropriate treatment and rehabilitation in a cost-effective manner. With the exception of acute/critical care, the claims management organisation makes the decisions regarding funding of health care for injured workers with accepted workers' compensation claims. Health care professionals are considered to have an important role in the rehabilitation and RTW process, as an advisor to the worker, the claims manager and the employer regarding reasonable and necessary treatment. The claims management function is the primary interface between the workers' compensation and health care systems.

Claims management

Claims management (also known as injury management or case management) is a critical component in all workers' compensation systems. **Claims managers** have a decision-making role regarding payments for treatment, income replacement and the provision of health care and other services to the injured person. There is now substantial evidence that certain approaches to claims management can have positive impacts on recovery (e.g. Arnetz et al. 2003) and that other approaches can substantially impede recovery or lead to exacerbation of mental health concerns in some injured people (Kilgour et al. 2015a; Lippel 2007). Effective and efficient claims management is also considered critical to maintaining the financial viability of the injury compensation systems, and ensuring a positive experience for injured persons and employers engaging with the system. There is relatively little research evidence regarding the features of an effective claims management approach. However, it is commonly accepted in the sector that a holistic approach that engages the multiple parties involved in worker rehabilitation is desirable, with a focus on engaging health care providers, employers and the injured person in developing common treatment and occupational goals.

Claims management within workers' compensation systems is distinct from case management in related systems such as health and disability services. Claims managers act for, or on behalf of, the compensation authority or insurer, and have a dual objective of facilitating the recovery of the injured person while minimising the costs of rehabilitation for the insurer. They do not represent the injured person in their interactions with health care and social policy agencies.

A recent Australian qualitative study identified that claims managers experienced their role as highly stressful, with multiple competing priorities from within their own organisations and from external parties (Newnam et al. 2014). These findings are consistent with anecdotal reports of a high level of staff turnover in claims management organisations (up to 29% per annum) and challenges in embedding good practice and appropriate training and education for those at the 'front line'.

There are many different approaches to claims management within the workers' compensation sector in Australia. At a macro level, some jurisdictions outsource claims management services to private sector insurers; others provide claims management services directly. At a more micro level, there is substantial variation between jurisdictions and between claims management organisations with respect to critical issues such as identification of complex cases (or claims 'triage'), education and training of claims managers, segmentation of cases according to complexity or client needs, and use of independent medical examiners to aid decision-making (Kosny et al. 2013).

Treatment versus assessment

Workers' compensation systems utilise health care services for two distinct purposes. The primary role of health care practitioners in the workers' compensation systems is to provide diagnostic, treatment and rehabilitation services to injured workers. Combined, Australia's workers' compensation systems spend more than $2 billion annually on payments for health care services. The most common services are provided by medical practitioners, including GPs and physical therapists. Other major categories include psychology, occupational therapy and rehabilitation counsellors.

Many Australian workers' compensation systems provide guidance to health care providers about their expectations regarding what constitutes reasonable treatment. These include policies outlining what services the workers' compensation system will (and at times will not) pay. Emerging from Victoria, but now in place in many jurisdictions, there is also the *Clinical framework for the provision of health services* (Transport Accident Commission and WorkSafe Victoria 2012). This framework outlines a set of five guiding principles for the delivery of health services in workers' compensation and motor vehicle accident compensation systems. The principles have the support of peak health care practitioner groups, and focus on measuring the progress of treatment to determine effectiveness, adopting a biopsychosocial approach to treatment, focusing on empowering the injured person to manage their injury and their recovery, developing and implementing treatment goals focused on optimising function, participation in activities and return to work, and using an evidence-based approach to treatment.

A secondary, but important, role for health care providers in workers' compensation systems is in the assessment of injured workers. Medical and allied health care practitioners may also perform the role of an independent medical assessor. These assessments are used by the claims management organisation as a means of reviewing an injured worker's injury status and progress throughout the claims process. Such assessment may be conducted to establish the work-relatedness of the injury, to identify treatment needs, to establish a worker's functional capacity for RTW purposes, or as a means of determining the degree of impairment once maximum medical progress has been achieved (Busse et al. 2014). These assessments can serve to reinforce the adversarial nature of the workers' compensation system, as assessments can be requested by both claims management organisations and lawyers (Busse et al. 2014) – at times with the purpose of disputing the other party's assessment.

The reliability of these assessments in fairly determining the existence of a health condition or the degree of impairment has been questioned. Typically, assessments are completed in one consultation and in most cases have no therapeutic purpose (Lax 2004). It has been reported that the vulnerability of the injured worker can be accentuated during assessment, and that the requirement to demonstrate illness symptoms to assessors may fuel the **iatrogenic nature** of the process (Tsushima et al. 1996). Numerous recent studies demonstrate that injured workers can find these **independent medical assessments (IMAs)** stressful, and that they can exacerbate underlying mental health conditions or lead to their onset (Grant et al. 2014; Kilgour et al. 2015a).

PAUSE
for
REFLECTION
...

Many Australian workers' compensation systems request that health care providers practise according to the *Clinical framework for the provision of health services*. The framework outlines a set of five guiding principles for the delivery of health services in workers' compensation and motor vehicle accident compensation systems. It is available at: http://www.vwa.vic.gov.au/forms-and-publications/forms-and-publications/clinical-framework-for-the-delivery-of-health-services (Transport Accident Commission and WorkSafe Victoria 2012).

Take time to review the framework. This is an attempt to influence clinical practice to conform to evidence-based principles in the specific context of workers' compensation.

Factors affecting health care provider engagement in workers' compensation

There is a growing body of evidence demonstrating that engagement in workers' compensation systems can affect the interaction between health care providers and their patients (injured workers) (Kilgour et al. 2015a). Although involvement in workers' compensation has the benefit of providing low-income workers with access to health care services that may otherwise be unaffordable, a number of negative consequences have been reported.

A systematic review found some injured workers experience bias by health care providers against workers' compensation clients, in some cases through declining to provide services. This was attributed to the providers' frustration with compensation system administrative demands, and delays with approvals and payment (Kilgour et al. 2015b).

Some conditions are less visible than others, including mental health and some musculoskeletal conditions such as back pain, which can contribute to detrimental interactions. In such cases, determining whether a condition is work-related – and thus eligible for compensation – is difficult. Without obvious physical manifestations, it is harder for injured workers to establish they have been injured. In arguing their case, injured workers must establish that they are unwell, which can contribute to the self-perception of being injured and impede future progress. Such workers are often long-term clients who show little improvement. They can be clinically challenging and may require lengthy consultations to address multiple health concerns, and can represent a significant administrative load for a busy health care provider, which may prevent them from seeing less-demanding clients.

System processes mean that claims managers can contest the health care provider's recommendations for treatment or medications. This can lead to frustration among health care providers, who may view this as disregard of their professional training and expertise.

In Canadian workers' compensation jurisdictions, similar impacts of claims management practices on health care providers have been observed (Kosny et al. 2011) and reported as resulting in a breakdown of trust between health care providers and the compensation system. This can have 'flow-on' effects to the injured people treated by those providers. These findings have been supported by studies of Australian GPs operating within the Victoria workers' compensation system (Brijnath et al. 2014).

System impact on worker health and well-being

Somewhat counter-intuitively, those who receive compensation for injury or disease have poorer injury recovery and RTW than those with matched injuries who do not receive compensation (Harris et al. 2005). Although most injured workers recover and return to work promptly, there is a minority with complex injuries whose claims are prolonged (Waddell & Burton 2006). Some research has proposed that injured workers may purposefully delay recovery owing to financial considerations and other secondary gains (Zelle et al. 2005); yet other research has suggested that the compensation process itself can exacerbate underlying health conditions or be an independent cause of disability (Kilgour et al. 2015b). Longer-term claimants who have delayed recovery with injuries that are not readily seen nor easily diagnosed are more likely to experience stigma and disbelief, attend multiple IMAs and subsequently develop adversarial relationships with claims management organisations and health care providers (Kilgour et al. 2015a, 2015b).

A number of Australian studies shed light on the mechanism by which this system-generated disability occurs. A systematic review of injured workers' experiences in workers' compensation systems has identified that case management practices can negatively influence the psychosocial function and mental health outcomes of injured workers. This review of 14 published qualitative studies identified that, in some instances, claims management practices contribute to a cyclical and pathogenic interaction between the compensation system and the injured person that can reduce access to health care, diminish social engagement and restrict the injured person's ability to participate in productive work (Kilgour et al. 2015b).

A long-term cohort study involving a group of seriously injured workers across three Australian states (Victoria, New South Wales and South Australia) identified that stressful claims experiences were highly prevalent, and that there were strong associations between stressful experiences during the claims process and poorer long-term mental and physical health and quality of life (Grant et al. 2014). Of note, this study identified a small number of specific claims management practices that those injured found particularly stressful.

Variation in policy between Australian workers' compensation systems appears to contribute to system level differences, from the length of the claim lodgement process (Lane et al. 2018a) to the duration of disability (Collie et al. 2015). Research from around the United States has identified a number of policy variations that may increase duration of disability, including longer retroactive periods (number of days since injury before a worker is eligible to claim), fee schedules (maximum reimbursement amount that a provider can claim) and choice in health care provider (Shraim et al. 2015).

The employment relationship – an important social determinant of health in injured workers

There are a number of accepted conceptual models of work disability that attempt to explain the biological, psychological and social factors that affect recovery from work injury. These include the biopsychosocial model of lower-back pain and disability, the WHO International Classification of Function, Disability and Health (WHO-ICF), the Institute of Medicine / National Research Council model of musculoskeletal disorders in the workplace and the Sherbrooke model of work disability prevention (Costa-Black et al. 2013). These models share some common features including an emphasis on the importance of social factors in work injury recovery and the prevention of ongoing disability.

The working environment and the injured worker's relationship with the employer are recognised as important social factors that influence recovery and RTW. Employer influence on injured worker outcomes starts as early as the moment of injury. Supervisors who respond to worker injury with sympathy, concern or support improve the likelihood of RTW (Jetha et al. 2018). High levels of social and supervisor support in the workplace have been associated with a reduction in work disability among those injured, whereas problems with colleagues and social isolation at work are associated with an increase in work disability (Shaw et al. 2013). In all of Australia's states and territories, employers are obliged to assist injured workers through the RTW process through interventions such as developing a RTW plan or providing a RTW coordinator, both of which can improve the likelihood of RTW (Gray et al. 2019; Lane et al. 2018b). Some of our recent work on this provides an interesting window on how workplace interventions could be targeted based on injured worker prognosis: the functional intervention (RTW plan) improved RTW outcomes in only shorter-duration claims, whereas the psychosocial intervention (low-stress interactions with a RTW coordinator) improved them only in longer-duration claims (Lane et al. 2018b). This aligns with existing research on the changing needs of injured workers over the course of the duration of a claim; injury factors such as severity are more important earlier, whereas psychosocial factors become increasingly important to RTW as the claim persists (Krause et al. 2001).

Within the working environment, there is a complex set of factors that can operate to either enhance or decrease a given individual's recovery or level of function. For example, job demands such as being involved in heavy physical work, being employed in a 'blue-collar' occupation and self-reported levels of high job stress and short job tenure (<2 years) have been reported as increasing the level of work disability (Shaw et al. 2013). The organisation of work and workplace support factors can also affect recovery.

The importance of workplace factors in recovery has led many RTW and work disability prevention intervention studies to focus on modifying workplace factors in efforts to improve RTW outcomes for injured workers. A recent systematic review concluded that workplace-based interventions had better evidence for effectiveness if they were multi-domain (i.e. accompanied by concurrent health- or communication-focused components) (Cullen et al. 2018).

This finding demonstrates that multiple factors, including the workplace, need to be addressed concurrently to improve RTW outcomes and reduce work disability in those injured at work.

Summary

- Work is good for health, and return to work can facilitate recovery after injury or illness. Prevention of work disability, promotion of RTW and effective management of workplace injury are central mandates of Australia's workers' compensation systems.
- Australia has a complex network of workers' compensation systems that provide health care and income replacement coverage for injured Australian workers.
- Benefits (payments for services) are provided to eligible workers and employers with a work-related injury or illness regardless of fault, and may include health care expenses, income replacement payments, costs of vocational rehabilitation and retraining, and in some cases lump-sum payments for workers with a permanent injury.
- All Australian workers' compensation jurisdictions now place substantial emphasis on returning to work as a primary goal of rehabilitation. Most jurisdictions encourage development of RTW plans for injured workers that identify the roles and responsibilities of employers, workers and health care providers in the RTW process.
- Claims management (also known as injury management or case management) is a critical component in all workers' compensation systems. Claims managers have a decision-making role regarding payments for treatment, income replacement and provision of health care and other services to the injured person.
- Workers' compensation systems utilise health care services for two distinct purposes. The primary role of health care practitioners is to provide diagnostic, treatment and rehabilitation services to injured workers. However, health care practitioners may also be requested to undertake independent medical assessments to assess workers' eligibility for system benefits or their work capacity.
- There is a body of evidence demonstrating that engagement in workers' compensation processes can affect the interaction between health care providers and their patients (injured workers), and that this can in some cases lead to slower recovery and RTW for the injured person.
- The working environment and the injured worker's relationship with their employer are important social factors that influence recovery and RTW.

Review Questions

1 How many workers' compensation systems are in operation in Australia?
2 What roles might health care providers be asked to undertake in workers' compensation systems?
3 Engagement in work and employment are important social determinants of health. How would being off work affect the health of an injured worker?

4 Workers' compensation system processes and procedures can have a major impact on health outcomes for injured workers in Australia. Can you identify the mechanisms by which these impacts might arise?

5 Considering Tuohy's economics of health care delivery, how does workers' compensation serve the 'agency' role between injured workers and health care providers?

References

Arnetz, B.B., Sjogren, B., Rydehn, B., et al., 2003. Early workplace intervention for employees with musculoskeletal-related absenteeism: a prospective controlled intervention study. J. Occup. Environ. Med. 45 (5), 499–506.

Brijnath, B., Mazza, D.S., Kosny, A., et al., 2014. Mental health claims management and return to work: qualitative insights from Melbourne, Australia. J. Occup. Rehabil. 24 (4), 766–776. doi:10.1007/s10926-014-9506-9.

Busse, J., Braun-Meyer, S., Ebrahim, S., et al., 2014. A 45-year-old-woman referred for an independent medical evaluation by her insurer. Can. Med. Assoc. J. 186 (16), E627–E630.

Collie, A., Gabbe, B., Fitzharris, M., 2015. Evaluation of a complex, population-based injury claims management intervention for improving injury outcomes: study protocol. BMJ Open. 5 (5), e006900.

Collie, A., Lane, T.J., Hassani-Mahmooei, B., et al., 2016. Does time off work after injury vary by jurisdiction? A comparative study of eight Australian workers' compensation systems. BMJ Open. 6 (5), e010910. doi:10.1136/bmjopen-2015-010910.

Collie, A., Di Donato, M., Iles, R., 2018. Work disability in Australia: an overview of prevalence, expenditure, support systems and services. J. Occup. Rehabil. doi:10.1007/s10926-018-9816-4. [Epub ahead of print].

Costa-Black, K.M., Feuerstein, M., Loisel, P., 2013. Work disability models: past and present. In: Loisel, P., Anema, J.R. (Eds.), Handbook of Work Disability Prevention and Management. Springer, New York.

Cullen, K.L., Irvin, E., Collie, A., et al., 2018. Effectiveness of workplace interventions in return-to-work for musculoskeletal, pain-related and mental health conditions: an update of the evidence and messages for practitioners. J. Occup. Rehabil. 28, 1.

Grant, G., O'Donnell, M., Spittal, M., et al., 2014. Relationship between stressfulness of claiming for injury compensation and long-term recovery. A prospective cohort study. JAMA Psychiatry 71 (4), 446–453.

Gray, S.E., Sheehan, L.R., Lane, T.J., et al., 2019. Concerns about claiming, post-claim support, and return to work planning. J. Occup. Environ. Med. 61, e139–e145.

Harris, I., Mulford, J., Soloman, M., et al., 2005. Association between compensation status and outcome after surgery – a meta analysis. J. Am. Med. Assoc. 293 (13), 1644–1652.

Jetha, A., LaMontagne, A.D., Lilley, R., et al., 2018. Workplace social system and sustained return-to-work: a study of supervisor and co-worker supportiveness and injury reaction. J. Occup. Rehabil. 28, 486–494.

Kilgour, E., Kosny, A., McKenzie, D., et al., 2015a. Healing or harming? Healthcare providers interactions with injured workers and insurers in workers' compensation systems. J. Occup. Rehabil. 25 (1), 220–239. doi:10.1007/s10926-014-9521-x.

Kilgour, E., Kosny, A., McKenzie, D., et al., 2015b. Interactions between injured workers and insurers in workers' compensation systems: a systematic review of qualitative research literature. J. Occup. Rehabil. 25 (1), 160–181. doi:10.1007/s10926-014-9513-x.

Kosny, A., MacEachen, E., Feerier, S., et al., 2011. The role of health care providers in long term and complicated workers' compensation claims. J. Occup. Rehabil. 21 (4), 582–590.

Kosny, A., Allen, A., Collie, A., 2013. Understanding independent medical assessments – a multi-jurisdictional analysis, Institute for Safety, Compensation and Recovery Research, Melbourne.

Krause, N., Dasinger, L.K., Deegan, L.J., et al., 2001. Psychosocial job factors and return-to-work after compensated low back injury: a disability phase-specific analysis. Am. J. Ind. Med. 40, 374–392.

Lane, T.J., Gray, S., Hassani-Mahmooei, B., et al., 2018a. Effectiveness of employer financial incentives in reducing time to report worker injury: an interrupted time series study of two Australian workers' compensation jurisdictions. BMC Public Health 18 (1), 100. doi:10.1186/s12889-017-4998-9.

Lane, T.J., Lilley, R., Hogg-Johnson, S., et al., 2018b. A prospective cohort study of the impact of return-to-work coordinators in getting injured workers back on the job. J. Occup. Rehabil. 28, 298–306.

Lax, M., 2004. Independent of what? The independent medical examination business. New Soluti. 14 (3), 219–251.

Lippel, K., 2007. Workers describe the effect of the workers' compensation process on their health: a Québec study. Int. J. Law Psychiatry 30, 427–443.

Marmot, M., 2005. Social determinants of health inequalities. Lancet 365, 1099–1104.

Newnam, S., Collie, A., Vogel, A.P., et al., 2014. The impacts of injury at the individual, community and societal levels: a systematic meta-review. Public Health 128 (7), 587–618. doi:10.1016/j.puhe.2014.04.004.

Rueda, S., Chambers, L., Wilson, M., et al., 2012. Association of returning to work with better health in working age adults: a systematic review. Am. J. Public Health 102, 541–556.

Safe Work Australia (SWA), 2016. The cost of work-related injury and illness for Australian employers, workers and the community: 2012–13. SWA, Canberra. https://www.safeworkaustralia.gov.au/system/files/documents/1702/cost-of-work-related-injury-and-disease-2012-13.docx.pdf.

Safe Work Australia (SWA), 2017. Australian workers' compensation statistics 2014–15. https://www.safeworkaustralia.gov.au/collection/australian-workers-compensation-statistics.

Safe Work Australia (SWA), 2018. Australian workers' compensation statistics 2015–16. https://www.safeworkaustralia.gov.au/collection/australian-workers-compensation-statistics.

Shaw, W.S., Kristman, V.L., Vezina, N., 2013. Workplace issues. In: Loisel, P., Anema, J.R. (Eds.), Handbook of Work Disability Prevention and Management. Springer, New York, pp. 163–183.

Shraim, M., Cifuentes, M., Willetts, J.L., et al., 2015. Length of disability and medical costs in low back pain: do state workers' compensation policies make a difference? J. Occup. Environ. Med. 57 (12), 1275–1283. doi:10.1097/JOM.0000000000000593.

Transport Accident Commission and WorkSafe Victoria, 2012. Clinical framework for the delivery of health services, Victorian WorkCover Authority and TAC, Melbourne. https://www.worksafe.vic.gov.au/resources/clinical-framework-delivery-health-services.

Tsushima, W., Foote, R., Merrill, T., et al., 1996. How independent are psychological examinations? A workers' compensation dilemma. Prof. Psychol. Res. Pr. 27 (6), 626–628.

Waddell, G., Burton, A., 2006. Is Work Good for Your Health and Well-being? The Stationery Office, London.

Zelle, B., Panzica, M., Vogt, M.T., et al., 2005. Influence of workers' compensation eligibility on functional recovery 10 to 28 years after polytrauma. Am. J. Surg. 190, 30–36.

Further Reading

Loisel, P., Anema, J., 2013. Handbook of Work Disability Prevention and Management. Springer, New York.

Safe Work Australia (SWA), 2013. Comparative performance monitoring report 15th edition: comparison of work health and safety and workers compensation in Australia and New Zealand, SWA, Canberra. http://www.safeworkaustralia.gov.au/sites/SWA/about/Publications/Documents/810/CPM-15.pdf.

Safe Work Australia (SWA), 2014. Comparison of workers' compensation arrangements in Australia and New Zealand, SWA, Canberra. http://www.safeworkaustralia.gov.au/sites/SWA/about/Publications/Documents/875/comparison-wc-aug-2014.pdf.

Online Resources

Heads of Workers' Compensation Authorities: www.hwca.org.au.

Insurance Work and Health Research Group: https://www.monash.edu/medicine/iwhgroup.

Personal Injury Education Foundation: www.pief.com.au.

Safe Work Australia: www.safework.gov.au.

CHAPTER 14

The complementary and alternative health care system in Australia

Julia Twohig

Key learning outcomes

When you finish this chapter you should be able to:

- describe complementary and alternative medicine (CAM) practices, their evidence base and their place in the Australian health system
- explain the holistic nature of CAM and the commonly used modalities
- discuss the increasing growth of and demand for CAM
- outline the current regulatory requirements and questions about statutory registration
- explain the change to natural therapies in the Private Health Insurance reforms
- comment on the current complaint before the Commonwealth Ombudsman

Key terms and abbreviations

allopathy
Australian Health Practitioner Regulation Agency (AHPRA)
Commonwealth Ombudsman
complementary and alternative medicine (CAM)
continuing professional development (CPD)
evidence-based medicine (EBM)
general practitioners (GPs)
holistic
modalities
National Health and Medical Research Council (NHMRC)
primary contact practices
Private Health Insurance (PHI)
randomised controlled trial (RCT)

Introduction

In Australia, **complementary and alternative medicine** (CAM) refers to a range of popular but diverse health care practices and products that exist parallel with, but are not regarded as part of, the mainstream biomedical system (McCabe 2005). However, this definition is rather wanting because it defines what CAM is not, rather than what it is (Coulter & Willis 2004). It is impossible to apply a single definition that covers all aspects of CAM. The variety of healing approaches that fall under the umbrella of CAM did not develop by force or persuasion but rather evolved out of a need and demand by people.

Even the name CAM is controversial, and it could even be argued that CAM is not always complementary to Western medicine and that for some people CAM is, in fact, an alternative (O'Brien 2004).

Common features of all CAM practices

Although many differences exist in their approaches to treatment, the **modalities** that comprise CAM do share some common features:

+ CAM takes a **holistic** view of the individual.
+ CAM places emphasis on individualising the treatment.
+ Most CAM approaches encourage a partnership approach to the consultation and management of the case.
+ Many of the CAM clinical approaches have an underlying belief that people heal themselves, given the right support and stimulus (Weir 2005).

What sets CAM apart from conventional medicine?

Most CAM practices have at their heart a concept of force or energy that is variously described as a *life force, vital force, vital energy, entelechy or élan vital:* this is a concept that has existed from the earliest days but was first referred to as *vitalism* in the early 19th century. In Traditional Chinese Medicine this concept is referred to as *ch'i* or *qi,* in Ayurvedic or traditional Indian medicine it is known as *prana,* and in homoeopathy it is referred to as the *vital force* or *life force.*

Conventional Western medicine does not include such a concept, instead embracing what is increasingly referred to as biomedicine. Although biomedicine has made enormous strides in treating disease, taken to extremes biomedicine can become a part of the reductionist scientific model, where only the parts can explain the whole. It is the opposite of a holistic approach, and can result in 'a never-ending search for causes within increasingly smaller parts' (Tesio 2010, p. 108). This approach is very beneficial when a 'part' can be repaired, but is somewhat lacking when it comes to complex issues such as chronic disease, mental health and problems of ageing and palliative care.

A particularly pertinent example of the deficiencies inherent in the reductionist model of medicine is the recent conclusion of cancer researchers that the majority of cancers are just 'bad luck' or, rather, random mutations in DNA replication of normal stem cells (Tomasetti & Vogelstein 2015, p. 78). Although it seems perfectly logical that many disease processes are not understood, it is rather surprising that this lack of understanding would be put down to 'bad luck'. If it is acceptable in the world of science to equate not knowing with luck, then might not CAM practitioners just as easily claim that cancer is a complex derangement of *ch'i* or *prana* or the life force?

Is a medical system that develops and operates without a concept of life energy very one sided? If this imbalance exists, does it result in a health system that is in the complete embrace of technology and pharmacology, encouraging a distancing from the individual and the human being who is sick (Dragos 2010)? Apart from anything else, could it be seen as an approach to health care that is wasteful of resources, very expensive to operate and often unrewarding for both patient and practitioner?

History of CAM in Australia

Many of the more established CAM practices have existed in Australia, in some form, since European settlement. Chinese medicine arrived with the early Chinese immigrants, and homoeopathy with early European migration. These practices were often carried out by lay practitioners or by medical doctors who were also homoeopaths. Homoeopathic hospitals were established in Melbourne in 1882 and in Sydney in 1901(Armstrong 2019).

The introduction of antibiotics, the rapid expansion of pharmaceutical treatments and greatly improved public health programs are widely credited with contributing to the decline of CAM, especially after World War II (Gray 2005). Since European settlement, CAM practitioners have often been marginalised by the dominant mainstream medical system; despite this, many practices have survived and even prospered, due in large part to the dedication and commitment of the practitioners and the demand of the followers.

Those who seek CAM

The increasing use of CAM by Australians mirrors the pattern of use in other Western industrialised countries. In a 2004 South Australian study, CAM was used by 52.2% of the study population, across a range of ages; the highest use was by well-educated, affluent women between the ages of 25 and

34 years, with the majority using CAM for maintenance of general health (MacLennan et al. 2006). In similar previous research, 57% of CAM users revealed that they did not tell their doctor that they were receiving CAM (MacLennan et al. 2002).

One group of patients who use CAM are those diagnosed with cancer. Individuals with cancer seek CAM treatments not only to treat the disease but also to treat the side-effects of some conventional treatments, including chemotherapy and radiation therapy; they also tend to seek out CAM when mainstream medicine has no treatments left to offer. The latter is a difficult situation for both patient and practitioner, as the disease is usually very advanced and the patient is also struggling with the debilitating side-effects of the medical treatment they have received.

In the first longitudinal study of its kind, a comparison was made between cancer patients under homoeopathic care and a similar group under conventional care (Rostock et al. 2011). The researchers found a significant and stable improvement in quality of life, including spiritual, mental and physical well-being, in the homoeopathic care group compared with the conventional care group. The improvement was clinically relevant and statistically significant (Rostock et al. 2011).

Trends in the rise of consumer confidence in CAM

Biomedicine, or allopathic medicine, did not emerge until the late 19th century. As **allopathy** became the dominant system of medicine, the other approaches declined until a resurgence in their popularity occurred in the 1960s (Gray 2005). The reasons why CAM is increasingly in demand are not fully understood nor fully researched, but what is apparent is that the rise in demand for CAM is a social phenomenon (Coulter & Willis 2004).

Globalisation and the rapid social changes that accompany it are regarded as part of the postmodern era in which we live. These changes have also seen a loss of faith in science, technology and medicine to provide all the solutions for living (Coulter & Willis 2007).

After World War II (1939–45), the introduction of antibiotics and immunisations resulted in a dramatic decline in infectious diseases. This decline has resulted in a drop in mortality, with the population in Western countries living longer. This in turn has shifted the pattern of disease from infections to chronic conditions. Chronic illnesses often have no quick-fix solutions and mainstream medicine, with its emphasis on biomedical solutions, may be able to alleviate some of the symptoms but not provide a cure. This has led some researchers to suggest that more emphasis needs to be placed on primary prevention strategies such as exercise (Booth et al. 2000). Living with a chronic disease often motivates patients to turn to CAM.

It has been confirmed that patients seek CAM because of an intuitive feeling that it could offer them a more appropriate medical model for their illness. Patients may therefore not be seeking proof of the efficacy of particular treatments, but instead meaning and context for their illness, thus allowing them the freedom to benefit from therapeutic consultations within their chosen milieu (Case study 14.1). 'Why should we [doctors] impose our medical model on patients? Their use of CAM may be their process of empowerment, which in turn allows them to contain and manage their chronic illness' (Lewith 2000, p. 102).

Case Study 14.1

A family seeking treatment for a chronic condition

A 16-year-old teenage boy presents, with his mother and father, for homoeopathic treatment of the inflammatory bowel disease Crohn's. The practitioner first negotiates who will be present in the interview. After an amicable discussion, the parents and the boy agree that the parents will remain in the consultation during the history-taking and then move to the waiting room so that the boy is able to speak freely.

History

The condition first developed when the boy was 14 and had returned to Australia with his family after living overseas for several years. Unlike the usual presentation of diarrhoea, this young man first presented to an emergency department with severe constipation, nausea and abdominal pain. Since his symptoms first appeared he has complained of continual tiredness, a poor appetite and, even though medicated, the constipation has remained a problem. There was nothing remarkable in the patient's history other than the parents relating that he was very badly affected by leaving his friends and returning to Australia, and found it difficult to establish new friends and begin at a new school. All agreed that the patient had a great reluctance to embrace change and often got himself 'in a state' over having to face new experiences.

Family history

Two members of the family have gluten intolerance, and a paternal uncle has ulcerative colitis. (Gluten is the protein in wheat and some other grains.)

Previous medical treatment

The patient had a colonoscopy, the first with a biopsy, which confirmed the diagnosis. He was, reluctantly, taking two anti-inflammatory drugs. The practitioner supported the doctor's prescription and recommended that he continue with these medications. If his symptoms improved with the homoeopathic treatment, the patient should raise the possibility of reducing the dose with his medical specialist at his next visit.

Physical symptoms

- Constipation with resulting haemorrhoids from straining
- Noisy flatulence
- Indigestion, which was better for burping
- Tiredness and lethargy
- Hungry, but a feeling of fullness after eating little
- Tenderness on palpation over the lower-right quadrant of the abdomen
- Nausea
- Sensitive to the cold but intolerant of being too warm

Continued

- 'Feeling anxiety' in his stomach
- A dislike of milk, cold food and drink, and oysters
- Cravings for sweet things, pastries and warm drinks
- Waking hungry during the night and getting up to eat

Mental symptoms
- Difficulty in adjusting to change and new situations
- Fear of heights, examinations, public speaking, being alone at home
- Unwilling to undertake anything unless he can do it perfectly
- Dreams: frightening and exhausting, although he cannot recall the detail

Treatment
After due consideration, a prescription was made of the homoeopathic medicine *Lycopodium*. This is a plant remedy with a similar symptom picture to that of the patient, and an excellent clinical reputation for treating inflammatory bowel disease.

A review of the patient's diet was made and advice given suggesting avoidance of the four grains containing gluten, with a gradual reintroduction as symptoms improved, beginning with oats. Alternatives to the grains were suggested. It was recommended that he eat six small meals spaced over the day, drink at least eight glasses of water a day, and have sufficient good-quality oil and fibre in his diet. The importance of his current exercise regimen was reinforced. A supplement of *Acidophilus* with fibre was also recommended as a gentle way of increasing levels of dietary fibre.

The patient was advised to contact the clinic if his symptoms worsened or if he developed any new symptoms. A follow-up appointment was made for 1 month ahead. The patient was also encouraged to keep in regular contact with his GP and gastroenterologist, and a referral was given to a specialist dietitian for further nutritional advice.

Follow-up 1 month later showed a steady improvement in the patient's symptoms. He was now able to move his bowels more easily and more often. He said that he felt happier and that his concentration had improved; he had also joined a band that a school friend had started. His mother commented that he seemed less anxious and had more energy.

Treatment continued unchanged. A further follow-up appointment was scheduled for 1 month ahead.

Research funding – how serious is it?

Given the high use of CAM in the Australian community the National Institute of Complementary Medicine (NICM) was established in 2007 and hosted by the University of Western Sydney at its Campbelltown campus. 'The National Institute of Complementary Medicine (NICM) was established to provide leadership and support for strategically directed research into complementary medicine and translation of evidence into clinical practice and relevant policy to benefit the health of all Australians' (National Institute of Complementary Medicine 2015, www.nicm.edu.au/about). Initial seed funding for the establishment of the NICM included (AU)$4 million from the Australian government and $0.6 million from the government of New South Wales (National Institute of Complementary

Medicine 2015). This support for CAM from the Australian government began to bring it in to line with international trends. The investment in Australian research looked positive for CAM until the Commonwealth government stopped funding the operations of the NICM in 2010. The institute is still hosted by the University of Western Sydney, but has had to drastically reduce its staff and operations and rely on substantial donations from the private sector, including CAM manufacturers (National Institute of Complementary Medicine 2015).

The NICM is responsible for two significant reports, *Cost effectiveness of complementary medicines* and *National research priorities in complementary medicine in Australia* (National Institute of Complementary Medicine 2010, 2013). The first report found that Australia could potentially save millions in health care costs without compromising patient outcomes if complementary medicine was more widely used. With more and more Australian consumers seeking out CAM, they would be entitled to ask why support for this institute has been withdrawn. The second report points out that Australians are among the highest users of CAM in the world, with two out of three people using some form of CAM. Despite expenditure of over $3.5 million each year, however, the research investment dollar for CAM is one of the lowest in the world. 'The report focuses on target areas that have a higher burden of disease, that accord with the Australian Government's National Health Priority Areas, and that have a greater probability of success' (National Institute of Complementary Medicine 2013, p. v). Rather than simply removing subsidies, perhaps a more positive outcome of the Review of Natural Therapies could have included increasing the funding of research in those areas (Wardle 2016a).

Integrative medicine – does it exist in Australia?

Moves to strengthen the integration of complementary medicine have occurred from within the medical profession. One such example is the formation of the Australasian Integrative Medicine Association (AIMA), which is an independent, not-for-profit group of medical practitioners whose mission statement is 'to lead and facilitate the development of integrative medical care as being core to the health and wellbeing of individuals and society as a whole' (Australasian Integrative Medicine Association 2011, https://www.aima.net.au/about/).

Why are CAM practitioners an under-utilised resource?

Australia's health 2018 is an extensive document developed by the Australian Institute of Health and Welfare (2018) on behalf of the Australian government. One of the questions this document aims to answer is 'Who does what in the health system?' – and yet this detailed account of the health of the nation does not make any mention of CAM, its statutorily *unregulated* practitioners, the services they offer, or the people who pay for these health services. Another example of this lack of inclusion is found in the Gratton Institute report *Access all areas: new solutions for GP shortages in rural Australia* (Duckett et al. 2013), which makes no mention of the rich resource of CAM health practitioners who are well equipped to make a contribution to a health system that is overtaxed and often understaffed.

Government reports rarely focus on the actual CAM workforce. Because there is no national government register of CAM practitioners, other than for chiropractors, osteopaths and practitioners of Chinese medicine, accurate numbers are difficult to establish, but figures from 2007 suggest that they are in the vicinity of 31,000 (Grace 2012). The increasing demand for CAM services is in complete contrast to the often-negative attitudes displayed towards them by some medical practitioners, other health professionals and even government policy-makers. For example, figures from the Australian Bureau of Statistics (ABS) tell us that the number of people visiting a complementary health professional increased by 51% in the 10 years to 2005. Almost 750,000 people had visited this type of practitioner in a 2-week period, and the number of people working as complementary health professionals nearly doubled from 4800 to 8600 in the 10 years to 2006 (Australian Bureau of Statistics 2008b).

Marginalisation of CAM

Ignoring the CAM workforce in government policies has been common practice until now, although **general practitioners (GPs)** can currently refer patients for a limited number of consultations with chiropractors and osteopaths. These patients are then entitled to claim a government rebate, under the Medicare Benefits Schedule, for a portion of these costs. This is the first time for many years that any CAM service has been included in government funding, even though to access it requires the oversight of a medical practitioner (see Chapter 7). The Australian government is also committed to a National E-Health Strategy (Australian Health Ministers' Conference 2008). This strategy is intended to streamline the movement of information, facilitate referrals and improve access to care. This system has been devised without the inclusion of CAM practitioners, thus further marginalising them from the Australian health care system (Grace 2012).

CAM practitioners are excluded from national registration despite this being the only real guarantee of securing best-practice and high educational standards, and enabling a legal system rigorous enough to afford protection to the consumer of CAM. **All unregistered CAM practitioners are regulated by systems of self-regulation**, operated by professional associations.

Education and training in CAM

Towards the close of the 20th century, many CAM professional associations participated in the development of a Health Training Package (Community Services and Health Industry Skills Council 2013), which ensured government endorsement and three nationally recognised components for CAM:

+ national competency standards
+ a national system of assessment
+ national qualifications.

Significant changes in CAM education

In 2014, as a result of a review of the Health Training Package, some CAM modalities believed that the knowledge and skills required for primary practice would be more accurately placed in the higher-education sector, and moved to increase the minimum practice standard to a Bachelor's degree (Steel & McEwen 2014). From 2018, homoeopathy, naturopathy, nutritional medicine and Western herbal medicine moved to the higher education sector, and now require a Bachelor's degree as the minimum entry level for practice.

Government-endorsed qualifications still exist for a variety of CAM modalities, however, ranging from Certificate IV to Advanced Diploma and including the following modalities:

◆ aromatherapy, Ayurvedic medicine, kinesiology, remedial massage, reflexology, shiatsu, Traditional Chinese Medicine, remedial massage.

PAUSE
for
REFLECTION
...

CAM practitioners are almost entirely involved in clinical care, the work of listening to and supporting people in their goal to wellness. Many of these health practitioners are extremely well educated, graduating with Bachelor degrees and higher qualifications.

Could these practitioners help to address the targets of such bodies as the National Health Workforce Taskforce, including increasing the numbers of health workers and reforming the health workforce (Australia's Health Workforce Online 2006), or is the ghostly absence of CAM workers in the Australian health workforce yet another example of the 'silences' illuminating their marginalisation (Bacchi 2012a, p. 21)?

Table 14.1 is a brief description of those CAMs that are **primary contact practices**: practices that accept patients directly, or without referral from another practitioner.

Problematising private health insurance rebates

'**Examining alternative therapy claims**' was identified by the **National Health and Medical Research Council** (NHMRC 2010) in their 2010–12 Strategic Plan as a major health issue that needed investigation. The resulting investigation, entitled 'The review of the Australian government rebate on private health insurance for natural therapies' (Baggoley 2015) set out to examine the evidence of clinical efficacy, cost-effectiveness, safety and quality of natural therapies. The review, chaired by the former Commonwealth Chief Medical Officer, found 'there is no clear evidence demonstrating the efficacy of the listed natural therapies' and resulted in 16 natural therapies losing 'the definition of private health insurance general treatment' and as a consequence from 1st April 2019 they no longer receive the **private health insurance (PHI)** rebate. The natural therapies affected are Alexander technique, aromatherapy, Bowen therapy, Buteyko, Feldenkrais, herbalism, homeopathy, iridology, kinesiology, naturopathy, Pilates, reflexology, Rolfing, shiatsu, tai chi and yoga (Australian Government 2018).

It should be noted that nutritional medicine and Ayurvedic medicine were not included in the review of natural therapies – nutrition because it was considered out of scope of the review and seen to be covered by dietitians already registered with the Australian Health Practitioner Regulation

TABLE 14.1 Principles of Primary Contact Practice Cams

Homeopathy	Based on the principle 'let like cure like', homeopathy stimulates the body's ability to fight infection, the susceptibility to disease and treats both acute and chronic disease
Naturopathy	Emphasises prevention, treatment and restoration of the body's natural balance with the use of a variety of natural, holistic approaches
Nutritional medicine	Nutrition is the central focus as a therapeutic tool to achieve and maintain good health
Western herbal medicine	Consultation and preparation of herbal remedies based on an individual's specific treatment needs
Indigenous medicine	A broad range of traditional approaches, such as the use of bush medicines, incorporated into healing practices

Agency (AHPRA), and Ayurveda because the necessary cooperation from the Indian Ministry did not occur (Baggoley 2015).

A limitation of the investigations into natural therapies was the single research design employed, which was a systematic review – in fact, a review of reviews (Bradbury 2017).

The private health insurance policy in Australia

Access to natural therapies is not available through Australia's universal health care scheme, Medicare. PHI has been available for natural therapies if consumers were prepared to pay the out-of-pocket costs of insurance and this gave them partial reimbursement for consultations (see Chapter 3 for more information on PHI). The PHI rebate covered a portion of the cost of a natural therapy consultation, allowing more people to afford to take out ancillary or 'extras' cover. It is estimated that PHI pays out around $90 million each year on natural therapies, the rebate covering one-third of this (Wardle 2016b). In the June quarter of 2018, benefits paid to natural therapies comprised 4.1% of the total ancillary benefits paid out. It is difficult to see how the withdrawal of natural therapies benefits will have a significant financial impact on PHI premiums (Australian Prudential Regulation Authority 2018). What we may see is a withdrawal from PHI by individuals who took out health insurance solely to support their use of natural therapies. Their potential withdrawal could result in an increase in premiums. The other possibility is that the removal of the partial rebate for natural therapies may create an increased demand on public health services and on general practice, systems which are already under great stress (Leach & Steel 2018).

The decision to remove private health insurance rebates for natural therapies is a change in government policy

In many ways this change in policy defies logic when CAM is increasingly in demand by a large proportion of the Australian population. Perhaps, as Tuohy suggests, not every policy change is entirely a 'rational choice', but it requires the passage of time to expose the broader political factions which seized the opportunity to carry out what seems a concerted attack on the CAM professions (Tuohy 1999). It is also something of an irony that this change, initially introduced by the Labor Government, has been enacted by a coalition government whose mantra has always been to support individual choice in healthcare services (Elliot 2006).

The Health Minister suggested the removal of the subsidy for natural therapies was necessary because the CAM professions are unregulated. The problem with this argument is that enforceable professional standards can be achieved only through statutory regulation with the Australian Health Practitioner Regulation Agency and yet every government, both state and federal and the current Council of Australian Governments, has so far refused all attempts at such regulation (Leach & Steel 2018).

Removal of natural therapies from private health insurance and the consequences

In order for a CAM practitioner to be allocated a provider number by a private health insurer they must meet strict requirements. They must belong to an accredited professional association or national register. All are required to have an adequate level of education, to work in an ethical way by adhering to their profession's standards of practice, to keep up to date with compulsory **continuing professional development (CPD)** requirements, to have adequate professional indemnity insurance and to have a current senior first aid certificate. Unless individuals met all of these requirements they were not eligible for a provider number.

Questioning the review process

In 2010, a draft position paper from the NHMRC was leaked to the media (NHMRC 2010). It described homoeopathy as *unethical* and *inefficacious*. In response to the wave of criticism and charges of bias and lack of scientific process the NHMRC initiated a formal investigation into homoeopathy. Their conclusions found very little in favour of homoeopathy (NHMRC 2013b).

The review resulted in the generation of many negative reports about homoeopathy (Davidson 2014) and has been used to inform anti-homoeopathy policies internationally (European Academies Science Advisory Council 2017). This has influenced Australian and international educators to withdraw their courses in homeopathy (4Homeopathy Group 2018).

In direct contradiction to the NHMRC finding, a press statement from the Swiss Government, in August 2017, confirms that complementary medical services including homoeopathy will be compensated by the Swiss Governments compulsory health care insurance in line with all other medical specialties (Federal Council 2017).

The difference between the positive Swiss findings (Bornhoft & Matthiesen 2012) and the negative findings of the Australian Homeopathic Review are in stark contrast. They have met with universal derision by the CAM community. This has resulted in an extensive public campaign by practitioners and consumers of natural medicine to draw attention to the flawed methods and therefore flawed findings of the review and to the potential loss of access to complementary medicines and services that may result (www.yourhealthyourchoice.com.au).

Researchers have found serious procedural and scientific anomalies in the review (Homeopathy Research Institute 2017). As a result, three of the leading natural medicine professional associations have submitted a complaint to the **Commonwealth Ombudsman** challenging the findings of the NHMRC (Complementary Medical Association (CMA) 2016).

Points raised in the complaint to the Commonwealth Ombudsman

- ◆ The NHMRC conducted two reviews of homeopathy but never released the first review, which presented positive evidence for the efficacy of homeopathy.
- ◆ The NHMRC refuses all freedom of information (FOI) requests to view the first review.
- ◆ The NHMRC outsourced the second review and changed the review protocols without notice, setting an unprecedented minimum number of participants to 150 and an unusually high quality standard, requiring 5 out of 5 on the 'Jadad' or equivalent quality rating scale.
- ◆ The above exclusion criteria resulted in only 5 trials of the 1863 studies presented being considered. The NHMRC decided that none of the 5 was effective.
- ◆ Agreeing on a research protocol which details the exact methods used to assess and interpret data is a well-accepted safeguard to protect against scientific bias.
- ◆ The NHMRC failed to disclose conflicts of interest of those involved in the review, and included members of the anti-homeopathy group Friends of Science in Medicine.
- ◆ The NHMRC failed to consult a single homeopathic expert or researcher.
- ◆ The NHMRC reviewed only studies conducted in native English, ignoring excellent research from countries such as Brazil, Italy, Portugal and Spain.

If the process and protocols that the NHMRC used to investigate homeopathy prove to be flawed, then their conclusions that it 'fails to demonstrate that homoeopathy is an effective treatment for any of the reported clinical condition in humans' (NHMRC 2015) must be questioned. If the review stands up to the scrutiny of the Ombudsman, does this imply that the increasing number of patients seeking homoeopathic treatment are entirely gullible and unable to make a judgment about efficacy of the treatment?

The problem of evidence for CAM

'Evidence-based medicine is the conscientious, explicit and judicious use of current best evidence in making decisions about the care of individual patients' (Sackett et al. 1996, p. 71). This sounds imminently sensible, for who would not want the best treatment for patients, but practising **evidence-based medicine (EBM)** requires a high degree of clinical expertise; a practitioner must be able to research, retrieve, interpret and then choose from various research findings what will be applied in busy clinical situations. This may prove difficult for any health practitioner, whether mainstream or from CAM. One of the disadvantages of EBM for CAM is that it is much more difficult to apply the research requirements to practice, which in turn diminishes acceptability. Randomised controlled trials (RCTs) remain the first choice for research in medicine, and are often conducted to meet the requirements for the registration of new drugs despite a plethora of information revealing that RCTs are often flawed and even corrupted by the vested interests of the pharmaceutical industry (Gøtzsche 2013). Chapter 7 explores the process for registering new drugs.

The questionable way that the NHMRC conducted reviews into CAM is a timely example of how such evidence gathering can be misused. Even the most elegantly designed trials with smart protocols for blinding and including a minimum of 150 participants only ever measure a narrow set of symptoms and effects. What seems glaringly absent from reviews of CAM is the fact that any production of sound scientific evidence must also be embedded in the social context, yet all investigations have actively excluded all reviews of qualitative evidence (Barry 2006).

The NHMRC, the national research institution for Australia, demonstrated a clear resistance to CAM not only by the unscientific way it conducted its reviews, but also by underfunding meaningful research and by not supporting CAM to develop appropriate research models (Clark-Grill 2007).

Problematising this approach to CAM raises some key political questions, such as whether biomedicine perceives the rise in demand for CAM as a threat to its long-standing dominance (Barry 2006). CAM organisations have challenged the findings of the review into their professions, and in doing so have shone a light on the politics of these marginalised, perhaps soon to be invisible, professions making the wide-ranging, ongoing negative effects on both practitioners and consumers visible (Bacchi 2012a).

The question remains whether this is either ethically or philosophically acceptable. Patients' increasingly positive experiences of CAM are too important to be dismissed and do 'deserve a truly scientific exploration of non-biomedical conceptualizations of health and illness' (Clark-Grill 2007, p. 21), and because 'regimes of truth' (Foucault 1977, p. 23) such as the evidence-based movement currently enjoy a privileged status, scholars have not only a scientific duty, but also an ethical obligation to deconstruct these regimes of power (Holmes et al. 2006).

Summary

This chapter:

- introduces the commonly used CAMs and gives a brief history of CAM in Australia, confirming the reality that many CAMs have been in existence for hundreds of years, and that what is mainstream biomedicine is, actually, a more recent development
- suggests that people who seek out CAM therapies are generally well educated and economically well-off and seeking to improve their general well-being, or are very sick with cancer or some other chronic disease and are looking for treatment options when mainstream medicine may have little to offer

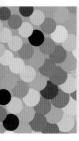

- outlines the benefits and disadvantages of government statutory regulation by registration for CAMs, and considers other models of regulation
- outlines how CAM is funded and the difficulties of conducting high-quality research without sufficient funding, and
- highlights the need to design research models that are suited to the multifaceted nature of CAM treatment.

An accompanying video exploring the themes of this chapter is hosted on Evolve: http://evolve.elsevier.com/AU/Willis/understanding/.

Review Questions

1   How is the problem of the PHI rebate represented?
2   One of the aims of the removal of the rebate was to reduce the premiums for private health insurance (Australian Government 2018), but has this occurred?
3   How has the perception of the problem been disseminated and how has it been resisted?
4   Will removing the natural therapies health rebate encourage practitioners to drop their professional memberships and to become lone, unregulated practitioners?
5   If Australia is a democracy, why are CAM therapies not available through the universal health scheme, Medicare?
6   Are patient's preferences and their right to choose being disregarded?
7   Which interest groups might oppose these changes to CAM, and which might support them? (Bacchi 2000, 2012a, 2012b; Tuohy 1999).
8   Does this change in government policy fly in the face of **international trends and directives for CAM?** Both the WHO Traditional Medicine Strategy 2014–2023 (WHO 2013) and the Beijing Declaration (WHO 2008) gave clear directions to their member nations, including Australia, that they should be doing all they could to improve patient access to natural medicine services and to support the integration of natural medicine into the health care system.

References

4Homeopathy Group 2018. Homeopathy course suspended on basis of European document citing SECOND Australian Report. https://releasethefirstreport.com/lille-faculty-medicine-suspends-homeopathy-diploma.

Armstrong, B., 2019. History of Homoeopathy in Australia, Melbourne. http://www.historyofhomeopathy.com.au/articles/item/185-homoeopathy-australian-colonies-early-knowledge.html.

Australasian Integrative Medicine Association (AIMA), 2011. About AIMA. https://www.aima.net.au/about/.

Australian Bureau of Statistics (ABS), 2008. Australian social trends, 2008 (media release; ABS cat. no. 4102.0). ABS, Canberra. www.abs.gov.au/AUSSTATS/abs@.nsf/Lookup/4102.0Main+Features12008.

Australian Government, 2018. Private health insurance reforms: changing coverage for some natural therapies. Australian Government, Canberra.

Australian Health Ministers' Conference (AHMC), 2008. National e-health strategy summary. AHMC, Sydney. www.ehealth.gov.au/Internet/ehealth/publishing.nsf/content/home.

Australian Institute of Health and Welfare (AIHW), 2018. Australia's health 2018. Cat. no. AUS 221. AIHW, Canberra. https://www.aihw.gov.au/reports/australias-health/australias-health-2018/contents/table -of-contents.

Australian Prudential Regulation Authority (APRA), 2018. Private health insurance statistical trends, PHI Publications, Sydney. https://www.apra.gov.au/publications/private-health-insurance-statistical-trends.

Australia's Health Workforce Online, 2006. National Health Workforce Taskforce. www.ahwo.gov.au/ nhwt.asp.

Bacchi, C., 2000. Policy as discourse: what does it mean? Where does it get us? Discourse 21 (1), 45–57.

Bacchi, C., 2012a. Why study problematizations? Making politics visible. Open J. Polit. Sci. 2 (1), 1–8.

Bacchi, C., 2012b. Introducing the 'What's the problem represented to be?' approach. In: Bletsas, A., Beasley, C. (Eds.), Engaging With Carol Bacchi: Strategic Interventions & Exchanges. University of Adelaide Press, Adelaide.

Baggoley, C., 2015. Review of the Australian government rebate on natural therapies for private health insurance, Australian Government, Canberra. http://www.health.gov.au/internet/main/publishing.nsf/ Content/4899F1657E19A6F4CA2583A50020140D/$File/Natural%20Therapies%20Overview%20Report %20Final%20with%20copyright%2011%20March.pdf.

Barry, C.A., 2006. The role of evidence in alternative medicine: contrasting biomedical and anthropological approaches. Soc. Sci. Med. 62 (11), 2646–2657.

Booth, F.W., Gordon, S.E., Carlson, C.J., et al., 2000. Waging war on modern chronic diseases: primary prevention through exercise biology. J. Appl. Physiol. 88 (2), 774–787.

Bornhoft, G., Matthiesen, P., 2012. Homeopathy in Healthcare: Effectiveness, Appropriateness, Safety, Costs. Springer, Herdecke.

Bradbury, J., Grace, S., Avila, C., 2017. N-of-1 trials: building the evidence for natural medicine, one patient at a time. J. Aust. Tradit. Med. Soc. 23 (1), 14–15.

Clark-Grill, M., 2007. Questionable gate-keeping: scientific evidence for complementary and alternative medicines (CAM): response to Malcolm Parker. J. Bioeth. Inq. 4 (1), 21–28.

Community Services and Health Industry Skills Council, 2013. Health training package HLT07. www.cshisc. com.au https://training.gov.au/Training/Details/HLT07.

Complementary Medical Association (CMA), 2016. CMA, AHA, ATMS executive summary: Complaint to the Commonwealth Ombudsman regarding the National Health and Medical Research Council (NHMRC) assessment of homeopathy, 2010–2015. https://www.hri-research.org/wp-content/uploads/2017/04/ Executive-Summary-to-Ombudsman-Complaint-re-NHMRC-Homeopathy-Review-FINAL.pdf.

Coulter, I.W., Willis, E., 2004. The rise and rise of complementary and alternative medicine: a sociological perspective. Med. J. Aust. 180 (11), 587–589.

Coulter, I., Willis, E., 2007. Explaining the growth of complementary and alternative medicine. Health Sociol. Rev. 16, 214–225.

Davidson, H., 2014. 'Homeopathy is bunk': study says, The Guardian – Australian Edition. https://www. theguardian.com/world/2014/apr/08/homeopathy-is-bunk-study-says.

Dragos, P., 2010. The Copernican Revolution in Homeopathy: The New Way of Dealing With Life Energy. Books on Demand GmbH, Norderstedt.

Duckett, S., Breadon, P., Ginnivan, L. 2013. Access all areas: new solutions for GP shortages in rural Australia. Grattan Institute, Melbourne.

Elliot, A., 2006. 'The best friend Medicare ever had'? Policy narratives and changes in Coalition health policy. Health Sociol. Rev. 15, 132–143.

European Academies Science Advisory Council, 2017, Homeopathic products and practices: assessing the evidence and ensuring consistency in regulating medical claims in the EU. EASAC, Halle.

Federal Council, 2017. Complementary medicine: regulations of new remuneration. https://www.admin.ch/gov/de/start/dokumentation/medienmitteilungen/bundesrat.msg-id-67050.html.

Foucault, M., 1977. Discipline and Punish: The Birth of the Prison. Vintage Books, New York.

Gøtzsche, P.C., 2013. Deadly Medicine and Organised Crime: How Big Pharma Has Corrupted Healthcare. Radcliffe, London.

Grace, S., 2012. CAM practitioners in the Australian health workforce: an underutilized resource. BMC Complement. Altern. Med. 12, 205.

Gray, D.E., 2005. Health Sociology: An Australian Perspective. Pearson Education, French's Forest, NSW.

Holmes, D., Murray, S.J., Perron, A., et al., 2006. Deconstructing the evidence-based discourse in health sciences: truth, power and fascism. Int. J. Evid. Based Healthc. 4 (3), 180–186.

Homeopathy Research Institute (HRI), 2017. World-renowned government research department misled scientists and the public over homeopathy. HRI, London. https://www.hri-research.org/wp-content/uploads/2017/04/20170405_HRI-NHMRC-PRESS-RELEASE-Full-Analysis.pdf.

Leach, M.J., Steel, A., 2018. The potential downstream effects of proposed changes in Australian private health insurance policy: the case for naturopathy. Adv. Integr. Med. 5 (2), 48–51.

Lewith, G., 2000. Complementary and alternative medicine: an educational, attitudinal, and research challenge. Med. J. Aust. 172, 102–103.

MacLennan, A., Wilson, D., Taylor, A., 2002. The escalating cost and prevalence of alternative medicine. Prev. Med. 35, 166–173.

MacLennan, A., Myers, S., Taylor, W., 2006. The continuing use of complementary and alternative medicine in South Australia: costs and beliefs in 2004. Med. J. Aust. 184 (1), 27.

McCabe, P., 2005. Complementary and alternative medicine in Australia: a contemporary overview. Complement. Ther. Clin. Pract. 11, 28–31.

National Health and Medical Research Council (NHMRC), 2010. Draft NHMRC public statement on homeopathy. NHMRC, Canberra.

National Health and Medical Research Council (NHMRC), 2013. Effectiveness of homeopathy for clinical conditions: evaluation of the evidence. Overview report prepared for the NHMRC Homeopathy Working Committee by Optum. NHMRC, Canberra. www.nhmrc.gov.au/_files_nhmrc/file/your_health/complementary_medicines/nhmrc_homeopathy_overview_report_october_2013_140407.pdf.

National Health and Medical Research Council (NHMRC), 2015. NHMRC statement: statement on homeopathy. NHMRC, Canberra. https://www.nhmrc.gov.au/about-us/publications/homeopathy#block-views-block-file-attachments-content-block-1.

National Institute of Complementary Medicine (NICM), 2010. Cost effectiveness of complementary medicines. Report prepared by Access Economics for the NICM, Penrith, NICM. www.westernsydney .edu.au/__data/assets/pdf_file/0006/537657/Cost_effectiveness_of_CM_2010.pdf.

National Institute of Complementary Medicine (NICM), 2013. Research priorities for complementary medicine in Australia, Penrith, NICM. www.nicm.edu.au/__data/assets/pdf_file/0009/537840/ Research_Priorities_for_CM.pdf.

National Institute of Complementary Medicine (NICM), 2015. About us, Penrith, NICM. https://www.nicm. edu.au/about_us/about_NICM.

O'Brien, K., 2004. Complementary and alternative medicine: the move into mainstream health care. Clin. Exp. Optom. 87 (2), 110.

Rostock, M., Naumann, J., Guethlin, C., et al., 2011. Classical homeopathy in the treatment of cancer patients – a prospective observational study of two independent cohorts. BMC Cancer 11 (19), 1–8.

Sackett, D., Rosenberg, W., Gray, J., et al., 1996. Evidence based medicine: what it is and what it isn't. BMJ 312, 71–72.

Steel, A., McEwen, B., 2014. The need for higher degrees by research for complementary medicine practitioners. Aust. J. Herbal Med. 26 (4), 136–140.

Tesio, L., 2010. The good-hearted and the clever: clinical medicine at the bottom of the barrel of science. J. Med. Person. 8 (3), 103–111.

Tomasetti, C., Vogelstein, B., 2015. Variation in cancer risk among tissues can be explained by the number of stem cell divisions. Science 347, 6217. www.sciencemag.org.

Tuohy, C., 1999. Accidental Logics: The Dynamics of Change in the Health Care Arena in the United States, Britain and Canada. OUP, Cary, NC.

Wardle, J., 2016a. More integrative research is needed: but where will it come from? Adv. Integr. Med. 3 (1), 1–2.

Wardle, J., 2016b. The Australian government review of natural therapies for private health insurance rebates: what does it say and what does it mean? Adv. Integr. Med. 3 (1), 3–10.

Weir, M., 2005. Alternative Medicine: A New Regulatory Model. Australian Scholarly, Melbourne, Australia.

World Health Organization (WHO), 2008. Beijing declaration. WHO Congress on Traditional Medicine, 7–9 November 2008, Beijing, China. WHO, Geneva. http://www.who.int/traditional-complementary-integrative-medicine/about/beijing-congress/en/index4.html.

World Health Organization (WHO), 2013. WHO Traditional Medicine Strategy 2014–2023. WHO, Geneva.

Further Reading

Baer, H., 2009. Complementary Medicine in Australia and New Zealand: Its Popularization, Legitimation, and Dilemmas. Verdant House, Australia.

Deans, M., 2004. The Trials of Homeopathy: Origins, Structure and Development. KVC–Verlag, Essen, Germany.

Kaptchuk, T., 2000. The Web That Has No Weaver: Understanding Chinese Medicine. St Martin's Press, New York.

Kennedy, I., 1981. The Unmasking of Medicine. Allen & Unwin, London.

Kotsirilos, V., Vitetta, L., Sali, A., 2011. A Guide to Evidence-Based Integrative and Complementary Medicine. Churchill Livingstone, Sydney.

Ninivaggi, F., 2001. An Elementary Textbook of Ayurveda Medicine With a Six Thousand Year Old Tradition. International Universities Psychosocial Press, Madison, CT.

Phelps, K., Hassed, C., 2010. The Integrative Approach. Churchill Livingstone, Sydney.

Pizzorno, J., Murray, M., 2005. Textbook of Natural Medicine, third ed. Churchill Livingstone, New York.

Schnaubelt, K., 1998. Advanced Aromatherapy: The Science of Essential Oil Therapy. Healing Arts Press, Rochester, Vermont.

Wood, M., 2004. The Practice of Traditional Western Herbalism: Basic Doctrine, Energetics and Classification. North Atlantic Books, Berkeley, CA.

Online Resources

Alliance of International Aromatherapists: www.alliance-aromatherapists.org.

Australian Homoeopathic Association – the national professional homoeopathic association in Australia: www.homeopathyoz.org.

Australian Natural Therapists Association (ANTA) – natural therapists' professional association covering multiple modalities: www.anta.com.au.

Australian Naturopathic Network (ANN): www.ann.com.au.

Australian Osteopathic Association: www.ozosteopathicsites.com.au.

Australian Register of Homoeopaths (AROH) – including their Code of Professional Conduct and Standards of Practice Regulations: www.aroh.com.au.

Australian Register of Naturopaths and Herbalists (ARONAH) – national register: www.aronah.org.

Australian Traditional Medicine Society (ATMS) – professional association covering multiple modalities: www.atms.com.au.

Ayurvedic medicine information and contacts: www.allayurveda.com.

Chinese medicine information: www.chinesemedicineboard.gov.au.

Chiropractors' Association of Australia – the peak body for chiropractic in Australia: www.chiropractors.asn.au.

Commonwealth Ombudsman – a government agency which assists members of the public with disputes: www.ombudsman.gov.au.

National Health and Medical Research Council (NHMRC) and research integrity: www.nhmrchomeopathy.com.

National Herbalists Association of Australia: www.nhaa.org.au.

Release the First Report: https://releasethefirstreport.com/.

Therapeutic Goods Administration – contains the TGA regulations governing natural medicines: www.tga.gov.au/complementary-medicines.

Your Health Your Choice: https://www.yourhealthyourchoice.com.au/.

CHAPTER 15

Oral health and dental services

Julie Satur

Key learning outcomes

When you finish this chapter you should be able to:

+ describe oral health in the context of overall health
+ briefly describe the features of the oral health care system and how it intersects with other aspects of the health system
+ describe the oral health and dental workforce and the range of activities they undertake, distinguishing between the different practitioners who work in oral health
+ describe the educational pathways to these professions
+ discuss the professional forces that have led to the current models of supply of dentistry and oral health practitioners
+ identify the issues this raises for future service delivery.

Key terms and abbreviations

Cleft Lip and Palate (CLP) Scheme
dental decay / dental caries
dentate
dental hygienist (DH)
dental prosthetists
dental therapists
dentist
edentulous
general practitioners (GPs)
oral health therapist (OHT)
oral health therapy practitioners
periodontal disease
public dental services
school dental services
Vocational Education and Training (VET)

Introduction

Dental disease is one of the most prevalent and costly diseases in our community. Oral health is fundamental to overall health, and supports peoples' ability to eat, sleep and socialise; in Australia, oral health is a significant marker of social inequality. Poor oral health erodes self-esteem and impacts on quality of life; it both affects people's ability to fully participate in society and is an outcome of low socio-economic status. Further, there is increasing evidence of its impact on general health, with links evident between chronic oral infections and stroke, premature births and low birthweight, heart and lung diseases and diabetes. Poor oral health is one of the chronic disease areas that our health service system does not deal with well, at least for those reliant on public-sector dental services. The private dental sector is world class and offers high-quality care to those who can afford it, and indeed around 88% of Australia's dental services are provided through private-sector dentistry. But, for around half of our population who are not able to participate in market-delivered services and instead rely on public-sector services, access to care is poor (Chrisopoulos & Harford 2013; Council of Australian Governments Health Council 2015; National Advisory Council on Dental Health 2012; Productivity Commission 2018; Sanders 2007; Spencer 2011).

This chapter will show that there is a need to deal with the problem of unmet need for care among low-income people and those at high risk of oral disease and at its interface with chronic disease and ageing. It will also discuss some ideas about how to increase the supply of services to those who currently have poor or no access to care, and reduce demand through much more preventively oriented oral health care and better use of the existing workforce.

Snapshot of population oral health and disease

Oral diseases, including **dental decay / dental caries** and **periodontal disease** (of gum and supporting tissues), are among the most prevalent diseases in Australia and rank as the second most costly disease to treat (Australian Institute of Health and Welfare (AIHW) 2014a). Dental trauma, developmental disorders such as cleft lip and palate, and oral cancers also contribute to the (AU)$10.1 billion spent on oral disease and disorders each year (AIHW 2018a). Although disease rates among school children have declined significantly since the 1970s, they are again increasing; in 2010, 48% of 5-year-olds, 69% of 9-year-olds and 64% of 14-year-olds had tooth decay, and children in low-income families had 50%–70% more decay-affected teeth than those in the most advantaged families (Chrisopoulos et al. 2016).

Dental decay is a disease of cumulative effects, and among adults continues to follow patterns of social inequality. Among all Australians over the age of 18 there are differences in disease experience: on average, low-income adults have 15 teeth affected by decay, with those on higher incomes having 13.3 teeth affected; for those over the age of 65, decay has affected 24 teeth on average. However, when looking at untreated decay the gap is wider: around 40% of low-income people have untreated decay compared with only around 17% of high-income people (Chrisopoulos et al. 2016).

People living in rural and remote areas had higher levels of untreated decay (38%), as did those without dental insurance (31%). In 2010, 65% of people aged 5 years and over had a dental visit in the previous year, ranging from 78% of 5- to 14-year-olds to 57% of adults. Among people aged 25–44 years, 17% reported having a toothache in the past year, with lower-income people being twice as likely to both experience toothache and to receive an extraction as treatment. Among older people, 29% reported feeling uncomfortable about their dental appearance, and 35% of those aged 45–65 years had moderate to severe periodontal disease, with 20% losing teeth as a result. For those over age 65, these figures were 16% and 20% respectively, with 21% edentulous (having no natural teeth). Edentulism is, however, decreasing over time – an outcome that will increase demand for dental services as our population ages (Chrisopoulos & Harford 2013; Chrisopoulos et al. 2016; Council of Australian Governments Health Council 2015).

The consequences of poor access to oral health care increase in significance and impact on general health in the elderly (Case study 15.1). Oral cancer, for example, is the eighth most common

Case Study 15.1

Oral health in the setting of residential aged care

A bed-bound, immobile, high-care patient is not eating and her health is deteriorating. The nursing-home staff finally determine that toothache is the problem but cannot get the patient to a dentist. The mobile public dental service is booked out and waiting lists are 2 years long. The busy local dentist is fully booked for several months, but finally attends and extracts a tooth for the patient. The staff of the nursing home realise that several of their patients are in need of dental care, and become aware that poor oral health can contribute to poor nutrition, inhalation pneumonia and other quality-of-life compromises for their residents. The local dentist does not have the time or resources to meet the needs of this group of residents. Investigations by the Director of Nursing reveal that there is a funded program operating in South Australia, the Better Oral Health in Residential Care (BOHRC) program (South Australian Department of Health 2014), which covers oral health checks when new residents are admitted and uses the residential aged-care hairdressing salon for dental checks. A study undertaken in Victoria by Hopcraft et al. (2008, 2011) found that dental hygienists can examine, diagnose and provide simple oral health care to the same standard as a dentist for dependent older people in residential aged-care settings, and can reliably identify and refer conditions beyond their scope to dentists and specialists. This study resulted in a change in dental practice regulation in 2000, to allow hygienists and oral health therapists to work in this way. Unfortunately, this model of service still relies on private funding.

Case study questions

1. What are the barriers to oral health for these residents?
2. Who is responsible for their oral health?
3. Which dental practitioners could provide care?
4. What sort of models of care would work in this setting?

cancer and, often as a consequence of late diagnoses (5091 diagnoses and 1034 deaths in 2018; AIHW 2018b), can result in higher mortality than many other cancers. Only 61% of **dentate** individuals (those with teeth) and 16% of **edentulous** (those without teeth) individuals over 60 years of age had visited a dentist in the past 12 months. These issues are exacerbated among nursing home residents whose access to care is complicated by immobility, dependence, multiple and chronic medical conditions and medications, and poor oral hygiene (Council of Australian Governments Health Council 2015; Productivity Commission 2018; Spencer 2011; Spencer & Harford 2008). This situation will worsen as our population ages and people increasingly retain their teeth.

Socio-economic circumstances are clearly related to risk status for dental disease, with the highest levels of disease prevalence occurring in those least able to access care. People from low-income families, refugees, people in rural areas, Aboriginal and Torres Strait Islander people, the elderly, the home-bound and the disabled and those with mental health problems all demonstrate higher levels of dental disease and greater difficulty in accessing dental care (Council of Australian Governments Health Council 2015). The most recent survey of Australia's oral health and dental visiting patterns describe two worlds of dental care. The 39% of adults who inhabit one world have favourable dental visiting patterns (regular check-ups with the same practice and access to timely care) and better oral health. The second world constitutes the majority – some 61% – who have unfavourable (29%) or intermittent (32%) patterns of dental visiting (less than yearly and problem related) and poorer oral health. These people have more untreated oral disease, and their delayed treatment leads to people in pain seeking emergency rather than general care. Further, this second group, who receive many times more tooth extractions, also receive fewer preventive services (Council of Australian Governments Health Council 2015; Productivity Commission 2018).

In summary, there are three key aspects to the community's needs for dental care. First, there is the issue of the high levels of disease prevalence across the whole community that require greater attention to oral health promotion and preventive care. Second, there is the issue of unmet need for services that is largely concentrated in lower-income groups and others least able to access services. Third, there are the cohort patterns associated with fluoridation and increasing retention of teeth among an ageing population, which results in a greater need for lower-technology services among the young to middle-aged and an increasing need for higher-technology services among middle-aged and older adults. Our existing system, while providing excellent care for some, is not meeting the needs of all and is not reducing oral disease levels (Council of Australian Governments Health Council 2015, Productivity Commission 2018).

The problem of service delivery system policy

Dental care sits at the interface between a market model and the welfare state, in that it is excluded from Medicare but is increasingly recognised as being integral to general health and therefore due for broader health policy consideration. The Rudd and Gillard Labor Governments moved to enable this consideration by generating proposals to begin the process of finding more universal approaches to providing services with public funding. The (now-ceased) Chronic Dental Disease Program initiated by the Howard Liberal Government in 2007 was the first of these initiatives, followed in 2012 by the

Child Dental Benefits Scheme which represented something of a revolution in public dental funding, 'looking a lot like the much talked about Denticare' (Dooland 2014, p. 20).

In the 1990s, Lewis and Satur both evaluated the policy environment against Alford's (1975) model of structural interests (dominant interests – professional monopolists, challenging interests – corporate rationalists, and repressed interests – equal health advocates), arguing that the exclusion of dental care from universal health insurance models had preserved the professional hierarchies and power of the market model (for further explanation of these ideas, please see Chapter 1.). Dentists (in private practice) had a monopoly over the market and thus the freedom to set prices, dominate regulatory systems and protect their sovereignty through professional dominance. This model has served those who can afford to participate in the market well, but excluded many, and mostly those with the highest needs for care such as those unable to access (pay for) private dental care (lower income / SES, Indigenous, dependent elderly, new migrants, those with mental or physical health challenges, etc.) (Lewis 2000; Satur 2002).

The National Health Strategy of the early 1990s recognised the high levels of dental disease and included dental care in the reform agenda, driving the consideration of oral health as a social welfare issue and offering opportunities to make proposals that cut across the division of market and welfare models (Dooland 1992). In 1995, for the first time since the development of universal school dental services in the 1970s, the Commonwealth government invested funding in a public dental program (Parliament of Australia 2008), providing services for adults using both public and private clinics. Sadly, this program was de-funded in the first Liberal Government Budget of 1996 (Lewis 2000) presenting a problem for public dental providers who now had visible demand for care from a previously undefined and underserved population group. The de-funding of this scheme set an agenda that drew on the emergence of 'new public management' to drive new models of care, with several states expanding access to adult care through the use of co-payment mechanisms.

The emergence of the National Competition Policy and managerialism challenged and shifted the landscape to redefine the problem as one of powerful interests groups limiting the ability to develop more innovative service models and workforces. This national agenda enabled a change process that diluted the absolute power of the dentist professional monopolists, allowing dental corporate rationalists and equal health advocates to align and challenge the policy monopoly of the dentists (Bacchi 2016; Lewis 2000; National Advisory Committee on Oral Health 2004; Satur 2002; Spencer 2004). In the 2000s, the application of the National Competition Policy and later the development of the National Regulation and Accreditation Scheme and Health Workforce Australia furthered this agenda, resulting in proposals to include dental care in Medicare and enabling challenges to traditional workforce professional hierarchies (see Chapter 1) (Health Workforce Australia 2011; National Advisory Committee on Oral Health 2004; National Advisory Council on Dental Health 2012; Parliament of Australia 2013). Ultimately, the problem with the various interest groups and the current health policy is that a majority (85%+) of dental care is provided through a market-based private business model that benefits business owners but fails to provide for those who are unable to participate in the market. This model of health care delivery has been replaced by Medicare for all other aspects of health care, but the mouth has been excluded and those who benefit from this market-based delivery continue to work to protect their interests.

Dental services: funding and services overview

Under Section 51 xxiii(a) of the Australian Constitution, the Commonwealth government has the power to legislate for 'the provision of pharmaceutical, sickness and hospital benefits, medical and dental services'; however, the state and territory governments have traditionally been responsible for delivering public oral health services (Commonwealth of Australia 2010, p. 15). In 2016–17, total expenditure on dental services in Australia was $10.1 billion, representing 5.6% of total health expenditure – a proportion that has remained relatively unchanged since 2004. Around three-quarters of the expenditure on dental services is borne by individual consumers, compared with just 12% of the expenditure on other health services; this is displayed in Fig. 15.1 (AIHW 2018c; Council of Australian Governments Health Council 2015).

Private-sector services

In Australia, the vast majority of services (88%) are delivered through private dental practices under self-funded (or self-insured) arrangements. The private sector offers care on a fee-for-service basis to all children and adults, including emergency, general and specialist care, with access to technology and evidence-based practice that is equivalent to the best international standards. Fees are set on a competitive market basis, and specialist services do not require referral but often involve one. In

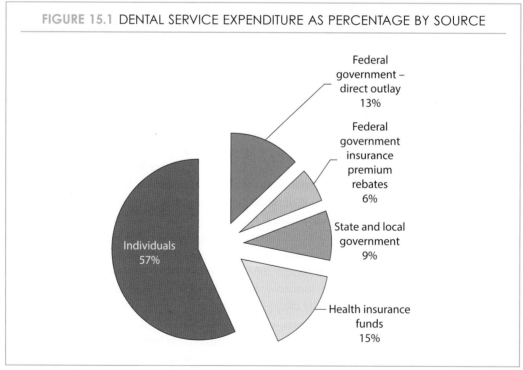

FIGURE 15.1 DENTAL SERVICE EXPENDITURE AS PERCENTAGE BY SOURCE

Federal government – direct outlay 13%

Federal government insurance premium rebates 6%

State and local government 9%

Individuals 57%

Health insurance funds 15%

Source: Adapted from Council of Australian Governments Health Council (2015)

2013, 50% of Australians had some level of private health insurance that included dental benefits; 77% of these policies contributed to dental services but did not entirely cover their cost (Chrisopoulos et al. 2016). Some health insurance funds own practices and provide care directly to their fund-holders, and the Commonwealth government also rebates private health insurance fees through taxation mechanisms.

Public-sector services

After the state dental hospitals, school dental services have been the longest-running **public dental services** in Australia and New Zealand. Australian **school dental services** have, since their expansion under the Whitlam Government in the 1970s, offered dental care to all primary school children and eligible adolescents, through fixed and mobile dental clinics. Funded largely by state and territory governments, this service has continued since that time, although eligibility and service delivery models vary from state to state. For example, Victoria, New South Wales and the Australian Capital Territory (ACT) provide services predominantly through community-based clinics with some outreach mobile clinics. Western Australia, Queensland and South Australia have dedicated school dental program clinics (both fixed and mobile), and the Northern Territory uses a mixed model consisting of community-based services and school dental clinics with outreach to remote communities (Council of Australian Governments Health Council 2015).

Eligibility also varies, from primary and secondary school children in some states to all children and young people aged 0–18 years regardless of school enrolment. Dental care is free (government funded) for all eligible children and adolescents in most states and territories, with Victoria, ACT and South Australia charging a co-payment for those without concession cards (National Advisory Council on Dental Health 2012). Children are seen as a priority population in the public dental services with no significant waiting periods, but if they require inpatient hospital care then waiting periods can be long (Council of Australian Governments Health Council 2015).

In 2014, following on from the recommendations of the National Advisory Council on Dental Health (NACDH), the Commonwealth government commenced the Child Dental Benefits Scheme, which provides a capped $1000 worth of dental care over a 2-year period to each child eligible for Family Tax Benefit A (around 80% of children). Under the scheme, children between 2 and 17 years old receive basic dental services such as examinations, x-rays, cleaning, fissure sealing, fillings, root canals and extractions. Benefits are not available for orthodontic or cosmetic dental work and cannot be paid for any services provided in a hospital. Services can be provided through private practices and public practices using a fixed scale of items and fees which are rebated through Medicare (Dooland 2014; Department of Health 2017, Productivity Commission 2018).

Public dental services for adults have been characterised over many years by inadequacy; around 36% of Australians are eligible for public dental care; however, current funding for public oral health services allows only around 10% of means-tested adults who are eligible for dental care (those with concession cards and other benefits) to receive care in any one year (AIHW 2018d; National Advisory Council on Dental Health 2012; Productivity Commission 2018). For low-income Australians, the impact of dental disease is magnified because they are unable to afford private care and instead choose public-sector care, which usually means being placed on a waiting list. The long wait for care worsens their dental conditions, resulting in problems that could have been fixed relatively easily becoming more complex and costly: prevention becomes a filling, a filling becomes an extraction; local infections become systemic; a problem becomes pain (Case study 15.2). Despite the investment in a range of programs (see Table 15.1), the 'safety net' is inadequate; this results in some services being overwhelmed by 'emergency' visits for pain and infections, and in the need for prioritising of care for particularly vulnerable people (e.g. Aboriginal and Torres Strait Islander people, pregnant women, those with mental health problems and disabilities, those who are homeless, and refugees and asylum seekers). Others simply miss out because they are not eligible for care in the public sector and cannot afford care in the private sector.

Case Study 15.2

Oral health for a low-income / working-poor family

Gerrard is a father of four and works as a cleaner; he earns too much to qualify for a Health Care Card or public dental care, but not enough to be able to afford regular dental care. His children see the school dental service, but there is simply not enough money left at the end of the week to afford health insurance or for private dental care for himself or his wife. He has had a hole in his tooth for some time, which has started to ache, but he has been too scared to go to a dentist because he knows there are several teeth needing treatment and fears the embarrassment of being unable to pay. He puts up with toothache until it becomes overwhelming, and finally goes to see his general practitioner and is given antibiotics (bulk-billed to Medicare). This resolves the problem temporarily, but it recurs and a swelling around his neck starts to make it hard to breathe. Gerrard, unable to breathe properly or sleep, finally goes to a hospital emergency department with an infection that is compromising his airway. He requires tracheotomy to maintain his airway and extraction of the tooth under general anaesthesia. Gerrard loses 3 days' work and another tooth.

Case study questions

1 What are the costs to Gerrard, the health system and his family?
2 How do you think this affects Gerrard's quality of life?
3 Can you think of better ways to deal with Gerrard's situation? How could this be funded?

Delays in being able to access preventive or urgent dental care shifts, compounds and creates other problems for non-dental health services. A downstream effect is that people often seek relief of pain and infections through other services, such as public and private hospitals, hospital outpatient clinics and general practitioners (GPs). In 2015–16, around 67,000 Australians were hospitalised for acute preventable dental conditions (up from 63,000 in 2012–13), the third highest cause of potentially preventable hospitalisations after kidney infections and dehydration / gastroenteritis. Young children have the highest rates of hospitalisations; in 2012, some 8000 children aged 0–4 years and 14,000 aged 5–9 years were admitted to hospital for dental conditions (Council of Australian Governments

TABLE 15.1 SUMMARY OF COMMONWEALTH-FUNDED DENTAL PROGRAMS

Period	Program	Scope
	Veterans' Affairs programs	Members of Australian Defence Force, Army Reserve and eligible veterans
	Aboriginal Community Controlled Dental Services	Dental services provided through Aboriginal Community Controlled Health Services
	Cleft Lip and Palate (CLP) Scheme	For children 0–18 years of age diagnosed with CLP
	Oral health services for prisoners and asylum seekers in community detention	People in detention facilities and community detention have access to free oral health care but may face long waiting times
1999–	Private Health Insurance Rebate	30%–40% rebate provided to people with private health insurance which includes dental services ($606 million in 2012–13)
2004–07	Enhanced Primary Care Program	People with specific chronic disease impacting on or impacted by their oral health
2007–12	Medicare Chronic Disease Dental Scheme	People with GP-managed chronic disease whose oral health is, or is likely to, impact on their oral health
2008–13	Medicare Teen Dental Program	Children aged 12–17 years receiving Family Tax Benefit A and other income support payments – examination and preventive services only
2013–15	Voluntary Dental Graduate Year Program	Provision of practice experience, professional development and mentoring to new graduate dentists in under-served areas
2014–15	Oral Health Therapist (OHT) Graduate Year Program	Provision of practice experience, professional development and mentoring to new graduate OHTs in under-served areas
2013–14	Dental relocation and infrastructure program	To encourage and support dentists to relocate to regional and remote areas (workforce redistribution)

Continued

TABLE 15.1 SUMMARY OF COMMONWEALTH-FUNDED DENTAL PROGRAMS—cont'd

Period	Program	Scope
2012/13–2021/22	Stronger Futures in the Northern Territory and National Partnership Agreement oral health implementation	Oral health services program for Aboriginal and Torres Strait Islander children under 16 years of age, with a focus on remote communities
2013–15	National Partnership Agreement – treating more public dental patients	Reduction of public dental waiting lists – tied grants allocated to state and territory public dental programs
2014–	Child Dental Benefits Scheme	Basic dental care for children aged 12–17 years receiving Family Tax Benefit A and other income support payments

Sources: Adapted from Council of Australian Governments Health Council (2015), National Advisory Council on Dental Health (2012), Department of Health (2017), Chrisopoulos et al. (2016)

Health Council 2015, Productivity Commission 2018). This downstream problem represents a significant cost-shift arising out of poor access to care, and a considerable cost to the health system and the economy through days lost at work and school.

> PAUSE
> *for*
> REFLECTION
> …
>
> Should the government include dental care in Medicare? Why do you think it is not included at present?

Current workforce or practitioner groups and roles

The dental and oral health workforce comprises registered dental practitioners (dentists, specialist dentists, dental therapists, hygienists and oral health therapists, and dental prosthetists) alongside dental assistants and dental technicians who are not registered (see Table 15.2). Prior to 2004, there was a projected shortage in the workforce which has resulted in considerable increases in education intakes for dentists and in the immigration of overseas-qualified dentists, resulting in workforce growth of almost 100% for dentists between 2007 and 2012 (Health Workforce Australia 2014). Some recent analyses show that there is an over-supply of dentists (arising out of both graduate and immigration pathways) in relation to market demand (Health Workforce Australia 2011;

TABLE 15.2 DENTAL AND ORAL HEALTH PRACTITIONER ROLE DESCRIPTIONS

Role		Description
Dentist	✓	Dentists practise all parts of dentistry, including assessment, diagnosis, treatment, management and preventive services for patients of all ages
Dental therapist	✓	Dental therapists provide oral health assessment, diagnosis, treatment, management and preventive services for children, adolescents and young adults (and, with additional education, for all adults) within a preventive philosophy. They provide fillings and tooth removal, additional oral care, and oral health education and promotion for individuals and communities. Dental therapists are autonomous practitioners who work in collaborative and referral relationships with dentists
Dental hygienist	✓	Dental hygienists provide oral health assessment, diagnosis, treatment, management and education for the prevention of oral disease to promote oral health for people of all ages. They provide periodontal/gum treatment, preventive services and other oral care. Dental hygienists are autonomous practitioners who work in a collaborative and referral relationship with dentists
Oral health therapist	✓	Oral health therapists are qualified as *both* a dental therapist and a dental hygienist and provide all the services of both. Like dental therapists and hygienists, they work with dentists and specialists providing orthodontic treatment, specialist periodontal and paediatric treatment, and dental care for other high-needs people
Dental prosthetist	✓	Dental prosthetists provide assessment, treatment, management and provision of removable dentures and mouth-guards used for sporting activities. With additional education and a written referral from a dentist, they also provide various types of splints, sleep apnoea devices, anti-snoring devices, immediate dentures and additions to existing dentures
Dental assistant		A dental assistant supports the provision of clinical dental care by preparing patients and assisting dentists, dental specialists, dental hygienists, therapists and oral health therapists in providing care and treatment. They may also carry out reception and administration work and, with additional training, are able to take X-rays and provide oral health education

Continued

Role		Description
Dental technician		A dental technician constructs and repairs dentures and other dental appliances, working closely with a dentist or dental prosthetist and usually having no patient contact
Specialist areas of dentistry	✓	Registered dental specialists are dentists who have completed additional postgraduate studies and preparation and limit their practice to a specific branch of dentistry, in one of the following areas: dental–maxillofacial radiology, endodontics, oral and maxillofacial surgery, oral medicine, oral pathology, oral surgery, orthodontics, paediatric dentistry, periodontics, prosthodontics, public health dentistry, special needs dentistry, forensic odontology

TABLE 15.2 DENTAL AND ORAL HEALTH PRACTITIONER ROLE DESCRIPTIONS—cont'd

✓ indicates those registered for practice with the Australian Health Practitioner Regulation Agency (Dental Board of Australia).

Sources: Adapted from Dental Board of Australia (2014) and Health Workforce Australia (2011)

Insight Economics 2012; Olive 2014). However, the Australian National Oral Health Plan (2015) states that there are still unresolved service distribution issues for rural and remote communities, and considerable unmet need in many at-risk population groups, and that current workforce numbers represent an opportunity to address unmet need and improve equity (Council of Australian Governments Health Council 2015). There have also been changes in the oral health practitioner workforce, although largely related to the phasing-out of dental therapy and dental hygiene courses and their replacement with oral health therapist courses. Workforce modelling for these professions is hampered by a lack of data on their practice activity and of sound evidence to inform modelling for workforce mix (Health Workforce Australia 2011; Council of Australian Governments Health Council 2015).

In 2013, a majority of dentists worked in the private sector (79.5%), with 34.4% working part-time. The majority of dentists work in major cities, resulting in dentist-to-population ratios of 63 per 100,000 people as compared with 38 per 100,000 people in outer regional and 26 per 100,000 people in remote areas. **Dental therapists** are the only practitioner group who are more evenly distributed, with 2.9 per 100,000 people in major cities, and 4.4 per 100,000 and 5.1 per 100,000 in outer regional and remote settings respectively. **Dental hygienist (DH)** distribution is similar to that of dentists; that of oral health therapists ranges from 3.4 per 100,000 people in cities to 0.7 per 100 000 people in remote settings (AIHW 2016). **Dental prosthetists**, who also mostly work in the private sector (78.2%), have a similar distribution to dentists; in 2013 there were 1195 registered dental prosthetists, with an average ratio of 5 per 100 000 people (AIHW 2016). In recent years, the Commonwealth government has put in place some initiatives in an effort to remediate this misdistribution (see Table 15.1). Table 15.3 shows

TABLE 15.3 ROLES AND NUMBERS OF DENTAL PRACTITIONERS IN AUSTRALIA

Practitioner type	Number of registered practitioners 2018[a] (% total workforce)	Number of registered (% total workforce) in 2012[b]	Practitioner: population ratio (/100,000)[b]	% Female[b]
Dentist	17,240 (74.6%)	14,687 (75.5%)	64.7	36.5
Specialist dentist	1743 (7.5%)	1330		
Dental therapist	934 (4%)	1276 (6.6%)	5.6	96.9
Dental hygienist	1463 (6.3%)	1600 (8.2%)	7.0	94.6
Oral health therapist	2139 (9.2%)	738 (3.8%)	3.2	84.7
Dental prosthetist	1255 (5.4%)	1161 (6%)	5.4	14.7
TOTAL dental practitioners	23,093	19,462	Growth 2012–18= 3631 (15.7%)	
Dental technician		3000		30.7
Dental assistant		19,000		98.2

Sources: a. Dental Board of Australia (2018).
b. Australian Institute of Health and Welfare (2014b).

the dental and oral health workforce characteristics as of 2018, and the workforce growth compared with 2012.

Estimating dental technician and dental assistant numbers is difficult as they are not registered practitioners and because very little reliable data is collected other than self-reported census data. There are perceived shortages of dental assistants reported by the professions and the state and territory governments. Dental assistants may undertake Certificate III or IV courses in dental assisting through the Vocational Education and Training (VET) sector, although training is not currently mandatory and career paths are limited (Health Workforce Australia 2014). Dental technicians undertake workplace-based training or apprenticeship, completing a 2-year VET-sector Diploma of Dental Technology. There has been considerable growth in the dental technician workforce, with graduate numbers almost doubling since 2007.

In recent years there has been an increasing recognition among general health practitioners and others outside the dental sector of the impact of oral disease. Oral disease recognition and referral and preventive advice have been incorporated into the practices of maternal and child health nurses, Aboriginal health workers, community and aged-care nurses and mental health case workers, among others. The contributions made to oral health promotion and individual care goes largely unmeasured but is an important element of holistic health care and promotion (National Advisory Committee on Oral Health 2004; Council of Australian Governments Health Council 2015). There is considerable opportunity to develop inter-professional practice approaches to oral health around the common disease risk factors such as diet, smoking, trauma and cancer prevention and through collaborative health promotion approaches.

Dentists and other oral health practitioners

Dentists, who practise all parts of dentistry, including assessment, diagnosis, treatment, management and preventive services for patients of all ages, are the most readily recognised type of dental practitioner, but not the only one. **Dental prosthetists** work largely from private practices (78.4%) but also in the public sector, providing dentures, mouth guards and other appliances through consulting directly with patients. Dental prosthetists originally train as dental technicians to manufacture dentures and dental appliances (through a VET-sector apprenticeship), and then complete additional training to enable registration for practice in direct patient care. Tasmania, in 1957, was the first jurisdiction to regulate the practice and title for prosthetists, who in some places are referred to as clinical dental technicians (Australian Dental Prosthetists Association 2015).

In Australia, **dental therapists** have practised for over 50 years, providing diagnostic, preventive, restorative and health promotion services to children and adolescents in a collaborative and referral relationship with dentists. Like their New Zealand counterparts (where they have practised for almost 100 years), dental therapists have been responsible for their own diagnosis and treatment planning and have referred to dentists those patients with treatment needs beyond their scope of practice. Dental therapists have been the backbone of school dental services Australia-wide, working in metropolitan, regional, rural and remote settings with some of the population groups with the highest needs, including those with poor access to health services. Until 2000, dental therapists were limited to employment with school dental services, but today they practise in the public and private sectors, community health, hospitals and outreach programs. Likewise, **dental hygienists** have practised in Australia since the early 1970s (internationally for 100 years), providing preventive and periodontal (gum disease) services to people of all ages, mostly in private practice. They have traditionally practised in private practice settings in close collaboration with dentists; however, in recent years they too have moved into all areas that have needs matching their skills. Both of these types of practitioner originally developed to address areas of dental practice that were not being well served (children and prevention), in collaborative models of care designed to extend the capacity of dentists. More recently, a combination of the two has evolved to produce the **oral health therapist**. Australia currently has approximately 4500 oral health practitioners (see Table 15.3).

Dental therapists and dental hygienists provide primary health care services (dental examinations, diagnosis, treatment planning, preventive and health promotion services), with therapists providing restorative services (fillings and simple extractions), and hygienists providing maintenance care for periodontal conditions; these are the most common dental services required in the population. Oral health therapists are able to provide all of these services;. Importantly, as autonomous practitioners who collaborate with dentists and refer people with needs beyond their scope of practice to a dentist (or other health practitioner), **oral health therapy practitioners** (dental hygienists, dental and oral health therapists) make an important contribution to the dental and oral health workforce (Case study 15.3). Research over many years has produced evidence that they provide services (within their scope) to the same quality as dentists, reliably recognise the boundaries of their practice and refer, can diagnose and plan treatment care in the most complex patients (including those with complex medical conditions and medications), and provide care that is acceptable to patients (Calache et al. 2009; Dooland 2014; Health Workforce Australia 2011; Hopcraft et al. 2008, 2011; Satur 2002; Satur et al. 2009).

Case Study 15.3

Oral health care in a remote Aboriginal community

Debbie is a dental therapist who has worked for 30 years providing remote-area oral health services in remote communities. She provides clinical dental services (check-ups, fillings, extractions and preventive treatments) for 0- to 18–year-olds and oral health promotion from a community-based clinic. She also provides outreach care for smaller, more remote communities, referring back to her own clinic in town for treatment services. Debbie works with the local Aboriginal health workers to ensure that all the eligible children and adolescents in her area receive care, collaborating with community nurses, elders and teachers and referring to a local GP for antibiotics when needed. She manages rheumatic heart and other complex issues locally, using the telephone or Skype when advice is required. There is a shortage of dentists up north, and a dentist employed by the public sector visits once every 2–3 months to handle cases beyond Debbie's scope of practice.

Mary, a 26-year-old mother of one of Debbie's patients (whom Debbie's routinely treated up until she was 18), presents with toothache – an acute and painful infection with swelling under the area of her lower jaw – asking for help. There is no dentist in the town, and due to staff shortages one will not visit for 6 weeks. The permanent tooth needs extracting (which Debbie was allowed to do up until 1990 before the regulations changed); antibiotics will reduce the infection, but the tooth needs to come out to allow the area to heal properly. Under current regulation and policy, Debbie cannot treat Mary in her clinic, and so Mary is evacuated by air to Darwin to have the tooth extracted at a cost of several thousand dollars.

Case study questions

1 What are some of the solutions for a situation like this?
2 Why are there not enough dental practitioners in remote areas?
3 Is this a private or a state/Commonwealth government problem?
4 What are the barriers to oral health for rural and remote residents?

Models of care for oral health therapy practitioners

The practice of oral health therapists is situated in a primary health care/public health paradigm that emphasises prevention and health promotion, offering the opportunity to re-orient oral health services into more preventive models of care given the appropriate funding models. They graduate 'practice-ready' after completing three-year undergraduate Bachelor's degrees in oral health at university dental or health science faculties and, like dentists, are registered for practice by the Australian Health Practitioner Regulation Agency through the Dental Board of Australia (DBA 2018). Their courses are accredited, again like dentists, by the Australian Dental Council (2016). Where dentists may spend five or even seven years (via graduate-entry models) preparing for practice, oral health therapists offer lower-cost models of care through shorter practice preparation and lower salaries. They are more likely to work in rural and remote settings and outreach programs, and offer the opportunity to free up dentists to focus on higher-technology and more complex care.

Oral health therapy practitioners offer considerable scope to extend the capacity of the dental care system by increasing the supply of services, and by working to reduce disease (demand) and extend the reach of public dental services into high-needs populations through these lower-cost models of care. Research in aged-care settings has shown that dental hygienists can reliably diagnose and plan oral health treatment for dependent people living in residential aged-care settings with high care needs (Hopcraft et al. 2008, 2011), offering the capacity to increase services to an ageing population (see Case study 15.1). Public-sector research has demonstrated that dental therapists can provide restorative care to both children (their traditional patient group) and adults (a more recent development) at the same level of quality and acceptability as dentists (Calache et al. 2009), and many studies have demonstrated their ability to appropriately refer people with needs beyond their scope of practice. Indeed, research over many years in many countries has provided evidence of the quality of care of both dental therapists and dental hygienists (Galloway et al. 2002; Nash et al. 2012; Satur 2002). Increasingly in Australia, they are also working in dental specialist practices including pedodontic, periodontic, prosthodontics and orthodontic practices, and in hospital and special-needs settings including cancer, cleft lip and palate, and HIV specialist units, and in outreach and remote communities.

In traditional private dental practice settings, dentists have been the first provider a patient would see, and they might then be referred to a hygienist or therapist for some components of care. In the public-sector school dental services, dental therapists have traditionally been the first practitioner to examine and treat patients, and only those with needs beyond the therapist's scope would be referred to a dentist. In recent times, some public-sector agencies have moved to utilising the dental or oral health therapist as the primary provider for all patients, with referral to dentists where needed. This model offers increased primary prevention for all patients with lower-cost care, and uses dentists' higher-level training for more complex care. Indeed, this model was recommended over 25 years ago by the World Health Organization (1990) and has been established as the main model of care in the Netherlands in recent years (Institute of Medicine of the National Academies 2009). The real benefit (yet to be realised) would be a reduction in the costs of care and extension of services for high-needs and under-served population groups and patients by enabling team dentistry approaches.

In addition to the clinical scope of practice, oral health therapy practitioners undertake preparation in the social sciences, behavioural sciences and health promotion (Australian Dental Council 2016).

This preparation is designed to enable interprofessional practice and a focus on the social determinants of health, to achieve improved oral health for the community. The vision is that these practitioners represent the capacity to 'un-silo' dentistry and integrate oral health in holistic ways. Collaboration with practitioners in the community, mental health, disability, nursing and welfare sectors is important to improving health generally, and oral health specifically (Council of Australian Governments Health Council 2015). The challenge, as with all health problems, is to re-orient health services and achieve a balance between clinical care and health promotion activity.

Debates around oral health therapy practice

There are, of course, some current debates around the practice models of oral health therapists. Originally, the practice of dental therapists and hygienists was tightly tied to that of dentists, with regulations requiring dentist supervision of such practice. The problem then is served by the professionally dominant monopolistic models of dentistry during their years of establishment, and there are discourses from vested interests that would return to these models (Australian Dental Association 2013, 2018). Many of the arguments applied will be familiar to nurse practitioners. Contemporary health workforce frameworks have now largely been applied to oral health therapy practice, although vestiges of the old rhetoric remain.

One issue held over from past practices relates to the age limit of people who can receive restorative services from dental and oral health therapists (in some states, only people over 5 and under 18 years old), arising from old school dental service models which remain despite national regulation (Health Workforce Australia 2011; National Advisory Council on Dental Health 2012). There is evidence from Victoria and elsewhere that dental and oral health therapists provide excellent-quality services to preschoolers and young adults and, with appropriate training, can provide restorative services to all adults (Calache et al. 2009; Calache & Hopcraft 2012; Nash et al. 2012). Indeed, Health Workforce Australia and the Commonwealth government have both recognised this and note that this would significantly increase public-sector capacity and translate the successes of the school dental service across the adult population (Australian Health Ministers' Advisory Council 1996; Health Workforce Australia 2011, Productivity Commission 2018).

Despite their autonomous practice, oral health practitioners are in many cases unable to charge directly for their services. Oral health practitioners do not have provider numbers, so their ability to directly bill funding organisations such as insurance companies and Medicare for their services is problematic. Their services are currently billed under dentists' provider numbers, which imposes a cost layer to billing and creates a bundled service model. As an example, dental therapists, dental hygienists and oral health therapists can prescribe, interpret and expose X-rays but cannot bill for them – a dentist must sign the prescription. Insurance companies will not rebate services provided in private practices by dental hygienists or dental and oral health therapists – they must use a dentist's provider number (Department of Health 2017; Health Workforce Australia 2011; Parliament of Australia 2013). This results, in many cases, in people receiving services from an oral health therapy practitioner and being charged for those of a dentist. Commonwealth dental services for veterans have also used the same funding models (Department of Veterans' Affairs 2014). A further problem is that this conceals the true data about their contribution to service provision.

PAUSE
for
REFLECTION
...

What is independent practice? What does it mean to be an independent practitioner? Is this different to autonomous practice?

Workforce numbers in the oral health professions are low, and there are arguments to support the notion that increasing the numbers of oral health therapy graduates and decreasing those of dentists to achieve greater numerical parity would offer better service orientation in line with community needs. In our current climate of health sector innovation and reform, oral health therapists, dental therapists, dental hygienists and dental prosthetists offer significant opportunities to improve the way we deliver oral health services and can contribute to increasing access to oral health care, particularly for under-served populations and in the public sector. While the voice of dentists is the loudest and most obvious, the need to consider new ways of providing oral health care means that prevention and health promotion, full utilisation of the workforce, and collaborative teamwork can re-orient our approaches to oral health and improve access to care.

Summary

- Dental diseases are among the most prevalent and costly in our community.
- The Commonwealth government funds only around 16% of dental services.
- Only about 40% of Australians have good access to oral health care.
- There is a range of dental practitioners other than dentists.
- There is potential to utilise oral health practitioners much more widely to improve access to care.

Review Questions

1 Think about the range of dental practitioners and consider why dentists are the most visible. Why do you think the other practitioner types have developed?

2 Why do you think dental and oral health therapists were originally limited to providing fillings for people up to the age of 25? (Note: permanent teeth begin to come through at the age of 6, and by the age of 14 people have most of their permanent teeth.)

3 If 88% of dental services are provided from private practices, how do we ensure the provision of preventive services and health promotion? Will individuals pay for this? What sorts of programs and funding mechanisms do we need to encourage health professionals to provide health promotion services for individuals and communities?

4 How can we increase access to regular dental care for low-income people? Are there better models of care available to address dental diseases?

5   What inter-professional collaborative practice opportunities exist to improve oral health? How could oral health and general health practitioners work together given the barriers imposed by funding and service models?

References

Alford, R., 1975. Health Care Politics: Ideological and Interest Group Barriers to Reform. University of Chicago Press, Chicago.

Australian Dental Association (ADA), 2013. Hope for Scope Campaign, ADA, Sydney.

Australian Dental Association (ADA), 2018. ADA, Sydney. https://www.ada.org.au/.

Australian Dental Council (ADC), 2016. Program accreditation standards and competencies. ADC, Melbourne. https://www.adc.org.au/Program-Accrediation.

Australian Dental Prosthetists Association (ADPA), 2015. What is a dental prosthetist. ADPA, Melbourne. https://www.adpa.com.au/dentalprosthetistsandyou/what-is-a-dental-prosthetist.

Australian Health Ministers Advisory Council (AHMAC), 1996. Project to pilot a dental auxiliary. Background paper, AHMAC, Sydney, September 1996.

Australian Institute of Health and Welfare (AIHW), 2014a. Australia's health 2014 (Australia's Health series no. 14; AIHW cat. no. AUS 178). AIHW, Canberra.

Australian Institute of Health and Welfare (AIHW), 2014b. Dental workforce, 2012. National Health Workforce Series no. 7. Cat no. HWL 53, AIHW, Canberra.

Australian Institute of Health and Welfare (AIHW), 2016. Oral health and dental care. AIHW, Canberra. https://www.aihw.gov.au/getmedia/57922dca-62f3-4bf7-9ddc-6d8e550c7c58/19000.pdf. aspx?inline=true.

Australian Institute of Health and Welfare (AIHW), 2018a. Australia's health 2018. Australia's health series no. 16. AUS221. AIHW, Canberra. https://www.aihw.gov.au/getmedia/7c42913d-295f-4bc9-9c24 -4e44eff4a04a/aihw-aus-221.pdf.aspx?inline=true.

Australian Institute of Health and Welfare (AIHW), 2018b. Cancer data in Australia 2018. Cancer Compendium. Cat. no. CAN 122. AIHW, Canberra. https://www.aihw.gov.au/reports/cancer/ cancer-data-in-australia/contents/summary.

Australian Institute of Health and Welfare (AIHW), 2018c. Health expenditure Australia 2016–17. Cat. no. HWE 74. AIHW, Canberra. https://www.aihw.gov.au/getmedia/ e8d37b7d-2b52-4662-a85f-01eb176f6844/aihw-hwe-74.pdf.aspx?inline=true.

Australian Institute of Health and Welfare (AIHW), 2018d. A discussion of public dental waiting times information in Australia: 2013–14 to 2016–17. Cat. no. DEN 230. AIHW, Canberra. https://www.aihw .gov.au/getmedia/df234a9a-5c47-4483-9cf7-15ce162d3461/aihw-den-230.pdf.aspx?inline=true.

Bacchi, C., 2016. Problematizations in health policy: questioning how "problems" are constituted in policies. Paper presented at the ASSA (Academy of the Social Sciences)-funded Workshop on Understanding Australian Policies on Public Health, Flinders University.

Calache, H., Hopcraft, M., 2012. Provision of oral health care to adult patients by dental therapists without the prescription of a dentist. J. Public Health Dent. 72, 19–27.

Calache, H., Shaw, J., Groves, V., et al., 2009. The capacity of dental therapists to provide direct restorative care to adults. Aust. N. Z. J. Public Health 33 (5), 424–429.

Chrisopoulos, S., Harford, J.E., 2013. Oral health and dental care in Australia: key facts and figures 2012. Cat. no. DEN 224. AIHW, Canberra.

Chrisopoulos, S., Harford, J.E., Ellershaw, A., 2016. Oral health and dental care in Australia: key facts and figures 2015. Cat. no. DEN 229. AIHW, Canberra.

Commonwealth of Australia, 2010. Australia's Constitution, AGPS Canberra. https://www.aph.gov.au/About_Parliament/Senate/Powers_practice_n_procedures/Constitution.aspx.

Council of Australian Governments (COAG) Health Council, 2015. Healthy Mouths Healthy Lives: Australia's National Oral Health Plan 2015–2024, prepared by the National Oral Health Monitoring Committee, for AHMAC, Canberra. http://www.coaghealthcouncil.gov.au/Portals/0/Australia%27s%20National%20Oral%20Health%20Plan%202015-2024_uploaded%20170216.pdf.

Dental Board of Australia (DBA), 2014. Guidelines for scope of practice, AHPRA, Melbourne. https://www.dentalboard.gov.au/Codes-Guidelines/Policies-Codes-Guidelines/Guidelines-Scope-of-practice.aspx.

Dental Board of Australia (DBA), 2018. Registrant data April 2018–June 2018, AHPRA, Melbourne. https://www.dentalboard.gov.au/About-the-Board/Statistics.aspx.

Department of Health, 2017. Guide to the Child Dental Benefits Schedule. Department of Health, Canberra. https://health.gov.au/internet/main/publishing.nsf/Content/42FC28F2797C4A10CA257BF0001A35F6/$File/Guide%20to%20the%20Child%20Dental%20Benefits%20Schedule.pdf.

Department of Veterans' Affairs, 2014. Fee schedule of dental services for dentists and dental specialists, effective 1 June 2014. Based on Australian Schedule of Dental Services and Glossary, tenth ed. Commonwealth of Australia, Canberra. www.dva.gov.au/sites/default/files/files/providers/dental/DentalFeeSched.pdf.

Dooland, M., 1992. Improving dental health in Australia. Background paper no. 9, National Health Strategy, Department of Health Housing and Community Services, AGPS, Canberra.

Dooland, M., 2014. Revolutionising public dental health, The Health Advocate. Australian Health and Hospitals Association, Canberra.

Galloway, J., Gorham, J., Lambert, M., et al., 2002. The professionals complementary to dentistry: systematic review and synthesis. University College London, Eastman Dental Hospital, Dental Team Studies Unit, London.

Health Workforce Australia, 2011. Scope of practice review – oral health practitioners, HWA, Adelaide.

Health Workforce Australia, 2014. Australia's future health workforce – oral health (detailed report). Commonwealth Department of Health, Canberra.

Hopcraft, M.S., Morgan, M.V., Satur, J.G., et al., 2008. Dental service provision in Victorian residential aged care facilities. Aust. Dent. J. 53 (3), 239–245.

Hopcraft, M.S., Morgan, M.V., Satur, J.G., et al., 2011. Utilizing dental hygienists to undertake dental examination and referral in residential aged care facilities. Community Dent. Oral Epidemiol. 39 (4), 378–384.

Insight Economics, 2012. Review of dental workforce supply to 2020. Australian Dental Association, St Leonards. www.ada.org.au/publications/dwreview.aspx.

Institute of Medicine of the National Academies (IOM), 2009. The U.S. Oral Health Workforce in the Coming Decade: Workshop Summary. National Academies Press, Washington USA.

Lewis, J., 2000. From 'fightback' to 'biteback': the rise and fall of a national dental program. Aust. J. Pub. Admin. 59 (1), 60–72.

Nash, D.A., Friedman, J.W., Mathu-Muju, K.M., et al., 2012. A Review of the Global Literature on Dental Therapists: In the Context of the Movement to Add Therapists to the Oral Health Workforce in the United States. The Kellogg Foundation, Battle Creek, MI.

National Advisory Committee on Oral Health, 2004. Healthy Mouths Healthy Lives: Australia's National Oral Health Plan 2004–2013. South Australian Department of Health, Adelaide.

National Advisory Council on Dental Health (NACDH), 2012. Report of the National Advisory Council on Dental Health, Commonwealth Department of Health, Canberra.

Olive, R., 2014. Long awaited Health Workforce Australia report confirms national oversupply of dentists. ADA media release. ADA, Sydney.

Parliament of Australia (PoA), 2008. Overview of Commonwealth involvement in funding dental care. Research paper no.1, 2008–09, Biggs A, Social Policy Section, Parliament of Australia. http://www.aph. gov.au/About_Parliament/Parliamentary_Departments/Parliamentary_Library/pubs/rp/ rp0809/09rp01#Dental.

Parliament of Australia (PoA), 2013. Bridging the dental gap: report on the inquiry into adult dental services, House of Representatives Standing Committee on Health and Ageing, (Chair, J. Hill), Commonwealth of Australia, Canberra.

Productivity Commission, 2018. Report on government services 2018. Part E, Chapter 10 Primary and community health. https://www.pc.gov.au/research/ongoing/report-on-government-services/2018/ health/primary-and-community-health.

Sanders, A.E., 2007. Social determinants of oral health: conditions linked to socioeconomic inequalities in oral health and in the Australian population. Cat. no. POH 7. AIHW, Canberra.

Satur, J., 2002. Australian dental policy reform and the utilisation of dental therapists and hygienists, PhD thesis, Deakin University, Melbourne.

Satur, J., Gussy, M., Mariño, R., et al., 2009. Patterns of dental therapists' scope of practice and employment in Victoria, Australia. J. Dent. Educ. 73 (3), 416–425.

South Australian Department of Health, 2014. Better oral health in residential care program, South Australian Department of Health, Adelaide. https://www.sahealth.sa.gov.au/wps/wcm/connect/ public+content/sa+health+internet/clinical+resources/clinical+topics/oral+health+care+for+older +people/better+oral+health+in+residential+care.

Spencer, A.J., 2004. Narrowing the inequality gap in oral health and dental care in Australia. Commissioned paper series 2004. Australian Health Policy Institute, University of Sydney.

Spencer, A.J., 2011. Oral health and dental services in Australia. Presentation to the National Advisory Council on Dental Health.

Spencer, A.J., Harford, J., 2008. Improving oral health and dental care for Australians. Prepared for the National Health and Hospitals Reform Commission. Australian Research Centre for Population Oral Health, The University of Adelaide.

World Health Organization (WHO) Expert Committee on Educational Imperatives for Oral Health Workforce, 1990. Change or Decay? Educational imperatives for oral health workforce. Report of a WHO Expert Committee, Technical Report Series 794, WHO, Geneva.

Further Reading

Brotherhood of St Laurence – End the decay: www.bsl.org.au/services/dental-care.

Council of Australian Governments (COAG) Health Council, 2015. Australian National Oral Health Plan 2015–2024, COAG Health Council, Canberra. www.nds.org.au/asset/view_document/979323603 (draft version).

Health Workforce Australia (HWA), 2011. Scope of practice review – oral health practitioners, HWA, Adelaide. www.hwa.gov.au/sites/uploads/hwa-oral-health-review-report-201208.pdf.

House Standing Committee on Health and Ageing, 2013. Bridging the dental gap: report on the inquiry into adult dental services in Australia, Parliament of Australia, Canberra. www.aph.gov.au/ parliamentary_business/committees/house_of_representatives_committees?url=haa/dental/ report.htm.

National Advisory Council on Dental Health, 2012. Final report of the National Advisory Council on Dental Health, Department of Health, Canberra. www.health.gov.au/internet/main/publishing.nsf/Content/ final-report-of-national-advisory-council-on-dental-health.htm.

Productivity Commission, 2017. Introducing competition and informed user choice into human services: reforms to human services. Report no. 85, Canberra. (Chapter 12: Public dental services) https:// www.pc.gov.au/inquiries/completed/human-services/reforms/report.

Online Resources

ADOHTA – Australian Dental and Oral Health Therapists' Association: www.adohta.net.au.

Dental Hygienists' Association of Australia: www.dhaa.info.

CHAPTER 16

Digital health and the divide

Sandeep Reddy

Key learning outcomes

When you finish this chapter you should be able to:

- describe the digital health landscape in Australia
- understand the importance of electronic health records in digital health strategy
- identify various digital health applications to improve health outcomes
- recognise the digital divide separating urban and regional Australia
- examine the role digital health plays in the Indigenous health context in Australia.

Key terms and abbreviations

Australian Digital Health Agency (ADHA)
digital divide
electronic health record (EHR)
mobile-driven health service delivery
My Health Record (MHR)
National Broadband Network (NBN)
Personally Controlled Electronic Health Record (PCEHR)
telehealth

Introduction

Australians are increasingly spending time online and utilising various forms of digital technology. The Digital Inclusion Index, which considers access, affordability and digital ability, went up from 52.7 in 2014 to 60.2 in 2018 for Australia (Thomas et al. 2018); 80% of Australians now own smartphones and 73% of Australians use the internet to research health issues. The network readiness of Australia was ranked as high as 18 in a list of 139 countries in 2016. As digital technologies achieve scale, the cost of deploying them has decreased. Organisations that invested early in digital technologies have begun to see the benefits of the investment in the form of labour and process cost savings (Blackburn et al. 2017; Thomas et al. 2018).

Digital health

The advent of internet and digital technologies has also led to new avenues for engaging patients to adopt healthy lifestyles and to be more involved with health services (Blackburn et al. 2017; Meskó et al. 2017). Coupled with this the proliferation of smart devices that collect health data and delivery of health care through online services has presented new options for treatment and management of diseases. This approach of utilising digital technology to deliver health care so that different points of care are electronically securely connected has been termed digital health (Australian Digital Health Agency (ADHA) 2017). More formally, digital health has been defined as 'the cultural transformation of how disruptive technologies that provide digital and objective data accessible to both caregivers and patients leads to an equal level doctor–patient relationship with shared decision-making and democratization of care' (Meskó et al. 2017, p. 1).

Incorporating digital technologies in health care enables automation and simplification of some processes, facilitates better connectivity amongst different parts of the health system and assists in better reporting with use of advanced analytics (ADHA 2017; Blackburn et al. 2017; National E-Health Transition Authority 2016). Also, adoption of digital technologies is said to improve access to health care to currently disadvantaged communities by enabling new models of care delivery and improving health literacy (ADHA 2017; Blackburn et al. 2017). These aspects will be explored further into the chapter. It has been stated that digitisation of health care delivery can reduce overall health care expenditure in Australia by 8%–12% and considerably improve the quality of health care by reducing adverse drug events, duplication of tests and re-admissions (Blackburn et al. 2017). On the other hand, movement to digital health can bring problems of its own such as exacerbating access to care for those who do not have access to digital infrastructure (discussed further in a later section), risks to privacy and security of data (Australian Association of Practice Management 2017). While privacy and inappropriate access is a concern even for non-digitally enabled health records, the risks accentuate with a digital health system.

PAUSE
for
REFLECTION
...

It has been stated that digitisation of health care can reduce health care costs and enable democratisation of care. How do you think this occurs?

Electronic health record

Electronic health records (EHRs) are considered to be the flagship application of a digital health strategy. An electronic health record has been described as a longitudinal compilation of health information about individual patients and population stored electronically (Gunter & Terry 2005). National EHRs provide a platform for integrating health care information currently collected through several sources thus enabling improvement in quality of care. Such health data repositories provide opportunities for research and analysis of the aggregated data such that evidence-based health care strategies can be adopted by governments and health care providers. Also, increased efficiency in health care delivery can be achieved through improved data sharing, reduced medical errors, improved data security, patient empowerment and time saving for staff (ADHA 2017).

In Australia, the National E-Health Transition Authority (NEHTA) was set up in 2005 to implement a national EHR (National E-Health Transition Authority 2016). The other objectives of NEHTA were to hasten the adoption of e-health by delivering required integration infrastructure and health information standards and lead the development of a security framework to enable authorised only access to data. In 2011, the NEHTA initiated a national EHR application termed '**Personally Controlled Electronic Health Record (PCEHR)**' (Morrison et al. 2011; Pearce & Bainbridge 2014). PCEHR was based on a previous 'Better Patient Management' model, which was an Australia-wide secure electronic system for medication management. With PCEHR, patients were to have a secure access portal through which they could view their medical history supplied by various health care providers they had visited. The PCEHR portal would display the patient's health summary, demographic information, medical conditions, medications and allergies (Pearce & Bainbridge 2014). An index and search function would yield a range of personal health care information including referrals, test results and prescriptions (Fig. 16.1).

In 2013, the Australian Government commissioned a review of the progress with the implementation of the PCEHR system (National E-Health Transition Authority 2016). Based on the recommendations from the review, which outlined the need of a dedicated digital health agency to drive the national EHR implementation and strengthen digital health infrastructure in the nation, the 2015–2016 budget allocated funding to establish a national digital health entity (ADHA 2018a). In July 2016, the **Australian Digital Health Agency (ADHA)** commenced operations as a statutory authority reporting to the states and territories health ministers. The ADHA was tasked to improve the health outcomes of all Australians by setting up a national EHR, improving the digital health infrastructure and pursuing the national digital health strategy.

A key objective of the ADHA was to transition the PCEHR to a national '**My Health Record (MHR)**'(National E-Health Transision Authority 2016). The record would by the end of 2018 be created for everyone unless they choose not to do so (Australian Healthcare and Hospitals Association (AHHA) 2018). It was expected that approximately 98% of Australians would have a health record after 2018. An opt-out period would be available for anyone who would not choose to have their medical records saved on the MHR system. This means a child born in 2018 and whose parents have chosen to retain the medical records of the child on the MHR system would potentially many years later have all their health information accessible from one place. The ADHA would partner with the

FIGURE 16.1 PCEHR SYSTEM

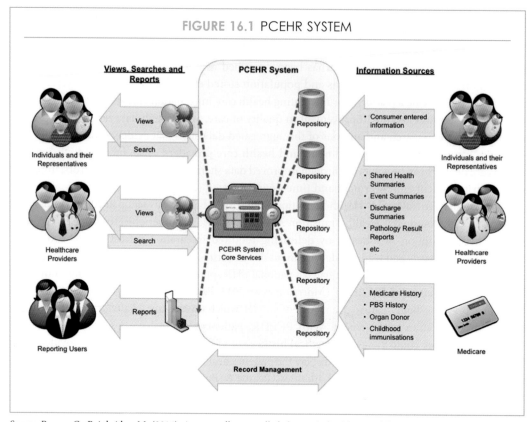

Source: Pearce, C., Bainbridge, M. (2014). A personally controlled electronic health record for Australia. J. Am. Med. Inform. Assoc. 21(4), 707–713.

31 Primary Health Networks and other Healthcare Clinical Information System Providers to source medical information of patients. The MHR is to enable secure health information exchange, better availability and access to prescriptions and medicine information, and drive digital enabled models of care. Just as with the PCEHR, a shared health summary, event summary, discharge summary, referral letters, and prescription records can be accessed via a national consumer portal viewed through a compatible web browser (Fig. 16.2).

While many medical, professional and consumer bodies have welcomed the introduction of a national EHR system and the opt-out approach bearing in mind the significant delays it took to implement the PCEHR, many quarters of the society have raised concerns about the opt-out process and privacy aspects of the stored information (ABC Science 2018). The Australian Government and ADHA have reacted to the concerns by extending the previously designated period to opt-out and by progressing legislative amendments as to who can access the MHR data and highlighting the sophisticated cyber-security protection mechanism and regular audit processes (ADHA 2018b).

FIGURE 16.2 MY HEALTH RECORD PATIENT PORTAL

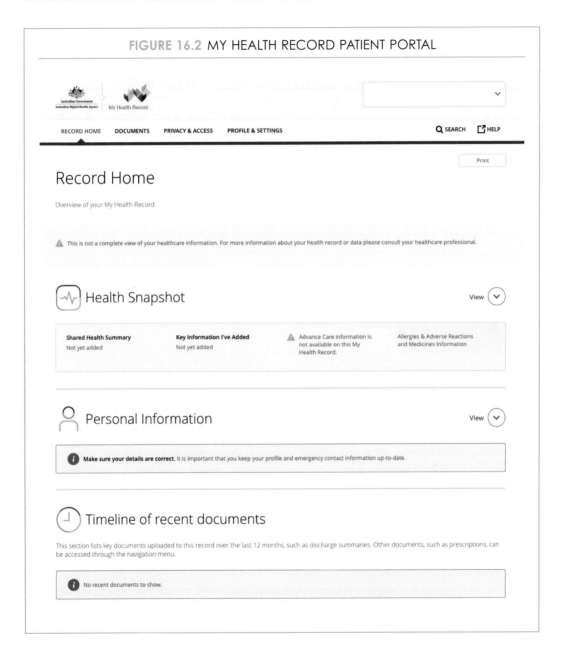

Bacchi discusses in her 'What's the problem represented to be' approach, how policies have problem representations contained within them (Bacchi 2016). If we adopt this line of thinking, it is easy to foresee the tensions between the government and the patient community over privacy concerns continue and ongoing amendments or updated policies issued to address these concerns.

PAUSE
for
REFLECTION
...

While EHRs have demonstrated improvement in quality of clinical care and communication, some have questioned whether benefits can be realised without related changes in the health system such as introduction of appropriate models of care and adequate funding. There are also barriers such as resistance to adoption of the EHR by clinicians. What other barriers do you foresee with the implementation of a national EHR?

Case study 16.1 examines digital health care delivery in acute care settings.

Case Study 16.1

Establishing the First Digital Tertiary Hospital in Australia

Digital health care delivery is well established in primary health care settings but not so much in acute care settings. Princess Alexandra Hospital is a major adult teaching hospital in Queensland with 6529 staff and 833 overnight beds (Sullivan et al. 2016). In 2016, the hospital was chosen to become Australia's first tertiary digital hospital. Becoming a digital hospital in this context included establishing an EHR system and enabling integrated digital vital sign monitoring, digital medication management and digital ECG records. The digital implementation process took place over an 18-month period, but the digital conversion occurred rapidly over the last 2 weeks. To achieve the objectives, an implementation team including practising clinicians was established. Large amount of training (approximately 32,000 hours) was provided to relevant staff including practice of scenarios before and after digitisation occurred. Also, an independent patient safety team was established to monitor adverse events during the course of implementation.

The main technical challenges the implementation team faced included reconciling the legacy and new systems, disruption of normal workflow, slowing down of procedural efficiencies and ensuring clinicians could retrieve significant amount of clinical data for their patients from the new EHR system (Sullivan et al. 2016). The benefits of the implementation were that patient records were now readily available throughout the hospital, digital recording of vital signs and ECGs were more accessible, there was improved clinical decision support and electronic data audits could now be conducted. It was also found that there was a 50% reduction in the rate of cost growth, a 14% reduction in medication incidents, 17% fewer emergency readmissions and a 19% reduction in medical imaging (AHHA 2018).

Other digital health applications in Australia

The national digital health strategy alongside driving the implementation of a national EHR intends to establish digital enabled models of health care that improve accessibility, quality, safety and efficiency of clinical care. One of the digital health approaches that can enable this in the Australian geographical context is '**telehealth**' (Australian Telehealth Society 2017). Telehealth is described as health care delivery or related processes utilising digital technologies to participants separated by distance. Healthcare delivery is slowly starting to see a shift from traditional face-to-face appointments to remote consultations, which are of lower cost and easier access. Almost every known medical specialty in Australia is now using telehealth approaches (e.g. Case study 16.2). Of the medical specialties, the image-focused specialties such as radiology, dermatology and pathology have the most mature telehealth applications. Other clinical activities that can be supported by telehealth models include health promotion, diagnosis, treatment and monitoring of chronic conditions, and team-based health care delivery. States and territories in Australia have adopted telehealth programs for many years now with Queensland, Northern Territory and Western Australia having advanced models. Also, the roll-out of the **National Broadband Network (NBN)** across Australia presents a promising opportunity for a broader telehealth network to be achieved. Though, the varied access to appropriate digital equipment amongst health providers to deliver telehealth services means this digital health approach is yet to achieve its full potential (Ellis 2004).

Mobile devices are playing a huge role in the digital economy with mobile devices exceeding the human population (Rich & Miah 2014). Consequently, the role of mobile devices and application in health is rapidly increasing. **Mobile-driven health service delivery** can operate where there is no cabled infrastructure. Health and technology entities are increasingly releasing mobile applications

Case Study 16.2

The Royal Institute for Deaf and Blind Children (RIDBC) Teleschool

The RIDBC Teleschool established in 2005 provides education and therapy for children with vision and hearing impairment across regional and remote Australia (Telstra 2017). Research has identified children with such impairments benefit from early intervention and specialist support. The Teleschool utilises various digital technologies to provide high-end and in-home video-conferencing services to involved children and families. RIDBC specialist support involves audiology, speech pathology, occupational therapy, physiotherapy and psychology support. Services from the Teleschool includes assessments, individual sessions, group parent sessions, spoken language development and transition to school support. These services are delivered through a combination of video-conferencing, web-based multimedia programs, mobile applications and face-to-face meetings. Parents have stated the programs offered by the Teleschool have not only benefited their children but also improved their confidence and knowledge of the impairments their children have.

whereby individual patient's health information is collected, recorded and shared with health providers (Meskó et al. 2017; Park et al. 2016). The health data is then used by health providers to variously monitor and manage health conditions. Mobile medical applications, which are defined by the Therapeutic Goods Administration as health-related applications that intend to diagnose or provide therapy are increasingly used by Australian health care providers in various domains such as preventive health, chronic disease management and mental health (Blackburn et al. 2017) (Case study 16.3). Mobile health applications have potential to reach vulnerable populations and communities where otherwise other digital technologies cannot be utilised. However, a barrier to wider spread of mobile health is the presence of 'blackspots' (areas with limited or no mobile coverage) (Perlgut 2011; Telstra 2017). While there is a rectification process underway, the vast geographical nature of Australia means there will always be areas where limited mobile coverage abounds.

Case Study 16.3

Mobile Application to Screen Chronic Diseases

The Brisbane North Primary Heath Network (then Metro North Brisbane Medicare Local) launched a mobile application called 'HealthNavigator' in 2014 to provide chronic disease risk assessment, linkage to local general practitioners and access to lifestyle programs and a personalised health report (Seneviratne et al. 2018). The assessments were to be conducted by community health workers or self-administered. The Primary Health Network through an initiative targeted ethnically diverse communities and over a period of 12 months, 2013 assessments were recorded. Of the recorded assessments a total of 41.3% of subjects reported a birthplace outside Australia. Subjects screened by the facilitators were found to have a higher risk of cardiovascular and type 2 diabetes scores compared with the subjects who undertook self-administered assessments. However, there were no significant differences in socio-economic profile of participants screened by facilitated assessments compared with participants undertaking self-administered ones. Evaluation of the mobile application indicates embedding mobile applications in community screening implementation helps with rapid assessments of community risk profiles and translate national guidelines into personalised recommendations.

The digital divide

Australia's growth in overall digitisation is because of increase in digital usage and digital labour. However, the digitisation is uneven across Australia and there has been slow growth in digital infrastructure (Telstra 2017; Willis & Tranter 2006). While the NBN has been the highest profile digital infrastructure program by the government, its aims of connecting all Australians and bridging the **digital divide** has been at best sluggish (Perlgut 2011). The current uneven spread, limitations of technology systems, and access to internet and digital technology has contributed to the digital divide in Australia. National digital connectivity is not only imperative to economic success and positive social dynamics but also important for achieving high-quality health care especially for rural and regional communities and Indigenous Australians (Blackburn et al. 2017; Thomas et al. 2018). Yet, it seems problems lie within the government's current NBN policies and plans where the objective is not so much to improve the bandwidth of internet access but ensure all Australian are connected to broadband internet (Bacchi 2016). This policy may not address the technical requirements for digital health delivery, which relies on large bandwidth and fast internet speeds (ADHA 2017; Australian Telehealth Society 2017; National E-Health Transision Authority 2016).

Digital health in rural and remote Australia

The degree of remoteness and other geographical and resource indicators impact on the cost and delivery of health services. It has been found rural and remote communities in Australia have lesser access to health services compared to their urban counterparts and consequently face poorer health outcomes (Rural Doctors Association of Australia 2017). Digital technologies have an important role in addressing these gaps by enabling affordable access to health care services. While a digital divide exists between city and country, development of the national digital health strategy and the roll-out of the NBN provides an opportunity to reverse the widening digital divide and aid improved diagnostic, treatment and management of health conditions for rural and remote communities (ADHA 2017; Blackburn et al. 2017).

The national digital health strategy outlines the digital divide can be addressed through use of appropriate technology and information services to improve access to care and support appropriate models of care, sustainable workforce and collaborative partnerships (ADHA 2017). A pragmatic step is to leverage the existing infrastructure to enhance adoption of digital health technologies to overcome the challenge of distance. Of the technologies, telehealth is a leading option (Australian Telehealth Society 2017). However, the telehealth services have to be designed for the rural consumer with input from clinicians / health care providers for the services to be user appropriate and sustainable (Ellis 2004). Also, digital health care delivery has to consider current technological limitations so appropriate designs are incorporated in delivery. This bespoke approach ensures development of models of care appropriate to the rural and remote setting. The Northern Territory and South Australian health services have actively used telehealth services to increase attendance at their rural and remote clinics, foster collegial decision making and encourage knowledge sharing between urban and rural clinicians (ADHA 2017; Blackburn et al. 2017).

Digital health In the Indigenous health context

The poorer health status of Indigenous Australians compared with non-Indigenous Australians is well known (Commonwealth of Australia 2017). The 2017 Closing the Gap Prime Minister's report while outlining the health of Indigenous Australians was slowly improving the current rate of progress in lessening the gap was insufficient. This gap is exacerbated for Indigenous Australians living in rural and remote areas. In addition to the geographical disadvantage, language and culture can be additional barriers. Studies have identified that digital technologies can be used as a cost-effective approach to overcome Indigenous disadvantage by affirming the Indigenous identity and providing culturally relevant information (Smith & Mcquire 2016).

In the context of health, cultural identity is important for Indigenous Australians. Digital technologies have been found to be useful in reinvigorating Indigenous cultural practices (Smith & Mcquire 2016).

There is potential for the digital infrastructure that is being rolled out in regional and rural areas to build strong health literacy for Indigenous Australians. Digital health services can be used as a creative and cost-effective opportunity to increase engagement of Indigenous Australians through provision of culturally appropriate and evidence-based interventions (Dingwall et al. 2015; Smith & Mcquire 2016).

The take-up of the MHR system has the potential to improve Indigenous health outcomes through the process of improved Indigenous health data collection and analysis of the same such that Indigenous health programs can be evidence based and informed by research (ADHA 2017). Further, the national digital health strategy states telehealth could be an important medium in ensuring timely access to health care services for Indigenous Australians enabling early diagnosis and early intervention. In addition, mobile applications have also been found to be effective in improving access to various health services for rural and remote Indigenous Australia (Dingwall et al. 2015). These digital health initiatives incorporating inclusive design principles can be an important factor in closing the health gap for Indigenous Australians.

PAUSE *for* **REFLECTION** ...

The establishment of the Australian Digital Health Agency and the roll out of the National Broadband Infrastructure present opportunities to increase delivery of health care through digital technologies. However, with poor access to internet in rural communities and poor health literacy and engagement amongst Indigenous Australians the digital divide may be harder to address. What measures could the government and health providers adopt to enhance the impact of digital health in these populations?

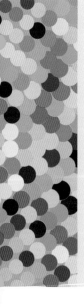

Summary

- Australian organisations and services are increasingly becoming digitised.
- The advent of various digital technologies has presented an opportunity to harness them to deliver health care services.
- Of the various forms of digital health applications being used to deliver health care in Australia are EHRs, telehealth services and mobile health applications.
- The Australian Digital Health Agency is leading the implementation of a national EHR process (MHR) and the national digital health strategy.
- While the prevalence of digital infrastructure is increasing, there exists a digital divide between the city and country populations. The non-uniform spread of digital infrastructure means different digital health delivery models have to be explored.
- Also, there exists a digital health divide between the rest of Australia, and regional and rural communities and Indigenous Australians. Yet, digital health has great prospects in contributing to the health of these disadvantaged communities.

Review Questions

1 What benefits does incorporation of digital technologies in delivery of health care bring?
2 How do Electronic Health Records increase quality and efficiency in health care delivery?
3 What has led to a digital divide in Australia? How can this be addressed?
4 How can digital health improve the health outcomes of rural and Indigenous Australians?

References

ABC Science, 2018. My Health Record opt-out period begins, but privacy concerns remain. https://www.abc.net.au/news/science/2018-07-16/my-health-record-experts-say-its-safe-privacy-concerns-remain/9981658.

Australian Association of Practice Management, 2017. Digital health for better health: the role of practice managers. December, 1–9. AAPM, Melbourne.

Australian Digital Health Agency (ADHA), 2017. Safe, seamless and secure| evolving health and care to meet the needs of modern Australia. National Digital Health Strategy, 1–63. https://conversation.digitalhealth.gov.au/sites/default/files/adha-strategy-doc-2ndaug_0_1.pdf.

Australian Digital Health Agency (ADHA), 2018a. About the Agency. https://www.digitalhealth.gov.au/about-the-agency.

Australian Digital Health Agency (ADHA), 2018b. Opt out of My Health Record. Media release. https://www.digitalhealth.gov.au/search/query:Opt%20out%20of%20My%20Health%20Record.

Australian Healthcare and Hospitals Association (AHHA), 2018. Digital healthcare. Health Advocate, (June), 1–44. https://ahha.asn.au/system/files/docs/publications/jun2018_tha_web_0.pdf.

Australian Telehealth Society, 2017. National digital health strategy-a submission to the Australian Digital Health Agency. https://conversation.digitalhealth.gov.au/sites/default/files/2017-05/Australasian%20Telehealth%20Society%20-%20Your%20Health%20Your%20Say%20Submission%202017.pdf.

Bacchi, C., 2016. Problematizations in health policy: questioning how "problems" are constituted in policies. SAGE Open 6 (2), 1–16. doi:10.1177/2158244016653986.

Blackburn, S., Freeland, M., Gartner, D., 2017. Digital Australia: seizing the opportunity from the Fourth Industrial Revolution. Digital Australia, McKinsey. https://www.mckinsey.com/featured-insights/asia-pacific/digital-australia-seizing-opportunity-from-the-fourth-industrial-revolution.

Commonwealth of Australia, 2017. Closing the Gap Prime Minister's report 2017. Commonwealth of Australia, Department of the Prime Minister and Cabinet, p.112. doi:10.5117/9789053565742.

Dingwall, K.M., Puszka, S., Sweet, M., et al., 2015. Evaluation of a culturally adapted training course in Indigenous e-mental health. Australas. Psychiatry 23 (6), 630–635. doi:10.1177/1039856215608282.

Ellis, I., 2004. Is telehealth the right tool for remote communities? Improving health status in rural Australia. Contemp. Nurse 16 (3), 163–168.

Gunter, T.D., Terry, N.P., 2005. The emergence of national electronic health record architectures in the United States and Australia: models, costs, and questions. J. Med. Internet Res. 7 (1), 1–11. doi:10.2196/jmir.7.1.e3.

Meskó, B., Drobni, Z., Bényei, É., et al., 2017. Digital health is a cultural transformation of traditional healthcare. Mhealth 3, 38. doi:10.21037/mhealth.2017.08.07.

Morrison, Z., Robertson, A., Cresswell, K., et al., 2011. Understanding contrasting approaches to nationwide implementations of electronic health record systems: England, the USA and Australia. J. Healthc. Eng. 2 (1), 25–42.

National E-Health Transition Authority, 2016. Evolution of eHealth in Australia. Achievements, lessons, and opportunities, (April), 1–70. https://www.digitalhealth.gov.au/about-the-agency/publications/reports/benefit-and-evaluation-reports/evolution-of-ehealth-in-australia-achievements-lessons-and-opportunities/Evolution of eHealth in Australia_Publication_20160517.pdf.

Park, S., Burford, S., Lee, J.Y., et al., 2016. Mobile health: empowering people with type 2 diabetes using digital tools. News and Media Research Centre, University of Canberra, 1–54. doi:10.1007/978-3-319-12817-7.

Pearce, C., Bainbridge, M., 2014. A personally controlled electronic health record for Australia. J. Am. Med. Inform. Assoc. 21 (4), 707–713. doi:10.1136/amiajnl-2013-002068.

Perlgut, D., 2011. Digital inclusion in the broadband world: challenges for Australia. In: Communications Policy and Research Forum. pp. 1–13.

Rich, E., Miah, A., 2014. Understanding digital health as public pedagogy: a critical framework. Societies 4 (2), 296–315. doi:10.3390/soc4020296.

Rural Doctors Association of Australia, 2017. Digital health strategy submission, January, 1–16. https://www.rdaa.com.au/documents/item/16.

Seneviratne, M., Hersch, F., Peiris, D.P., 2018. HealthNavigator: a mobile application for chronic disease screening and linkage to services at an urban Primary Health Network. Aust. J. Prim. Health 24 (2), 116–122. doi:10.1071/PY17070.

Smith, K., Chenhall, R., McQuire, S., et al., 2016. Digital futures in Indigenous communities to community hubs. https://www.researchgate.net/publication/306378878_Digital_Futures_in_Indigenous_Communities_From_Health_Kiosks_to_Community_Hubs.

Sullivan, C., Staib, A., Ayre, S., et al., 2016. Pioneering digital disruption: Australia's first integrated digital tertiary hospital. Med. J. Aust. 205 (9), 386–389. doi:10.5694/mja16.00476.

Telstra, 2017. Measuring Australia's digital divide: Australian Digital Inclusion Index 2017. https://digitalinclusionindex.org.au/wp-content/uploads/2018/03/Australian-Digital-Inclusion-Index-2017_v2.pdf.

Thomas, J., Barraket, J., Wilson, C.K., et al., 2018. Measuring Australia's digital divide: the Australian Digital Inclusion Index. RMIT University, Melbourne, Australia. https://researchbank.rmit.edu.au/view/rmit:45478.

Willis, S., Tranter, B., 2006. Beyond the "digital divide": internet diffusion and inequality in Australia. Journal of Sociology 42 (1), 43–59. doi:10.1177/1440783306061352.

Further Reading

Rich, E., Miah, A., 2014. Understanding digital health as public pedagogy: a critical framework. Societies 4, 296–315. doi:10.3990/soc4020296.

NEHTA, 2016. Evolution of eHealth in Australia: Achievements, Lessons and Opportunities. National E-Health Transition Authority, Sydney.

Gunter, T.D., Terry, N.P., 2005. The emergence of national electronic health record architectures in the United States and Australia: models, costs, and questions. J. Med. Internet Res. 7 (1), e3.

Willis, S., Tanter, B., 2006. Beyond the 'digital divide': internet diffusion and inequality in Australia. Journal of Sociology 42 (1), 43–59. doi:10.1177/1440783306061352.

Online Resources

Australian Digital Health Agency (ADHA), 2018. Australia's national digital health strategy: https://conversation.digitalhealth.gov.au/sites/default/files/adha-strategy-doc-2ndaug_0_1.pdf.

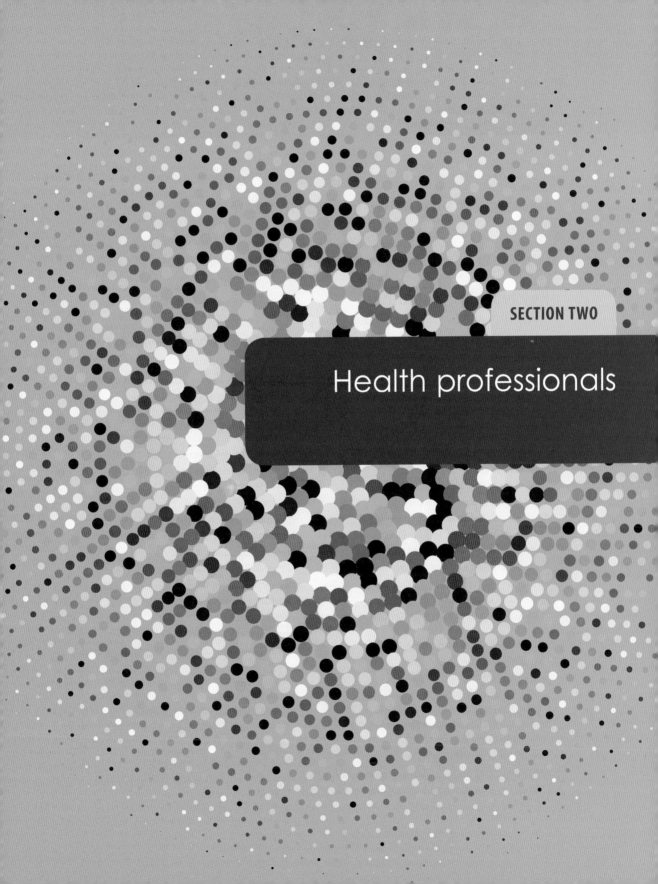

Health professionals

CHAPTER 17

Australia's health workforce

Keith Sutton, Anthony Smith and Susan Waller

Key learning outcomes

When you finish this chapter you should be able to:

+ briefly describe the distribution of the health workforce and how it is organised
+ explain the roles of health professionals and how they contribute to the health care system
+ describe the function of registration and accreditation in the health workforce
+ discuss trends and issues that affect the organisation of the health workforce.

Key terms and abbreviations

Aboriginal and Torres Strait Islander (ATSI)
advanced practice
alcohol and other drug (AOD)
allied health professionals (AHPs)
Allied Health Professions Australia (AHPA)
Australian Association of Social Workers (AASW)
Australian Bureau of Statistics (ABS)
Australian College of Critical Care Nurses (ACCN)
Australian College of Nurse Practitioners (ACNP)
Australian College of Nursing (ACN)
Australian Health Practitioner Regulation Agency (AHPRA)
Australian Medical Association (AMA)
Australian Medical Council (AMC)
Australian Nursing and Midwifery Accreditation Council (ANMAC)
Australian Physiotherapy Association (APA)
Australian Psychology Accreditation Council (APAC)
clinical nurse consultant (CNC)
clinical nurse specialist (CNS)
complementary and alternative medicine (CAM)
Council on Chiropractic Education Australasia (CCEA)

Department of Veterans' Affairs (DVA)
Dietitians Association of Australia (DAA)
extended scope of practice
fee-for-service
general practitioners (GPs)
interprofessional education and practice
National Disability Insurance Scheme (NDIS)
National Rural Health Alliance (NRHA)
non-government organisations (NGOs)
not-for-profit (NFP)
primary care
resident medical officers (RMOs)
Royal Australian College of Dental Surgeons (RACDS)
scope of practice
secondary care
Speech Pathology Australia (SPA)
technical and further education (TAFE)
tertiary care
value-based health care (VBHC)
Vocational Education and Training (VET)

Introduction

This chapter describes the health workforce and the contexts in which health professionals work. Sharing some common characteristics and competencies, different health professions have different core or expert knowledge, skills and abilities, complementing each other's roles. While the contexts and the services provided are diverse, they share a common focus on improving the health and well-being of individuals and the population. Optimal health outcomes are achieved when health professionals from different disciplines work together.

A broad perspective of the workforce is covered before considering the various practice environments, structural elements, and mechanisms organising and regulating practice. Potential changes for the future workforce are also presented.

Overview of the Australian health workforce

The health workforce includes all those who are employed in providing health and welfare services, in public, government-funded, private and non-government organisations. Increasingly, volunteers and carers are also included.

Size and distribution

More than one million Australians are employed providing health and welfare services (Australian Institute of Health and Welfare (AIHW) 2015). Table 17.1 lists by profession the 2016 census data of practitioners required by law to be registered by the **Australian Health Practitioner Regulation Agency (AHPRA)**. Paramedicine is also a registered profession but is not included as the requirement for registration commenced after 2016. Fig. 17.1 shows the comparative size of the registered professions. Nursing and midwifery is by far the largest, representing almost 60% of the registered health workforce. Medicine has many specialties, making up more than 60% of medical practitioners (Medical Board of Australia 2018). Not shown are the health professions not required to have AHPRA national registration, including audiologists, dietitians, exercise physiologists, social workers and speech pathologists. Reliable data are not available for those occupations, nor for providers of **complementary and alternative medicine (CAM)**. Table 17.1 illustrates that the number of practitioners decreases markedly from major cities to remote regions, except for Aboriginal and Torres Strait Islander (ATSI) health practitioners, whose numbers are much higher in RA5 compared with RA1 locations. Considering that about one-third of the Australian population lives outside major cities, the table also illustrates the health workforce imbalance between urban communities and rural and remote communities.

Organisation of the health workforce

This section provides an overview of workforce across the primary, secondary and tertiary levels of health services. Additional factors that also contribute to workforce organisation are funding, care setting and type of intervention; however, a range of other factors also influence how the health workforce is structured and operates.

TABLE 17.1 NUMBER OF REGISTERED PRACTITIONERS, WITH PROPORTIONS IN PROFESSIONAL SUB-GROUPS AND BY THE ASGC-RA CATEGORY

Health Professionals	Location by ASGC-RA Category					Total
	RA1	RA2	RA3	RA4	RA5	
Allied health practitioners						
ATSI health practitioners	63	58	148	90	115	474
Chinese Medicine practitioners	3454	408	112	NP	NP	3983
Chiropractors	3472	801	268	39	9	4589
Medical radiation practice	10,361	2015	673	76	26	13,156
Diagnostic radiographers	Proportion of medical radiation practitioners =					77.4%
Nuclear medicine scientists	"					5.7%
Radiation therapists	"					15.3%
Occupational therapists	12,273	2414	1,079	117	44	15,928
Optometrists	3,738	722	237	27	10	4734
Osteopaths	1,536	323	52	NP	NP	1914
Pharmacists	18,391	3559	1595	211	85	23,842
Community pharmacists[a]	Proportion of pharmacists =					63.1%
Hospital pharmacists[a]	"					17.6%
Other + non-clinical[a]	"					19.3%
Physiotherapists	19,621	3189	1222	154	79	24,271
Podiatrists	3262	789	235	29	11	4327
Psychologists	20,914	3110	1035	109	47	25,219
Dental health	15,394	2755	1159	131	46	19,490
Dentists	Proportion of dental health practitioners =					74.7%
Dental hygienists / therapists	"					13.0%
Dental prosthetists	"					5.7%
Oral health therapists	"					6.6%
Medical practitioners	72,304	12,422	5299	865	376	91,341
General practitioners	Proportion of medical practitioners =					31.0%

TABLE 17.1 NUMBER OF REGISTERED PRACTITIONERS, WITH PROPORTIONS IN PROFESSIONAL SUB-GROUPS AND BY THE ASGC-RA CATEGORY—cont'd

Health Professionals	Location by ASGC-RA Category					
	RA1	RA2	RA3	RA4	RA5	Total
Hospital non-specialists	"					10.6%
Specialists	"					33.5%
Specialists in training	"					17.7%
Other + non-clinical	"					7.2%
Nurses and midwives[b]	221,541	62,712	25,841	3151	1576	315,137
Registered nurses	Proportion of nurses and midwives =					75.2%
Enrolled nurses	"					16.3%
Registered nurses & midwives	"					7.4%
Midwives	"					1.1%
Total health professionals	**406,324**	**95,277**	**38,955**	**4999**	**2424**	**548,405**
Proportion of health professionals	**74.1%**	**17.4%**	**7.1%**	**0.9%**	**0.4%**	**100%**

Abbreviations: ASGC-RA=Australian Standard Geographical Classification – Remoteness Area; ATSI=Aboriginal and Torres Strait Islander; NP=not published; RA1=major cities; RA2=inner regional; RA3=outer regional; RA4=remote; RA5=very remote. http://www.abs.gov.au/ausstats/abs@.nsf/mf/1270.0.55.005.

Main data source: Australian Government Department of Health (2016) Health workforce data. http://www.health.gov.au/internet/main/publishing.nsf/content/health_workforce_data

Supplementary data sources:

[a]Health Workforce Australia (2014) Australia's health workforce series – *Pharmacists in focus*. http://iaha.com.au/wp-content/uploads/2014/03/HWA_Australia-Health-Workforce-Series_Pharmacists-in-focus_vF_LR.pdf

[b]RA category data derived from Australian Bureau of Statistics (2016) Census table builder. http://www.abs.gov.au/websitedbs/D3310114.nsf/Home/2016%20TableBuilder

Health care funding

Governments are the largest health funder. Smaller commitments come from private health insurance and direct payments by consumers (gap and **fee-for-service** payments). Commonwealth funding includes the Medical Benefits Scheme (MBS), Pharmaceutical Benefits Scheme (PBS) (see Chapter 7), Department of Veterans' Affairs (DVA), National Disability Insurance Scheme (NDIS), My Aged Care and grants for ATSI health, primary mental health care and alcohol and other drug (AOD)

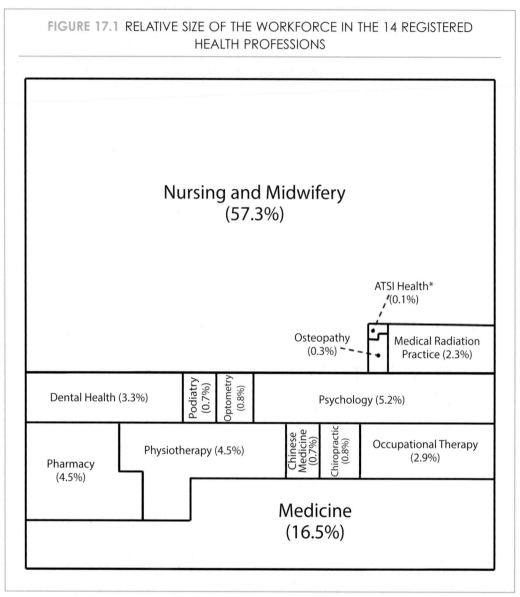

FIGURE 17.1 RELATIVE SIZE OF THE WORKFORCE IN THE 14 REGISTERED HEALTH PROFESSIONS

ATSI = Aboriginal and Torres Strait Islander

Source: Based on data from Australian Health Practitioner Registration Agency (AHPRA) 2016 / 17 National Board summaries, http://www.ahpra.gov.au/annualreport/2017/downloads.html

services. State and territory governments fund public health services, including hospitals, mental health, alcohol and drug, dental, community health and preventive health services. Services funded by private health insurance include private inpatient care, dental care, optometry services, allied health and some CAM.

The majority of health professionals in the public system work in hospitals. States and Territories directly manage public health services and contract some service delivery to non-government organisations (NGOs) and private providers. Other health professionals operate as private practitioners. Pharmacists are primarily funded via the PBS for handling and dispensing medications. General practitioners (GPs), medical specialists and some allied health professionals (AHPs) and nurse practitioners can receive payment through MBS and private health insurance. Dentists are primarily remunerated through private health insurance. Private practitioners may also register as providers through other Commonwealth programs and state-based rehabilitation schemes. They may operate as sole providers, or be organised as small businesses or large publicly owned companies. The sector includes both for-profit and not-for-profit (NFP) entities where practitioners work on a fee-for-service basis or as salaried employees in both health professional and administrative roles.

Primary and community care

Generally, the primary health sector cares for the more common health problems. Consumers can directly access primary and community care without referral. GPs are central to **primary care** and 'gate-keepers' to secondary and tertiary services. They assess, manage and refer patients to other services and practitioners to support diagnosis (pathology and imaging) and treatment (medical specialists and AHPs). Practice nurses in GP clinics provide services such as health screening, immunisations and wound care. GP services are predominately available on weekdays, with extended hours of services on evenings and weekends. Coordination of after-hours GP services is the responsibility of local Primary Health Networks (PHNs) (see Chapter 6).

Consumers may directly access primary care from AHPs practising privately or in community-based health services. Optometrists and most psychologists and podiatrists operate only in private practice. However, other disciplines (e.g. occupational therapists, physiotherapists and speech pathologists) work in either the public or the private sector, with services available only on weekdays during business hours.

For many people, the first point of primary care is their local pharmacy. Over 80% of pharmacists either own or work in community pharmacies (Table 17.1). Community pharmacy (see Chapter 26) income is derived from handling and dispensing medications, and selling over-the-counter medications and retail products. Some pharmacists offer vaccinations and health checks.

Like pharmacists, most dentists are in private practice, although some also service the public sector (see Chapter 15). Publicly funded dental clinics are accessible for people on low incomes and for children, the latter as part of school-based health care. Dental health services commonly employ dental nurses, dental hygienists and oral health therapists, in both the private and the public sectors.

Providers of CAM are private practitioners and earn income through fee-for-service payments. Reimbursement is possible from private health insurance but arrangements are limited and government has increasingly restricted rebates for these services (you can read more about their role in Chapter 14).

Secondary referral services

Secondary care services manage conditions requiring more specialised care and access is by referral. Specialist medical practitioners (e.g. cardiologists, psychiatrists, etc.) are the main secondary care providers. Medical specialists may be private practitioners who also provide services to public hospitals as visiting consultants, or may be employed as salaried hospital staff specialists.

Diagnostic services, such as pathology and medical imaging, are a component of secondary care and operate in both the public and the private sectors. Referrals are made to specialist pathologists or radiologists from other specialists or GPs, although a limited range of services can be requested by physiotherapists, nurse practitioners, osteopaths, podiatrists and chiropractors. In medical imaging and pathology the workforce includes AHPs and nurses, diagnostic radiographers, nuclear medicine scientists, sonographers, medical laboratory scientists, radiology nurses and nurse phlebotomists.

Other services with a specialist focus are mental health and AOD services. Private services are mostly provided by psychiatrists, psychologists and GPs; however, mental health nurses and social workers are a growing component of this sector. Most services are state funded and operate during core business hours; however, some intensive outreach services operate 7 days a week, including 24-hour phone services. Public services may be accessed directly or by referral and community-based services may refer consumers to residential and hospital services.

Community mental health teams include nurses (the largest occupation), psychiatrists, psychologists, occupational therapists and social workers. The NGO-managed psychosocial rehabilitation services workforce includes both degree-qualified health professionals and workers with Vocational Education and Training (VET) qualifications (Community Mental Health Australia 2015). People with a lived experience of mental illness have also become an important part of the mental health workforce; however, formal qualifications for this role are only now emerging. Most AOD services are delivered by the NFP sector and are principally provided by nurses and VET-qualified practitioners.

Rehabilitation services are provided by AHPs, medical specialists and nurses working in multidisciplinary teams (MDTs). Some AHPs, doctors and nurses undertake advanced training to become specialists in particular aspects of rehabilitation. Rehabilitation services are provided in hospitals, residential and day rehabilitation facilities and increasingly in the home. If unable to manage independent living in the community, individuals may be admitted to a residential care facility.

Funded by the Commonwealth, aged-care services aim to enable older people to remain in their home for as long as they are able, while residential aged care is for those who can no longer live at home. Services range from help in the home with daily tasks and personal care to 24-hour nursing care. Aged-care services are delivered by a range of providers including NFP, private and public-sector organisations. Day-to-day care and support is provided by personal care assistants and enrolled nurses under supervision by registered nurses, while activities are organised by diversional therapists. Allied health and medical services are generally provided by private practitioners in aged care. (See Chapter 8 for more information on aged care.)

Tertiary referral services

Tertiary care services are for more complex and/or acute conditions requiring intensive support and treatment. Care is provided in hospitals that integrate general and specialist assessment, treatment and support services. Most staff in hospitals, apart from visiting consultant medical specialists, are salaried employees. They are organised into MDTs. Nurses are the mainstay of hospital care and, working together with resident medical officers (RMOs) and other health professionals, care is provided 24 hours a day, 7 days a week.

Commonly, medical specialists admit patients into hospital; however, in smaller rural hospitals GPs have admitting rights and provide inpatient medical care. Another admission pathway is via the emergency department (ED). This usually involves patients who are experiencing painful, disabling, distressing or potentially life-threatening conditions, including trauma (e.g. a motor vehicle accident) and acute illness (e.g. pneumonia). Ambulance service paramedics are usually the first health professionals to respond in emergencies. They provide immediate care to stabilise or begin treatment of patients at the scene and then transport them to the emergency department. The majority of paramedics are employed by state ambulance services and their role is outlined in Chapter 25.

Hospital services are organised into wards, departments and specialised units (e.g. coronary care, psychiatric unit, etc.). Health professionals working in these units often undertake advanced training in their field as an employment prerequisite. Allied health, medical imaging, pathology and pharmacy services are usually centralised departments supporting an entire hospital or group of hospitals. Hospitals are dependent upon a range of ancillary services such as patient transport, administration, laundry and maintenance services.

Follow-up care after discharge may involve intensive support with the person's home, which is also known as 'hospital-in-the-home'. People who are terminally ill may be admitted to a palliative care service, at home or in a hospice. These services include specialist doctors, nurses and AHPs, who collaborate to ensure that death is humane, dignified and painless, and that relatives and friends are supported through the process.

PAUSE
for
REFLECTION
...

1 Reflect on the varying size and distribution of the registered health professions shown in Table 17.1 and Fig. 17.1 and the implications for health service delivery.

2 Visit the Department of Health site regarding Chronic Disease Management-Individual Allied Health Services under Medicare – Provider Information (see Online Resources).

a. Explore what services are funded, and the requirements for funding.

b. Identify the registered and accredited professions that come under this provision.

c. How might the requirements enhance or hinder interprofessional care?

3 A GP can refer a patient to a physiotherapist, chiropractor, osteopath or exercise physiologist for chronic musculoskeletal conditions. How would the GP choose?

Take your reflections on these questions to the next tutorial class or raise them at your tutorial.

Governance and regulation of the health workforce

The right to practise is governed through processes which accredit educational / training programs and determine who may practise (i.e. registration). Professional associations advocate for their members in relation to these matters.

Education and accreditation

Most health professional courses have three broad components:

- ◆ foundation knowledge about the human body and disease, social and individual determinants of health, and the context of health and illness
- ◆ specialist knowledge, skills and attitudes related to practice of specific professions, including observation and simulation, and
- ◆ supervised practice of professional competencies with patients / clients in appropriate settings.

Bodies established by the professions set standards and carry out accreditation reviews. Accreditation standards specify the necessary educational processes, graduate competencies and professional experiences. Accreditation bodies also specify the requirements of obtaining and maintaining accreditation, published as guidelines for universities and other educational providers. When applying for accreditation or renewal, education providers must submit comprehensive documentation on relevant curricula and undergo a review process that usually involves site visits to check staff competencies, facilities, administrative processes, selection procedures, professional placements and governance. Accredited courses are regularly reviewed to ensure standards are maintained and reflect contemporary developments.

Accreditation requirements dictate practice education. For example, student nurses complete 800 hours of clinical practice, while occupational therapy students complete 1000 hours of practice-based education. Accreditation requirements are continuously re-evaluated and evolve under the influence of professional boards in response to developments and demands in the health care system.

Universities and vocational colleges of technical and further education (TAFEs) must demonstrate that their courses meet specified professional accreditation standards, ensuring graduates are safe and competent to practise. Overall, AHPRA has responsibility for accreditation of programs in the registered professions but can delegate that authority to a committee of the national professional board or to an external body approved by AHPRA. Examples of accrediting authorities include the Australian Nursing and Midwifery Accreditation Council (ANMAC), the Australian Medical Council (AMC) and the Australian Psychology Accreditation Council (APAC). In non-registered professions, accreditation is carried out under the auspices of the relevant professional association such as the Dietitians Association of Australia (DAA) or Speech Pathology Australia (SPA). Registration and / or licensure to practise requires graduates to provide evidence of having completed an accredited education program.

In 2015, the AMC, in collaboration with the Australian Pharmacy Council (APC), ANMAC, and the Council on Chiropractic Education Australasia (CCEA), held a workshop titled 'Collaborating for patient care – interprofessional learning for interprofessional practice' (AMC, CCEA, APC,

ANMAC 2015). The workshop brought together delegates from a broad range of health sector stakeholder groups to discuss changes that are driving an increasing need for team-based care. Subsequently, accreditation authorities agreed to a common definition of interprofessional education, defined common learning outcomes, and committed to investigate further opportunities for additional interprofessional accreditation practices. In October 2018, AHPRA welcomed the release of the Accreditation Systems Review final report. Recommended reforms are aimed at improved efficiency of the regulation function to contribute to the safety and quality of the Australian health system. The report specifically referred to the requirement for **interprofessional education and practice** to support efficient team-based and coordinated care (Australian Health Practitioner Regulation Agency (AHPRA) 2018).

Registration

The national body that regulates and registers health professionals in Australia is the APHRA, having replaced a system of state and territory registration bodies in 2010. Responsibilities of the AHPRA include setting requirements for entry into professions, listing and monitoring who is eligible to practise, determining practice standards, managing complaints, disciplining practitioners where required and providing advice to government on matters relevant to regulation. Each registered profession has its own registration board, which includes experts from the profession, consumers and lawyers. Registration protects individual consumers and the community against sub-optimal health care.

Professional associations

With payment of an annual fee, all health professionals can join a professional body or association. Membership is not mandatory and it is common that a minority, rather than a majority, of practitioners are members of their professional body. Some examples of professional associations are the Australian College of Nursing (ACN), the Australian Medical Association (AMA), the Australian Physiotherapists Association (APA) and the Australian Association of Social Workers (AASW). Many professional associations have specialist sub-groups, as well as state and local branches.

Professional associations offer members a range of benefits, such as subscription to a professional journal and newsletter, free career advice and access to 'positions vacant' directories, discounted conference registration and, in some cases, professional indemnity insurance at reduced corporate rates. They also provide members with continuing education, which may include access to online, self-directed learning and webinars, as well as face-to-face conferences, symposia or workshops. Through continuing education, professional bodies can influence change and members can maintain currency of practice and thus meet registration requirements.

The collective power of professional associations enables an important advocacy role on behalf of members. The associations also uphold core professional values of the profession and executive members of professional bodies sometimes represent the profession in the public arena. They may influence government policy by lobbying politicians and informing policy debate on behalf of the profession. There is a vested interest in them garnering political support and, if possible, gaining preferential treatment.

Where they have common interests, professional organisations may band together and form alliances. Alliances advocate for members and provide a platform for education and interprofessional collaboration. For example:

◆ the **National Rural Health Alliance (NRHA)** (http://ruralhealth.org.au/about), which includes 35 member bodies, representing the interests of health professionals, consumers, students and educators in rural and remote areas

◆ the **Allied Health Professions Australia (AHPA)** (https://ahpa.com.au/), which is an alliance of AHPs bodies, with 20 member organisations.

PAUSE
for
REFLECTION
...

1 To understand the governance of your profession visit the AHPRA website and / or your professional association's website. Explore the registration requirements of your profession. Search for the 'code of ethics', 'code of conduct', 'code of practice' or similar. In a few sentences, summarise the key messages of that code.

2 Visit the website of another national board or professional association and explore that profession's governance requirements. In what ways, if any, do they differ from your profession? Why may this be?

Specialisation, advanced practice and extended scope of practice

Health professionals may choose to specialise, which usually requires further study and qualifications in a particular field. Most medical practitioners specialise or sub-specialise. Colleges administer specialist medical education and successful candidates become Fellows of the Colleges. While training, Fellowship candidates work in hospitals or in GP clinics as 'registrars', gaining experience while providing specialist services under supervision.

Dentistry and nursing also have a number of specialties, with their own professional sub-groups and certification. Examples include the Royal Australian College of Dental Surgeons (RACDS), the Australian College of Critical Care Nurses (ACCN) and the Australian College of Nurse Practitioners (ACNP). The ACNP's industrial award also permits nurses to be employed as a clinical nurse consultant (CNC) or a clinical nurse specialist (CNS) providing specialised services in particular fields, although positions are based mainly on experience rather than additional qualifications. Other health professions also have specialties, which, though not necessarily marked by additional qualifications or industrial award categories, may afford membership of specialist sub-groups.

Overlapping with specialisation and bearing similar characteristics is the concept of **advanced practice** in allied health and nursing. This is 'a state of professional maturity in which the individual demonstrates a level of integrated knowledge, skill and competence that challenges the accepted boundaries of practice' (McGee & Castledine 2003, p. 24). Advanced practitioners are experts in their field, recognised by some professional associations through advanced practitioner membership, and acknowledging the ability to provide more-complex clinical services.

The **scope of practice** of health professionals includes a range of fundamental knowledge, skills and abilities. Some are generic and common to all health professions, such as communication and collaborative skills. Others are profession specific and it is these that largely set the boundaries to scope of practice. The CanMEDS 2015 Physician Competency Framework (see Online Resources) includes seven practice domains, of which that of 'Expert' defines the particular competencies that graduates are expected to possess and apply in practice (Frank et al. 2015). Each health profession has such a domain of expert knowledge and skills fundamental to their role.

Health professions sometimes extend their scope of practice to adopt knowledge, skills and abilities that traditionally belong in the expert domain of another profession (e.g. nurse practitioners). Where **extended scope of practice** occurs, it is common to find interprofessional tension, as each profession lays claim to legitimacy, authenticity or ownership over the roles or tasks in question. Notwithstanding such challenges, new models of care, therapies, procedures and roles, including extended scope of practice, can be safely introduced with guidance by frameworks such as the credentialling, competency and capability framework (see Online Resources).

PAUSE
for
REFLECTION
...

1 Approach a tutor and have a discussion about scope of practice in your profession and how it relates to other professions and practice context.
2 Visit the CanMEDS 2015 website (see Online Resources).
   a. Open the 'CanMEDS 2015 Physician Competency Framework' at the top of the page.
   b. Open the role of 'Medical Expert' (p. 3), including the table of competencies (p. 4). Consider how you would reword the statements to reflect your own expert health professional role.

Emerging trends and issues in the health workforce

A bit after 11 pm on 6th August 2018, the Australian Bureau of Statistics (ABS) Population Clock ticked over to 25 million (ABS, 2018). One of the challenges in the future is to provide health services for an expanding and ageing population. Projections are that the proportion of the population aged 65 years or over will increase at a faster rate than that of working age Australians (between 15 and 64 years), thereby widening the gap between the proportion of the population needing care and the proportion in the health care workforce. Using the 'What's the problem represented to be' (WPR) approach enables practitioners, researchers and policy-makers to critically analyse the implicit assumptions and implications of health policy solutions designed to address complex and challenging issues such as this (Bacchi 2016).

The policy shift towards personalised care funding packages (e.g. NDIS, My Aged Care), which aim to ensure consumer involvement in decisions about their health and care needs and choice of provider, is impacting upon how care is organised and delivered. These policy initiatives present individualised funding as the solution to the 'problem' of enabling better outcomes through individuals directing their own care. However, a tension exists between these policy shifts and the capacity of the health workforce to adapt to consumer demands. Care and support roles are changing rapidly as organisations adopt new business models and ways of interacting with consumers in order to remain competitive, flexible and responsive. Implications for the workforce are demonstrated in the reported increase in casual employment arrangements and, for some AHPs, fixed-term employment contracts in the disability sector (National Disability Services 2018).

National and international studies and reports have highlighted the need to change the way health care is delivered. A Grattan Institute report stated that 'too many health professionals squander their valuable skills on work that other people could do' (Duckett et al. 2014, overview p. 3). Some innovations have already occurred but shifting professional boundaries is often fraught, the greatest barrier being issues of professional status and hierarchy (O'Meara et al. 2015). In rural Canada, the introduction 'of a broader primary health care role for community paramedics' met surprise and curiosity from the traditional health workforce as they struggled to understand how to work together and maximise service delivery (O'Meara et al. 2015). New and evolving roles are negotiated within the context of historical professional boundaries shaped by educational, regulatory and organisational histories.

Technological change is creating greater efficiencies and diversifying roles, tasks and duties. New practices, roles and even entire occupations will develop around large-scale data storage and management. Most patients already have an electronic health record, improving the capacity to share data between providers. Problems of distance, geographical remoteness and a lack of health service providers will be increasingly addressed with information technology. Policies being developed to address these challenges represent implicit representations of the universal right to equitable health care. Individual policy initiatives will 'problematise' specific aspects related to access to health care (Bacchi 2016). With local health care coordinators 'on-site', who may be volunteers or assistant practitioners, health professionals can be based remotely from where the care is provided. Remote robotic surgery using virtual reality is already feasible. It is hard to predict how such technologies will alter future workforce development and clinical practice (Chapter 16 outlines the digital potential).

Models of funding health care may also change. Funding of health care is generally represented as a problem of limited resources allocated according to evidenced-based medicine and dedicated to managing increasing need. As referred to by Bacchi (2016), reflecting on the 'problem' implicit in specific policy solutions should form part of the policy development process. For example, **value-based health care (VBHC)** is a funding model that balances health care benefit against costs. Providers are held accountable for both quality and outcomes of care and remunerated accordingly. Thus, the best-performing, lowest-cost providers with the highest levels of patient satisfaction are most rewarded. The model also rewards integration of care. More-collaborative models of care will develop, where consumers access a range of services at a single location. Efficiency and better health outcomes will be achieved with MDTs of health professionals co-located, sharing patients and consulting with each other to diagnose and treat the increasingly common chronic morbidities of ageing. The emphasis will be on keeping people out of hospital, with greater collaborative, interprofessional teamwork to provide community-oriented, home-based care. Case study 17.1 demonstrates some of these points.

Case Study 17.1

Scenario 1

John's wife wheels John into the ED late on Friday evening. A receptionist asks for contact details and John's age. An ED nurse in the waiting room asks a few more questions. Another nurse wheels John into a cubicle and conducts an assessment. He notes that John has some weakness, is drowsy and cannot speak clearly. He tells John's wife that a registrar will be along shortly.

The registrar completes her own checklist. A stroke possibly accounts for John's presentation. Immediate care is addressed by the registrar. Early next morning John is admitted to the general ward when a prostate-specific antigen is available.

Breakfast is delivered. Reviewing the ED notes, a nurse notes difficulty in swallowing. The dietitian on call recommends both nil-by-mouth until John has the consultant review on Monday and a speech pathology assessment; however these staff members don't work on the weekend.

On Monday morning, the consultant requests a scan as she is concerned about John's cough and pallor. On Monday afternoon the speech pathologist assesses John and recommends videofluoroscopy. A radiographer does this on Tuesday.

John spends 3 weeks in hospital, with aspirational pneumonia and malnutrition. John's stroke is mild but diabetes is also diagnosed. On discharge, John is referred to social work and physiotherapy for ongoing care, but is re-admitted to hospital 2 weeks later after collapsing at home.

But it could have been like this …

Scenario 2

The ED is designed around what it is there for, rather than what health care workers do in it. Health care team composition is around client groups. John is immediately part of the older persons' team, and a range of skills are linked to care at the outset. Dietitians, speech pathologists and radiographers are supported and authorised to share specific skills across roles/traditional domains of care. Performance and accountability is both individually and team based. John and family collaborate with the team to plan his care and discharge.

John recovers at home, supported by the older persons' team care liaison, his GP, a physiotherapist and a diabetes educator. John becomes a volunteer community advocate with the older persons' team.

Case study questions

1. In the first scenario, what factors contributed to John's re-admission to hospital?
2. What resources do health care practitioners require to support John in the model of care described in scenario 2?
3. How would interprofessional education during pre-qualification study support this model of care?

A final commentary

The Australian health workforce is dynamic and must be responsive to change. Motivation for change can be problematic, intrinsically and extrinsically, including changing patient needs and expectations, implementation of new models of care or funding, dynamics of interprofessional collaboration, and demands of continuing professional education and development, or the unending advance of technology. Health care consumers are better informed than ever before. They have greater access to information about their health, enabling them to have a central role in decision-making, so that patient-centric, rather than professional-centric, care is the optimal practice model.

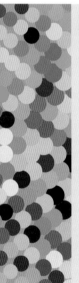

Summary

- The Australian health workforce includes many different occupations, the largest being nursing and midwifery, constituting nearly 60% of registered practitioners. The various AHPs and medical and dental practitioners make up the bulk of the rest, although there are several other occupations.
- The health workforce is organised around the structural elements of the health care environment, including in primary, secondary and tertiary settings. Health professionals often practise across multiple settings, independently or in teams.
- Health professions are governed and regulated via various mechanisms. Tertiary education and course accreditation are primary means of establishing scopes of practice, which may change with specialisation or advanced and extended roles. Professional bodies have an advocacy as well as a continuing educational role and may influence change.
- Health professional practice is changing under a variety of influences, not least of which is the rapid growth and ageing of the patient population. Responses are required to maintain optimal quality care.

Review Questions

1. Reflect on the distribution of the health workforce and the potential impact upon access to health care in different communities.
2. Compare the composition of the health workforce in the primary and secondary health sectors. What are the differences and the similarities?
3. You are part of a multidisciplinary team. What are the characteristics of the team that will support interprofessional practice?
4. Explore the ways in which the cost of health care is presented through media. What factors influence this public discourse?
5. An interprofessional allied health practitioner has been appointed to work in the emergency department. What might be the drivers of this new role and appointment?

References

AMC, CCEA, APC, ANMAC, 2015. Workshop report: Collaborating for patient care – interprofessional learning for interprofessional practice. https://www.amc.org.au/workshop-report-collaborating-for-p atient-care-interprofessional-learning-for-interprofessional-practice/.

Australian Bureau of Statistics (ABS), 2016. Feature article: Population by age and sex, Australia, states and territories. Australian demographic statistics 3101.0, June. http://www.abs.gov.au/AUSSTATS/abs@.nsf/Previousproducts/3101.0Feature%20Article1Jun%202016.

Australian Bureau of Statistics (ABS), 2018. Australia's population to reach 25 million, media release. ABS, Canberra, 7 August. https://www.abs.gov.au/ausstats/abs%40.nsf/mediareleasesbyCatalogue/C3315F5 2F6219DE9CA2582E1001BC66A?OpenDocument'.

Australian Health Practitioner Regulation Agency (AHPRA), 2018. AHPRA welcomes release of the accreditation systems review final report. https://www.healthreform.org.au/wp-content/uploads/2018/02/AHCRA-Position-Paper-Workforce-FINAL-DEC-2017.pdf.

Australian Institute of Health and Welfare (AIHW), 2015. Workforce overview 2015. https://www.aihw.gov.au/reports-data/health-welfare-services/workforce/overview.

Bacchi, C., 2016. Problematizations in health policy: questioning how 'problems' are constituted in policies. Sage Open April–June, 1–16. doi:10.1177/2158244016653986.

Community Mental Health Australia, 2015. Developing the Workforce: Community Managed Mental Health Sector National Disability Insurance Scheme Workforce Development Scoping Paper Project. Mental Health Coordinating Council, Sydney. https://www.aph.gov.au/DocumentStore.ashx?id=7875dc67-4813-4412-a93f-8ad3471007fb&subId=464070.

Department of Health & Human Services, 2016. Bridging allied health roles for better patient outcomes. Victoria State Government, Melbourne. https://www2.health.vic.gov.au/about/publications/researchandreports/bridging-allied-health-roles-for-better-patient-outcomes.

Duckett, S., Breadon, P., Farmer, J., 2014. Unlocking Skills in Hospitals: Better Jobs, More Care. Grattan Institute, Melbourne.

Frank, J.R., Snell, L., Sherbino, J., 2015. CanMEDS 2015 Physician competency framework. Royal College of Physicians and Surgeons of Canada, Ottawa. http://canmeds.royalcollege.ca/en/framework.

McGee, P., Castledine, G., 2003. Advanced Nursing Practice, second ed. Blackwell Science, Oxford.

Medical Board of Australia, 2018. Registration data table – March. http://www.medicalboard.gov.au/News/Statistics.aspx.

National Disability Services, 2018. Australian disability workforce report – February. https://www.nds.org.au/policy/australian-disability-workforce-report-second-edition-highlights-workforce-risks1.

O'Meara, P., Stirling, C., Ruest, M., et al., 2015. Community paramedicine model of care: an observational, ethnographic case study. BMC Health Serv. Res. 16 (1), 39.

Further Reading

Australian Healthcare Reform Alliance, 2017. Policy position paper: health workforce. December. https://www.healthreform.org.au/wp-content/uploads/2018/02/AHCRA-Position-Paper-Workforce-FINAL-DEC-2017.pdf.

Online Resources

Australia's health is released biennially on the Australian Institute of Health and Welfare website: https://www.aihw.gov.au/reports-statistics/health-welfare-overview/australias-health/overview

Australian Government Department of Health – Chronic disease management – individual allied health services under Medicare – provider information: https://www.health.gov.au/internet/main/publishing.nsf/Content/health-medicare-health_pro-gp-pdf-allied-cnt.htm

Australian Government Department of Health's health workforce data provide resources to investigate the nature of the Australian health workforce: http://hwd.health.gov.au/publications.html

Australian Health Practitioner Regulation Authority National Boards: http://www.ahpra.gov.au/National-Boards.aspx

CanMEDS 2015 describes seven characteristics and related competencies expected of physicians: http://canmeds.royalcollege.ca/uploads/en/framework/CanMEDS%202015%20Framework_EN_Reduced.pdf

CanMEDS 2015 also provides an overview of the framework and related competencies expected of physicians: http://www.royalcollege.ca/rcsite/canmeds/canmeds-framework-e

Credentialling, competency and capability framework: https://www2.health.vic.gov.au/health-workforce/allied-health-workforce/allied-health-ccc-framework

CHAPTER 18

Clinical exercise physiology in the Australian health care system

Steve Selig, Melainie Cameron and Kirsty Rawlings[a]

Key learning outcomes

When you finish this chapter you should be able to:

- summarise the evolution of clinical exercise physiology practice in Australia
- describe the roles of an Accredited Exercise Physiologist (AEP) and the scope of practice for AEPs
- describe the roles of Exercise & Sports Science Australia (ESSA), the National Alliance of Self-Regulating Health Professionals (NASRHP) and the ESSA Course Accreditation Program for the accreditation of AEPs
- discuss ways in which AEPs and other health professionals collaborate in multidisciplinary service provision
- demonstrate, through the presentation of case material, an understanding of how AEPs practise.

Key terms and abbreviations

Accredited Exercise Physiologist (AEP)
Accredited Exercise Scientist (AES)
activities of daily living (ADLs)
Australian Health Practitioner Regulation Agency (AHPRA)
Exercise & Sports Science Australia (ESSA)
National Alliance of Self-Regulating Health Professionals (NASRHP)

[a]We acknowledge the contribution by Steve Fraser to the chapter in the 3rd edition of this book.

Introduction

In this chapter we describe the scope of practice, education, and regulation of Accredited Exercise Physiologists (AEPs) in Australia. Regulation occurs through a national university course accreditation scheme administered by **Exercise & Sports Science Australia (ESSA)**. We outline the education and development of clinical competencies aligned to the scope of practice of AEPs, summarise where AEPs fit within the health care system and indicate how AEPs may engage in multidisciplinary practice. Because exercise physiology is one of the newer entrants into allied health, we also provide a brief history of the profession. We touch on some evidence supporting the therapeutic benefits of exercise, and conclude by demonstrating these scientific bases for the profession through case examples.

What is an Accredited Exercise Physiologist?

An **Accredited Exercise Physiologist (AEP)** is a university-educated allied health professional who designs and implements individualised exercise and physical activity interventions for people living with acute, sub-acute and chronic health conditions, disabilities or injuries. AEPs are registered in Australia under a national accreditation scheme administered by ESSA. An **Accredited Exercise Scientist (AES)** is the foundational accreditation for clinical exercise physiology. An AES is trained to provide exercise services for clientele with no known medical conditions, disabilities or injuries, or working under the guidance of an AEP for the delivery of clinical exercise services. Typically, AEPs undertake 4-year undergraduate courses at AQF Level 7 (Bachelor degree) or AQF Level 8 (Honours degree) in exercise sciences and clinical exercise physiology, or complete graduate entry courses in clinical exercise physiology (AQF Level 9) – the latter for individuals who are already eligible for AES accreditation on entry to postgraduate programs.

The primary goals of exercise interventions developed by AEPs for clients with chronic conditions are threefold. The first goal is to apply appropriate intensities, volumes and modes of exercise to improve clinical status and alleviate symptoms, while considering client presentations and medical treatments, the available scientific evidence and the client's individual needs and situations. 'Improvement' in clinical status refers to retarding natural progression of a condition or to promoting regression of a condition, and these outcomes are known collectively as 'secondary prevention'. In contrast, AESs provide services related to 'primary prevention' such as risk factor amelioration and prevention of new disease. Secondly, AEPs work with their clients to improve fitness and function, including the capacity to work or perform activities of daily living (ADLs). The capacity to perform ADLs predicts long-term independence and the ability to live independently (Mlinac & Feng 2016). Thirdly, interventions are designed to improve quality of life including reducing symptoms of depression or anxiety (Strohle 2009) and other co-morbid conditions. A key component of an AEP intervention is to move beyond the often-reinforced social construct that an individual is at fault if they have a lifestyle-related disease or are not fit (Bacchi, 2016) and consider enablers and barriers to a client making long-term lifestyle changes, including social (e.g. socio-economic status, family dynamics, social expectations, access to support services, time and availability) and environmental factors (such as urban design, geographical location and accessibility to services), and to work with clients to plan an appropriate program that considers these factors and will continue to support them to operate in this construct.

For all three of these domains (clinical, functional and psychosocial), there is extensive evidence supporting the efficacy of exercise as either a stand-alone (independent) intervention or combined with other lifestyle interventions such as diet or mental health interventions across a wide range of pathologies (see the excellent review by Pedersen & Saltin (2015)). AEPs within university, hospital and private settings contribute extensively to the research and knowledge bases regarding the effectiveness of exercise to support the prevention of and management of medical conditions, injuries and disabilities. For instance, many AEPs in Australia have contributed to pathology-specific position statements, clinical practice guidelines and joint position statements with other professions.

Regulation of exercise physiology practice in Australia

ESSA is the national self-regulating membership body responsible for the accreditation of AEPs. ESSA is a foundation member of the **National Alliance of Self-Regulating Health Professions (NASRHP)**, which is committed to providing assurance to consumers, government and other entities regarding the safety and quality of self-regulating health services through an evidence-based national framework of regulatory standards. To date, NASRHP membership covers clinical exercise physiologists, dietitians, speech pathologists, sonographers, perfusionists, orthotists / prosthetists, social workers and audiologists. AEPs are required not only to meet the minimum academic standards, as regulated by ESSA, but also to adhere to NASRHP standards and requirements pertaining to professional conduct, ethical practice, complaint management and recency of professional practice. Other allied health professionals are regulated by the Australian Health Practitioner Regulation Authority (AHPRA) and the respective professional boards, which include professions such as physiotherapy, occupational therapy, medicine, nursing and pharmacy.

The accreditation of AEPs is restricted to graduates of ESSA-accredited programs. In 2005, just five universities were accredited for clinical exercise physiology programs; this has since increased to 23 universities in 2018 out of a total of 43 public and private universities in Australia. There were approximately 450 AEPs across Australia in 2006, with rapid growth from then to 4626 AEPs in Australia in 2017 (*ESSA annual report 2017*; https://www.essa.org.au/wp-content/uploads/2018/03/ESSA-2017-annual-report_final1.pdf).

In addition, there are accreditation pathways available to individuals with overseas qualifications who meet the education and practice criteria required for an AEP, and to individuals wishing to return to practise as an AEP after an extended time away from practice.

Professional standards of the AEP

The AEP professional standards are competency based and build on the underpinning AES Standards. The AEP standards are organised into 13 study areas, with generic standards 1 to 5 broadly describing practice of the profession. These comprise foundational knowledge, professional practice, referrals, screening and assessments, and design of individualised exercise interventions and implementation of exercise interventions. Standards 6 to 13 comprise pathology-specific domains of cancers and cardiovascular, renal, respiratory/pulmonary, mental health, musculoskeletal, neurological and metabolic conditions. Taken together, the standards describe sets of knowledge and competencies that are needed to provide safe and effective exercise services for various broad-based pathology domains and they include the capacity to practise across multiple co-existing pathology domains with a single client (i.e. co-morbidities and complex situations).

Historical perspective

In 2004, the Australian Department of Health released a range of Medicare Australia chronic disease management (CDM) items for allied health professionals, including AEPs, to support individuals with one or more chronic disease/s. This change in policy was in response to the increasing incidence and prevalence in chronic disease in the Australian population, particularly those aged 45 years and above, the increasing cost of managing chronic disease in terms of the national health expenditure, and the perceived lack of ability of an individual to self-manage their chronic conditions without intervention or support (Bacchi 2016). AEPs were funded to deliver clinical exercise services and behavioural change counselling for individuals with chronic medical conditions and complex care needs who had a CDM plan. Since 2006, other schemes have been approved for AEPs to provide exercise for people injured in traffic accidents or at work, returned service personnel and those with private health insurance. Elsewhere in the world there are compensable schemes and professional opportunities for clinical exercise physiologists, but the recognition of the AEP as an independent provider of clinical exercise services under the breadth and depth of schemes in Australia is without equal. In 2007, the Australian Department of Health released further item numbers through Medicare Australia for AEPs (and dietitians and diabetes educators) to assess suitability for and delivery of group exercise sessions for individuals who had been diagnosed with type 2 diabetes. For the period 2013–17, as the AEP profession has matured, the provision of exercise services under the relevant AEP Medicare item 10953 has grown by 52% compared with 37% for the related general practitioner (GP) item 721 (preparing a management plan for a patient who has a chronic medical condition) (Department of Human Services 2019). This growth in services aligns with corresponding increases over the decade in the number of accredited university courses, new graduates, practising AEPs and full members of ESSA. This growth has been echoed in the other allied health professions recognised to deliver support to individuals with chronic disease/s, with the provision of occupational therapy and physiotherapy under their respective Medicare Australia CDM item numbers also increasing steadily since 2004, and with the annual number of physiotherapy services delivered in 2017/18 sitting at over 2.5 million. Using Bacchi's 'What's the problem?' (WPR) framework (Bacchi 2016; see Chapter 1), it might be argued that this policy response was steeped significantly in the increasing prevalence of lifestyle-related chronic diseases in the Australian population aged 45 years and over; however, it did not recognise fully the level of service required to support an individual with changing and maintaining significant lifestyle change (with the number of Medicare Australia sessions being limited to five allied health sessions per individual per calendar year); also it was not supported with changes required in an individual's environment to support lifestyle change, such as a corresponding increase in policy or funding in urban design to support health, or health promotion and literacy.

The curricula for clinical exercise physiology within Australia evolved from physical education (in the 1970s), human movement (in the 1980s), sports science (in the 1990s), exercise science (in the 2000s) and, more recently, clinical exercise science and practice. These evolutions have created challenges and opportunities for universities, the profession and the professional association, ESSA. As a direct consequence of the inclusion of AEP services in the Medicare Benefits Schedule and other schemes, universities recognised the need to align their programs with the new knowledge and competency bases required of AEPs to work effectively within allied health. The education and accreditation systems for AEPs are distinct from those of the professions of physical education, sports science and exercise science, and it is the only profession within this cluster that is regulated for access to the allied health domain. In addition, personal trainers and other fitness industry-trained professionals do not have access to any of the compensable schemes available to AEPs.

Career pathways for exercise physiologists in Australia

There are a number of career pathways across a broad range of settings available to AEPs. These opportunities include public or private hospital settings (both inpatient and outpatient care) and government-funded community, primary and ambulatory care centres, where AEPs support CDM and lifestyle behavioural change often within a multidisciplinary team environment. Opportunities for AEPs within private-practice settings have been steadily increasing, with AEPs practising under schemes including Medicare, Department of Veterans' Affairs and workers' compensation schemes and third-party insurance schemes. AEPs work independently in private clinics and as part of multidisciplinary care teams, collaborating with other health professionals including general practitioners, physiotherapists, dietitians, podiatrists, diabetes educators, nurses and psychologists. Other opportunities include occupational rehabilitation and insurance work, which see AEPs provide rehabilitation services and / or case management services to clients injured at work or on the road. AEPs also work in aged-care settings including day therapy / respite centres, patients' homes or in residential aged-care facilities. Other areas of work include health planning and policy, health services and practice management, sporting organisations, corporate health promotion and academic teaching, clinical education and research. Opportunities are also emerging for AEPs seeking to work with clients with mental health conditions, pain management and disabilities, including under the National Disability Insurance Scheme (NDIS).

The scope of practice for AEPs

AEPs design, implement and evaluate exercise interventions for individuals with acute, sub-acute and chronic conditions, injuries and disabilities. AEPs provide their services using a clinical reasoning model (see Fig. 18.1) (Maiorana et al. 2018), under which they may receive referrals from other

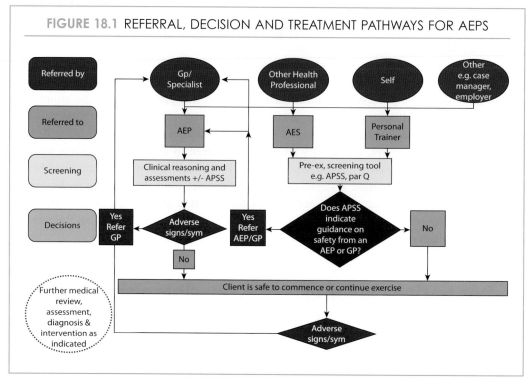

FIGURE 18.1 REFERRAL, DECISION AND TREATMENT PATHWAYS FOR AEPS

Source: Adapted from Maiorana, A.J., Williams, A.D., Askew, C.D., et al. (2018). Exercise professionals with advanced clinical training should be afforded greater responsibility in pre-participation exercise screening: a new collaborative model between exercise professionals and physicians. Sports Med. 48, 1293–1302

health professionals including general and specialist medical practitioners. One of the critical elements of this model is that, at the point of referral, the referrer transfers the risk of exercise participation to the AEP. In other words, the GP is not required to deem that the patient is safe for exercise participation, but rather refers the patient to the AEP and, in so doing, consciously transfers the decision-making regarding the risks of exercise participation to the AEP. This is quite distinct from the situation for exercise physiologists in other parts of the world (e.g. UK, USA, South Africa) where the medical practitioner retains the overall responsibility to make an assessment as to the risks of exercise participation for their patient. In Australia, AEPs are equipped through education and advanced development of clinical competencies to make those decisions independently, triangulating the referral information (presenting medical conditions, treatments and interventions), the patient's story and the published evidence with the results of examination, screening and exercise testing undertaken by the AEP.

As part of the process to design and develop individualised and evidence-based exercise interventions, AEPs conduct scientifically based exercise and functional assessments appropriate to the individual and the situation. A core component of AEP services is to design interventions that are safe and effective, both in the immediate sense and for the longer term. AEPs are expected to provide these services incorporating behavioural change strategies in order to increase the likelihood of long-term participation in physical activity and exercise.

AEPs need to collect, record, interpret and report back to the referrer any exercise-related information or data that may contribute to diagnoses, in turn leading to possible changes to treatments, interventions or management strategies. This is just one way in which the AEP may contribute to improvement in a client's clinical status, along with the therapeutic benefits flowing from exercise interventions. AEPs collaborate with other health professionals when clients need advice or treatments from other health disciplines or to ensure that their intervention is in line with the client's overall treatment plan, to clarify any concerns relating to the client's clinical condition or medication usage (see Fig. 18.1) (Maiorana et al. 2018). Like other health professionals, AEPs have a responsibility to understand and practise within their knowledge bases and competencies, and ensure that their clients are receiving other care when appropriate. AEPs must practise in accord with the ESSA code of professional conduct and ethical practice. They must also understand and adhere to standards established through legislation, regulations and common law.

AEPs are accredited to practise across a range of 'target conditions' on the basis that the condition (i) has significant national incidence and prevalence, and / or (ii) is costly in terms of national health expenditure, and (iii) there is scientific evidence supporting the therapeutic benefits of exercise for that condition (see below). The current list of 'target conditions' that satisfy these three criteria includes, but is not restricted to: (i) cardiovascular (high blood pressure, ischaemic heart disease, peripheral arterial disease, heart failure, cardiac valve disease, cardiac rhythm disturbances, pacemakers), (ii) respiratory / pulmonary (asthma, chronic obstructive pulmonary disease, cystic fibrosis), (iii) metabolic (obesity, excessive blood fat or glucose, diabetes), (iv) renal (stages of kidney failure), (v) musculoskeletal (arthritis, osteoporosis, sprains and strains, and other musculoskeletal causes of pain and poor function), (vi) neurological / neuromuscular (stroke, spinal cord injury, acquired brain injury, Parkinson's disease, multiple sclerosis, dementia), (vii) cancers (especially breast, colorectal, prostate) and (viii) mental health conditions (particularly depression and anxiety disorders).

Brief evidence supporting efficacy of exercise as a therapeutic intervention

In 2011 in Australia, 4.5 million disability-adjusted life-years (DALYs) were lost owing to illness or premature death; coronary heart disease, other musculoskeletal disease, back pain, chronic obstructive pulmonary disease (COPD) and lung cancer were the five leading contributors to the national burden of disease and injury (Australian Institute of Health and Welfare (AIHW) 2018, p. 83). Exercise has been shown to confer benefits such as reduced rates of hospitalisation, reduced need for prescribed medications and improvements in symptoms for a long list of conditions including coronary artery disease (Winzer et al. 2018), heart failure (O'Connor et al. 2009; Sagar et al. 2015), type 2 diabetes (T2DM) (Dunstan et al. 2002; Kirwan et al. 2017; McCarthy 2015), cancers including breast, prostate and colorectal cancers (Ballard-Barbash et al. 2012; Cormie et al. 2017) and depressive and anxiety disorders (Carek et al. 2011; Rosenbaum et al. 2014; Strohle 2009).

PAUSE
for
REFLECTION
...

Compare the development of the profession of exercise physiology and its relatively recent entry into allied health with some of the more established allied health professions. Why do you think AEPs were recognised as allied health providers at the same time as the introduction of Medicare Australia CDM allied health item numbers? Discuss the challenges that lie ahead for AEPs in a crowded allied health domain, where other professions also provide exercise services. Consider whether there are niche areas of expertise and practice that distinguish AEPs from other professions.

The risk of adverse signs and symptoms during exercise: the 'exercise paradox'

The benefits of exercise for clients with a wide range of chronic conditions are undeniable, but there is an acknowledged increased risk of adverse signs or symptoms, and even (very rarely) sudden cardiac death while clients with chronic conditions are exercising (Franklin et al. 1997). This increased risk during exercise stands in contrast to the reduced risk for the rest of the day, and is known as the 'exercise paradox'. AEPs have a primary responsibility to be able to design and implement exercise interventions that are safe during actual exercise participation, yet efficacious in terms of clinical benefits during the 'rest of the day and year'.

Assessment of clients to inform the exercise prescription

A very important competency of the AEP is to be able to properly assess clients before the commencement of exercise training, in order to inform the exercise prescription. Assessments are also valuable for documenting changes in status (e.g. improvement) and are repeated at specific time-points, such as following an acute medical event, changes to prescribed medications, interventions or treatments, or surgery, before the patient returns to exercise training.

AEPs should be competent to design and use fatigue-, sign- and symptom-limited incremental exercise tests to assess the risk of participation in exercise, and to use the results to prescribe exercise scientifically. Cardiologists and other physicians conducting 'stress tests' often proceed beyond the onset of adverse signs or symptoms and use exercise to provoke signs or symptoms for the purpose of diagnosis. In contrast, AEP-led exercise tests are used to determine a safe range of exercise intensities, and these tests are stopped at either fatigue or the onset of adverse signs or symptoms (Fig. 18.2). Very few clients are referred to AEPs following a recent (and therefore reliable) cardiologist-supervised stress test; thus it is important that AEPs conduct their own exercise assessments at the commencement of an exercise intervention. Most referrals to AEPs come from GPs and other health professionals, not cardiologists. It is impracticable, and would cause significant over-servicing, if every client who presented to an AEP for exercise first underwent a cardiologist-supervised stress test (Maiorana et al. 2018).

FIGURE 18.2 GENERIC MODEL FOR EXERCISE ASSESSMENTS BY AEPS

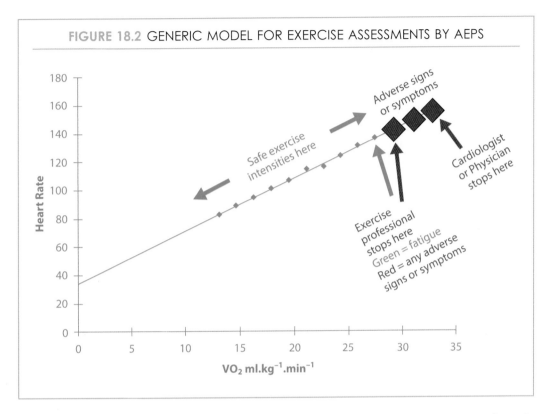

It is important that AEPs are competent in recognising and taking appropriate and timely (sometimes immediate) action when adverse signs or symptoms arise during exercise. Adverse signs or symptoms may arise months after the initial assessment, so AEPs need to be vigilant whenever seeing a client, and appropriately report adverse signs or symptoms to the referring health professional (Fig. 18.1). This has an additional feed-forward benefit for the exercising client, who then can often return to exercise in better condition than previously and so derive more benefit from exercise.

Multidisciplinary practice: how AEPs work with other health professionals

Exercise physiologists are not the only allied health practitioners who value exercise: dietitians, physiotherapists, podiatrists, diabetes educators, occupational therapists, osteopaths, chiropractors, psychologists and social workers might be expected to encourage patients to exercise, become more active or maintain ongoing involvement in sport and physical pastimes. Exercise physiologists are distinguished from their colleagues by their sharp focus on exercise and physical activity as the *primary* clinical intervention, and the detail and depth in which they plan, deliver, monitor, refine and progress exercise with clients. AEPs promote and support lifestyle behavioural change as core to AEP interventions, and understand the influence of complex primary and co-morbidities on clients' capacity to exercise.

It might seem intuitively reasonable that interdisciplinary care serves patients better than single-practitioner care; however, the evidence for this assertion is somewhat mixed. For example, a client with osteoarthritis of the knees who has become less physically active due to pain when walking, and overweight as a result of reduced activity, might be equally well served by consulting with a dietitian to modify their diet for weight loss, or an exercise physiologist to plan safe and pain-free exercise, or an occupational therapist to be fitted for walking aids. A Cochrane systematic review of multidisciplinary rehabilitation for older people with hip fractures found no statistically significant difference between multidisciplinary and usual care when considering pooled data from 11 trials in hospital settings for key outcomes including mortality (pooled relative risk (RR) 0.90, 95% confidence interval (CI) 0.76–1.07) and hospital re-admission (reported in six trials only; pooled RR 0.99, 95% CI 0.82–1.19) (Handoll et al. 2009). These results speak to the blunt reality of interdisciplinary rehabilitation: that it may be expensive, complex and time-consuming to deliver, that it may improve patients' functional capacity and quality of life and appears to do no harm, but that we really do not know whether it keeps people out of hospital in the long term or reduces mortality.

Naylor et al. (2017) conducted a propensity score analysis to explore the value of inpatient rehabilitation in 258 people (129 matched pairs) following total knee replacement (TKR) surgery. Their study was specific to the Australian health care context, conducted across 12 Australian hospitals. All participants were privately insured, so interventions were not capped owing to limited public funds – all participants received rehabilitation services as required. Further, participants with surgical complications, who may be referred to inpatient rehabilitation to allow close clinical monitoring, were excluded from the study. The only significant difference between groups was that at day 35 (7 weeks post-surgery) patients discharged to home reported higher quality-of-life (EuroQoL) scores, which is indicative of better overall health and quality of life than their inpatient counterparts. At 90 and at 365 days after surgery, participants in both groups were similar on measures of knee function (Oxford knee score) and general well-being (EuroQoL).

Inpatient rehabilitation is multidisciplinary and complex, requiring collaboration among practitioners to deliver a range of health care interventions, as well as ongoing nursing care and medical oversight. Further, it is considerably more expensive than home-based care. Naylor et al. (2017) reported that in 2015, at the commencement of their study, inpatient rehabilitation for TKR typically required 12 nights of hospital stay at an average cost to the insurer of (AU)$8400 (patient out-of-pocket expenses not reported). Yet these layers of complexity, interdisciplinarity and cost do not appear to return notably improved outcomes for 'uncomplicated' patients.

The lack of clarity in the research on the comparative efficacy of interdisciplinary care versus solo-practitioner care, and inpatient versus home-based care, also speaks to the reality of AEP work. AEPs can work constructively with other allied health professionals who value exercise, but sometimes the professional boundaries overlap and it may be difficult to ascertain which interventions are of most value to patients. For example, there is a growing body of evidence that exercise is beneficial for improving mental health, including reducing the symptoms of depression and schizophrenia (Rosenbaum et al. 2014) and anxiety disorders (Stubbs et al. 2017). The effects of exercise on components of these disorders and the dose–response relationships between exercise and outcomes are gradually becoming better understood, such that we can now say that even low doses of exercise, which would be insufficient to meet national guidelines for the general population, can still produce symptom-reducing benefits in people with mental health conditions (Rosenbaum et al. 2014). Mental health conditions, particularly depression, may occur co-morbidly with other chronic illnesses such that exercise interventions pre-scribed primarily for chronic complaints may also produce beneficial effects on concurrent depressive symptoms (Herring et al. 2012). AEPs working with clients to improve mental health conditions are not psychologists, but they need to be able to speak the language of psychology and work with clients to set exercise goals that psychologists and other mental health professionals could support and share. Further, AEPs need to be aware of the limitations of their knowledge and skills in any domain, and seek help from other practitioners when they approach their own professional boundaries.

Unexplored in the study by Naylor et al. (2017) are the reasons why simpler, home-based rehabilitation appears to afford comparable outcomes to complex, multidisciplinary, inpatient care. Regardless, this study serves as a sage reminder to AEPs not to be seduced by the glamour of complex care delivery, and to ensure that their contributions to any care team serve patients first of all.

PAUSE
for
REFLECTION
...

Consider and discuss each of the following clinical scenarios. Ask where the professional boundaries might be approached, and where the AEP scope of practice overlaps with those of practitioners in other disciplines. Identify the potential points of dispute with colleagues as well as the points of commonality. Consider how the client might be best served in each scenario.

1 Anne had a total hip joint replacement yesterday. The prosthesis is uncemented. Anne needs to be mobilised out of bed as soon as possible to promote bone growth to secure the prosthesis in place. An AEP or a physiotherapist could guide and monitor Anne through this physical activity.

2 Brian has prostate cancer. Because Brian is taking androgen-suppressing medication, his bone density is likely to decline. His oncologist has suggested that he would benefit from an exercise program to maintain his bone mineral density through jumping, skipping and other weight-bearing exercises. The oncologist values exercise but lacks sufficient time or the skills to plan an exercise intervention, so refers to an AEP to design a suitable program for Brian.

3 Casey has battled with depression for most of her adolescence. Her GP has prescribed antidepressants. Casey refuses to see a psychologist because she is concerned about the stigma of being labelled as mentally unwell. Her GP recommends that Casey become more physically active, and offers her a referral to an AEP.

4 Deidre has been discharged home after 3 weeks in hospital following a fall in which she lacerated her legs and fractured a wrist and three ribs. A social worker has assessed Deidre as mentally prepared to return home, but highly apprehensive about using the stairs at the front and rear of her Queenslander-style house. The social worker has invited an AEP and an occupational therapist to a case conference to discuss options for Deidre's stair use at home.

Case study 18.1 considers AEP collaboration with medical professionals in heart rhythm disturbance.

Cyclist with a heart rhythm disturbance: interdisciplinary case study involving an AEP, a GP and a cardiologist

Paul is a 51-year-old recreational cyclist with previously very high levels of fitness and performance. Recently, Paul has experienced breathlessness, fatigue, light-headedness and feelings of a 'racing heart rate' during and after exercise. Paul's GP referred him to an AEP for an assessment of the safety of exercise participation and to fine-tune Paul's exercise regimen. Paul's GP had previously prescribed medications to relieve, control and prevent his asthma symptoms, but Paul confessed to being lax with medication compliance. The medications consisted of a combination puffer containing an anti-inflammatory (preventer) and a long-acting bronchodilator (symptom controller) and another puffer containing a short-acting bronchodilator (symptom reliever). Nevertheless, the AEP assessed his lung function at rest as more than adequate, with his large- and medium-sized airways both functioning at well over 100% of predicted values.

The AEP measured Paul's breathing and monitored his self-reported levels of breathlessness during a fatigue-, sign- and symptom-limited incremental cycle ergometer test. Heart rate and rhythm were monitored using electrocardiography, and haemoglobin oxygen saturation ($HbO_{2sat\%}$) and blood pressure were also monitored. Although Paul's lung function fell below predicted values during exercise, his $HbO_{2sat\%}$ did not fall and his level of breathlessness was subjectively in line with his level of exertion. At peak exercise, his heart rate (HR) was normal for his age ($HR_{peak} = 166$ beats / min) and his aerobic fitness was exceptional. The exercise test was uneventful, but at 45 seconds of recovery Paul's HR suddenly accelerated to 252 beats / min for a period of 10 seconds before falling to a near-constant HR of 184 beats / min for the following 3 minutes, and then falling again to a constant 134 beats / min for a further 3 minutes. Paul was experiencing a post-exercise supraventricular tachycardia (very high heart rate). Attempts at reverting this arrhythmia to normal sinus rhythm using a Valsalva 'straining' manoeuvre failed and the AEP did not want to apply carotid artery massage (which is a method that can interrupt this rhythm disturbance). Fortunately, Paul spontaneously reverted to normal sinus rhythm at 6:50 minutes of passive recovery.

The AEP continued to observe and monitor Paul for a further 20 minutes before permitting him to drive home. He was in sinus rhythm throughout the remainder of his recovery. Paul was advised to avoid high-intensity exercise until his tachycardia could be followed up. A report on the exercise assessment was provided to the GP within 24 hours. The GP then referred Paul to a cardiologist together with copies of the exercise and recovery ECG traces. The cardiologist subsequently referred Paul to a specialised cardiologist known as an electrophysiologist who was able to induce (reproduce) the arrhythmia and diagnose the arrhythmia to be dependent on an atrioventricular nodal re-entrant pathway. The pathway was ablated during the same procedure and the arrhythmia was no longer inducible.

Paul then returned to the AEP for a subsequent exercise assessment. His HR and rhythm responses to high-intensity exercise were normal and he was free from symptoms apart from normal fatigue. In the following 12 months, his symptoms did not recur and his anxiety levels concerning participation in high-intensity and high-volume exercise plummeted. Paul is extremely grateful for the overall services offered by his GP, the AEP and the cardiologists and is now enjoying symptom-free participation in high-intensity cycling.

Case study questions

1   Was the exercise test stopped due to fatigue or to the arrhythmia?

2   The rhythm disturbance reverted to normal sinus rhythm at about 7 minutes, and the client never lost consciousness and was actually unaware of his high heart rate. Do you think that an ambulance should have been called?

3   How should an AEP deal with poor medication compliance?

4   Suppose this client also had coronary artery disease with exercise-induced chest pain that needed anti-anginal medication for relief. How could poor asthma management make his chest pain (angina) worse during exercise? (Hints: (i) explain how poor asthma management can cause falls in $HbO_{2sat\%}$. (ii) Use the Fick law of the heart to explain why decreased $HbO_{2sat\%}$ can impact negatively on oxygen supply to the heart and can therefore make angina worse in individuals with CAD.)

5   Referring to Fig. 18.1, comment on the appropriateness of the referral pathways that occurred between the GP, the AEP and the cardiologists.

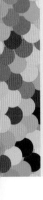

Summary

In this chapter, we have considered a number of factors that affect health service provision by AEPs including independent roles and as part of multidisciplinary teams.

- AEPs design and deliver exercise services with the primary goals of improving the clinical, functional and psychosocial status of clients.

- AEPs accept referrals from medical practitioners and other health professionals and are responsible for assessing and managing the safety of exercise interventions based on a clinical reasoning model.

- Clinical exercise physiology education and accreditation are regulated by the professional association, Exercise and Sport Science Australia (ESSA), and the National Alliance of Self-Regulating Health Professionals (NASRHP).

Continued

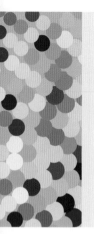

- ESSA also provides the important roles of professional advocacy, member support and professional development for its members.
- AEPs work broadly across the public and private health care systems.
- It is important that health professionals understand the services provided by other health professionals if interdisciplinary care is to be effective.
- Although there is some overlap of the professional roles of the AEP with those of other allied health professionals, the sharp focus on exercise and physical activity as their primary clinical intervention, with emphasis on individualised, safe and effective exercise for all clients, distinguishes AEPs from other allied health professions that also value and promote exercise. AEPs are also focused on helping their clients to better long-term health behaviours through counselling and appropriate exercise interventions.

Review Questions

1. What is an Accredited Exercise Physiologist? Outline the scope of practice for AEPs.
2. For clients with chronic disease and complex care needs, suggest some common and/or interdisciplinary approaches that dietitians and AEPs may use to improve lifestyle and self-management of clients' health.
3. Suppose you are a health professional in a community health setting. How are you going to promote increased exercise and physical activity participation in clients with chronic disease and complex care needs?
4. Reflect on the issues relating to the comparative effectiveness of interdisciplinary care, independent care by AEPs and 'usual care' for clients with chronic disease and complex care needs.
5. Compare and contrast the accreditation arrangements for AEPs and dietitians who are accredited via their respective professional associations and NASRHP with the professions of physiotherapy and occupational therapy that accredit via their respective registration boards and the Australian Health Practitioner Regulation Agency (AHPRA).

References

Australian Institute of Health and Welfare (AIHW), 2018. Australia's health 2018, Cat. no. AUS 221. AIHW, Canberra. https://www.aihw.gov.au/reports/australias-health/australias-health-2018/contents/table-of-contents.

Bacchi, C., 2016. Problematizations in health policy: questioning how "problems" are constituted in policies. SAGE Open 1–16.

Ballard-Barbash, R., Friedenreich, C.M., Courneya, K.S., et al., 2012. Physical activity, biomarkers, and disease outcomes in cancer survivors: a systematic review. J. Natl. Cancer Inst. 104, 815–840.

Carek, P.J., Laibstain, S.E., Carek, S.M., 2011. Exercise for the treatment of depression and anxiety. Int. J. Psychiatry Med. 41, 15–28.

Cormie, P., Zopf, E.M., Zhang, X., et al., 2017. The impact of exercise on cancer mortality, recurrence, and treatment-related adverse effects. Epidemiol. Rev. 39, 71–92.

Department of Human Services, 2019. Medicare Australia statistics item report. http://medicarestatistics. humanservices.gov.au/statistics/mbs_item.jsp.

Dunstan, D.W., Daly, R.M., Owen, N., et al., 2002. High-intensity resistance training improves glycemic control in older patients with type 2 diabetes. Diabetes Care 25, 1729–1736.

Exercise & Sports Science Australia (ESSA), 2018. Annual report 2017. https://www.essa.org.au/ wp-content/uploads/2018/03/ESSA-2017-annual-report_final1.pdf.

Franklin, B.A., Fletcher, G.F., Gordon, N.F., et al., 1997. Cardiovascular evaluation of the athlete. Issues regarding performance, screening and sudden cardiac death. Sports Med. 24, 97–119.

Handoll, H.H., Cameron, I.D., Mak, J.C., et al., 2009. Multidisciplinary rehabilitation for older people with hip fractures. Cochrane Database Syst. Rev. (4), CD007125.

Herring, M.P., Puetz, T.W., O'Connor, P.J., et al., 2012. Effect of exercise training on depressive symptoms among patients with a chronic illness: a systematic review and meta-analysis of randomized controlled trials. Arch. Intern. Med. 172, 101–111.

Kirwan, J.P., Sacks, J., Nieuwoudt, S., 2017. The essential role of exercise in the management of type 2 diabetes. Cleve. Clin. J. Med. 84, S15–S21.

Maiorana, A.J., Williams, A.D., Askew, C.D., et al., 2018. Exercise professionals with advanced clinical training should be afforded greater responsibility in pre-participation exercise screening: a new collaborative model between exercise professionals and physicians. Sports Med. 48, 1293–1302.

McCarthy, M., 2015. Diet and exercise are effective in preventing type 2 diabetes, task force finds. BMJ 351, h3785.

Mlinac, M.E., Feng, M.C., 2016. Assessment of activities of daily living, self-care, and independence. Arch. Clin. Neuropsychol. 31, 506–516.

Naylor, J.M., Hart, A., Mittal, R., et al., 2017. The value of inpatient rehabilitation after uncomplicated knee arthroplasty: a propensity score analysis. Med. J. Aust. 207, 250–255.

O'Connor, C.M., Whellan, D.J., Lee, K.L., et al., 2009. Efficacy and safety of exercise training in patients with chronic heart failure: HF-ACTION randomized controlled trial. J. Am. Med. Assoc. 301, 1439–1450.

Pedersen, B.K., Saltin, B., 2015. Exercise as medicine – evidence for prescribing exercise as therapy in 26 different chronic diseases. Scand. J. Med. Sci. Sports 25 (Suppl. 3), 1–72.

Rosenbaum, S., Tiedemann, A., Sherrington, C., et al., 2014. Physical activity interventions for people with mental illness: a systematic review and meta-analysis. J. Clin. Psychiatry 75, 964–974.

Sagar, V.A., Davies, E.J., Briscoe, S., et al., 2015. Exercise-based rehabilitation for heart failure: systematic review and meta-analysis. Open Heart 2, e000163.

Strohle, A., 2009. Physical activity, exercise, depression and anxiety disorders. J. Neural Transm. (Vienna) 116, 777–784.

Stubbs, B., Vancampfort, D., Rosenbaum, S., et al., 2017. An examination of the anxiolytic effects of exercise for people with anxiety and stress-related disorders: a meta-analysis. Psychiatry Res. 249, 102–108.

Winzer, E.B., Woitek, F., Linke, A., 2018. Physical activity in the prevention and treatment of coronary artery disease. J. Am. Heart Assoc. 7 (4), e007725.

Further Reading

Cameron, M., Hemphill, D., Selig, S. (Eds.), 2011. Clinical Exercise: A Case-Based Approach. Elsevier, Chatswood, NSW.

Coombes, J., Skinner, T. (Eds.), 2014. ESSA's Student Manual for Health, Exercise and Sport Assessment. Mosby Elsevier, Sydney.

Dietitians Association of Australia (DAA), 2011. Manual for Accreditation of Dietetic Education Programs, version 1.2. DAA, Deakin, ACT.

Online Resources

Accredited Exercise Physiologist professional standards: www.essa.org.au/wp-content/uploads/2016/12/AEPProfessional-Standards-with-coverpage_approved.pdf.

Accredited Exercise Scientist scope of practice: www.essa.org.au/wp-content/uploads/2018/04/Accredited-Exercise-Scientist-Scope-of-Practice_2018.pdf.

Australian Institute of Health and Welfare: www.aihw.gov.au.

Changes in healthcare professions' scope of practice: legislative considerations. 2006, revised 2012: https://www.ncsbn.org/Scope_of_Practice_2012.pdf.

Exercise & Sports Science Australia – accreditation: https://www.essa.org.au/Public/EDUCATION_PROVIDERS/Public/EDUCATION_PROVIDERS/Education_Providers.aspx?hkey=3ef6f181-dbfa-407b-a4b8-53a55de8ecf4.

Exercise & Sports Science Australia – code of professional conduct and ethical practice, version 2: https://www.essa.org.au/wp-content/uploads/2011/08/Code-of-Ethics-and-Professional-Conduct.pdf.

Exercise & Sports Science Australia – position statements: https://www.essa.org.au/for-media/position-statements.

Exercise & Sports Science Australia – professional development: https://www.essa.org.au/members-home/professional-development.

Exercise & Sports Science Australia – scope of practice policy: https://www.essa.org.au/Public/Professional_Standards/ESSA_Scope_of_Practice_documents.aspx.

Exercise & Sports Science Australia / Sports Medicine Australia joint pre-exercise screening tool: https://www.essa.org.au/for-gps/adult-pre-exercise-screening-system.

The joint position statement for ESSA, Dietitians Association of Australia (DAA) and Australian Psychological Society (APS): https://www.essa.org.au/Public/Advocacy/Position_Statements/Public/Advocacy/Position_Statements.aspx?hkey=c2c01874-ffdc-4a20-adb9-42e6d3d020a7.

When to refer: www.essa.org.au/wpcontent/uploads/2015/09/When-to-refer_With-Links_v2-ESSA-Dropboxs-conflicted-copy-2015-07-20.pdf.

CHAPTER 19

Nutrition and dietetics: promoting health for all Australians

Louisa Matwiejczyk, Marian McAllister and Iris Lindemann[a]

Key learning outcomes

When you finish this chapter you should be able to:

- briefly outline the development of nutrition and dietetics as a profession
- describe the range of roles of the dietitian and nutritionist within the Australian health care system
- identify some of the key nutrition disorders and nutrition-related public health issues impacting on the health of Australians
- describe how dietitians and nutritionists are involved in interprofessional practice.
- identify some of the government policies directing the nutrition and dietetics profession in promoting health for all Australians, including the Australian Dietary Guidelines
- describe how various health reforms have impacted on nutrition-related practice

Key terms and abbreviations

accredited practising dietitian (APD)
Australian Dietary Guidelines (ADGs)
Australian Health Practitioner Regulation Agency (AHPRA)
Commonwealth Scientific and Industrial Research Organisation (CSIRO)
dietitian
Dietitians Association of Australia (DAA)
food insecurity
general practitioners (GPs)
general practitioner management plans (GPMPs)

medical nutrition therapy
national competency standards
non-communicable diseases (NCDs)
Nutrition Society of Australia (NSA)
nutritionist
obesity epidemic
obesogenic environment
public health nutrition
registered nutritionist (RNutr)
social model of health

[a]We acknowledge the contribution by Amanda Wray to the chapter in the 3rd edition of this book.

Introduction

Almost all of us are interested in food. We may enjoy selecting food, cooking favourite dishes and sharing food with family and friends. Many of us also have definite ideas about the types of food we consider crucial in our lives and, as such, food can play an important role in defining who we are (Ogden 2010). Food, however, plays a much broader role than the social and cultural practices evident in everyday life. It provides our bodies with nutrients essential for normal functioning and is key to our state of health (National Health and Medical Research Council (NHMRC) 2013a). As early as 400 BCE the link between food and health was already well known – 'Let food be thy medicine and let thy medicine be food' (Hippocrates 460–377 BCE).

Dietitians and nutritionists are health professionals who are trained to understand the functions and roles played by food in our lives and in our communities. These nutrition-related professions use this understanding to enhance the nutritional health of individuals, groups and populations through promoting health-enhancing changes to food practices and the food environment (Dietitians Association of Australia (DAA) 2018a; Nutrition Society Australia (NSA) 2018a).

Nutrition and dietetics in Australia

A **dietitian** is an allied health professional who is expert in the nutritional treatment of illness and prevention of disease in individuals and communities. Accredited practising dietitians (APDs) have completed a minimum 4-year accredited Bachelor degree in nutrition and dietetics, or a relevant undergraduate degree followed by an accredited postgraduate qualification in nutrition and dietetics. APDs have the skills to modify diets to assist in the management of various diseases and conditions using **medical nutrition therapy**. The clinical management of patients is what distinguishes the dietitian from the accredited nutritionist (Health Workforce Australia 2014). An accredited **nutritionist** will be trained in human nutrition but will not have undertaken the extra coursework, professional practice placements or assessment in medical nutrition therapy, community **public health nutrition** and food service management. Dietitians may refer to themselves as nutritionists to reflect their broader, non-clinical role, but a nutritionist cannot use the title 'dietitian'.

A nutritionist provides advice on matters relating to food and how it impacts on health. Nutritionists can design, implement, coordinate and evaluate population-level interventions which promote positive health outcomes through food and nutrition. Other nutrition-related areas nutritionists work in include consultancy, research, public health and food-related industries as nutritionists, food technologists and nutrition scientists (NSA 2018a).

Nutritional and dietetic services are delivered across the continuum of health care, from primary prevention and early intervention to management of a disease. What people eat can increase their risk of developing **non-communicable diseases (NCDs)** such as cardiovascular disease, strokes, diabetes and some cancers (NHMRC 2013b). These account for 87% of all deaths in Australia (Australian Institute of Health and Welfare (AIHW) 2018) and 70% of deaths worldwide (World Health Organization (WHO) 2017). Globally, more than 75% of cardiovascular diseases, stroke and diabetes and 40% of cancers can be prevented or delayed by reducing the behavioural risk factors such as poor nutrition, physical inactivity, smoking and harmful alcohol intake (WHO 2013). Dietitians and nutritionists are instrumental in preventing NCDs and in treating and supporting people with diet-related diseases and conditions.

NCD's are increasingly prevalent with an ageing population and rising risk factors including obesity (AIHW 2016). Many nutrition-related diseases occur later in life, although food preferences are determined early in life (Birch 1999; Skinner et al. 2002) and will track through into adulthood (Singh et al. 2008). This means a 'whole of life-span' approach is needed, with prevention focused on children and the people who support them, and treatment targeted at adults with NCD risk factors and existing chronic disease.

Dietetics in Australia

Dietetics is a relatively new profession in Australia, starting in the 1930s as hospital-based internships (Nash 1989). The **Dietitians Association of Australia (DAA)** is the peak professional body for dietitians and membership has almost doubled since 2008 to more than 6000 members (DAA 2016). It is female dominated, 93.7% of nutrition professionals being women (Australian Bureau of Statistics (ABS) 2016). Despite the increasing prevalence of nutrition-related NCD and risk factors, it remains a relatively small allied health profession, comparable in numbers to podiatry and optometry (Health Workforce Australia, 2014).

Dietetic university programs are reviewed regularly by the DAA to ensure that training meets the **national competency standards** for dietitians in Australia (DAA 2015). These competency-based standards cover four domains including practising professionally, positively influencing health, applying critical thinking into practice, and collaborating with clients and stakeholders. These domains are described in detail in the standards and their interpretation is supported with observable or measurable actions to assist in assessment of students and dietitians in practice. To become a DAA member, dietitians must graduate from a DAA-accredited university program (DAA 2018a). The Commissioner's standards for employment recognises that a person must be eligible for DAA membership to be employed as a dietitian (Commissioner of Public Employment 2007). Currently 15 Australian universities offer accredited training programs, including undergraduate (4 years) and postgraduate (18 months–2 years) programs (DAA 2018b). Curricula must meet content requirements in biochemistry, human physiology and food and nutrition science (DAA 2018c). Specialist subject areas also include food and nutritional science, medical nutrition therapy, community and public health nutrition practice, research skills, communication skills, food service and the sociology of food and nutrition.

Dietitians in Australia are eligible to become APDs with the DAA after completing a defined and ongoing professional development program and at least 1 year of mentorship (DAA 2018d). APDs are committed to the DAA *code of professional conduct* and to undertaking continuing professional development. After at least 5 years of experience, dietitians can apply to become Advanced APDs by demonstrating expertise in many competencies. A few dietitians have progressed to become Fellows of the DAA (FDAA), who are dietitians who are proactive leaders (DAA 2018e).

Australian dietetic qualifications are accepted in the UK, some countries in Asia and the Middle East and some states in Canada (DAA 2018f). New-Zealand-registered dietitians with an annual practising certificate are also eligible to apply to work in Australia. For accredited dietitians wanting to be recognised as specialists in the field of sports nutrition, Sports Dietitians Australia (2018) offers membership and accreditation options. However, in Australia, dietetic and nutrition practice is not regulated by the government. Reforms implemented through the **Australian Health Practitioner Regulation Agency (AHPRA)** do not currently include dietitians or nutritionists (Australian Health Practitioner Regulation Agency 2014), as nutrition-related activities are not thought to pose a risk of harm to the public.

Nutritionists in Australia

Founded in 1975, the **Nutrition Society of Australia (NSA)** was formed by scientists working in the field of nutrition (including physiology, biochemistry, agriculture, medicine, sociology, economics and public health). The NSA comprises qualified practising scientists and educators from diverse backgrounds interested in increasing and communicating the scientific value and relevance of nutrition science in Australia. For nutritionists wanting to be accredited, the Nutrition Society of Australia has developed a voluntary register of nutritionists (NSA 2018b). This register ensures the quality and safety of practice by approving appropriately qualified individuals who have received an approved level of training and experience. At a minimum, nutritionists have a Bachelor degree majoring in nutrition to become an Associate Nutritionist. Following 3 years of relevant experience (or further study) a nutritionist can apply to become a **registered nutritionist (RNutr).** To maintain this, the RNutr undertakes continuing professional development and must meet minimum competency standards as deemed essential by the NSA and the *Code of conduct* (NSA 2018b).

PAUSE
for
REFLECTION
...

Much of the work delivered by clinically trained dietitians and nutritionists in the community setting may be similar. How might the two roles be differentiated? Can you foresee how these two professions can work in a complementary way in a community-based setting such as community health? At what stages of the human life-span could intervention by a nutritional and dietetic professional be of benefit?

Where do dietitians and nutritionists work?

In 2011, most dietitians worked in health care and social assistance industries (86%), with over half (53%) working in hospitals. Dietitians were found to be employed evenly across the public and private sectors, including non-government organisations (Health Workforce Australia 2014).

Clinical dietetics

Clinical dietetics usually involves the day-to-day management of clinical conditions such as diabetes, heart disease, cancer, renal disease, gastrointestinal diseases and other disorders using medical nutrition therapy consistent with the biomedical model of care. Dietitians prescribe individualised and specific dietary regimens that will assist in improving the health of the patient. They consider the type, amount and consistency of foods in dietary prescriptions and may provide additional high-energy, high-protein supplements to ensure that nutritional needs are met. Clinical dietitians often specialise in a particular disorder (e.g. diabetes, renal diseases, liver diseases, eating disorders). They may also become specialists in the management of acute care food service systems, ensuring quality and efficiency of delivery of both standard and therapeutic diets. Clinical dietitians predominately work in acute settings such as hospitals, but with health reform in several sectors this work is increasingly provided in community-based settings and private practice. In hospital settings the *National safety and quality health standards* detail quality standards for improving quality of care and protecting the health of consumers (Australian Commission for Safety and Quality in Health Care, 2017). This now requires the implementation of comprehensive systems delivering nutrition-related screening and monitoring and evidenced-based nutrition care plans complemented with the provision of food and fluids.

Community-based dietetics

Community-based dietitians work in primary health care sites such as community health centres, GP Plus Centres, non-government organisations and publicly funded community services such as domiciliary care in metropolitan, rural and remote areas. Non-government organisations include Diabetes Australia and aged-care organisations such as Helping Hand Inc. Community-based dietitians work within a primary health care model or a **social model of health**. Many community dietitians are increasingly involved in clinical care pathways to assist individual patients re-entering the community from acute care settings. The development of GP Plus Health Centres and Superclinics constituted a key strategy of the federal and some state governments to increase integration of the private and public health systems aiming to improve management of chronic diseases (Department of Health, 2013).

Dietitians also focus on public health nutrition issues that affect populations, such as the **obesity epidemic,** or nutritional issues impacting on vulnerable sub-groups, such as people living in rural and remote areas, people from low socio-economic areas and Indigenous peoples. In a health environment with limited funding and resources, competition for resources between interest groups representing the dominant medically oriented clinical services and broader public health groups continues to be a feature of the health system. In 2013–14, only 1.5% of the national health budget of (AU)$154.6 billion was directed towards public health (AIHW 2015).

Interprofessional practice

Dietitians are not new to interprofessional practice, as they commonly work with other health professionals to improve the health care of patients and populations. Within a clinical interprofessional setting, for example, dietitians work closely with speech therapists, social workers and medical doctors to maximise safe food intake and hydration for people with swallowing disorders. In a community and public health setting, dietitians collaborate with a range of allied health and other professionals, including teachers, general practitioners (GPs), and researchers. They work with government and non-government departments and industry, to deliver individual, group and population nutrition services (Hughes 2004).

Case study 19.1 outlines an interprofessional approach for dietetic involvement in the care of a patient admitted to a tertiary hospital. The case study questions ask you to consider what can go wrong, in this setting, in the provision of an interprofessional approach to client-centred care.

Case Study 19.1

Shared care in nutrition and dietetics

Barbara is a 76-year-old woman living alone. Her daughter rings for an ambulance after finding Barbara collapsed at home after suffering a cardiac arrest. She is taken to the local emergency department and admitted into the cardiac unit for further investigation and bypass surgery.

Barbara's case is discussed at the team meeting with the medical, nursing and allied health teams. Barbara's diagnosis has come as a shock to her and her daughter, who weren't aware that her blood cholesterol levels and blood pressure are high. Barbara's care includes education from the dietitian and the cardiac nurse about the management of her condition post-surgery.

Before discharge, the dietitian gathers information about Barbara's past medical history, her weight history, social situation and usual food and beverage intake. The dietitian assesses the adequacy of the diet and, based on her dietary assessment, provides individualised dietary education for Barbara that will assist her to improve her blood cholesterol levels and achieve a healthy weight. It becomes obvious during the interview that Barbara lives alone with limited social support and that she has difficulty with shopping and cooking. A social worker also sees Barbara during her admission and negotiates additional support for Barbara at home, such as Meals on Wheels and basic cleaning.

Before Barbara goes home, the cardiac rehabilitation nurse arranges for Barbara and her daughter to attend the next 'My Heart, My Life' group. This group is facilitated by several health professionals, including a nurse, a dietitian, an exercise physiologist, a pharmacist and a social worker. Coordinated care between the hospital cardiologist and Barbara's GP will ensure her relevant medical care is continued in the community. With Barbara's permission, the hospital dietitian liaises with the community dietitian to support ongoing care in the community

Barbara attends the cardiac group, learning more about her condition, and meeting others with similar experiences. This motivates her to manage her cholesterol and weight and quit smoking. Barbara has regular reviews with her GP and appointments with a community dietitian, and commences an exercise program supported by the exercise physiologist. Barbara continues to have Meals on Wheels, and her daughter supports her with meal preparation at weekends.

Case study questions

1   This is an ideal situation where the dietitian is a key member of an interprofessional team and the clinical pathway from the acute care setting to the community setting is fluent and effective. Consider the financial, social and other resource issues within the complexity of a

health care system which may cause this pathway to be less effective or even ineffective for Barbara's care.

2   Do you think the Australian health care system can deliver such ideal management from the acute to community settings? Consider the reasons for your answer.

3   How different do you think Barbara's care would be if she were an Indigenous woman living in a rural and remote community such as Esperance in Western Australia? How is your rationale supported by Duckett's (2014) perspective of Australian health care?

Private practice

Private practice is an area of growth within the dietetics profession, representing nearly a third of total DAA membership (Ball et al. 2013). This increase has been enabled by health reform changes to Medicare which fund more effective partnerships between GPs and private-practice dietitians, especially in the areas of chronic disease management, **general practitioner management plans (GPMPs)** and team care (Department of Health 2014). If patients have private health insurance then other referral types will be partly funded by these insurers. Private-practice dietitians may work with medical specialists in specialised clinical areas such as radiotherapy and cancer treatment, gastrointestinal disease and weight loss surgery. They also work as consultants in a broad range of settings, including food services, private hospitals and aged-care facilities.

Other areas of employment for nutritionists and dietitians

Other areas of employment for nutrition-related professions include the following:

◆ Government and health departments, where nutrition-related professionals work to maintain and improve the health of populations, including advising health ministers on appropriate nutrition policy and industry on food regulation and food standards. Examples include front-of-pack labelling, the health star rating of packaged food, and the Healthy Food Partnership with the food industry to change their products so that they are healthier. The environmental impact and the sustainability of food production, packaging and distribution have received increasing attention over recent years, both in Australia and globally (Friel et al. 2014; Lang & Barling 2013). Issues of concern relate to the security, sustainability and quality of the Australian food supply, and work with government and industry partners to discuss the long-term impacts of policy changes to agriculture, development and planning. There have been calls for further research into diets that sustain both healthy populations and healthy environments (Macdiarmid 2013). Others are encouraging an expanded view of the effect of national food guidelines, to include not just health and well-being but also the impact of these guidelines on the finite agriculture and aquaculture resources and on waste production (Selvey & Carey 2013).

◆ Non-government organisations such as the Heart Foundation, and education and research organisations such as universities and the **Commonwealth Scientific and Industrial Research Organisation (CSIRO)**. New discoveries in nutrition and nutrition-related trials create many opportunities for Nutrition Scientists.

♦ The food industry, with many opportunities for new food product development, new food technologies, innovation, marketing and health promotion.

♦ Media, corporations, workplaces and enterprises.

Government priorities in health are driving growth in areas such as private practice, dietetic services supporting the transition from acute care to home, healthy ageing, disability (particularly with the National Disability Insurance Scheme), Aboriginal and Torres Strait Islander health, and diabetes. Population interest in sustainable, healthy behaviours is driving changes in our food supply, food demand and interest in healthy eating. Many more nutritionists are being employed in these areas of public engagement.

With a shift towards more neoliberal government policies, and with increasing budget pressures on health, nutritional health promotion has been de-funded at both the national and the state level. This has resulted in a shift towards non-government, private industries, enterprises and local government sectors to provide this type of work. This will be an area of growth for dietitians and nutritionists, particularly with the existing *Public Health Acts* in South Australia (SA) and Victoria including the prevention of NCDs as a priority (Government of South Australia, Attorney-General's Department 2018).

Dietary advice in Australia for health for all

The **Australian Dietary Guidelines (ADGs)** are the national guidelines for healthy eating in Australia (NHMRC 2013a). The ADGs provide evidence-based recommendations that aim to meet the population's immediate dietary needs and to prevent chronic disease. Complementing the ADGs is a food selection guide which visually represents the proportion of the five food groups recommended for consumption each day. The Australian Guide to Healthy Eating has been developed for various age groups and specifies daily minimum serves of food from each of the food groups (NHMRC 2013b).

Cardiovascular disease is the most significant cause of death for Australians (AIHW 2016) and has also been directly linked to low levels of fruit and vegetable intake (NHMRC 2013a). Other dietary factors, such as high intakes of fat and salt, influence cholesterol levels and blood pressure, two of the major biomedical risk factors for cardiovascular disease (NHMRC 2013a). According to the Australian Health Survey 2011–2012, one in three adults (32.8%) has abnormal or elevated cholesterol levels, but only 10% of people are aware of this (ABS 2013). As many as 30%–35% of cancer cases, another leading cause of death in Australia, are attributed to overweight and obesity, physical inactivity, poor diet and consumption of alcohol (Aggarwai et al. 2008). Similarly, diabetes is a major cause of death and disability in Australia and is rising. According to the 2011–2012 National Health Medical Survey, 5.1% of Australians have diabetes with a further 3.1% at very high risk of having the condition (ABS 2013). Obesity is known to increase the risk of developing diabetes, with obese adults five times more likely to have diabetes (ABS 2018).

Overweight and obesity rates are continuing to rise in Australia, with almost two in three adults overweight or obese (67%) (ABS 2018). Nearly 1 in 4 (26%) children aged 5–14 and nearly 4 in 10 (37%) young people aged 15–24 are overweight or obese (ABS 2018). These figures are alarming when we consider that excessive body weight contributes to chronic diseases, is very difficult to treat and incurs substantial economic costs in health care and lost productivity (Leung & Funder 2014).

The government has invested considerable public health effort to address the burden of disease, including the development of public health national and state-level policies. These statistics, however, suggest that the majority of adults in Australia are unaware of their health condition or do not consider it a problem. This prompts us to consider Bacchi's (2016) proposition of 'What's the problem represented to be?' from the perspective of the government and from the perspective of those living with these conditions, the public.

An example of a policy which would benefit from an interrogation using Bacchi's (2016) 'What's the problem represented to be?' framework is the ADGs. As a population, we struggle to meet the ADGs. The majority of adults (95%) do not consume enough recommended protective fruit and vegetables, and children fare worse, with 98% of children not consuming the recommended serves of fruit and vegetables and 41% of their total daily energy intake coming from discretionary foods which are low in nutrients but high in energy and/or fat, added sugar and salt (ABS 2014, 2018). Dietitians and nutritionists have a role in changing this. Yet, despite government efforts with policy and social marketing messages, the statistics for nutrition-related risk factors and nutrition-related chronic diseases continue to rise (ABS 2018; AIHW 2018). Deconstructing the ADGs and examining what the underpinning 'problems' are, addressed from the perspective of the different levels of government, the public and the food industry, is insightful. From the public's perspective there are many examples of how people are confused with government-endorsed nutrition messages and a disconnect between what is promoted as evidence based and cultural food-related practices, beliefs and social norms (Lindsay 2010).

Food and nutrition policy in Australia

Contemporary dietary advice and nutrition services and interventions provided to the Australian public are directed by national and international nutrition policy. Since 1992, Australia has had a national food and nutrition policy and federal government funding for strategies to reduce obesity and promote preventive health. With a change in government in 2013 to one that is neoliberal and favours a small government with a focus on the private sector, these policy-driven initiatives were de-funded. Consequently the states and territories followed by decreasing funding for diet-related initiatives. Led by the Obesity Policy Coalition (2017), leading public health, medical and academic organisations called for the federal government to address obesity and provided key elements for a national strategy. In 2019 the outcomes of the Australian Parliamentary Select Committee into the obesity epidemic is expected to be published and actioned. In the mean time, joint Australian, state and territory government initiatives have been developed with industry, public health and consumers. The 'Health Star Rating' is a voluntary front-of-pack food labelling initiative which complements the work of the Healthy Food Partnership where government, the public health sector and the food industry make positive food-related changes. The involvement of multiple levels of government, policy-makers, food industry, legislators, advocacy groups and other stakeholders suggests a tension between interest groups, particularly government, food industry and consumer groups where change can be perceived as slow based on 'evidence', or threatening. This situation warrants an interrogation of what the problems are represented to be using Bacchi's (2016) framework to provide an understanding of the tensions.

Other examples of policy which involve several stakeholders including government, the private industry and consumers include the Aged Care Quality Standards and National Quality Standards (ACECQA 2018), which are national benchmarks for the provision of food and nutrition in aged-care facilities and residential care, early childhood education and care services and outside-school-hours services.

Nutrition and dietetic professionals are crucial in the development and implementation of national, state and territory policies which provide direction and guidelines for healthy nutrition promotion strategies in everyday practice and to populations.

Current issues in nutrition in Australia

Obesity – an individual's or government responsibility?

The dominant paradigms in the Australian health system include the medical and behavioural approaches to health care, which promote curing illness and the promotion of lifestyle changes with emphasis on the individual being responsible for their health and food behaviour. Less attention is given to the multitude of social, cultural and environmental factors that influence food choice in Australia and can limit the effectiveness of medical care and the capacity of the individual to make changes (Swinburn et al. 2011).

This is most evident in the debate surrounding the **obesity epidemic**. Australian culture allows an abundance of cheap high-energy, nutrient-poor foods that are affordable, readily available and heavily marketed (Gortmaker et al. 2011; Swinburn et al. 2011; Watson et al. 2014). Advertising and marketing abounds, promoting the kinds of food not recommended by health authorities (Watson et al. 2014), and the location, type and number of takeaway and fast-food outlets allow these high-fat, high-sugar, high-salt food options to become familiar, desirable and all too easily accessible (Gortmaker et al. 2011; Swinburn et al. 2011).

Calls for changes to the **obesogenic environment** (Gortmaker et al. 2011) continue to attract limited funding, with the bulk of public money going into initiatives to address the problem once it already exists. An obesogenic environment refers to a built, physical, social and food environment that encourages overconsumption, unhealthy eating, sedentary behaviour and a lack of physical activity. Many dietitians and nutritionists advocate for a greater emphasis on broader public health initiatives that recognise the influence of social, environmental and cultural factors on food choice and seek to address nutritional health issues more holistically.

Food insecurity and an ecological paradigm

Paradoxically, while overconsumption of food contributes to Australia's poor health and burgeoning health costs (Leung & Funder 2014), not having enough food affects a significant number of Australians and transcends age, social class and geographical location (McCrindle 2017). **Food insecurity** is when people at all times do not have physical, social and economic access to sufficient, safe and nutritious food (Gallegos et al. 2017). The cause is multifaceted relating to the individual, social, economic, political and environmental factors. Given that food insecurity has a cultural dimension, it is valuable to examine food security policies against Bacchi's (2016) framework, discussed in Chapter 1, as to what the problem is represented to be and from whose perspective.

Public health concerns also extend to the sustainability of our food supply given food wastage, the challenges of climate warming on our food supply and demand for food requiring unsustainable food production practices (Lang & Barling 2013). These concerns have led to an alternative paradigm for solutions. The ecological paradigm takes a holistic, food system literacy approach which considers factors at all levels of influence (Kickbusch 2010; Wilkins et al. 2010). This has implications for future dietitians and nutritionists and our work towards preventive health.

PAUSE
for
REFLECTION
...

Dietitians and nutritionists represent one interest group. What other interest groups have a stake in food consumption? At an individual level, we are responsible for what we eat and how much. However, are we? Who is responsible for the proliferation of factors in our environment which nudges us to over-consume? Who is responsible for the regulation of these influencing factors? What about children who do not have the knowledge or agency to be responsible for food consumption? Using Bacchi's (2016) model described in Chapter 1, 'What's the problem represented to be?', analyse either the ADGs against the six proposed questions or policies developed by welfare groups, or local government addressing food security.

Summary

This chapter has outlined key information about the nutrition and dietetic profession in the Australian health care system:

- The roles of dietitians and nutritionists are diverse and include a range of settings and roles. Within the health care system this ranges from the clinical biomedical treatment of patients to primary health care and health promotion advocacy work.
- The nutrition and dietetics professions in Australia have been described as small but growing professions within the allied health sector.
- The primary health issues of concern include NCDs such as cardiovascular disease, cancer and diabetes, and their risk factors such as obesity. These are all affected by dietary intake and so are an important preventive and treatment focus for the nutrition and dietetic profession, particularly as the major causes of morbidity and mortality in Australia relate to these conditions.
- Key nutrition policies and guidelines that inform nutrition practice in Australia are a particular focus of governments.

Review Questions

1 Identify where dietitians and nutritionists are employed within the Australian health care system, and list the diversity of roles undertaken by nutrition and dietetic professionals.

2 Currently, the numbers of nutrition and dietetic professionals employed within the community remain small; however, the demand for nutrition and dietetic services is increasing. How might the work of dietitians and nutritionists change as they move to create environments that make healthy food choices easier choices?

3 In 1992, the first National Food Policy was developed. Why do you think this was important for Australians and nutrition and dietetic professionals working within the Australian health care system?

4 Outline the structural changes that have been introduced into Medicare that allow dietitians, physiotherapists and others to work with GPs in providing multidisciplinary primary care. Can these changes be explained according to frameworks for policy development introduced by Tuohy (see Chapter 1)?

5 Food choices are often seen as individual choices, and there is a belief that individuals should be responsible for changing their behaviour. What structural/environmental factors influence food choices that are beyond an individual's direct control or behaviour? How do you think policy could respond to addressing these factors affecting food choices?

References

Australian Children's Education and Care Quality Authority (ACECQA), 2018. National quality standard. https://www.acecqa.gov.au/nqf/national-quality-standard.

Aggarwai, B.B., Anand, P., Harikumar, K.B., et al., 2008. Cancer is a preventable disease that requires major lifestyle changes. Pharm. Res. 25 (9), 2097–2116.

Australian Bureau of Statistics (ABS), 2013. Australian Health Survey: biomedical results for chronic disease 2011–12. Cat no. 4364.0.55.005. ABS, Canberra.

Australian Bureau of Statistics (ABS), 2014. National Health Survey – first results 2014–2015. Cat. no. 4364.0,55,007. ABS, Canberra.

Australian Bureau of Statistics (ABS), 2016. Census of population and housing. 2016 table builder – employment, income and education data. ABS, Canberra.

Australian Bureau of Statistics (ABS), 2018. National Health Survey: first results, 2017–18. Cat no. 4364.0.55.001. ABS, Canberra.

Australian Commission of Safety and Quality in Health Care, 2017. National safety and quality health service standards, second ed. ACSQHC, Sydney.

Australian Health Practitioner Regulation Agency (AHPRA), 2014. Regulating health practitioners in the public interest – annual report 2012/2013. AHPRA, Melbourne. https://www.ahpra.gov.au/Publications/Annual-reports/Annual-report-archive.aspx.

Australian Institute of Health and Welfare (AIHW), 2015. Health expenditure Australia 2013–14. Health and welfare expenditure series no. 54. Cat. no. HWE 63. AIHW, Canberra.

Australian Institute of Health and Welfare (AIHW), 2016. Australia's health 2016. Australia's health series no. 15, Cat. no. AUS 199. AIHW, Canberra.

Australian Institute of Health and Welfare (AIHW), 2018. Australia's health 2018. Cat. no. AUS 221. AIHW, Canberra. https://www.aihw.gov.au/reports/australias-health/australias-health-2018/contents/table-of-contents.

Bacchi, C., 2016. Problematizations in health policy: questioning how "problems" are constituted in policies. SAGE Open doi:10.1177/2158244016653986.

Ball, L., Larsson, R., Gerathy, R., et al., 2013. Working profile of Australian private practice accredited practising dietitians. Nutr. Diet. 70 (3), 196–205. doi:10.1111/1747-0080.12015.

Birch, L., 1999. Development of food preferences. Annu. Rev. Nutr. 19, 41–62.

Commissioner of Public Employment, 2007. Quality staffing: about commissioners standards. https://publicsector.sa.gov.au/wp-content/uploads/20070301-Standard-2-Quality-staffing.pdf.

Department of Health, 2013. About the GP Super Clinics programme. Department of Health, Canberra. http://www.health.gov.au/internet/main/publishing.nsf/Content/pacd-gpsuperclinic-about.

Department of Health, 2014. Chronic disease management individual allied health services under Medicare. Patient information, February. Department of Health, Canberra. https://health.gov.au/internet/main/publishing.nsf/Content/74EB0CF19603E7B7CA257BF0001FA204/$File/Fact%20Sheet%20-%20CDM%20-%20Individual%20Allied%20Health%20Services%20-%20Patient%20Info.pdf.

Dietitians Association of Australia (DAA), 2015. National competency standards for dietitians in Australia 2015 (version with guide). DAA, Deakin. https://daa.asn.au/wp-content/uploads/2017/01/NCS-Dietitians-Australia-with-guide-1.0.pdf.

Dietitians Association of Australia (DAA), 2016. President's report. DAA, Deakin. https://daa.asn.au/wp-content/uploads/2017/02/DAA04763_AnnualSummary_170426.pdf.

Dietitians Association of Australia (DAA), 2018a. Becoming a dietitian in Australia. DAA, Deakin. https://daa.asn.au/becoming-a-dietitian-in-australia/.

Dietitians Association of Australia (DAA), 2018b. Accredited dietetics education programs. DAA, Deakin. https://daa.asn.au/becoming-a-dietitian-in-australia/currently-accredited-dietetic-programs/.

Dietitians Association of Australia (DAA), 2018c. Accreditation standards and processes, accreditation standards, summary of key changes to the standards. DAA, Deakin. https://daa.asn.au/becoming-a-dietitian-in-australia/accreditation-of-dietetics-education-programs/accreditation-standards-and-processes/.

Dietitians Association of Australia (DAA), 2018d. How to join the APD program. DAA, Deakin. https://daa.asn.au/apd-program/joining-the-apd-program/.

Dietitians Association of Australia (DAA), 2018e. Fellow of DAA. DAA, Deakin. https://daa.asn.au/apd-program/apd-program-handbook/fellow-of-apd/.

Dietitians Association of Australia (DAA), 2018f. Mutual recognition. DAA, Deakin. https://daa.asn.au/becoming-a-dietitian-in-australia/mutual-recognition/.

Duckett, S., 2014. The need for a regulatory rethink: a perspective from Australia. Future Hosp. J. 1 (2), 117–121.

Friel, S., Barosh, L.J., Lawrence, M., 2014. Towards health and sustainable food consumption: an Australian case study. Public Health Nutr. 17 (5), 1156–1166.

Gallegos, D., Booth, S., Cleve, S., et al., 2017. Food insecurity in Australian households from charity to entitlement. In: Germov, J., Williams, L. (Eds.), A Sociology of Food and Nutrition, fourth ed. OUP, Melbourne, Chapter 4.

Gortmaker, S., Swinburn, B., Levy, D., et al., 2011. Changing the future of obesity: science, policy and action. Lancet 378, 834–837.

Government of South Australia, Attorney-General's Department, 2018. South Australian Public Health Act 2011, part 8. https://www.legislation.sa.gov.au/LZ/C/A/SOUTH%20AUSTRALIAN%20PUBLIC%20 HEALTH%20ACT%202011.aspx.

Health Workforce Australia, 2014. Australia's health workforce series. Dietitians in focus (March). http:// iaha.com.au/wp-content/uploads/2014/03/HWA_Australias-Health-Workforc e-Series_Dietitians-in-focus_vF_LR.pdf.

Hughes, R., 2004. Work practices of the community and public health nutrition workforce in Australia. Nutr. Diet. 61 (1), 38–45.

Kickbusch, I., 2010. The food system: a prism of present and future challenges for health promotion and sustainable development. Health Promotion Switzerland. http://www.ilonakickbusch.com/kickbusch -wAssets/docs/White-Paper—The-Food-System.pdf.

Lang, T., Barling, D., 2013. Nutrition and sustainability: an emerging food policy discourse. Proc. Nutr. Soc. 72 (1), 1–12.

Leung, J., Funder, J. 2014. Obesity: a national epidemic and its impact on Australia. Report by Obesity Australia. pp. 1–33. https://static1.squarespace.com/static/57e9ebb16a4963ef7adfafdb/ t/580ec0679de4bb7cf16ffb9a/1477361771570/NTTW%2BReport.pdf.

Lindsay, J., 2010. Healthy living guidelines and the disconnect with everyday life. Crit. Public Health 20 (4), 475–487.

Macdiarmid, J.I., 2013. Is a healthy diet an environmentally sustainable diet? Proc. Nutr. Soc. 72 (01), 13–20.

McCrindle, 2017. Food bank hunger report 2017 by McCrindle. Foodbank Australia. https://mccrindle .com.au/wp-content/uploads/2018/04/Foodbank_HungerReport_McCrindle_Oct2017_Digital.pdf.

Nash, H., 1989. The History of Dietetics in Australia. DAA, Deakin.

National Health and Medical Research Council (NHMRC), 2013a. Australian Dietary Guidelines. NHMRC, Canberra.

National Health and Medical Research RCouncil (NHMRC), 2013b. Australian Dietary Guidelines; providing the scientific evidence for healthier Australian diets. NHMRC, Canberra. https://www.nhmrc.gov.au/ about-us/publications/australian-dietary-guidelines.

Nutrition Society of Australia (NSA), 2018a. Home page. http://nsa.asn.au.

Nutrition Society of Australia (NSA), 2018b. NSA registration. http://nsa.asn.au/nsa-registration/.

Obesity Policy Coalition, 2017. Tipping the Scales: Australian Obesity Coalition Consensus. Obesity Policy Coalition and Global Obesity Centre, Australia, pp. 1–20.

Ogden, J., 2010. The meaning of food. In: Ogden, J. (Ed.), The Psychology of Eating, second ed. Wiley-Blackwell, Oxford, (Chapter 4).

Selvey, L.A., Carey, M.G., 2013. Australia's dietary guidelines and the environmental impact of food "from paddock to plate". Med. J. Aust. 198 (1), 18–19.

Singh, A.S., Mulder, C., Twisk, J.W.R., et al., 2008. Tracking of childhood overweight into adulthood: a systematic review of the literature. Obes. Rev. 9 (5), 474–488.

Skinner, J., Carruth, B., Bounds, W., et al., 2002. Children's food preferences: a longitudinal analysis. J. Am. Diet. Assoc. 102 (11), 1638–1647.

Sports Dietitians Australia, 2018. Sports nutrition course. https://www.sportsdietitians.com.au/courses-events/sports-nutrition-course/.

Swinburn, B., Sack, G., Hall, K., et al., 2011. The obesity pandemic: shaped by global drivers and local environments. Lancet 378, 804–814.

Watson, W., Johnston, A., Hughes, C., et al., 2014. Children's Health or Corporate Wealth? The Battleground for Kid's Hearts, Minds and Tummies. Cancer Council NSW, Sydney.

Wilkins, J., Lapp, J., Tagtow, A., et al., 2010. Beyond eating right: the emergence of civic dietetics to foster health and sustainability through food system change. J. Hunger Environ. Nutr. 5 (1), 2–12.

World Health Organization (WHO), 2013. Global action plan for the prevention and control of noncommunicable diseases 2013–2020. WHO, Geneva.

World Health Organization (WHO), 2017. Noncommunicable diseases progress monitor, 2017. Licence: CC BY-NC-SA 3.0 IGO. WHO, Geneva.

Further Reading

Croxford, S., Itsiopoulos, C., Forsyth, A., et al., 2015. Food and Nutrition Throughout Life. Allen & Unwin, Sydney.

Saxelby, C., 2018. Catherine Saxelby's Complete Food and Nutrition Companion: The Ultimate A–Z Guide. Hardie Grant Books, Sydney.

Wahlqvist, M.L. (Ed.), 2011. Food and Nutrition: Food and Health Systems in Australia and New Zealand, third ed. Allen & Unwin, Sydney.

Online Resources

Department of Health – national nutrition policy: http://www.health.gov.au/internet/main/publishing.nsf/Content/phd-nutrition-health

Dietitians Association of Australia – smart eating; nutrition information, tips and recipes written by accredited practising dietitians, with topics listed alphabetically A–Z: https://daa.asn.au/smart-eating-for-you/

Eat for Health (national dietary guidelines) – detailed information on the Australian Dietary Guidelines plus advice, tips, resources, recipes and calculators; extensive scientific background information on each of the guidelines can be found in the Eat for Health educator guide – information for nutrition educators: http://www.eatforhealth.gov.au

Heart Foundation – non-government, not-for-profit organisation providing information for health professionals, including information on healthy eating and the dietary management of cardiovascular-related diseases and risk factors: https://www.heartfoundation.org.au/for-professionals

Nutrition Australia – this independent, member organisation aims to promote the health and wellbeing of all Australians and has a number of resources available: http://www.nutritionaustralia.org

CHAPTER 20

Health care managers in a changing system

Janny Maddern, Anne Cahill Lambert and Judith Dwyer

Key learning outcomes

When you finish this chapter you should be able to:

- ◆ describe the role of managers in health care organisations, and their main professional profiles
- ◆ outline the skills and knowledge that managers need to be successful
- ◆ identify the sources of tension between managers and clinicians
- ◆ understand the links between politics and health care management
- ◆ name the main sources of change in the challenges facing health care managers
- ◆ understand the impact of recent health care reforms on the role of health care managers
- ◆ critically explore your own interest in a management career.

Key terms and abbreviations

ambulance ramping
Australasian College of Health Service Management (ACHSM)
blame-shifting
chief executive officers (CEOs)
chief financial officer (CFO)
chief information officer (CIO)
chief operating officer (COO)
clinical stream
cost-shifting
health information manager (HIM)
interprofessional practice (IPP)
Local Hospital Networks (LHNs)
management
organisational politics
Primary Health Networks (PHNs)
restrictive practices
Royal Australasian College of Medical Administrators (RACMA)

Introduction

Health care managers come from diverse professions and backgrounds. Their roles and responsibilities vary enormously from one context to another, and are significantly affected by health reforms and changes in the policy and political environments. This chapter discusses the nature of health care management, the changes and challenges experienced and the knowledge and skills required.

Managers, management and organisations

Management is often defined as getting things done through other people (Iles 1997, pp. 1–16). This is a good shorthand definition, but it needs a second element – the manager needs to be responsible for, and have authority over, the work of those other people. When doctors write prescriptions, they are not managing the pharmacists. The pharmacist who dispenses the medicine is obliged to follow the instructions of the doctor about that particular prescription, but the doctor is not held responsible for the work of the pharmacist. So management is getting things done through other people with the authority to direct them and responsibility for the results of their work. One of the earliest ways of defining the functions of management is summed up as 'plan, organise, lead, control (POLC)' (based on Fayol 1949).

A third important element is that management is done in the context of a company, organisation or team. Authority is part of the job – the manager's mandate to control or coordinate the work of others is included in the position description and often laid out in an organisation chart. It is the organisation that defines and sets the limits of managers' authority, sometimes called delegations. For example, a nurse manager will usually have responsibility as a supervisor of staff and the authority, or a delegation, to order supplies and equipment to a certain monetary value. Of course, the limits of authority are also set by the laws and regulations of the society and the industry. For example, your boss cannot direct you to do something illegal, something that is unsafe for you or others, or something that is not part of the manager's responsibility as a manager. These three elements – getting things done through others, taking responsibility for their work, and doing it within an organisation – define management in the health and community services industries.

While some clinicians and politicians have wondered whether managers are needed, they are essential in all but the smallest of organisations (e.g. a self-employed therapist with a receptionist and a book-keeper). Managers are needed because the work of organisations must be divided up into job roles, and then the work of the individuals in those jobs must be coordinated in order to achieve the organisation's purposes or goals (Weber 1947). The underlying goal of most organisations can be stated as some version of 'to deliver services or products that meet consumer needs at the required standards and costs'. Government health authorities may define this as 'to provide policy advice and administer programs in accordance with government policies', even this is a specialised version of the general statement. All organisations of any size – rural or metropolitan, network, hospital or community – need managers to coordinate the work ('organise'), to solve problems ('control'), to adapt the organisation to changes in the environment ('plan'), and to enable staff to work collaboratively towards achieving the organisation's goals as effectively as possible ('lead').

PAUSE

for

REFLECTION

...

How much do management and being the captain or coach of a sports team have in common?

Managers and management in health care

Management in health care is both similar to management generally – for example, managing people is usually the most challenging task in any industry (Griffin et al. 2016) – and different in important ways. First, health care organisations tend to be more complex than other organisations of equivalent size. The complexity arises from the complicated nature of illness and injury, the wide range and technological complexity of treatments and other interventions, and the fact that the work is done by many different and highly skilled professionals, who need to coordinate their work for the patient. There is less predictability and certainty in most activities and outcomes in such complex systems (McDaniel 2007).

The current focus on developing **interprofessional practice (IPP)** (see Chapter 1) and changes to the scope of practice of health workers – for example, for nurses, paramedics and physiotherapists (see Chapter 17) – bring helpful changes in the way the work is coordinated, but also introduce further complexities to the management task. First, the national health reforms agreed by the federal and state/territory governments (see Chapters 1, 2 and 6) have added further levels of complexity.

Second, decision-making power in health care organisations is often shared among more people. If you are the senior manager of a business that makes shoes, you will take advice from your line managers and from your own experts in materials, finance, logistics, design and marketing. They will expect you to set the direction and in the end to make the hard decisions. Should the business move its production offshore? This is a decision that will be made after much investigation and consideration, but the boss will make the call.

However, if you are a senior health care manager you are more like the mayor of a small town than the boss of a factory. Mayors can get their preferences implemented only if they can get the support of other councillors. Health care managers often have only as much real power to set directions as they have support from important internal and external stakeholders. The number and diversity of those stakeholders (e.g. doctors, nurses, allied health professionals, accountants and community advocates) together with the expectations of patients make this a complicated process indeed.

Third, health policy is one of the most important responsibilities for governments. In practice, this means that almost everything health care organisations, and their managers, want to do or change has some sort of policy or political dimension. Difficulties arise when there is a conflict between management attempts to deal with a problem and political goals of ensuring that voters are happy with their access to, or the quality of, their health services. This is more likely to be the case in the public sector, but even private-sector organisations are influenced in their management by this kind of interaction with the political world.

PAUSE
for
REFLECTION
...

Think about how often you see media stories about people having to wait for a health care service, **ambulance ramping** or hospital bypass, a government minister over-ruling the decision of a hospital to close beds or stop a service to save money, or a shortage of general practitioners to meet particular needs. Do the ideas above about tension between the goals of managers and those of politicians help with understanding how the issue emerged in the media?

Who are the managers?

To understand the current management workforce, a little history about the role of professional and general managers is useful. The departments within health organisations were traditionally defined according to professional groups (e.g. a social work department). So, one of the career paths for all health professional groups was through the management stream within their disciplines – for example, chief orderly, or head **health information manager (HIM)** (formerly 'head of medical records'). Although some of these roles are still important, since the late 20th century there have been moves to make management structures more interprofessional. Influenced by general business models, health care organisations have largely moved from having primarily discipline-based structures to more functional structures – that is, clinical units or business units.

The professional backgrounds of **chief executive officers (CEOs)** have become more diverse. There has also been increasing emphasis on postgraduate health care management and business qualifications. New positions have also emerged, such as **chief operating officer (COO)**, **chief financial officer (CFO)**, general counsel and **chief information officer (CIO)**, as well as new management and policy roles in peak health bodies and regional services.

Similarly, there has been a shift in the way that staff groups are organised to deliver care, towards multidisciplinary teams that can address the multiple clinical needs of patients; for example, maternity patients need access to midwives, sometimes obstetricians and physiotherapists, ultrasound, and so on. Those with an interest in management in all the professions and occupations have thus had some opportunities to broaden their scope, and to take on the management of, for example, operating theatres or laboratories, a community health team, a division of allied health, or a **clinical stream**. With the introduction of national health care reforms in Australia, a number of health care facilities became part of networks (see Chapter 2), thus opening up new opportunities for clinical streams to operate across hospitals and other health services in a region. Hospital and health network organisational structures vary considerably, but the structure shown in Fig. 20.1 is typical.

Credentialling and networking with peers

Although there is no national registration system in Australia for health care managers, there are two major professional associations. The **Australasian College of Health Service Management (ACHSM)**, founded in 1945, is the professional body for health and aged-care managers (Australasian

FIGURE 20.1 EXAMPLE OF A POSSIBLE ORGANISATIONAL STRUCTURE FOR A LARGE HEALTH SERVICE

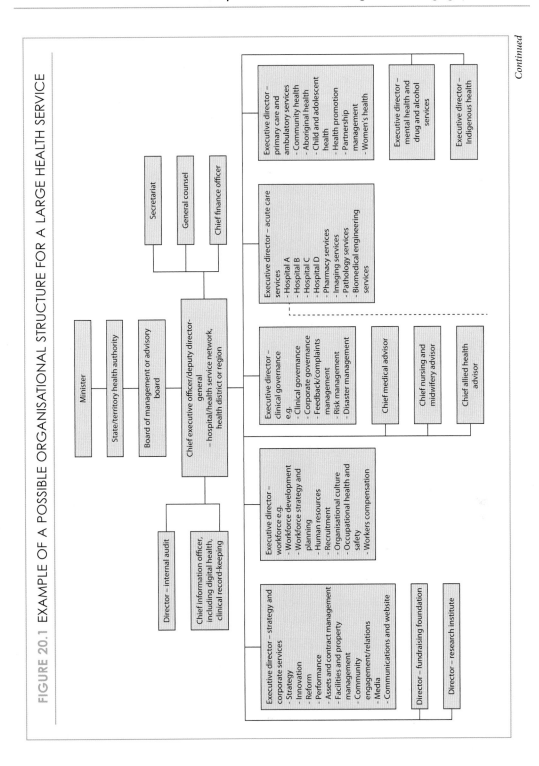

Continued

FIGURE 20.1, cont'd

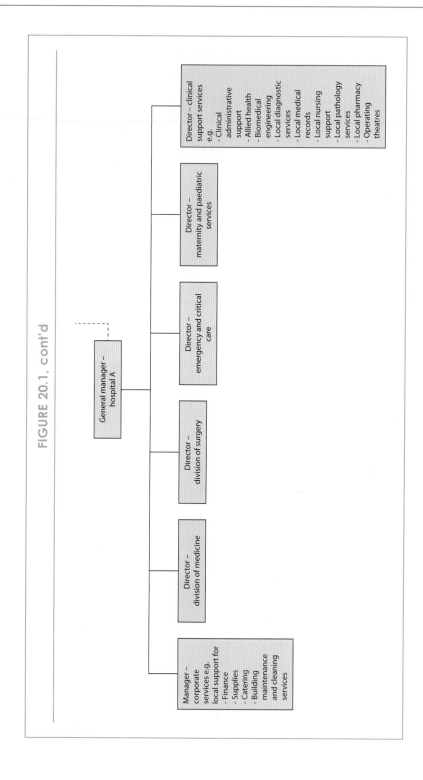

General manager – hospital A

Manager – corporate services e.g. local support for
- Finance
- Supplies
- Catering
- Building maintenance and cleaning services

Director – division of medicine

Director – division of surgery

Director – emergency and critical care

Director – maternity and paediatric services

Director – clinical support services e.g.
- Clinical administrative support
- Allied health
- Biomedical engineering
- Local diagnostic services
- Local medical records
- Local nursing support
- Local pathology services
- Local pharmacy services
- Operating theatres

College of Health Service Management 2018). Membership categories cover health care management students as well as those with a recognised qualification in health care management and/or management experience. The membership profile of the College includes the full range of disciplines working in health care, and a fairly even balance of women and men.

The **Royal Australasian College of Medical Administrators (RACMA)**, founded in 1968, is the professional body for medical managers in public and private health service organisations (Royal Australasian College of Medical Administrators 2018). Fellowship is recognised as a medical specialist qualification. These colleges provide ongoing professional development and networking opportunities for their members, an annual conference and an assessment process for advancement to fellowship. Both of these bodies accredit health care management education programs to ensure that they address the required knowledge and competencies for membership (and for career success).

What makes a good manager?

Although there are many different kinds of management jobs requiring different skills and knowledge, there are some common elements that all managers need. The first thing to understand is the debate about leadership and management. In his well-known argument that separates leadership from management, Kotter (2012) says that things such as planning, organising, budgeting and controlling are management, but to inspire and motivate staff to work well together towards a common goal and succeed in making change you need **leadership**. You may have known people who were good at budgeting, for example, but had no chance of getting staff to agree on a strategic direction.

We would argue that while you can be a good leader without being a manager, at least in health care, you cannot be a good manager without being a leader as well. This is because, in this field, management success largely depends on managing people well, and that requires leadership (Griffin et al. 2016).

Liang et al. (2018) have studied this question, and have identified six kinds of knowledge, skill and attitudes, or 'core competencies', that good health care managers need. They are:

♦ evidence-informed decision-making
♦ operations, administration and resource management
♦ knowledge of the health care environment and the organisation
♦ interpersonal and communication qualities and relationship management
♦ leading people and organisations
♦ enabling and managing change.

The relative importance of each of these competencies depends on the level at which a manager is employed. Senior managers are expected to demonstrate strategic skills and greater leadership competence, whereas middle managers need to use their interpersonal and relationship management skills to facilitate teamwork, manage operations and monitor service quality.

Some of these competencies, such as operations, administration and resource management, and knowledge of the health care environment and the organisation, are perhaps the easiest to understand – they are the kinds of thing you can learn from formal study and from working in the field in any capacity. The role of middle managers in leading change is important and challenging (Balogun et al.

2015; Buchanan et al. 2013; Hyde et al. 2013). Middle managers must make sense of changes imposed from above and work with their colleagues, staff and professional networks to translate them into feasible and constructive change processes. At the same time, they must maintain the safety and quality of existing services. There is also substantial 'emotion' work (Clarke et al. 2007) in maintaining a positive approach and supporting and encouraging staff, colleagues and other stakeholders through the changes.

Leadership, incorporating skills such as judgement, adaptability of managerial styles for different situations (Kolb 1984) and ethical practice to honour responsibilities and avoid doing harm to staff, patients or the community (Legge et al. 2006), is a little more complex and mysterious. **Judgement** is the ability to correctly see a situation, its underlying causes and the potential directions that can be taken: to know when to trust the information at hand, when to act decisively and when to watch and wait. Good judgement arises partly from self-knowledge – you need to have insight into your own prejudices and tendencies and to recognise, for example, when you are just doing what you are comfortable doing rather than the best thing in the situation. A knowledge of theory helps in the task of putting the pieces of the picture together correctly in order to make the right judgement or the best decision.

Using **managerial styles** correctly (e.g. coercion when strong direction is required or coaching to help people improve) requires judgement, and the skill of emotional intelligence (Goleman & Boyatzis 2017) also requires judgement. The manager must decide what kind of approach is required to lead, support, guide or direct in a given situation, in 'real time' as it unfolds, and to be able to enact that knowledge in a genuine way to give the response or take the initiative that will work.

Ethical practice is essential for any professional whose job requires them to act in good faith on behalf of others. For example, we all rely on doctors, nurses, dentists, lawyers and accountants to act in our interests when they are giving us advice, and we call this requirement *professional ethics*. Managers also apply professional ethics. They must act in the interests of their organisation, their staff and their clients or patients and must strive not to simply act in their own self-interest. An ethical framework, and an intention to act ethically, will help managers to recognise ethical dilemmas when they arise, and to 'see' the potential conflict between self-interest and professional ethics. This will not guarantee that they will act ethically, but it will make it more likely.

PAUSE *for* REFLECTION ...

Managers are called on every day to find ways of reconciling the requirements of their jobs with their commitment to values – such as staff participation or community benefit – and perhaps the ability to do this is part of what we all want from leaders. Think about a manager you have known who demonstrated ethical practice: what were the conflicts of interest that person had to manage? Or maybe you have known an unethical manager: what did they do wrong, and do you think they were aware of the ethical dilemma?

Challenges in a changing health care system

Health care is always changing, and so too is the role of the health care manager. Some of the underlying reasons for change in health care were explained in earlier chapters. A number of significant reforms that began in 2010 (see Chapters 1, 2 and 6) have impacted on the role of managers, including:

- the restructuring of health services, including primary care, through the establishment of hospital and health service networks, **Local Hospital Networks (LHNs)** and **Primary Health Networks (PHNs)**
- ongoing changes to the methods and mix of funding in health care, with shifts between casemix (Diagnosis Related Groups) and other 'activity-based' funding methods on the one hand and population-based funding on the other
- shifts in the way funding is provided by national and jurisdictional governments.

The idea behind LHNs was to enable local clinicians and managers to have more say over the running of their health services, thus 'moving decision-making closer to the bedside'. The PHNs are about greater integration of care across service providers, especially in management of chronic conditions and making primary care services more responsive and targeted for local communities.

The split of responsibility for health care between the national and the state/territory governments creates opportunities for health care organisations to engage in **cost-shifting** (activities aimed at making a health care service eligible for funding by a different level of government than is currently involved), and leads governments to engage in the related activity of **blame-shifting** (i.e. trying to blame the other level of government if things are not working well, see Chapter 2). While governments argue it out, patients, health service managers and organisations are left with the problems.

For example, the states and territories pay for public hospitals, but the Commonwealth government pays for nursing-home beds and other services that aim to enable people to have the support they need to stay at home, which most people prefer. There has been a long-term problem with the timely transfer of older and frail patients out of acute hospital beds when they no longer need acute treatment funded by states/territories, and into either residential or home care funded by the Commonwealth. It often falls to patients and their families to negotiate with many different professionals and organisations to get the range of services they need. Many health care providers hope that this issue will be resolved through changes in the way both acute and aged-care services are funded. Nevertheless, the system will still face the challenge of finding ways to enable continuity of care and to reduce the burden on patients and their families in navigating the system. This is one of the critical challenges that health care managers need to solve, working with their clinical colleagues.

Health and aged-care managers face the constant dilemma of attempting to meet the ever-increasing demand for services and at the same time improving service quality, safety and access within tight financial constraints and workforce shortages.

The manager–clinician relationship

It is traditional for managers and clinicians to see things differently. Some clinicians would say 'We just want to do the best for our patients, if only the managers would stop getting in the way – they should simply make sure the system supports us and we have the resources we need.' Some managers would say 'Clinicians just want to have as many resources as possible for themselves and their own work; they don't have to worry about making the money last or about making sure all patients get a fair share. Why can't they be more reasonable?' It is this very conflict that has led to some of the reforms itemised above.

In many ways, it is ideal for health care managers to have some kind of clinical background. However, when clinicians become managers without management training or experience, they can find their new roles and responsibilities very difficult. People in this situation are the largest single group in most postgraduate health care management courses.

The gap in understanding between managers and clinicians has always been a problem, because clinicians and managers have always needed to work together – and have also often been allies. There are even more reasons for working together now. For example, a big challenge for the health system is to change the way it works with people who have chronic conditions. When there is no cure, patients need to be able to understand and take an active role in managing their conditions, and they need to work with a team of health care professionals over the long term.

The kinds of change needed to achieve a shift towards multidisciplinary teamwork and IPP (see Chapter 1) and to ensure more continuity in care relationships are only partly changes in clinical processes. We also need changes in the way that care is organised (e.g. changing the role of outpatient clinics and the communication between primary and secondary, urban and rural providers). These are management questions and the best solutions are not yet known. Managers and clinicians have to understand each other's concerns and talk the same language to meet these challenges.

Patients (or 'consumers' or 'clients') are also more questioning of the quality of health care, for several reasons. Increasingly, CEOs are being held accountable for poor outcomes; a number of scandals have occurred in Australia (see Case study 20.1) and overseas that highlight the importance of clinicians and managers working closely together. (For more information about these major scandals, see the Online Resources section at the end of this chapter.)

Case Study 20.1

Oakden Aged Care
....

Late in 2016, South Australia's chief psychiatrist, Dr Aaron Groves, was asked to urgently review Oakden because the CEO of the North Adelaide Local Health Network (NALHN) was concerned about the level of clinical care. The review was instigated following a patient's family raising concerns about unexplained bruising which required a hospital admission. There had been a number of warnings, including the death of a patient, allegedly as a result of an assault by another patient.

Oakden was an older persons' mental health service that opened in 1982. Over the years, governance responsibility was shifted between South Australia (SA), the Commonwealth and local area health services. It seems that during this time very little capital was invested in improving or maintaining the facilities at Oakden. Neither was there a commitment to spend on human resources.

Dr Groves provided his report in April 2017. Despite the short time frame for review, Dr Groves's findings are comprehensive and address models of care, staffing levels, quality and safety of care, culture and **restrictive practices** (restraining patients physically or with medication). The Review found significant shortcomings that were inconsistent with good clinical practice; indeed, Oakden was found to be 'more like a mental institution from the middle of the last century than a modern Older Person's Mental Health Facility' (Groves et al. 2017, p. 57). The photographs in Dr Groves's report show dilapidated facilities and an institutional rather than domestic style. The report concludes that the dominant culture among Oakden staff was inward-looking, and characterised by poor morale, disrespect, secrecy and a sense of entitlement and indifference; and that the result was a loss of dignity and rights for both consumers and staff (p. 100). The review also found that the use of restrictive practices 'contravened legislation, national standards, state policy and local procedures and [was] likely implemented for staff convenience and or used as punishment' (p. 113).

Subsequently, the SA Coroner reopened an inquest into the death of one of Oakden's residents (Donnellan & Gage 2017) and the SA Independent Commissioner Against Corruption investigated maladministration at Oakden. The Commissioner made findings against five individuals (Lander 2018) and recommendations concerning governance, the role of the Chief Psychiatrist and the community visitor scheme. It also recommended a review of the physical condition of all government mental health facilities. Interestingly, the report was critical of Dr Groves as chief psychiatrist for having visited Oakden only once between 2015 and 2017, prior to being asked to review the facility.

The patients were gradually moved out of the facility from April 2017 and it was finally shut down in September 2017.

Case study questions

1 What are the main issues in this case study?
2 Consider the difficulties with different funding agencies and frequent changes in the governance arrangements. How would these impact on the quality of care provided to patients?
3 What are the pitfalls in ignoring accreditation reports and complaints from patients and their families?
4 How would you go about ensuring appropriate resourcing and governance for an area in the health sector that is not considered as needy?
5 If you were a manager at Oakden, how might your ethical framework have affected your actions, and what consequences would you be prepared to bear?

Management and politics

Organisational politics is the term for the ways in which individuals and groups within an organisation get and use power or influence, usually to protect or enhance their position. More broadly, 'politics' is the term we use for the structure and use of power to make public policy and allocate resources (Jones 2013, pp. 407–412). Health care is so important to any community and the health industry is so large that managers in health care find it hard to escape getting caught up in the politics of their community or jurisdiction.

Managers ignore organisational politics at their peril. While there will always be alliances and interest groups and informal structures within organisations, managers can act to minimise the space available for these activities to either impede change or determine the direction the organisation takes. Those who study organisational politics emphasise the importance of active leadership and strategy, so that workforce concerns are surfaced and addressed, rather than ignored and there is less room for vested interests to engage in internal politics. Leaders need to work with interest groups, and understand what is going on by taking an open and inclusive approach to managing and being aware of shifting alliances and concerns (Egan 1994). 'Management by walking around' will often elicit more real information about an organisation than an in-depth formal organisational review by consultants – but managers need to have a good instinct for informally sifting the material they gather.

Managing organisational politics is not as difficult as it sounds, but can be time-consuming. Much of the practice of change management, and in health care this often means project management, is aimed at assisting the manager to handle stakeholder interests (staff, community, funders and regulators) and organisational politics constructively (Dwyer et al. 2013).

PAUSE
for
REFLECTION
…

The health care reforms that commenced in 2010 were described as aiming to give clinicians more of a say in how health care is delivered. The Commonwealth government took lead responsibility for this reform through the provision of specific funds for LHNs and PHNs. States and territories are still responsible for hospitals and other aspects of the health care system. What do you think are the pros and cons of these reforms, and how effective have they been in ending cost-shifting and blame-shifting?

Career development

For those with an interest in management, it might be helpful to consider how people get into it and make their careers. Some people look at those who appear to be good and ethical managers, and review their practice and career paths. It is also a good idea to take some management and policy-related topics in undergraduate studies.

There are some steps that new entrants to the workforce can take to help them get into management. Managers and leaders learn from experience, so opportunities to extend practice and knowledge can be valuable – for example, by 'acting' in more senior positions or becoming engaged in project work to redesign care processes or reform health programs. Many senior managers report the value of encouragement and advice given by mentors, usually senior people in their field who took an interest in their development.

Increasingly, postgraduate management qualifications are becoming the 'gold standard' for management careers. It is also a good idea to join one of the professional colleges as a student member and take advantage of opportunities for networking with peers and leaders.

For those who are serious about working in management or in health policy, we would make some final suggestions. Learn to look behind the issues you confront at work; try to understand the causes of problems and the range of stakeholder interests involved. Learn to analyse the available options for resolving problems, and to think through the strategies needed to achieve resolution. In other words, aspiring managers and policy-makers need to see the big picture.

Summary

In this chapter, we have outlined these points:

- Management is getting things done through other people.
- Health care management is complicated because of the complexity of the health care system.
- Leaders are not necessarily good managers, but in the health system it is difficult to be a good manager without being a good leader because management in health care is all about people.
- Health care managers come from a range of backgrounds, including clinical or business/accounting.
- It is critical for health care managers, whatever their background, and clinicians to work together, given the increased complexity of the health system and the accountability standards required by patients.
- Health care managers need a strong ethical framework.
- Cost-shifting and blame-shifting are common tools of trade for those who seek more resources, particularly when dealing with patients with chronic illness.
- Health politics are important in understanding organisation and system relationships in the health care system.

Review Questions

1. What is the difference between a manager and a leader?
2. Compare the role of the CEO of a health service with that of the mayor of your local council or the manager of a local supermarket. What are the differences?
3. What tensions exist between clinicians and managers, and how might these tensions be overcome?

4 Managers and leaders must often deal with 'wicked problems' that don't have a single right answer, or where none of the options seem like safe choices.

  a. How do you deal with situations like that in your personal, family, study or work life?

  b. What strengths, and what strategies, would you bring to this challenge if you were a health care manager?

References

Australasian College of Health Service Management, 2018. Home page. Australasian College of Health Service Management, Sydney. www.achsm.org.au.

Balogun, J., Hope-Hailey, V., Cleaver, I., et al., 2015. Landing transformational change: closing the gap between theory and practice. Research report, Chartered Institute of Personnel and Development, London, England. https://www.cipd.co.uk/knowledge/strategy/change/theory-practice-report.

Buchanan, D.A., Denyer, D., Jaina, J., et al., 2013. How do they manage? A qualitative study of the realities of middle and front-line management work in health care. Health Services and Delivery Research, 1.4.

Clarke, C., Hope-Hailey, V., Kelliher, C., 2007. Being real or really being someone else? Change, managers and emotion work. Eur. Manag. J. 25 (2), 92–103.

Donnellan, A., Gage, N., 2017. Oakden nursing home killing of Graham Rollbusch to be probed by coroner, ABC News 13 April. http://www.abc.net.au/news/2017-04-13/graham-rollbusch-nursing-home-death-to-be-investigated/8443996.

Dwyer, J., Liang, Z., Thiessen, V., et al., 2013. Project Management in Health and Community Services: Getting Good Ideas to Work, second ed. Allen & Unwin, Sydney.

Egan, G., 1994. Working the Shadow Side. Jossey-Bass, San Francisco.

Fayol, H., 1949. General and Industrial Management (C. Storrs, Trans.). Pitman, London.

Goleman, D., Boyatzis, R.E., 2017. Emotional intelligence has 12 elements. Which do you need to work on? Harvard Business Review Digital Articles, 6 February, 2-5. https://hbr.org/2017/02/emotional-intelligence-has-12-elements-which-do-you-need-to-work-on.

Griffin, R.W., Phillips, J.M., Gully, S.M., 2016. Organizational Behavior: Managing People and Organizations, twelfth ed. Cengage Learning, Boston, MA.

Groves, A., Thomson, D., McKellar, D., et al., 2017. The Oakden Report. Adelaide, South Australia, SA Health, Department for Health and Ageing.

Hyde, P., Granter, E., Hassard, J., et al., 2013. Roles and behaviours of middle and junior managers: managing new organisational forms of healthcare, NIHR Service Delivery and Organization Programme, Southampton, England. https://www.journalslibrary.nihr.ac.uk/programmes/hsdr/081808241/#/.

Iles, V., 1997. Really Managing Health Care. Open University Press, Buckingham, England.

Jones, G.R., 2013. Organizational Theory, Design and Change, seventh ed. Pearson, Boston, MA.

Kolb, D., 1984. Experiential Learning: Experience as the Source of Learning and Development. Prentice Hall, New Jersey.

Kotter, J.P., 2012. Leading Change. Harvard Business Press, Boston, MA.

Lander, B., 2018. Oakden: a shameful chapter in South Australia's history, Independent Commission Against Corruption, Adelaide.

Legge, D., Stanton, P., Smyth, A., 2006. Learning management (and managing your own learning). In: Harris, M.G., Society for Health Administration Programs in Education.; Australian College of Health Service Executives (Eds.), Managing Health Services: Concepts and Practice, second ed. Elsevier, Sydney, pp. 1–24.

Liang, Z., Howard, P., Leggat, S., et al., 2018. Development and validation of health service management competencies. J. Health Organ. Manag. 32 (2), 157–175.

McDaniel, R.R., 2007. Management strategies for complex adaptive systems: sensemaking, learning, and improvisation. Perform. Improv. Q. 20 (2), 21–42.

Royal Australasian College of Medical Administrators, 2018. Home page. http://www.racma.edu.au.

Weber, M., 1947. In: Parsons, T. (Ed.), The Theory of Social and Economic Organization (A.M. Henderson, T. Parsons, Trans.). Free Press, New York.

Further Reading

Cohn, K., 2007. Collaborate for Success! Breakthrough Strategies for Engaging Physicians, Nurses and Hospital Executives. American College of Healthcare Executives Management Series. Health Administration Press, Chicago.

Day, G.E., Leggat, S.G. (Eds.), 2015. Leading and Managing Health Services: An Australian Perspective. CUP, Port Melbourne, Victoria.

Degeling, P., Zhang, K., Coyle, B., et al., 2006. Clinicians and the governance of hospitals: a cross-cultural perspective on relations between profession and management. Soc. Sci. Med. 63 (3), 757–775.

Goleman, D., Boyatzis, R.E., McKee, A., 2013. Primal Leadership: Unleashing the Power of Emotional Intelligence. Harvard Business Review Press, Boston, MA.

Mintzberg, H., 2013. Simply Managing: What Managers Do – and Can Do Better. Berrett-Koehler, San Francisco, CA.

Mintzberg, H., 2017. Managing the Myths of Health Care: Bridging the Separations Between Care, Cure, Control and Community. Berrett-Koehler, Oakland, CA.

Online Resources

Australasian College of Health Service Management website: www.achsm.org.au.

Australian Commission on Safety and Quality in Health Care website: www.safetyandquality.gov.au.

Council of Australian Governments website: https://www.coag.gov.au.

Council of Australian Governments, 2011. National Health Reform Agreement, July 2011. http://www.federalfinancialrelations.gov.au/content/national_health_reform.aspx.

Council of Australian Governments, 2018. Heads of Agreement between the Commonwealth and the States and Territories on Public Hospital Funding and Health Reform. https://www.coag.gov.au/about-coag/agreements/heads-agreement-between-commonwealth-and-states-and-territories-public-0.

Council on Federal Financial Relations website: www.federalfinancialrelations.gov.au/Default.aspx.

Department of Health (Australia), 2010. A National Health and Hospitals Network for Australia's future: delivering better health and better hospitals. https://apo.org.au/node/20570.

National Health and Hospitals Reform Commission, 2008. Beyond the Blame Game: accountability and performance benchmarks for the next australian health care agreements. http://pandora.nla.gov.au/pan/104821/20140113-1636/www.health.gov.au/internet/nhhrc/publishing.nsf/Content/commission-1lp.html.

National Health and Hospitals Reform Commission, 2009. A healthier future for all Australians – final report of the National Health and Hospitals Reform Commission, June 2009. http://pandora.nla.gov.au/pan/104821/20140113-1636/www.health.gov.au/internet/nhhrc/publishing.nsf/Content/nhhrc-report.html.

Royal Australasian College of Medical Administrators website: www.racma.edu.au.

Swerissen, H., Duckett, S., Moran, G., 2018. Mapping primary care in Australia, Grattan Institute, Melbourne. https://grattan.edu.au/report/mapping-primary-care-in-australia/.

The Grattan Institute – health website (independent reports and commentary on health policies and system reform): https://grattan.edu.au/home/health.

Websites of the health departments in each state also provide information on state-level health reforms and how Commonwealth health reforms have been interpreted.

The following reports outline the findings of inquiries into medical misadventure that give some insight into the need for managers to work in close collaboration with medical staff to reduce patient risk (if links have changed, enter the title of the inquiry into your search engine):

ACT Audit Office, 2018. ACT Health's management of allegations of misconduct and complaints about inappropriate workplace behavior: report No. 9/2018. https://www.audit.act.gov.au/__data/assets/pdf_file/0004/1229530/Report-No.-9-of-2018-ACT-Healths-management-of-allegations-of-misconduct-and-complaints-about-inappropriate.pdf.

ACT Auditor-General's Office, 2012. Emergency department performance information: report no. 6/2012. https://www.audit.act.gov.au/__data/assets/pdf_file/0014/1205330/Report-6-2012-Emergency_Department_Performance_Information.pdf.

Australian Council for Safety and Quality in Health Care, 2002. Lessons from the Inquiry into Obstetrics and Gynaecological Services at King Edward Memorial Hospital 1990–2000, Sydney, NSW, ACSQHC. https://www.safetyandquality.gov.au/former-publications/lessons-from-the-inquiry-into-obstetrics-and-gynaecological-services-at-king-edward-memorial-hospital-1990-2000-pdf-653-kb/.

Davies, G., 2005. Queensland public hospitals commission of inquiry report, Brisbane, Queensland Government. http://www.qphci.qld.gov.au.

Francis, R., 2013. Report of the Mid Staffordshire NHS Foundation Trust public inquiry. http://webarchive.nationalarchives.gov.uk/20150407084003/http://www.midstaffspublicinquiry.com/.

Groves, A., Thomson, D., McKellar, D., et al., 2017. The Oakden report. https://www.sahealth.sa.gov.au/wps/wcm/connect/Public+Content/SA+Health+Internet/About+us/Reviews+and+consultation/Review+of+the+Oakden+Older+Persons+Mental+Health+Service.

Kennedy, I., 2001. The report of the public inquiry into children's heart surgery at the Bristol Royal Infirmary 1984–1995 learning from Bristol (Cm 5207(I)). http://webarchive.nationalarchives.gov.uk/20060802133451/http://www.bristol-inquiry.org.uk/final_report/report/index.htm.

Lander, B., 2018. Oakden: a shameful chapter in South Australia's history. https://icac.sa.gov.au/system/files/ICAC_Report_Oakden.pdf.

Picone, D., Pehm, K., 2015. Review of the Department of Health and Human Services management of a critical issue at Djerriwarrh Health Services. https://www2.health.vic.gov.au/about/publications/ResearchAndReports/review-dhhs-management-djerriwarrh-health-services.

CHAPTER 21

The medical profession in Australia

E Michael Shanahan

Key learning outcomes

When you finish this chapter you should be able to:

- understand how the profession of medicine Australia is organised, funded and delivered
- understand the training pathways to becoming a medical practitioner in Australia
- understand what it means to be a medical professional and how this notion is evolving and changing over time
- understand current issues regarding the medical workforce and how this impacts on the delivery of good health care in Australia.

Key terms and abbreviations

Australian Commission on Safety and Quality in Health Care (ACSQHC)

Australian Health Practitioner Regulation Agency (AHPRA)

Australian Medical Council (AMC)

bulk-billing

code of conduct

constructivist

contextual learning

continuing professional development (CPD)

corporatised

economic rationalism

evidence-based practice

fee for service

gap fee

National Safety and Quality Health Service (NSQHS)

neoliberalism

proceduralists

programmatic assessment

reflective learners

registered medical officers (RMOs)

trainee medical officers (TMOs)

Introduction: What is a medical practitioner?

While acknowledging that in Australian Indigenous culture there is a long tradition of the delivery of medical care, this chapter will focus on the practice of medicine in Australia provided by those practitioners educated in the 'Western' practice of medicine. Medicine in Australia has been practised by individuals trained in this manner since the beginning of White settlement in the latter part of the 18th century, with the arrival of several doctors on the first fleet in 1788 (Lewis 2014).

Modern medical training in Australia has its roots in what is considered to be largely western European traditions. For example, in the early 19th century any qualified doctors practising in Australia were graduates from (mainly) British medical schools, with Australian apprentices being sent to Britain to obtain formal qualifications. The first medical school in Australia was established in 1862 at the University of Melbourne; however, it wasn't until 1900 that the *Medical Practitioners (Amendment) Act 1900* (Act No. 33, 1900) was passed. This imposed penalties on persons using titles including surgeon or physician if they were not appropriately registered (Lewis 2014).

So what is the definition of a medical practitioner in Australia? The Australian Bureau of Statistics (ABS) *Standard Classification of Occupations* defines medical practitioners as individuals who diagnose physical and mental illnesses, disorders and injuries, provide medical care to patients and prescribe and perform medical and surgical treatments to promote and restore good health (Australian Bureau of Statistics (ABS) 2006). A medical practitioner as defined by the *Health Practitioner Regulation National Law Act 2009* is an individual who is registered with the Medical Board of Australia. The Medical Board acts under the umbrella of the **Australian Health Practitioner Regulation Agency (AHPRA)**, which is responsible for a suite of health practitioner registration authorities. The role of the Medical Board is to maintain the medical register, to decide the requirements for registration and to approve accredited programs of study as providing qualifications for registration. The **Australian Medical Council (AMC)** is the organisation charged by the Medical Board with the responsibility to approve and reaccredit programs licensed to deliver medical education. Students successfully undertaking such programs can then be registered as medical practitioners in Australia.

In addition, the AMC sets the standards for medical practitioners trained outside Australia who wish to work in Australia. Those international medical graduates wishing to work in Australia usually have to undergo assessments arranged by the AMC and undertake a period of supervised work prior to achieving full registration.

Medical education in Australia

Prior to the mid 1860s, all legitimate medical practitioners in Australia had undertaken their assessments and licensure through medical schools and colleges outside of Australasia, mainly in Britain. From the 1860s, medical schools began to develop in Australia. By 1900 there were three schools (Melbourne, Sydney and Adelaide), with a further five schools added up until the mid 1960s (Geffen 2014). Medical education in Australia until the 1960s followed in the tradition of medical education on the model of Flexner – namely an undergraduate preclinical education followed by a period of clinical emersion. Since the mid 1960s there has been a steady expansion in the numbers and types of medical schools. Since 2000, in response to perceived current and future shortages of medical practitioners in Australia, there has been a rapid expansion in the numbers of medical schools and students. Currently there are 20 medical schools in Australia, with a further one under discussion (Table 21.1). In 2018 there were over 17,000 students enrolled in medical schools in Australia, which represents an increase of approximately 100% since the year 2000.

Medical education has also changed markedly since the 1960s. The majority of medical students in Australia are now in postgraduate programs (Medical Schools Outcomes Database (MSOD) 2017).

TABLE 21.1 MEDICAL PROGRAMS IN AUSTRALIA 2018		
Medical school	**Year opened**	**Enrolment (2018)**
University of Melbourne	1862	1391
University of Sydney	1883	1168
University of Adelaide	1885	959
University of Western Australia	1956	850
University of Tasmania	1965	589
Monash University	1958	1823
University of NSW	1960	1635
Flinders University	1974	626
Newcastle University	1978	1049
Deakin University	2008	577
Griffith University	2004	665
University of Wollongong	2006	326
University of Notre Dame (Sydney and Fremantle)	2008	905
Bond University	2005	547
Australian National University	2004	417
James Cook University	2000	1132
University of Queensland	1936	1580
Western Sydney University	2007	630
Curtin	2017	133
Macquarie	2018	50

Source: Medical Deans Australia and New Zealand.

The style of education delivery has moved from traditional lecture format to more modern adult learning approaches emphasising **constructivist**, collaborative and **contextual learning** approaches. The aim of developing self-directed learners, with emphasis on **reflective learners** capable of developing into self-correcting practitioners, is now emphasised. To facilitate this, forms of **programmatic assessment** for learning are increasingly underpinning the assessment processes in medical courses as traditional formal examination-based assessments are becoming less central to student progress. What continues to be central to medical education, however, is the clinical immersive experience with its cognitive apprenticeship-style learning approaches underpinned by increasingly sophisticated forms of workplace-based assessments.

Increasingly, the process of medical education is seen as a continuum whereby skills are developed over many years from novice to expert, with the medical school providing only the first step in the process. Medical school graduate students obtain provisional registration with the medical board (internship). They then generally enter training programs run by the medical colleges in order to differentiate into various areas of specialty (including family medicine or 'general practice'). During this period of medical practitioners' training, they generally work under supervision in hospital- or community-based employment and are known as **trainee medical officers (TMOs)** – either **registered medical officers (RMOs)** or registrars. Usually the term 'registrar' is reserved for the more senior TMOs, but the meaning of this title is not defined and does not imply any particular level of qualification such as passing a specialist examination.

Developing into a specialist independent practitioner takes a number of years through the different pathways. Following medical school and internship, further training generally takes a minimum of 4–6 years, depending on the trainee's progress and the specialty pathway chosen. Additionally, because of a bottleneck at the level of entering programs, a doctor might wait for several years, generally undertaking RMO or 'service' positions prior to being accepted into the program of their choice. Their progress can be further impeded by their success or otherwise with the rigorous exams (set by the colleges) that they are required to pass. Then, following the completion of the program, if an individual wishes to work in a staff position in the public or academic environment often a higher degree (such as a PhD) is undertaken. This may take a further 3–5 years to complete. Therefore, it is not uncommon for specialists to have taken 20 years or more to complete the training process from the commencement of medical school to working as an independent consultant. The personal and community investment in the training of these individuals is considerable. Following the completion of their formal education, all medical practitioners now undertake some form of **continuing professional development (CPD)**, again usually under the umbrella of their specialist college. The maintenance of professional education is now mandated by the AHPRA and the continued medical registration of the practitioner is dependent on being part of a continuing educational program.

The modern medical professional

The medical profession is often seen as the archetypical professional group (Willis 1989). But what does being a medical professional mean in the 21st century? Generally, the understanding of being a professional implies a control over one's work (Freidson 1970). According to Freidson, elements of being a professional include having a strong service ethic, having a professional monopoly over an area of knowledge and having autonomy of practice (including a capacity to set one's own price for one's work). The responsibility to self-regulate is also said to be central to the notation of being a professional (see Chapter 1).

In modern medical practice a number of these concepts no longer hold true, or are under significant threat. Nonetheless at many levels the modern medical practitioner would identify as a professional and would be regarded as such by the majority of the community in Australia.

> **PAUSE**
> *for*
> **REFLECTION**
> ...
>
> How does the development of a professional identity come about, and what does it mean to be a medical professional in Australia?

Professionalism is a required core competency for medical practitioners. Increasingly, the development of a medical professional identity among medical students is considered to be a central task of medical schools (Byyny 2015). The development of a true professional identity involves the development of a mindset and attitude that transcends rules and means an individual will seek to do 'the right thing' in a situation whether or not they have previously encountered it. The fully formed professional is habitually faithful to professional values in highly complex situations. Sustaining professionalism is considered to be a complex adaptive problem that defies easy definition where the rules are constantly changing (Lucey 2015). It involves a deep understanding of ethics, the law and community values as well as high-level interpersonal skills. Despite the difficulties, most medical schools in Australia have developed, or are developing, an explicit thread of professionalism within their curricula (Parker et al. 2008). These curricula are sometimes supported by explicit codes of conduct and mechanisms to correct aberrant behaviour (including progression impediment), with the ultimate sanction being exclusion from the medical school. Although a separate code of conduct for Australian medical students has yet to be developed, a number of these codes do exist around the world (e.g. UK, Ireland). A **code of conduct** for doctors that describes what is expected of all doctors registered to practise medicine in Australia has been developed by the Australian Medical Council (2009). So, what are the fundamental principles expounded by these curricula and the doctors' code of practice? Byyny (2015) has recently outlined these principles as follows:

- Adhere to high ethical standards: do right, avoid wrong and do no harm.
- Subordinate your own interests to those of your patients.
- Avoid business, financial and organisational conflicts of interest.
- Honour the social contract you have undertaken with patients and communities.
- Understand the non-biological determinants of poor health and the economic, psychological, social and cultural factors that contribute to health and illness.
- Care for patients who are unable to pay; advocate for the medically under-served.

- ◆ Be accountable, both ethically and financially.
- ◆ Be thoughtful, compassionate and collegial.
- ◆ Continue to learn, increase your competence and strive for excellence.
- ◆ Work to advance the field of medicine, and share knowledge for the benefit of others.
- ◆ Reflect dispassionately on your own actions, behaviours and decisions to improve your knowledge, skills, judgement, decision-making, accountability and professionalism.

All modern Australian medical practitioners would be expected to adhere to these standards. The standards would also be part of every medical curriculum in the country, and indeed in most medical courses in the world. They are certainly explicitly articulated in the code of conduct produced by the AMC.

> **PAUSE**
> *for*
> **REFLECTION**
> ...
>
> In an era of tight resource allocation, where do some of the tensions lie in medical practice? How does a practitioner provide the best care for their individual patient while balancing this against the need to conserve the community resources?

What about the sociological notions of medical professionalism? How well do these notions hold up when considering medical practice in Australia? Willis (2006) argues that a number of challenges to the profession since the 1960s have radically reshaped the concept of professionalism as relating to the medical profession. These include challenges to medical dominance posed by **neoliberalism** and **economic rationalism**, a growth in consumerism and associated litigiousness, the change from a cottage industry basis to mass marketing as medicine has become industrialised, the rise of complementary medicine and the changing roles of health care professionals (Willis 2006).

1 The concept of autonomy of practice

Increasingly medicine is not being practised in the autonomous way it once was. Practice guidelines and restrictions on prescribing (often because of cost to the community or considerations of patient safety) are part of every medical practitioner's way of life. Guidelines are promulgated in the interests of safety and consistency of practice and are often developed under the guise of 'evidence-based practice'. There is, however, considerable push-back on these guidelines with the increasing understanding that the evidence base upon which they are derived can be flimsy and the application of population-based evidence to the individual circumstance contains a flawed logic (Lenzer 2013). There is clear evidence that the application of practice guidelines amongst experienced medical practitioners is at best limited (Mafi et al. 2013). Nonetheless, the push for such guidelines is continuing and is likely to increase, especially when they can be used for cost containment. There are a number of other restrictions on the autonomy of medical practice becoming obvious in daily medical practice. Some of these are generated by directives from the **Australian Commission on Safety and Quality in Health Care (ACSQHC)** who audit medical practice against the **National Safety and Quality Health Service**

(NSQHS) standards (Australian Commission on Safety and Quality in Health Care (ACSQHC) 2017). These processes are often seen as burdensome but are the reality of modern medical practice.

The roll-out of electronic medical records and electronic prescribing also has the potential to limit the autonomy of medical practice. Although on balance these developments are seen to be advantageous in terms of patient safety, they also hold the potential to restrict the ordering of what might be considered to be unnecessary tests or 'off-label' medical prescribing. ('Off-label' is the term used when medication is prescribed for indications other than those approved by the pharmaceutical benefits scheme.)

2 The notion of self-regulation

Increasingly in Australia the notion that professions can be self-regulating has been disabused. The primary regulatory authorities for the medical profession, the AHPRA and the Medical Boards, have significant community, non-medical representation. With respect to currency of practice, although the maintenance of professional education continues to be delivered by the profession through the colleges, this is now linked to the practitioner's registration though the Medical Board. Medical practitioners are subject to audit with respect to their education through both their colleges and the AHPRA.

3 The notion of price setting

The remuneration of medical practitioners in Australia is complex and many models exist (see below). Suffice to say that, for many practitioners (such as those on public salaries), there is no possibility of setting a price directly for the service provided. For others there is still (theoretically) considerably autonomy, although there are many practical restrictions on setting very high fees. For some in the profession, however, this remains a jealously guarded right and privilege.

4 The notion of a monopoly of a body of knowledge

Increasingly, medical knowledge in itself is becoming widely accessible. Almost-universal access to computers with increasing sophisticated search engines and diagnostic algorithms means the role of the doctor as the repository of medical knowledge is rapidly declining (Ieraci 2018). What it is increasingly being replaced with is the ability to apply this knowledge to the individual's situation. This can only come with the perspective that experience brings, and demands the development of high-level communication and cognitive skills. Technical skills (such as surgical skills) are also being facilitated with (but not replaced by) robotics. These changes are being reflected in the changing content of medical school curricula and training programs. Despite the prediction of some futurists, however, the likelihood of the profession of medicine being replaced by artificial intelligence remains low.

5 A strong service ethic

Although most medical practitioners have a strong service ethic in the sense of considering the primacy of their patient's needs, the implications of this commitment are increasingly being seen by the profession as potentially unhealthy for the individuals in the system. Long hours of work and the personal psychological toll of many years of training and the burden of medical responsibility have seen individuals pay a heavy price. Suicide rates in the medical profession (including among junior medical staff and medical students) exceed the national average. There is considerable discussion about how this might be addressed (beyondblue 2013), but possible solutions may include reducing the hours of work and increasing the flexibility of work practice. There is evidence that this is starting to occur (Munir 2018).

PAUSE
for
REFLECTION
...

Given these increasingly tight restrictions on medical practice, how well does the concept of 'medical dominance' still hold true in this century?

The medical workforce in Australia

There were 111,166 medical practitioners and 20,057 medical students registered with the Medical Board in 2016/17 – just under 400 doctors per 100,000 population (Medical Board of Australia 2017). The number of doctors registered has grown consistently at rate of 3.9% from 2005 to 2015, reflecting the significant increase in the numbers of medical student places in Australia from around the year 2000. Excluding provisionally registered practitioners, the number of registered doctors in Australia increased from 67,890 to 97,466 during this period. In 2015, 88,040 registered practitioners were employed in medicine and 95% of these worked in a clinical role; one in every four was aged 55 or over, and two in five were women (Australian Institute of Health and Welfare (AIHW) 2015). The percentage of women as a total of the workforce continues to increase, reflecting the increase in the percentage of women in medical schools over the last two decades. In 2016/17, women made up 42% of the workforce and 57% of doctors under the age of 30 (Medical Board of Australia 2017). In addition, women made up over half of all clinician specialists in training. Despite this change, there are large disparities in some disciplines of medicine such as orthopaedic surgery, where women make up only 3.3% of the total workforce, and women still only make up 25% of the specialist workforce overall (up from 20% 5 years previously). The average hours of work for medical practitioners in Australia were 42 hours per week. The largest proportion of clinicians was specialists (35%) followed by general practitioners (33.1%), specialists in training (18.0%) and hospital non-specialists (11.6%). The supply of GPs was stable between 2012 and 2015 (around 110 FTE per 100,000) and the supply of specialists increased from 128 to 134 per 100,000 population (AIHW 2015).

Under-serviced groups

Estimates of the numbers of doctors identifying as Indigenous vary, but may be around 300. This is an approximate doubling since 2004, but estimates suggest approximately 10 times that number would be required if the proportion were to reflect the numbers of Indigenous people in the community. In 2013 there were over 300 medical students who identified as Indigenous (Australian Indigenous Doctors' Association 2014; see Chapter 10).

Major cities continue to have the highest rate of supply of registered medical practitioners, with the supply of medical practitioners overall lowest in remote / very remote areas. Paradoxically, in 2015 the supply of general practitioners in remote / very remote areas was the highest per capita (136 full-time equivalent per 100,000) but the AIHW (2015) cautions against suggesting this reflects adequate servicing, pointing out that service delivery models vary radically in urban compared with remote areas (see Chapter 9 for a discussion on rural health). Of the non-clinician medical practitioners, the majority worked in areas of medical administration (1490 or 34.6%), as researchers (24.5%) or as teachers (AIHW 2015).

Employment and remuneration

Traditionally in Australia, employment levels in registered medical practitioners have been very high. The employment arrangements and subsequent remuneration vary widely – as would be expected given the enormous variety in medical practice and the complexities of delivering a medical service in a country such as Australia. As in many countries, various blends of 'public' and 'private' employment arrangements exist in medicine. Many practitioners derive their employment from a mixture of these. At one end of the 'public' spectrum are doctors fully employed by the state and remunerated via a fixed salary. This tends to be more the case with provisionally registered doctors and doctors in training. At the other end of the spectrum are doctors working fully 'in private'. These doctors set their own fee schedules, and are paid '**fee for service**'. The majority of these services, however, are still heavily underwritten by the public purse through the Medicare system (see Chapter 2). Those working in such arrangements have the opportunity to '**bulk-bill**' their patients and receive the fee determined by the item number attached to that service. Item number schedules are a hybrid of time-based and service-based items. Many practitioners charge above the scheduled fee, and the patient then encounters a '**gap fee**' at the point of delivery (the gap being the difference between the fee charged and the Medicare rebate). Increasingly, general practitioner services are becoming **corporatised**, where individual practitioners allow a company to take over the running of the 'business' of medicine and the doctors simply contract themselves to the organisation and receive a proportion of the takings that they generate (Erny-Albrecht & Bywood 2016).

The federal government uses various levers to try to control costs in the health care system. Among the most unpopular with the medical profession has been a freeze on Medicare rebates. This has had a negative effect on doctors' remuneration and led to much debate about doctors ceasing **bulk-billing** services. The logical effect of this behaviour is to cost shift the price of service delivery into pockets of patients.

There is considerable debate in the medical political literature about the most appropriate way to work, and of the various incentives that drive practice behaviours. For example, it is often stated that '**proceduralists**' are relatively well remunerated for the performance of individual procedures, which potentially encourages them to perform more procedures than may be otherwise considered medically necessary. Good examples of this in the Australian system include knee arthroscopy and shoulder ultrasound (Awerbach 2008; Harris et al. 2018). Despite the ongoing debates and tensions, however, doctors are still among the best-remunerated occupational group in Australia today.

The public view of the medical profession

Despite the occasional political portrayal of medical practitioners working in their own self-interest, confidence in the profession remains high. Most Australians visit their doctors each year (Australian Bureau of Statistics 2013) and most surveys put medical practitioners at or near the top of trustworthiness and satisfaction ratings, with 90% of the community trusting doctors. Patient complaints to AHPRA and disciplinary actions against medical practitioners remain low, with 5% of practitioners having complaints made about them in 2016/17 resulting in 0.6% having their registration suspended or cancelled (Australian Health Practitioner Regulation Agency (AHPRA) 2017). This would suggest that the commitment to the social contract between doctors and the community (part of being a professional) continues to be central to how doctors deliver their community responsibilities.

The future of the medical profession

The medical profession in the 21st century faces extraordinary challenges to achieve its primary role of delivering quality medical care to the Australian community. An almost inexorable increase in medical costs coupled with rising community expectations of care and improving technical ability to increasingly prolong life makes for a perfect storm with respect to resource allocation. The profession itself needs to be nimble enough to meet changing community expectations, and to continue to redefine and reshape what it means to be a medical professional. Educational institutions likewise need to be flexible enough to recognise and lead the changes. New technologies and artificial intelligence will certainly continue to redefine the role of a doctor. The maldistribution of medical services, in particular with a relative lack of service to rural and remote Australia, continues to be a major issue. Inequities in health care outcomes among Indigenous Australians and those of poorer socioeconomic status remain as major challenges to a fairer Australia in which the medical profession has a major role to play. Nonetheless the profession has shown itself to be robust and highly adaptable to changing environments and circumstances. There is every indication than new generations of Australian medical practitioners will have the skill and courage to continue with the necessary reforms to meet these and future challenges.

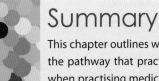

Summary

This chapter outlines what it means to be a medical practitioner in Australia in the 21st century. It discusses the pathway that practitioners take to become doctors, and then some of the responsibilities they have when practising medicine. The chapter also describes the concept of medical professionalism and how this has changed since the turn of the century. The demographics of the Australian medical workforce is briefly outlined, and some of the contemporary challenges facing current and future practice in Australia are discussed.

Review Questions

1 Outline the pathway for a medical practitioner to become a fully registered independent doctor. Do you think the community can continue to afford such a lengthy pathway, and how might the same outcome be achieved in a lesser time period?

2 A significant maldistribution of medical services still exists in Australia. How might this issue be addressed effectively?

3 Do you think that the continued development of artificial intelligence will make the role of the doctor largely redundant? If not, why not?

4 Over the last decade the Commonwealth Government offered a number of 'bonded' places to medical students to enter medical schools around Australia. Apply Bacchi's (2012) approach to try to examine why this policy was developed.

References

Australian Bureau of Statistics (ABS), 2006. Australian and New Zealand Standard Classification of Occupations, first ed. cat. no. 1220.0, ABS, Canberra.

Australian Bureau of Statistics, 2013. Patient experiences in Australia: summary of findings 2012–13. Cat. no. 4839.0. http://www.abs.gov.au/ausstats/abs@.nsf/Lookup /4839.0main+features32012-13.

Australian Commission on Safety and Quality in Health Care (ACSQHC), 2017. National Safety and Quality Health Service (NSQHS) standards, second ed. https://www.safetyandquality.gov.au/our-work/ assessment-to-the-nsqhs-standards/.

Australian Health Practitioner Regulation Agency (AHPRA), 2017. AHPRA annual report 2016/17. http:// www.ahpra.gov.au/annualreport/2017/downloads.html.

Australian Indigenous Doctors Association, 2014. Twice as many Indigenous doctors – media release. https://www.aida.org.au/wp-content/uploads/2018/03/1-Twice-as-many-Indigenous-doctors.pdf.

Australian Institute of Health and Welfare (AIHW), 2015. Medical practitioners workforce 2015. https:// www.aihw.gov.au/reports/workforce/medical-practitioners-workforce-2015/contents/how-man y-medical-practitioners-are-there.

Australian Medical Council, 2009. Good medical practice: a code of conduct for doctors in Australia. https://ama.com.au/sites/default/files/documents/AMC_Code_of_Conduct_July_2009.pdf.

Awerbach, M., 2008. The clinical utility of ultrasonography for rotator cuff disease, shoulder impingement syndrome and subacromial bursitis. Med. J. Aust. 188 (1), 50–53.

Bacchi, C., 2012. Introducing the 'What's the problem represented to be?' approach. In: Bletsas, A., Beasley, C. (Eds.), Engaging With Carol Bacchi: Strategic Interventions and Exchanges. University of Adelaide Press, Adelaide. https://www.adelaide.edu.au/carst/docs/wpr/wpr-summary.pdf.

beyondblue, 2013. National mental health survey of doctors and medical students. October. https:// www.beyondblue.org.au/docs/default-source/research-project-files/bl1132-report—nmhdmss-full- report_web.pdf?sfvrsn=4.

Byyny, R.L., 2015. Medical Professionalism: Best Practices. Alpha Omega Alpha Honor Medical Society, California.

Erny-Albrecht, K., Bywood, P., 2016. Corporatisation of general practice – impact and implications. PHCRIS policy issue review. Primary Health Care Research and Information Service, Adelaide. https://dspace.flinders.edu.au/xmlui/bitstream/handle/2328/38389/phcris_pub_8460.pdf?sequence=1&isAllowed=y.

Freidson, E., 1970. Profession of Medicine: A Study of the Sociology of Applied Knowledge. University of Chicago Press, Chicago.

Geffen, L., 2014. A brief history of medical education and training in Australia. Med. J. Aust. 201 (1), S19–S22.

Harris, I., O'Connor, D., Buchbinder, R., 2018. Needless procedures: knee arthroscopy is one of the most common but least effective surgeries. The Conversation. https://theconversation.com/needless-procedures-knee-arthroscopy-is-one-of-the-most-common-but-least-effective-surgeries-102705.

Health Practitioner Regulation National Law Act 2009. https://www.legislation.qld.gov.au/view/html/inforce/current/act-2009-045.

Ieraci, S., 2018. Redefining the physician's role in the era of online health information. Med. J. Aust. 209 (8), 340–341.

Lenzer, J., 2013. Why we can't trust clinical guidelines. BMJ 346, f3830.

Lewis, M.J., 2014. Medicine in colonial Australia 1788–1900. Med. J. Aust. 201 (1), S5–S10.

Lucey, C.R., 2015. The problem with professionalism. In: Byyny, R.L., Papadakis, M.A., Paauw, D.S. (Eds.), Medical Professionalism: Best Practices. Alpha Omega Alpha Honor Medical Society, California, pp. 9–21.

Mafi, J.N., McCarthy, E.P., Davis, R.B., et al., 2013. Worsening trends in the management and treatment of back pain. JAMA Intern. Med. 173 (17), 1573–1581. doi:10.1001/jamainternmed.2013.8992.

Medical Board of Australia, 2017. Annual report 2016/17. http://www.ahpra.gov.au/annualreport/2017/downloads.html.

Medical Practitioners (Amendment) Act 1900 (Act No 33, 1900). https://www.legislation.nsw.gov.au/acts/1915-33.pdf.

Medical Schools Outcomes Database (MSOD), 2017. Medical Schools Outcomes Database national data report 2017, Medical Deans Australia and New Zealand, Sydney. https://medicaldeans.org.au/md/2018/08/2017-MSOD-National-Data-Report-1.pdf.

Munir, V., 2018. MABEL: doctors shouldn't work in excess of 50 hours per week. InSight (6), https://insightplus.mja.com.au.

Parker, M., Luke, H., Zhang, J., et al., 2008. The 'pyramid of professionalism': seven years of experience with an integrated program of teaching, developing, and assessing professionalism among medical students. Acad. Med. 83 (8), 733–741. doi:10.1097/ACM.0b013e31817ec5e4.

Willis, E., 1983 revised ed. 1989. Medical Dominance. Allen & Unwin, Sydney.

Willis, E., 2006. Introduction: taking stock of medical dominance. Health Soc. Rev. 15 (5), 421–431.

Further Reading

Dent, J.A., Harden, R.M., 2013. A Practical Guide for Medical Teachers, fourth ed. Churchill Livingstone Elsevier, USA.

Groopman, J., 2007. How Doctors Think. Houghton Milfflin, Boston, MA.

Tai-Seale, M., Olson, C., Li, J., et al., 2017. The practice of medicine. Health Aff. (Millwood) 36(4), 655–662.

Online Resources

For a list of medical colleges go to: https://www.ahpra.gov.au/education/approved-programs-of-study.aspx?ref=medical%20practitioner&type=specialist.

CHAPTER 22

Midwifery in Australia

Jenny Gamble

Key learning outcomes

When you finish this chapter you should be able to:

+ describe maternity services reforms
+ explain the impact of evidence-based reforms on the role of the midwife
+ understand the legal, regulatory and evidence-based frameworks impacting midwifery including collaborative working relationships
+ critically analyse how redesigning maternity services to align with the evidence can improve maternal and infant outcomes.

Key terms and abbreviations

Australian College of Midwives (ACM)

Australian Health Practitioner Regulation Agency (AHPRA)

caesarean section (CS)

continuity of midwifery care (CoC)

endorsed midwife

International Confederation of Midwives (ICM)

Maternity Care Classification System (MaCCS)

Medicare Benefits Schedule (MBS)

midwifery group practice (MGP)

Nursing and Midwifery Board of Australia (NMBA)

Pharmaceutical Benefits Scheme (PBS)

professional indemnity insurance (PII)

Quality Maternal and Newborn Care (QMNC)

woman-centred care

Introduction

Since 1989 there have been at least ten national and state reviews of maternity services (e.g. Commonwealth of Australia 2009; Ministerial Task Force on Obstetric Services in New South Wales 1989; Senate Community Affairs Committee 1999). Maternity consumer activism has been a powerful influence in calls for change. Each review has consistently recommended demedicalising birth, changing to a social model of health and making better use of midwives' skills by freeing the midwife to work to their full scope of practice. These recommendations are consistent with international and global recommendations for maternity services globally. At the highest levels of global health policy (e.g. World Health Organization (WHO), International Confederation of Midwives (ICM), United Nations Children's Fund (UNICEF)), there is a shared understanding that the world needs more midwives and for them work to their full scope of practice, to advance the health of childbearing women and babies, achieve universal health coverage and prevent avoidable death and morbidity.

This chapter will discuss the impact of maternity services reform on midwifery, identify key quality and safety issues and frameworks, and explore how midwives work collaboratively. A case study will provide a 'real-life' example of maternity service redesign to reflect the evidence and promote **woman-centred care**.

Maternity services in Australia

In 2016 there were 310,247 births (Australian Institute of Health and Welfare (AIHW) 2018). Overall, Australia is one of the safest countries to give birth for mothers and babies. The maternal death ratio for 2012–14 was 6.8 per 100,000 women giving birth (AIHW 2017) and the perinatal death rate was 9 per 1000 births in 2016 (AIHW 2018). However, disparity in outcomes exists, with First Peoples mothers and babies experiencing poorer outcomes. The majority of women gave birth in hospitals (97%), with some women birthing in birth centres (1.8%) and a few at home (0.3%) (AIHW 2018). Women can access public maternity care, which is free at point of service, or use private-sector maternity care with a private (self-employed) midwife or doctor (usually an obstetrician). About 26% of women use private-sector care, mostly that of a private doctor (AIHW 2018). Out-of-pocket costs for women using private obstetric services have increased and in 2018 there was a 12% decline in women using the private sector (LaFrenz 2018). There has been a rapid decline in women using the private obstetric sector since 2010.

In addition to costs, there are other differences between private and publicly funded hospital-based maternity care. For example, in 2016, the **caesarean section (CS)** rate was 34%, an increase of 3% points in a decade (from 31% in 2006) and an 11% point increase since 2000 (AIHW 2018). The CS rate is consistently much higher in women who are cared for by private obstetricians and use private hospitals (46%) than in women accessing public hospitals (30%) (AIHW 2018). This high rate of CS is well above the WHO recommended rate of 10%–15%. As the graph in Fig. 22.1 shows, the increase in CS is not associated with an improvement in perinatal mortality. Similarly, many other medical interventions in birth are overused (relative to the evidence) – such as induction of labour and electronic fetal monitoring (Miller et al. 2016).

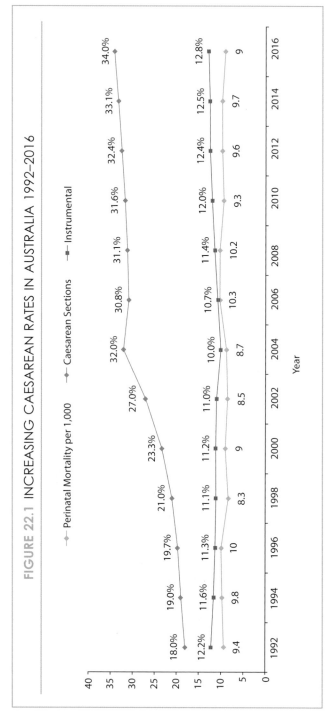

FIGURE 22.1 INCREASING CAESAREAN RATES IN AUSTRALIA 1992–2016

Source: Australian Institute of Health and Welfare (2018). Australia's mothers and babies 2016 – in brief. Perinatal statistics series no. 34. Cat. no. PER 97. AIHW, Canberra.

With a focus on pathology resulting from the dominance of the medical model of care, the ability of the health system to respond effectively to emerging population health issues such as rising rates of obesity and mental health issues is hampered (WHO 2017). Furthermore, the key role of maternity services in preventative health care is not being enacted through a social model of primary care. The following section describes models of maternity care in Australia and roles of key health professionals within them. The extent to which women 'know' and trust their care provider varies.

Models of maternity care

Maternity care is provided in a variety of settings, including at home, in community clinics, standalone birth centres, in birth centres attached to hospitals and in hospitals. There are different ways of organising maternity care services. This is referred to as 'models of care'. There are four main models of care in Australia. These main models are described here; however, a more detailed description of maternity care models has been developed and documented using the **Maternity Care Classification System (MaCCS)** (AIHW 2016).

- General practitioner (GP) shared care is where the GP provides the pregnancy care, and the labour and birth care is provided by hospital midwives and doctors. Sometimes the GP may also oversee labour care and be present for the birth. This model is more prevalent in rural areas. The GP remains in contact with the mother and baby, providing care for the family after birth and following discharge from hospital.

- Obstetric-led care is often referred to as a medical model of care. In this model, an obstetrician (i.e. a doctor who specialises in pregnancy and birth) provides or oversees pregnancy care. Labour is monitored by midwives, with the obstetrician usually attending the birth itself. There might be a 3- to 5-day hospital stay and very limited care following discharge from hospital.

- Hospital or clinic care involves attending a hospital or clinic for all care during pregnancy and birth, and seeing a wide variety of doctors and midwives – usually whoever is on duty that day. There is often a short hospital stay and sometimes a few home visits after the birth.

- Continuity of midwifery care (CoC) involves care from a known midwife. It is often referred to as **midwifery group practice (MGP)**. Women have the same midwife caring for them throughout pregnancy, labour and birth, and following birth, with the midwife involving other care providers if they are needed. This model of care is often extended for up to 6 weeks after the birth. Continuity of midwifery care reflects a social model of health based on a primary health care framework. A central feature is development of a trusting, supportive, long-term relationship between the midwife and a woman.

There is compelling evidence demonstrating that continuity of midwifery care produces significant physical benefits for mothers and babies, with no identified adverse effects compared with other models of maternity care (Sandall et al. 2016). In a systematic review of 461 studies 'midwifery was associated with improved efficient use of resources and outcomes when provided by midwives who were educated, trained, licensed, and regulated, with midwives being the most effective maternity carers when integrated into the health system' (Renfrew et al. 2014a, p. 1130). Reported outcomes from midwifery care include reduced maternal and neonatal mortality and fetal loss, reduced maternal and neonatal morbidity including preterm birth, reduced use of interventions, improved psychosocial outcomes, improved public health outcomes and improved organisational outcomes (Renfrew et al. 2014a, p. 1133). Furthermore, a systematic review and meta-analysis of more than 17,000 women (15 randomised controlled trials) demonstrated that women who received continuity of midwifery care (caseload midwifery) across pregnancy, labour and birth and postpartum were less likely to experience preterm births, to miscarry before 24 weeks or lose their fetuses after 24 weeks of pregnancy. Additionally, women were more likely to be satisfied with their birth in a continuity of midwifery care model compared with other models of maternity care (Sandall et al. 2016).

Continuity of midwifery care is good for midwives too. Studies in Australia and New Zealand showed that midwives providing continuity of care to a caseload of women had better emotional health and less burnout than midwives working in fragmented models of care (Dixon et al. 2017; Fenwick et al. 2018).

Importantly, continuity midwifery of care models costs less than standard, fragmented care (Donnellan-Fernandez, 2016; O'Brien et al. 2010; Toohill et al. 2012). The structures and processes used to design and provide maternity services are in need of reform. Change is necessary to enable the widespread implementation of evidence-based models of maternity care, consistently provide woman-centred care and maximise the role of the midwife.

PAUSE *for* REFLECTION ...

Key evidence of what works

We know that, compared with routine care, caseload midwifery produces improved clinical outcomes for women and babies, cost savings for the health system and high maternal satisfaction with care. However, only approximately 8% of Australian women are provided with caseload midwifery. What factors hinder the roll-out of caseload midwifery? What needs to change to enable universal access for women to caseload midwifery care?

The midwife

In Australia, midwifery is recognised legally as a profession and regulated by the **Australian Health Practitioner Regulation Agency (AHPRA)** through the **Nursing and Midwifery Board of Australia (NMBA)**. Midwives make up 4.9% of all registered health practitioners in Australia (Australian Health Practitioner Regulation Agency (AHPRA) 2017). As of 2018, there were 33,552 registered midwives and 98.3% were women (Nursing and Midwifery Board of Australia (NMBA) 2018a). The legal scope of practice of the midwife in Australia is consistent with the international definition of the midwife. The **International Confederation of Midwives (ICM)** (2017, n.p.) definition of the midwife states:

> A midwife is a person who has successfully completed a midwifery education programme that is based on the ICM Essential Competencies for Basic Midwifery Practice and the framework of the

ICM Global Standards for Midwifery Education and is recognized in the country where it is located; who has acquired the requisite qualifications to be registered and / or legally licensed to practise midwifery and use the title 'midwife'; and who demonstrates competency in the practice of midwifery.

Scope of Practice

The midwife is recognised as a responsible and accountable professional who works in partnership with women to give the necessary support, care and advice during pregnancy, labour and the postpartum period, to conduct births on the midwife's own responsibility and to provide care for the newborn and the infant. This care includes preventative measures, the promotion of normal birth, the detection of complications in mother and child, the accessing of medical care or other appropriate assistance and the carrying out of emergency measures.

The midwife has an important task in health counselling and education, not only for the woman, but also within the family and the community. This work should involve antenatal education and preparation for parenthood and may extend to women's health, sexual or reproductive health and child care. A midwife may practise in any setting including the home, community, hospitals, clinics or health units.

Frameworks for midwifery practice

As a regulated profession, various frameworks guide midwifery practice, including the ethical and legal boundaries of the work of a midwife, and scope of practice. The key frameworks applicable in Australia and the impact of these on midwifery practice are discussed in this section.

Nursing and Midwifery Board of Australia: registration

Midwives must be registered with the NMBA and meet its professional standards in order to practise in Australia. To remain registered, all midwives must undertake 20 hours of continuing professional development per year relevant to the midwife's context of practice. Professional standards and codes (NMBA 2018b) define the practice and behaviour of midwives and include:

◆ *Code of conduct for midwives*
◆ *Midwife standards for practice*, and
◆ *Code of ethics for midwives*.

The ICM *Code of ethics for midwives* (2008) is applicable to all midwives in Australia. The *Code of ethics* speaks to partnership with women, rights-based care and obligations to address inequity.

Nursing and Midwifery Board of Australia: endorsement

In addition to registration for midwives, NMBA has established pathways for midwives to apply for endorsement to prescribe scheduled medicines. An endorsed midwife can prescribe scheduled medications on the Pharmaceutical Benefits Scheme (PBS)-approved list for prescription by a midwife and order diagnostic and screening tests. The NMBA provides a formulary of scheduled medications and additional medications not on the PBS that endorsed midwives can prescribe. Midwives seeking endorsement are required to provide evidence of:

♦ registration as a midwife that is the equivalent of 3 years' full-time clinical practice (5000 hours) in the past 6 years (NMBA recognises three contexts of practice: antenatal, postnatal, or ante- and postnatal)

♦ successful completion of an NMBA-approved program of study leading to endorsement for scheduled medicines.

> **PAUSE** *for* REFLECTION ... If the scope of practice for all midwives in Australia is consistent with the international definition of a midwife, what is the benefit of requiring the equivalence of 3-years full time practice prior to being eligible for endorsement? Are there better mechanisms for ensuring quality and safety than years of experience? What alternative criteria leading to endorsement for midwives would you suggest?

The Australian Nursing and Midwifery Accreditation Council accredits programs that lead to registration and endorsement for midwives. Many Australian universities offer accredited programs leading to registration as a midwife and several universities offer programs for midwives to become eligible to apply for endorsement to prescribe scheduled medicines. Over 33,000 midwives are registered with AHPRA, yet, as of March 2018, only 407 midwives were endorsed to prescribe scheduled medications (NMBA, 2018a). Many more midwives meet the criteria and are eligible to apply for endorsement. Despite this, midwives employed in the public sector by state and territory health departments are not yet able to prescribe medications even when they meet all the criteria for endorsement to prescribe. As a result, midwives are not utilised to their full scope of practice within public-sector maternity services.

Once endorsed, midwives can apply for access to the **Medicare Benefits Schedule (MBS)** enabling women to receive a rebate for the fees charged by a midwife. To be eligible to provide services and receive a Medicare provider number, a midwife is required to: be working in private practice (self-employed), have professional indemnity insurance and have collaborative arrangements in place with a specified medical practitioner (Department of Health 2013).

The criteria that a 'collaborative arrangement' be established between a midwife and a specified medical practitioner is fraught with difficulty. The collaborative arrangement that must provide for includes consultation with an obstetric specified medical practitioner, referral of a woman to a specified medical practitioner and transfer of the woman's care to an obstetric specified medical practitioner as clinically relevant to ensure safe, high-quality maternity care. However, there is no onus on the medical practitioner to enter a collaborative arrangement with a midwife and no incentive for the medical practitioner. This is a major barrier to the roll-out of private midwifery services.

The formation of the AHPRA in July 2010 through the *Health Practitioner Regulation National Law Act* enabled national registration of health professionals. The Act included the requirement for all health professionals to have **professional indemnity insurance (PII)**. Employed midwives are covered by their employing agency; however, PII is problematic for self-employed (private) midwives. There is only one choice of indemnity insurance for private midwives – a Commonwealth-supported scheme that covers pregnancy, labour and birth, and postnatal care (Department of Human Services 2018); however, it does 'not cover the planned delivery of babies in the home' (NMBA 2017a, p. 5).

Midwives must be endorsed to prescribe scheduled medicines to access the PII scheme. PII is not available for self-employed (private) midwives providing homebirth care and the requirement to hold PII for this activity is covered by a PII exemption to enable them to attend homebirths provided that they have secured insurance for antenatal and postnatal care (NMBA 2017a). This exemption has been extended until 2019 but has not yet been resolved (Australian College of Midwives (ACM) 2018). Consequently, women giving birth at home with a private midwife are the only health care consumers not able to access the PII of their registered health professional in cases of negligence. Even qualifying for the exemption is complex. Private midwives must meet certain requirements of the NMBA, gain consent of the woman to not have insurance for labour and birth, submit data about each woman's care to the state/territory perinatal data agency and be able to demonstrate they are working within the NMBA's *Safety and quality guidelines for privately practising midwives* (NMBA 2017b).

PAUSE *for* REFLECTION ⋯

There are many barriers to private midwifery practice in Australia.

- Midwives require the equivalence of 3-years full-time practice prior to being eligible for endorsement to prescribe medicines.
- The government-sponsored PII scheme has been made available to self-employed (private) midwives providing labour and birth care in hospitals and birth centres, yet homebirth has been excluded.
- The criteria for a 'collaborative arrangement' between a midwifery and a medical practitioner practising obstetrics is problematic, with no onus on a medical practitioner to participate.

Why do you think these multiple barriers exist and have not been resolved?

National midwifery guidelines for consultation and referral

The *National midwifery guidelines for consultation and referral* (3rd ed.) (ACM 2013) facilitate collaboration between midwives and doctors in the care of individual women through guidance about consultation and referral indications to support integrated maternity care. They were developed by the **Australian College of Midwives (ACM)** and are endorsed by the Royal Australian and New Zealand College of Obstetricians and Gynaecologists and state and territory governments.

The guidelines are used in most maternity services across Australia and are embedded in practice at every level. The guidelines are used extensively by privately practising midwives, as well as medical consultants at tertiary hospitals. The adoption of the guidelines by all institutions and midwives who offer pregnant women midwifery care will help to ensure maternity services provide high-quality, safe and collaborative care to women and their babies.

Midwifery practice decision flowchart

The scope of an individual midwife's practice is dynamic and relative to a range of factors including context. To assist midwives' decision-making about their scope of practice the NMBA developed a *Midwifery practice decision flowchart* (NMBA 2013). A midwife is guided through a series of decisions or considerations. The first consideration is to identify benefit to the woman and / or newborn of undertaking the activity / practice. Once the midwife works through the flowchart, a decision can be made as to whether the midwife is the appropriate caregiver or whether there must be consultation with and / or referral to other health professionals. The *National midwifery guidelines for consultation and referral* as described above assist midwives in working through the practice decision flowchart.

Reform of maternity services and impact on midwifery

At the beginning of this chapter the three decades of effort to reform maternity services were described. This section outlines progress towards reform of maternity services at national and international levels. It also provides a real-life case study to demonstrate the impact of reform on the midwifery profession and midwives' practice.

National strategic approach to maternity services

Following a national review of maternity services in 2009, the Commonwealth Government published the *National Maternity Services Plan* (the Plan) in 2010 (Commonwealth of Australia 2010). The plan was endorsed by state, territory and Commonwealth governments for the 5-year period 2010–15. Slow progress on implementing some of the recommended reforms led to an extension of the plan until 30 June 2016. This extension did little to advance widespread access to continuity of midwifery care models, or reduce health inequalities experienced by First Peoples mothers and babies.

In September 2017 the Australian Health Ministers Advisory Council (AHMAC) agreed to start a new process to develop a National Strategic Approach to Maternity Services (NSAMS). The expected outcome for the NSAMS project is a document to guide national maternity services policy.

Framework for quality maternal and newborn care – The Lancet

In 2014, The Lancet published a series of papers on midwifery. A summary of these papers by Renfrew et al. (2014b) provided an evidence-based framework for **Quality Maternal and Newborn Care (QMNC)**. This framework details how maternity services should be designed and implemented to enable universal provision of quality maternal and newborn health services. Its component parts include practice categories depicting the type of care provided, the organisation of care, the values underpinning services, the philosophical approach to care and guidance on how care providers should work. The QMNC framework is illustrated in Fig. 22.2. It identifies that all women need the

FIGURE 22.2 FRAMEWORK FOR QUALITY MATERNAL AND NEWBORN CARE

	For all childbearing women and infants			For childbearing women and infants with complications	
Practice categories	Education Information Health promotion*	Assessment Screening Care planning†	Promotion of normal processes, prevention of complications‡	First-line management of complications§	Medical obstetric neonatal services
Organisation of care	Available, accessible, acceptable, good-quality services—adequate resources, competent workforce Continuity, services integrated across community and facilities				
Values	Respect, communication, community knowledge, and understanding Care tailored to women's circumstances and needs				
Philosophy	Optimising biological, psychological, social, and cultural processes; strengthening woman's capabilities Expectant management, using interventions only when indicated				
Care providers	Practitioners who combine clinical knowledge and skills with interpersonal and cultural competence Division of roles and responsibilities based on need, competencies, and resources				

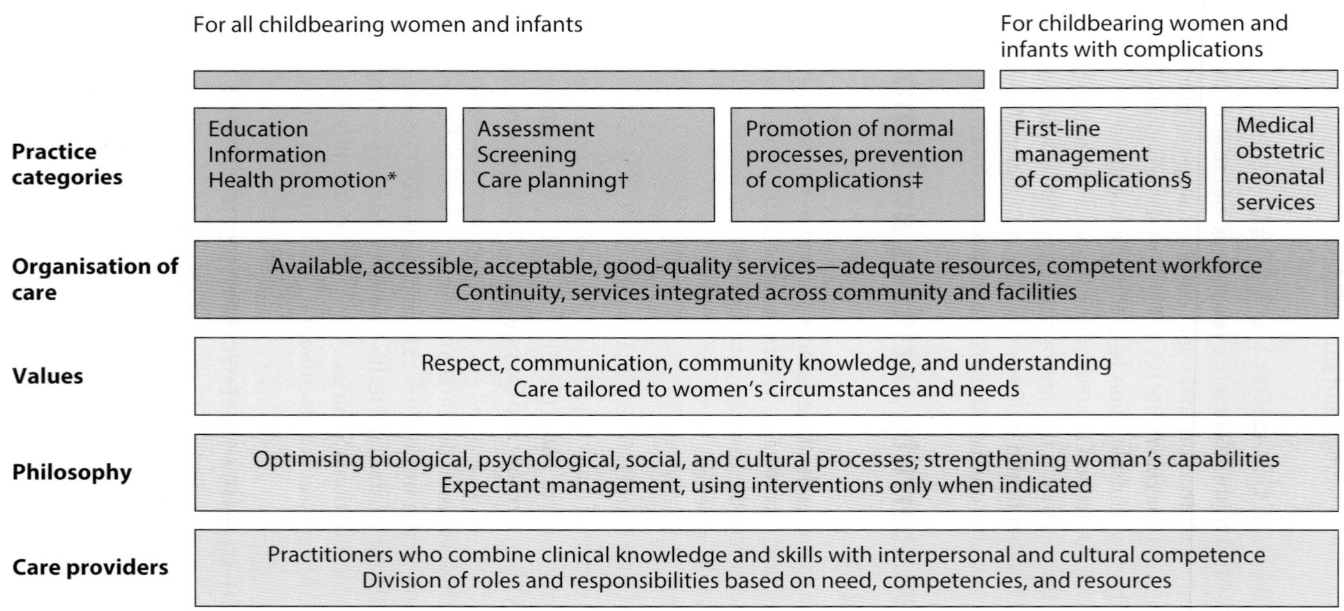

Source: Renfrew, M., McFadden, A., Bastos, M., Campbell, J., Channon, A., et al. (2014a). Midwifery and quality care: findings from a new evidence-informed framework for maternal and newborn care. Lancet, 384 (9948), 1129–1145

type of care provided by midwives: education, information, health promotion, assessment, screening, care planning, promotion of normal birth, prevention of complications and first-line management of complications, and that some women will need medical care and services of other health professionals.

Relationships and role clarity are the key to improving outcomes in every aspect of maternity care. Where care providers work together and create and sustain relationships based on trust and respect, everybody has a more satisfying experience and outcomes are improved. Relationships matter, at every level of care: women to midwife, midwife to midwife, and midwife to obstetrician and to other service providers within the hospital and community.

The 'integrality' model graphically represents woman-centred care and the organisation of health care providers and services around the woman and her baby (see Fig. 22.3). The services accessed by pregnant women and new mothers are diverse, highlighting the need for all services to be woman centred.

FIGURE 22.3 INTEGRALITY MODEL

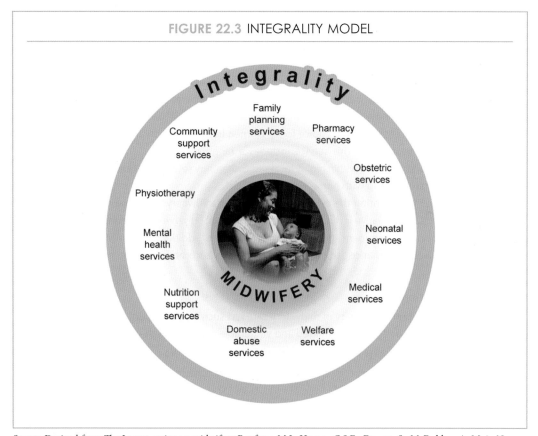

Source: Derived from The Lancet series on midwifery Renfrew, M.J., Homer, C.S.E., Downe, S., McFadden, A. Muir, N., et al. (2014b). Midwifery: an executive summary for The Lancet's series. Lancet 388, 1–8

Changing the system

Case study 22.1 in this section provides an example of changes that are occurring to implement evidence-based models of maternity care. The case study is about the development and implementation of community maternal and child health hubs, which were designed to reach socially disadvantaged and vulnerable women in need of a range of support services in addition to maternity care.

Case Study 22.1

Changing the system – community maternal and child health hubs

The Logan area in south-east Queensland has poorer birth outcomes than the rest of Queensland and Australia. Two key indicators demonstrate (1) a higher incidence of low-weight babies (over 9% compared with a 6.6% state average) and an increased number of preterm babies (over 15% in pockets of Logan compared with a 9.3% state average); and (2) higher incidence of babies admitted to special care nurseries – in some areas over 20% compared with a 17.9% state average (Logan Together 2018). These poor birth outcomes are associated with a lack of appropriate, accessible maternity services and support. Approximately 1 in 10 women have little or no contact with services during their pregnancy – about double the average for Queensland.

Partnership between service providers, community members and government representatives resulted in a co-design process, involving research, consultation, deliberation and negotiation to develop an evidence-informed, community-embedded, relationship-based, caseload midwifery model of care designed to improve access, care and choice for all women from early in pregnancy through birth to the end of the first year of life. This service includes a range of antenatal, intrapartum and post birth/transition support services within highly localised community settings that are currently accessed by parents in the target group with home visits as required.

In addition to implementing the evidence that caseload midwifery care improves outcomes for mothers and babies, this initiative includes three unique features: (1) services embedded in community settings are run by non-government agencies and offer a range of additional health and social services, (2) there is a shared governance structure, and (3) there is a community (not hospital) building component.

Case study questions

1. Why do you think continuity of midwifery care has such a strong positive effect on outcomes for socially disadvantaged and vulnerable women and their newborns?
2. What needs to change to enable universal access for women to caseload midwifery care?

The future

There are many challenges in the provision of quality maternity services in Australia. Challenges include high rates of medical intervention during pregnancy and birth, poorer health outcomes for First Peoples women and babies, poor access for women living in rural and remote areas and socially disadvantaged and vulnerable women, health service cultural issues, and structural funding and policy issues that limit the potential contribution of midwives to the wellbeing of childbearing women and families.

There is significant need to expand continuity of midwifery care and deliver better-integrated services in line with the evidence. Structural reforms to funding health and hospital services and funding of health providers through MBS will be needed to make continuity of midwifery care universally available. Freedom to practise to the full scope for midwives through cultural change within the health system is also required.

Pressure for change continues to build. Maternity consumer activism has been key, as has the activity of midwives. Increasingly there is multidisciplinary support for change and it is being reflected in health service policy at all levels.

Summary

This chapter has provided a snapshot of midwifery in Australia. The following key points illustrated the current and emerging position of midwifery in Australia:

- There is considerable evidence and consumer lobbying for maternity services to change to better meet the needs of women and families and to enable midwives to work to their full scope of practice.
- Midwifery is recognised legally as a profession separate from nursing; however, culture change within health services is still required to enable full utilisation of midwives as primary care providers for childbearing women and families.
- Even though the *National Maternity Services Plan* (2010) did not fully deliver the recommended changes, it did establish the agenda for change and momentum is building. The changes see a greater role for midwives.
- In keeping with the evidence-based framework for QMNC, every pregnant woman needs a midwife and some women need other services and health providers; however, this approach to design and delivery of maternity services is yet to be universally applied.
- Disparity in maternal and newborn outcomes between First Peoples and other Australians remains, and must be addressed through growing the First Peoples midwifery workforce and redesigning services.

Review Questions

1. Describe the models of maternity care and variation in the scope of practice of the midwife and interprofessional practice in each model.
2. Ask women to describe the role of the midwife and compare descriptions with the information provided in this chapter.

3 Describe how you would design a maternity service for women less than 20 years old using the framework for QMNC.

4 To what extent is women's access to continuity of midwifery care a feminist issue?

5 Using the guidelines by Bacchi (2012) what is your critique of current policies governing the delivery of woman-centred maternity care in Australia.

References

Australian College of Midwives (ACM), 2013. National Midwifery Guidelines for Consultation and Referral, issue 2, third ed. https://www.midwives.org.au/shop/national-midwifery-guidelines-consultation-and-referral-3rd-edition-issue-2-book.

Australian College of Midwives (ACM), 2018. Midwives and insurance. https://www.midwives.org.au/midwives-insurance.

Australian Health Practitioner Regulatory Authority, 2017. Annual report 2016/17. https://www.ahpra.gov.au/annualreport/2017/downloads.html.

Australian Institute of Health and Welfare, 2016. Maternity Care Classification System: maternity model of care data set specification. AIHW, Canberra.

Australian Institute of Health and Welfare, 2017. Maternal deaths in Australia 2012–2014. Cat. no. PER 92. AIHW, Canberra.

Australian Institute of Health and Welfare, 2018. Australia's mothers and babies 2016 – in brief. Perinatal statistics series no. 34. Cat. no. PER 97. AIHW, Canberra.

Bacchi, C., 2012. Introducing the 'What's the problem represented to be?' approach. In: Bletsas, A., Beasley, C. (Eds.), Engaging With Carol Bacchi: Strategic Interventions and Exchanges. University of Adelaide Press, Adelaide. https://www.adelaide.edu.au/carst/docs/wpr/wpr-summary.pdf.

Commonwealth of Australia, 2009. Improving maternity services in Australia: the report of the Maternity Services Review. Commonwealth of Australia, Canberra.

Commonwealth of Australia, 2010. National Maternity Services Plan. Commonwealth of Australia, Canberra.

Department of Health, 2013. Eligible midwives questions and answers. Commonwealth of Australia, Canberra. http://www.health.gov.au/internet/main/publishing.nsf/content/midwives-nurse-pract-qanda.

Department of Human Services, 2018. Midwife professional indemnity scheme. Commonwealth of Australia, Canberra. https://www.humanservices.gov.au/organisations/health-professionals/services/medicare/midwife-professional-indemnity-scheme.

Dixon, L., Guilliland, K., Pallant, J., et al., 2017. The emotional wellbeing of New Zealand midwives: comparing responses for midwives in caseloading and shift work settings. N. Z. Coll. Midwives J. 53, 5–14. doi:10.12784/nzcomjnl53.2017.1.5-14.

Donnellan-Fernandez, R.E. (2016). Proceed with caution – the strength and weakness in reported cost data in South Australia. Invited presentation for Enhancing performance and cost effectiveness in maternity and women's healthcare, Women's Healthcare Australasia. Women's Healthcare Australasia Annual Benchmarking Meeting, Northside Conference Centre, Sydney, NSW, 16 May.

Fenwick, J., Sidebotham, M., Gamble, J., et al., 2018. The emotional and professional wellbeing of Australian midwives: a comparison between those providing continuity of midwifery care and those not providing continuity. Women Birth 31 (1), 8–43. doi:10.1016/j.wombi.2017.06.013.

Health Practitioner Regulation National Law (SA) 2010. www.governmentgazette.sa.gov.au/2014/august/2014_060.pdf.

International Confederation of Midwives (ICM), 2008. Code of ethics for midwives. https://www.internationalmidwives.org/our-work/policy-and-practice/international-code-of-ethics-for-midwives.html.

International Confederation of Midwives. (ICM), 2017. English definition of the midwife. https://www.internationalmidwives.org/assets/files/definitions-files/2018/06/eng-definition_of_the_midwife-2017.pdf.

LaFrenz, C., 2018. Ramsay Health Care hurt by slump in maternity, rehab bookings, Australian Financial Review, 21 June. https://www.afr.com/business/health/hospitals-and-gps/ramsay-health-care-hurt-by-slump-in-maternity-rehab-bookings-20180621-h11opg.

Logan Together, 2018. The state of Logan's children and families: summary and update. Volume 3. Logan Together, Brisbane.

Miller, S., Abalos, E., Chamillard, M., et al., 2016. Beyond too little, too late and too much, too soon: a pathway towards evidence-based, respectful maternity care worldwide. Lancet 388 (10056), 2176–2192.

Ministerial Task Force on Obstetric Services in New South Wales, 1989. The Shearman report. Department of Health, Commonwealth of Australia, Sydney.

Nursing and Midwifery Board of Australia (NMBA), 2013. Midwifery practice decision flowchart. http://www.nursingmidwiferyboard.gov.au/Codes-Guidelines-Statements/Frameworks.aspx.

Nursing and Midwifery Board of Australia (NMBA), 2017a. Professional indemnity insurance arrangements for nurses and midwives, Appendix 1. www.nursingmidwiferyboard.gov.au/Codes-Guidelines-Statements/FAQ/Fact-sheet-PII.aspx.

Nursing and Midwifery Board of Australia (NMBA), 2017b. Safety and quality guidelines for privately practising midwives. http://www.nursingmidwiferyboard.gov.au/Codes-Guidelines-Statements/Codes-Guidelines.aspx.

Nursing and Midwifery Board of Australia (NMBA), 2018a. Registrant data. Reporting period: 1 January 2018–31 March 2018. https://www.nursingmidwiferyboard.gov.au/about/statistics.aspx.

Nursing and Midwifery Board of Australia (NMBA), 2018b. Professional codes and guidelines. https://www.nursingmidwiferyboard.gov.au/Codes-Guidelines-Statements/Professional-standards.aspx.

Renfrew, M., McFadden, A., Bastos, M., et al., 2014a. Midwifery and quality care: findings from a new evidence-informed framework for maternal and newborn care. Lancet 384 (9948), 1129–1145. doi:10.1016/S0140-6736(14)60789-3.

Renfrew, M.J., Homer, C.S.E., Downe, S., et al., 2014b. Midwifery: an executive summary for *The Lancet*'s series. Lancet 388, 1–8.

O'Brien, B., Harvey, S., Sommerfeldt, S., et al., 2010. Comparison of costs and associated outcomes between women choosing newly integrated autonomous midwifery care and matched controls: a pilot study. J. Obstet. Gynaecol. Can. 32 (7), 650–656.

Sandall, J., Soltani, H., Gates, S., et al., 2016. Midwife-led continuity models versus other models of care for childbearing women. Cochrane Database Syst. Rev. (4), CD004667, doi:10.1002/14651858.CD004667. pub5.

Senate Community Affairs Reference Committee, 1999. Rocking the cradle: a report into childbirth procedures. December. Commonwealth of Australia, Canberra. http://www.aph.gov.au/senate.

Toohill, J., Turkstra, E., Gamble, J., et al., 2012. A non-randomised trial investigating the cost-effectiveness of midwifery group practice compared with standard maternity care arrangements in one Australian hospital. Midwifery 28 (6), E874–E879. doi:10.1016/j.midw.2011.10.012.

World Health Organization (WHO), 2017. Depression and Other Common Mental Disorders: Global Health Estimate. WHO, Geneva.

Further Reading

Kildea, S., Lockey, R., Roberts, J., et al. (2016). Guiding Principles for Developing a Birthing on Country Service Model and Evaluation Framework, Phase 1. Mater Medical Research Unit and University of Queensland, Brisbane.

Miller, S., Abalos, E., Chamillard, M., et al., 2016. Beyond too little, too late and too much, too soon: a pathway towards evidence-based, respectful maternity care worldwide. Lancet 388 (10056), 2176–2192.

Renfrew, M., McFadden, A., Bastos, M., et al., 2014. Midwifery and quality care: findings from a new evidence-informed framework for maternal and newborn care. Lancet 384 (9948), 1129–1145.

Sandall, J., Soltani, H., Gates, S., et al., 2016. Midwife-led continuity models versus other models of care for childbearing women. Cochrane Database Syst. Rev. (4), CD004667, doi:10.1002/14651858.CD004667. pub5.

Online Resources

Australian College of Midwives – professional issues and news for midwives: www.midwives.org.au.

Australian Health Practitioners Regulation Agency – information on the regulation of midwifery: www.ahpra.gov.au.

Australian Institute of Health and Welfare (AIHW) *Australia's mothers and babies* reports: https://www.aihw.gov.au/reports-statistics/population-groups/mothers-babies/overview.

Australian Nursing and Midwifery Accreditation Council: www.anmac.org.au.

Nursing and Midwifery Board of Australia: www.nursingmidwiferyboard.gov.au.

CHAPTER 23

Advancing nursing in the Australian health care system

Trudy Rudge and Luisa Toffoli

Key learning outcomes

When you finish this chapter you should be able to:

+ demonstrate an understanding of where nursing fits in the health professional workforce
+ demonstrate an understanding of the scope of practice and roles of registered and enrolled nurses, advanced care nurses and nurse practitioners
+ identify how scope of practice varies according to context of care and level of nurse
+ identify different nursing responses to the development of IPP/IPE in models of care in different settings such as aged care, primary health care, mental health nursing and nurse practitioner practice.

Key terms and abbreviations

Australian Health Practitioner Regulation Agency (AHPRA)
Australian Nursing and Midwifery Accreditation Council (ANMAC)
enrolled nurse (EN)
International Council of Nurses (ICN)
interprofessional education (IPE)
interprofessional practice (IPP)
Medicare Benefits Schedule (MBS)
National Law
Nursing and Midwifery Board of Australia (NMBA)
nurse practitioners (NPs)
Pharmaceutical Benefits Scheme (PBS)
practice nurse
residential aged-care facilities (RACFs)
registered nurse (RN)
unlicensed health care worker

Introduction

Nursing has a long history of co-development alongside changes in health care, from its earliest role in nursing by religious women and men, through developments of hospitals, asylums and hospices in the 19th century, to the provision of health care in the community. From development of a 'professional' caring under women such as Florence Nightingale (Nelson & Rafferty 2010) to the development of educational programs in hospitals and in universities, nursing has worked to have its discipline (knowledge system), practice and work recognised on its own professional footing (see International Council of Nursing (ICN) 2019; Meleis 2016; Nelson & Gordon 2006). To accomplish such a footing, nursing has pre-eminently used self-regulation and codes of conduct and registration to bring its recognition as a profession and discipline (Freidson 2001).

Worldwide legislation exists to protect the title of 'nurse'. Here in Australia the nursing workforce is regulated by a series of Acts of Parliament at a national, state and territory level which support the functions of the **Nursing and Midwifery Board of Australia (NMBA)**. The NMBA is responsible for registering nurses and midwives, monitoring of nurse education through the accreditation of programs and institutions that provide such education (Australian Nursing and Midwifery Accreditation Council (ANMAC)), assessment of competencies of overseas-trained nurses to obtain their registration, development of standards of practice and codes of conduct as well as policies that deal with maintenance of registration and the endorsement of **nurse practitioners (NPs)**. Registering authorities are enacted by legislation to adjudicate cases of unsafe practice or unprofessional conduct brought before the Boards.

The chapter will discuss how the nursing discipline and workforce have undergone changes in the last decades, with a focus on scope of practice, changes in advanced practice and workforce as well as the effects of **interprofessional practice (IPP)** and **interprofessional education (IPE)** on nursing. The changing policy environment in health care will be explored for how problems are defined for nursing and its development.

The nursing workforce in Australia

Nursing is a self-regulating profession with a guaranteed level of education and practice, where to use the title 'nurse' a person must be registered or enrolled under the *Health Practitioner Regulation National Law Act 2009*, hereafter referred to as the **National Law** (Commonwealth of Australia 2009), that is in force in each state and territory. In this section, we discuss the workforce, its constituent characteristics and how descriptions of the workforce relate to policy concerns about nursing and accessibility of health care in the geographical complexities of Australia (see also Chapter 17).

The nursing workforce makes up the largest proportion of workers in the health care industry. The workforce is distributed across the states and territories of Australia (NMBA 2018a; see Table 23.1 registrant data), the distribution being largely in line with the population in each state or territory, and depending on the density of population in regional and remote Australia. The workforce is recognised as dominantly female, with the total registrations of female gender registrants at 89% and male registrants at 11%. This statistic has remained over time, despite recruitment programs for males and assumptions that more men would be recruited after the move into tertiary education occurring in the 1980s.

Previous workforce data collection focused on the number of nurses and shortages. However, currently how data are reported suggests that the ageing workforce (Australian Government 2019) and shortages in specific locations such as the state of NSW dominate (ABC 2018). The age of RNs, according to the NMBA (2018a) report for registrants in June 2018, is shown in Fig. 23.1. There is a reduction in the workforce of people in their 30s, then an increase in the 40s age group. However, numbers do not return to their former levels. This tallies with the movement out of the nursing

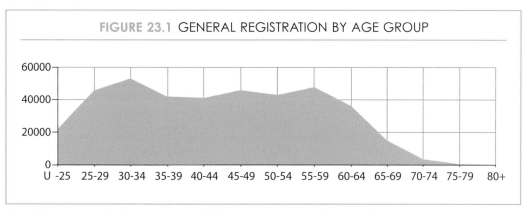

FIGURE 23.1 GENERAL REGISTRATION BY AGE GROUP

(Note: This graph includes <u>all</u> registrants with NMBA, without separation of midwives.)

Source: NMBA (2018a). Nursing and Midwifery Board of Australia: registrant data (reporting period: 1 April 2018–30 June 2018), p. 11. https://www.nursingmidwiferyboard.gov.au/documents/default.aspx?record=WD18%2f26398&dbid=AP&chksum=qNWDOD2t5jceAnYCnCrL1A%3d%3d

TABLE 23.1 GENERAL REGISTRATION BY PLACE OF PRACTICE (RNS, ENS and RNS / MW)[a]

	ACT	NSW	NT	Qld	SA	Tas	Vic	WA	No PPP[c]	Total
EN	708	13,833	429	13,515	7933	1589	20,966	5533	124	64,630
RN	4980	83,585	3526	58,211	22,335	7080	72,974	29,552	9821	292,064
EN and RN	88	1432	64	1645	826	81	2999	730	33	7898
Nurse / midwife[b]	508	7732	491	5730	1873	629	7499	2839	307	27,608

Notes

[a]Modified table from p. 6 of NMBA (2018a) – registered midwives only removed.

[b]Practitioners with a nurse and midwife qualification may hold registration as an EN and midwife, RN and midwife or EN and RN and midwife (see chapter text for discussion).

[c]No PPP means that survey respondent did not record working in Australia, or no permanent place of residence in Australia.

Source: NMBA (2018a). Nursing and Midwifery Board of Australia: registrant data (reporting period: 1 April 2018–30 June 2018). https://www.nursingmidwiferyboard.gov.au/documents/default.aspx?record=WD18%2f26398&dbid=AP&chksum=qNWDOD2t5jceAnYCnCrL1A%3d%3d

TABLE 23.2 NURSE WORKFORCE: REGISTERED IN AUSTRALIA – 2016 BY MODIFIED MONASH MODEL (MMM)

MMM[a]	Head count	Total FTE[a]	Av. age	Av. total hours
MMM 1	227,568	200,544	43.5	33.5
MMM2	30,929	27,250	44.8	33.5
MMM3	24,916	21,743	46.2	33.2
MMM4	11,802	10,049	47.5	32.4
MMM5	13,628	11,404	48.9	31.8
MMM6	3857	3734	45	36.8
MMM7	2400	2520	47.8	39.9
TOTAL	315,100	277,244	44.3	33.4

[a]MMM is a measure of geographical remoteness developed by McGrail & Humphries (2009) that discriminates the levels of access to medical care. This measure is usually about access to GPs in Australia. In 2016, the distribution of the nurse workforce was estimated using this geographical measure (Department of Health 2016).

Source: Department of Health (2016) Health workforce summaries – nursing. https://www.health.gov.au/internet/main/publishing. nsf/Content/health_workforce_data.

workforce during what are now reproductive years for women in Australia, and movement into other forms of employment.

The nursing workforce data provided by government (Department of Health 2016) concentrates on accessibility to health facilities and health professionals (particularly in regional and remote Australia (Table 23.2). (NB: This collection is available for 2016 only.) Table 23.2 shows that most nurses are in the MMM1 measure (following McGrail & Humphries 2009), where the measure (Modified Monash Model (MMM)) uses census data to classify remoteness.

The ABS has now updated their remoteness classification system to the Australian Statistical Geography Standard – Remoteness Areas (ASGS-RA), which uses the latest residential population data from the 2011 census to determine the five remoteness categories. The MMM uses the ASGS-RA as a base, and further differentiates areas in inner and outer regional Australia based on local town size (see http://www.doctorconnect.gov.au/internet/otd/publishing.nsf/Content/Classification-changes).

Location in MMM1 is to be expected and is in line with hospitals, public and private, being the majority employer of nurses on graduation. The measure MMM2 relates to cities in smaller states, as well as regional cities with larger hospitals. The most remote measure is MMM7, where nurses might be in remote West Australian community settings or in Central Australia with Aboriginal and Torres Strait Islander (ATSI) community health centres.

However, such a view of the distribution of nurses fails to take account of variations in specialisations, the variability of nursing employment over periods of budgetary constraint and how scope of practice of nurses makes a difference to quality and patient outcomes.

To get past this reliance on a rather narrow view of nursing, how to measure scope of practice is a 'problem' (see Bacchi 2012) that requires us to work out where nurses and nursing sit exactly in the health care system with certainty about what a nurse's scope of practice 'is' (Birks 2016). Scope of practice matters because, as Bender et al. (2018, p. 653) assert, nursing is 'the largest sector of the healthcare workforce … this provides a powerful incentive to fully leverage nursing scope of practice – the roles, responsibilities and functions that nurses are educated, competent and licensed to perform – into care models that … meet quality mandates'. Such an argument suggests how important using the nursing workforce to its maximum potential is an investment of economic import. In the following sections we explore scope of practice, and how the idea of scope of practice has been mobilised to deal with the complexities and changing dynamics of the Australian health care system.

The problem of scope of practice

We begin with a definition of nursing from international peak body for the nursing profession, the **International Council of Nursing (ICN)** (2019):

> Nursing encompasses autonomous and collaborative care of individuals of all ages, families, groups and communities, sick or well and in all settings. Nursing includes the promotion of health, prevention of illness, and the care of ill, disabled and dying people. Advocacy, promotion of a safe environment, research, participation in shaping health policy and in patient and health systems management, and education are also key nursing roles.

In Australia the nursing workforce is divided into three levels – that is, **registered nurses** and **enrolled nurses** based on their level of functioning, and **nurse practitioners** who have advanced certification with the NMBA (NMBA 2016a, 2016b, 2016c). This categorisation differentiates the nursing workforce according to their **scope of practice** and takes into account nurses' educational preparation, role activities and professional accountability as defined by legislation. Registered general nurses, midwives, nurse practitioners and enrolled nurses are identified on the register with the NMBA – the National Law – (Commonwealth of Australia 2009). There is supporting legislation with the states of New South Wales (NSW) and Queensland (Qld) (see NMBA 2018b, p. 3).

Nurses have an annual practising certificate where they guarantee safe and competent practice in the area in which they practise, with the understanding that each nurse practises within their scope, is of sound health and that they are of good character (e.g. they have not committed a criminal offence in the previous year, or they have not had limits put on their practice), and that they have undertaken the required mandatory hours of education or continuing professional education as set (NMBA 2016d, 2018b, 2018c). A recent change to this mandated education is that all RNs have to undertake cultural safety education to guarantee safe care to ATSI people in their care or culturally safe relationships with their ATSI colleagues (NMBA, 2019).

The report of the registrants (AHPRA 2018) does not differentiate whether nurses are working in clinical practice, education, research or administrative positions, nor their specialty areas (e.g. mental health). Nurses' registration status and details are published and are available for searching on the public register of the **Australian Health Practitioner Regulation Agency (AHPRA)** website (http://www.ahpra.gov.au/Registration/Registers-of-Practitioners.aspx). Statements about nursing practice on this website have an emphasis on the regulation of nursing as a profession; however, if we turn to an employment website such as Job Outlook under the Australian Government (2019) website, a different picture of nursing emerges (see below).

Nurses as employees

A **registered nurse** is authorised to practise without supervision and is accountable and responsible for the provision of nursing care. The registered nurse is accountable for assessment of patients and decisions in relation to delegation and supervision of **enrolled nurses** and **unlicensed health care workers.** Enrolled nurses practise under the supervision (direct and indirect) of a registered nurse; they remain responsible for their actions and are accountable to the registered nurse for all delegated decisions and functions. A final group of health care workers provide personal care, primarily for the aged-care industry, although increasingly these workers form part of a team in tertiary care institutions. Unlicensed health care workers are also known as assistants in nursing or personal care workers. They are not regulated by the National Board and are not, therefore, legally entitled to use the title of 'nurse'.

On the Australian government's Job Outlook website (https://joboutlook.gov.au/), the nurse's tasks are detailed. This website is used for recruitment by those looking for employment, international students and nurses who are wishing to migrate. It provides information about registration as well as nursing tasks, nursing specialisations and so on. It lists the tasks outlined for nursing as follows.

- assessing, planning, implementing and evaluating nursing care for patients according to accepted nursing practice and standards
- working in consultation with other health professionals and members of health teams, and coordinating the care of patients
- providing interventions, treatments and therapies such as medications, and monitoring responses to treatment and care plan
- promoting health and assisting in preventing ill health by participating in health education and other health promotion activities
- answering questions and providing information to patients and families about treatment and care
- supervising and coordinating the work of enrolled nurses and other health care workers.

(https://joboutlook.gov.au/occupation.aspx?code=2544)

In this approach to nursing, tasks are the role. Under these tasks is a list of nursing 'job titles' that makes distinctions between a variety of specialisations (that are not noted on the NMBA website or APRHA). The title of 'registered nurse' is protected legally, yet this government department confuses the issues for those who are looking at employment, migration or role expectations (Gardner et al. 2007). RNs on this website are divided into designations such as aged care, child and family health, community health, critical care and emergency, disability and rehabilitation, medical, medical practice nurse and mental health or psychiatric nurse. These specialties are not how a nurse obtains registration – that occurs on completion of a Bachelor degree from a university that guarantees the person has undertaken the education accredited by the **Australian Nursing and Midwifery Accreditation Council (ANMAC)** (and if trained overseas the NMBA website provides details how to obtain Australian registration).

Moreover, the qualities that they present as necessary to have as nurses are from a site on nursing networks from the USA,[a] not by reference to the regulatory body (NMBA) – where an interested person would get the registration information they need to register to work as a nurse in Australia. In Table 23.3 is an outline of the differences between an RN, an advanced nurse (someone with a qualification or specialty in nursing) and a nurse practitioner, which illustrates how all of these different RN roles work together with different scopes of practice.

PAUSE
for
REFLECTION
...

Scope of practice and employment

Compare the description of what a RN does between the ICN (2019) definition of a nurse, which is the legally presented understanding about the protected title of nurse; and the Job Outlook approach. Also given that specialisation is not recognised, how does this confuse issues of scope of practice and decision-making as this relates to employment? We will return to this review when we look at a nurse practitioner's work and then how scope of practice matters for interprofessional practice.

TABLE 23.3 SCOPE OF PRACTICE: COMPARISON ACROSS NURSING ROLES

	Registered nurse	Advanced practice nurse	Nurse practitioner
Legislation	Title protected General nurse registration	Title not protected No specialist registration Credentialling	Title protected Endorsement under Section 95 of National Law
Nomenclature	Registered nurse	Variations, clinical nurse specialist, clinical nurse consultant, advanced practice nurse, nurse manager	Nurse practitioner

Continued

[a]US Department of Labor, Employment and Training Administration. The importance ratings on this page are derived from the US Department of Labor O*NET Database version 21.2 (cited on Job Outlook – nursing https://joboutlook.gov.au/occupation?code=2544).

	Registered nurse	Advanced practice nurse	Nurse practitioner
TABLE 23.3 SCOPE OF PRACTICE: COMPARISON ACROSS NURSING ROLES—cont'd			
Education	Bachelor of Nursing	Bachelor of Nursing; while not essential a postgraduate qualification in a clinical nursing specialty is recommended	Bachelor of Nursing; postgraduate qualification in clinical nursing specialty, and completion of approved Master's degree in Nurse Practitioner Studies
Clinical experience	Not specified, but graduate nurse program after graduation – either general of specialist experience	2–4 years post-registration experience (specialty education in some cases)	10–12 years post-registration
Scope of practice	Set by *Registered nurse standards for practice* (NMBA, 2016a). General and/or specialist clinical activities as required for direct patient care; administration of medications by all routes. May need credentialling by hospital or context of care; ongoing mandated professional education	Set by hospital or ANMF with a position statement, and a level of remuneration about grade for RN. Advanced clinical activities, management, supervision, consultation, education and research components increased. Limited initiation and supply of medications under protocol; ongoing mandated professional education	Set by *Nurse practitioner standards for practice* (NMBA, 2018c). Advanced nursing practice in an area of clinical nursing specialty or therapy, plus expanded clinical activities that include advanced patient assessment; ordering and interpretation of diagnostic investigations and pathology; medications as per set by certification (state/territory variations). Mandated continuing education. Certification as per NMBA audit

Source: Adapted from NMBA (2016a, 2016c, 2016d, 2018b, 2018c); Parry & Grant (2016)

Nurse practitioner: a solution to deficits in health care access?

The nurse practitioner role has a 50-year history in the USA and was developed as a response to the numbers of people who were under-served in the country. Such problems emanate from lack of access to health care for those who were not working so were uninsured, not covered by government programs such as Medicare and Medicaid or unable to afford health care – hence the term 'under-served'. To provide health care to the under-served, nurses set up clinics for such populations and moved to have this practice recognised and regulated as an advanced form of nursing for the provision of health care (Fairman 2008). In Australia, nurses' professional bodies and some registration authorities set up working groups to bring the role of NP to the health care professional workforce in the 1990s. As with the US, Australia has many populations that do not have easy access to primary care physicians or access to the provision of timely care (Gardner et al. 2010).

The NP role is an innovative response to pressures caused by well-recognised health care service and workforce shortages (Klynveld Peat Marwick Goerdele (KPMG) 2009; Productivity Commission 2005, 2017). The presence of NPs are argued to overcome access issues, timeliness of care in remote and rural Australia, also timeliness for clients with complex and chronic health conditions and the development of collaborative relationships with other health professionals to improve health outcomes for vulnerable populations such as socially disadvantaged rural communities, mental health clients and those in aged-care facilities (Clark et al. 2013; Driscoll et al. 2005; Harvey et al. 2011; Kelly et al. 2017; Wand et al. 2012).

Despite international research showing that NPs deliver safe and effective care to patients, families and their communities (Horrocks et al. 2002; Laurant et al. 2008), there was resistance to bringing this new role into the Australian health care system (Pesce 2010), as well as concerns about whether clients would recognise the role (Allnut et al. 2010; Parker et al. 2013).

An NP is a registered nurse who has undertaken several years of nursing practice since graduation, sometimes in a specialty area such as mental health, emergency nursing, primary health care or other medical specialty. Often that has meant doing further study at graduate level with an education provider, usually a university School of Nursing. To qualify as a NP, though, a nurse must undertake a Master of Nursing (Nurse practitioner) through a course accredited with the ANMAC and approved by the NMBA (2018b; *Registration standard: endorsement as a nurse practitioner*, effective 2014, updated 2018). As with the RN title, the nurse practitioner is a legally protected title (see Table 23.3) through the NMBA registration standard for endorsement under s95 of the National Law (Commonwealth of Australia 2010a).

There is a range of different activities undertaken by NPs that are governed by the NMBA, and regularly updated; the *Nurse practitioner standards for practice – effective from 1 January 2014* (NMBA 2018b); *Code of conduct for nurses* (NMBA 2018c) and *Safety and quality guidelines for nurse practitioners* (NMBA 2016d) are a few of guidelines, which cover NP practice across Australia. There is state-based legislation that governs NP practice under legislation such as the Poisons and Therapeutic Goods Acts in each state. After legislation for practice and registration, NPs are then admitted as eligible Medicare providers with the ability to be in both the **Medicare Benefits Schedule (MBS)** and the **Pharmaceutical Benefits Scheme (PBS)** as enabled by the *Health Legislation Amendment (Midwives and NPs) Act* (Commonwealth of Australia 2010a, 2010b).

The scope of practice allows a NP to practise across four domains – clinical, educational, research and leadership. There are four standards of practice that cover assessment using diagnostic capability, planning care and engaging with others; prescribing and implementing therapeutic interventions; and evaluating outcomes and improving practice (NMBA 2016c, 2018c).

The scope of practice for an NP differs markedly from that of a RN; although its foundation is that of a registered nurse (NMBA 2016a), it covers the recent changes made to codes of conduct for nurses (NMBA 2018c), the need to follow guidelines for culturally safe practice as well as prepare and maintain a electronic practice portfolio for audit of practice with mandated continuing education (NMBA 2018b). Currently under a MBS Schedule Review (see Department of Health 2018), the Nurse Practitioner Reference Group has provided a report of the necessary changes to MBS and PBS access for NPs (Medicare Benefits Review Taskforce – NPRG 2018). The report obtained an immediate response from the Australian Medical Association (AMA) that 'called on the Government to immediately reject draft proposals that would expand the ability of nurse practitioners to provide Medicare funded services and remove the current requirement for them to collaborate with doctors in delivering care for patients' (Australian Medical Association, 2019). As NPs often find that GPs are not nearby, they recommend changes to the collaboration requirements. The Australian College of Nurse Practitioners (ACNP) website records that the report's recommendations are in the following areas:

◆ enabling much greater access to timely and appropriate care, especially in aged care and rural and remote areas
◆ enabling access to preventative care and early intervention in disease management
◆ enabling patients to access rebates for procedures and a wider range of services provided by nurse practitioners
◆ enabling nurse practitioners to work to full scope of practice, especially in areas of Australia where communities have poor, or reduced access to health services
◆ enabling nurse practitioners to integrate further into primary care
◆ reducing fragmentation of care, encouraging true collaboration between health professionals, and reducing delays, duplication of services and inefficiencies
◆ removal of artificial barriers to practice, which currently limit access to nurse practitioners' services.

(Media release, Australian College of Nurse Practitioners, 6 February 2019:
https://www.acnp.org.au/index.cfm?module=news&pagemode=indiv&page_id=83389)

PAUSE
for
REFLECTION
...

Over several decades, there has been a concerted media campaign and lobbying waged by what Tuohy (1999:15) refers to as 'professional collegial institutions' such as the AMA against nurses working in the NP role. These institutions argue that patients would be put at risk from a health care system that 'fragmented care'. To what extent is current policy surrounding NPs a product/outcome of the market? To what extent is it a product/outcome of contestation with professional collegial institutions such as the AMA?

Interprofessional practice and nursing

Case study 23.1 highlights issues that are very relevant to nursing and to the necessary changes in the modern health care system used by proponents of interprofessional practice and education to legitimise their case (Meleis 2016; WHO 2006).

Meleis asserts that 'without awareness and analysis of the power differential and gender divide in the health professions, the same ineffective, hierarchical system will continue to prevail' (2016, p. 110).

However, such a view relates to the need for health professional education to include contact with the health professional groups that are part of the health care workforce. As you will have seen from the case study in Chapter 17, outcomes for clients / patients can be affected by how professionals work together. A landmark report from a special commission into safety and quality in NSW (Garling 2008) asserted that there was a growing interdependence between groups, and that, unless work across professional groups improved, there would be consequent loss of quality and unsafe outcomes in acute care hospitals in that state. Other authors point to transition points such as discharge to home / facility, admission to acute care and moving from youth services to adult services, or adult services to aged-care facilities, were all problematic because there were deficiencies in communications (Curtis 2011; Wei et al. 2016). Concerns about NP practice has made collaboration with physicians' mandatory, despite a lack of GPs or physicians in the areas where nurse practitioners were to work (Australian College of Nurse Practitioners (ACNP) 2019) – this points to the validity of Meleis's (2016) argument above. The report also highlights resistance by physicians to making themselves available for collaboration (Medicare Benefits Taskforce Group – NPRG 2018). The AMA asserts that NPs lead to fragmentation of the health care system (AMA 2019), but without recognition of gaps and fragmentation that are caused by lack of GPs and failure to work with other health professionals when opportunities for collaboration are not maximised (Wei et al. 2016).

As you would have noted in Chapter 1, using nurses in navigation roles is a form of interprofessional practice viewed as a way of improving outcomes and providing a 'seamless' experience of the health care system for patients / clients / consumers that improves safety and quality of care (Allen 2015; Wilson et al. 2016). In nursing there are several developments that go across sectors or provide linked care in some settings such as general practice. The **practice nurse** and its development into the primary health care nurse could point in this direction (Lane et al. 2017). Practice nurses have been identified as not practising at their scope of practice (although this is difficult when not all practice nurses are RNs, and as we noted at the beginning of this chapter if the level of practice was constrained, and not at the full potential of the standards (NMBA 2016a). The practice nurse workforce cannot work to improve outcomes in the primary care network if nurses cannot leverage their scope of practice (Lane et al. 2017; McKittrick & McKenzie 2018).

Other treatment areas such as cancer care (e.g. breast care nurses), or transitions of care, or clients with complex and chronic conditions (such as mental health care), require coordination of their care across sectors (sometimes out of health care into education, housing or local government, as is often the case for vulnerable populations such as the homeless, aged or mentally ill). Handley and McAllister (2017) provide evidence of nurses working with teachers in a wellness / strength-based intervention in adolescent mental health as central to the success of the program.

Case Study 23.1

Residential aged-care facilities (RACFs)

Mark is an NP providing comprehensive clinical services to older people living in RACFs across the metropolitan area of Adelaide. He routinely sees residents who would not otherwise have access to timely primary care. A typical day may require Mark to assess, diagnose and treat minor or acute illnesses or injuries including infections, wounds, behavioural and psychological symptoms of dementia, musculoskeletal injuries and mental health episodes, or to provide end-of-life care. This can involve a range of interventions and care coordination; prescribing, titrating and/or ceasing medicines; ordering diagnostic investigations; and directly referring patients to other health professionals.

However, residents can experience delays in receiving necessary diagnostic investigations as current MBS rules do not enable NPs to initiate many common diagnostic imaging tests otherwise subsidised in primary health care, such as ultrasounds and X-rays. This leads to fragmented and unnecessary duplication of services, requiring either a second attendance by a GP or, worse, an unnecessary transfer to an emergency department.

Some residents may not have access to a GP who conducts comprehensive medical assessments or team care arrangements, including accessing allied health services. Residents then do not have their chronic health conditions proactively assessed and monitored for early signs of deterioration, increasing the incidence of acute events and hospitalisation or reducing their overall quality of life. Residents and RACF staff have asked Mark to assist in the provision of comprehensive health assessments, chronic disease management, case conferences and advance care planning. However, the allocated times for NP professional attendances (i.e. MBS items 82200–82215) are not practically useful for this care.

Case study questions
1 What are the problems that the NP is assisting with?
2 How does a NP provide care in this setting, as they are not part of the staff at the RACF?
3 What is the issue about attendance at emergency departments that would make this NP's role useful to the aged-care sector and also to local hospitals and GPs?
4 Would the NP work with other health professional groups to provide care (see case studies in Chapters 26 and 28)?

Source: Medicare Benefits Review Taskforce – Nurse Practitioner Reference Group (2018) Report from the Nurse Practitioner Reference Group, pp. 30–31. http://www.health.gov.au/internet/main/publishing.nsf/Content/58EFEA022C2B7C49CA2583960083C4EA/$File/NPRG%20Final%20Report%20-%20v2.pdf

Obtaining nursing's potential

As we highlighted at the beginning of this chapter, nursing is at a moment in its development where it could meet its full potential. But let us take a look at some of the challenges and the dynamics of the Australian health care system and what effect these challenges can have on any discipline's practice within the system. Dark et al. (2017) highlight what can happen to throw a project to reorganise mental health care predicted to improve outcomes in mental health into disorder. They write:

> Within the 3-year period of this study, a new Queensland state government was elected [in March 2012]. Health services were reorganized to establish local area health networks overseen by boards. The state health budget was reduced with the loss of 2754 staff. There were reductions in the Commonwealth Health Budget following a change of government in 2013 (Australian Budget 2014–2015) after which the Queensland Health budget was reduced by an estimated two billion dollars (Budget Estimates 2015–2016).
>
> *(Dark et al. 2017, p. 4)*

It is remarkable that the profession of nursing has been able to advance its cause in the implementation of advanced practice models given the dynamics of change seen above. Yet, as we see, reorganisation for improvement is at the mercy of changes external to the organisation and even to the health care system resulting from government changes, changes to the economic climate and to readings of the problems of nursing through lenses such as new public health management. Where budget constraints result in staff losses or bed closures, which amount to the same thing, we see problems defined by the shortcomings of nurses (Harvey et al. 2017) rather than as restraints put on nursing practice through standardisation and managerialist oversight (Cooke 2006). If nurses' work were leveraged to its maximum and nurses were practising to scope, would there be problems defined as 'missed care', or failures to provide safe care in aged care (see Chapter 20) that have led to a Royal Commission into Aged Care, or failures of compassion as described in the Francis Report (Francis 2013)?

Friedson (2001), in his analysis of professionalism, argues that the soul of professional practice is denied when professions are over-regulated and lacking autonomy in providing patient care. Molina-Mula et al. (2018) highlight how these effects largely emanate from the two sources: austerity (in their case in the financial situation in Spain) and managerialism that has not only limited practice, but also suppressed patient autonomy (see also Chapter 21 for these effects on medicine). Further advances in nursing require that nurses and their leaders critique and problematise the system that constrains nursing's advancement (Cooke 2009). The health care system needs nurses who can critique the system not only for what it does to their practice, but also for how it disrespects and disempowers the patients/clients/consumers of that system (Molina-Mula et al. 2018), providing navigating roles, working across sectors and challenging assumed hierarchies that limit manager capabilities of the nursing role (Allen 2015).

Summary

- The nursing workforce is described and current concerns about the location of nurses show what the government deems to be the problem with nursing labour and its geographical distribution in Australia. The population profile of nurses is also an issue; as the general population ages, the nursing workforce is looking at major retirements.
- There are differences in how nursing's scope of practice is defined, from a professional perspective that provides a broad definition of what nurses are expected to undertake in their practice. When

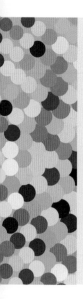

nurses are viewed as employees, to provide an understanding of nursing work the employing bodies talk about tasks. Such descriptions also confuse the protected title of nurse with 'job titles' that describe medical specialties.

- The development of advanced practice roles (such as care coordinators) and specialist roles has been used to develop other advanced roles such as the NP. The NP is also a protected title under legislation – legislating collaboration, prescribing, diagnostics, treatment interventions and ongoing evaluation of practice for continuous improvement.

- Interprofessional education (IPE) and interprofessional practice (IPP) are considered a solution to the fragmentation and treatment silos of the Australian health care system. Safety and quality are the main drivers to promote IPP in the clinic.

- It is important to ensure that nurses during their education have a chance to critique the health care systems and the assumptions on which policies are based, and that act as constraints, and to learn to speak out through peak bodies on the distribution of budgets to health care, and to vulnerable populations.

Review Questions

1   What is the difference in the scope of practice of RNs, advanced practice nurses and NPs?
2   NPs provide some services that are also provided by general practitioners. How does this impact on the relationship between medical practitioners and nurses?
3   What difficulties are highlighted in this chapter for advancing nursing roles? Are we there yet?
4   What role can you see for NPs as opposed to practice nurses in general practice settings? Can the two roles coexist?
5   Carol Bacchi (2012) has developed five questions we can use to ask what is the 'real' problem (see Chapter 1). Using her framework, is the problem that professions need IPE and IPP to direct their practice? How can we rethink this 'problem'?

References

Allen, D., 2015. The Invisible Work of Nurses: Hospitals, Organisation and Healthcare. Routledge, Oxford.

Allnut, J., Allnut, N., McMaster, R., et al., 2010. Client's understanding of the role of the nurse practitioner. Aust. Health Rev. 34, 59–65.

Australian Broadcasting Corporation, 2018. NSW on the verge of a nursing shortage. www.abc.net.au/news/2018-01-12/nsw-set-for-major-shortage…nurses…/9321464.

Australian College of Nurse Practitioners (ACNP), 2019. Media release on report from Nurse Practitioner Reference Group, Medicare Benefit Schedule Review Taskforce, February 6. https://www.acnp.org.au/index.cfm?module=news&pagemode=indiv&page_id=833890.

Australian Government, 2019. Registered nurses. https://joboutlook.gov.au/occupation?code=2544.

Australian Health Practitioner Regulation Authority (AHPRA), 2018. Registrant data (reporting period: 1 April 2018–30 June 2018). www.ahpra.gov.au/annualreport/2018/registration.html.

Australian Medical Association (AMA), 2019. Media release: Nurse practitioner proposals must be rejected. https://ama.com.au/media/nurse-practitioner-proposals-must-be-rejected.

Bacchi, C., 2012. Introducing the 'What's the problem represented to be?' approach. In: Bletsas, A., Beasley, C. (Eds.), Engaging with Carol Bacchi: Strategic Interventions and Exchanges. University of Adelaide Press, Adelaide, pp. 21–24. https://www.adelaide.edu.au/carst/docs/wpr/wpr-summary.pdf.

Bender, M., Spiva, L., Su, W., et al., 2018. Organising nursing practice into care models that catalyse quality: a clinical nurse leader case study. J. Nurs. Manag. 26, 653–662.

Birks, M., Davis, J., Smithson, J., et al., 2016. Registered nurse scope of practice in Australia: an integrative review of the literature. Contemp. Nurse 52 (5), 522–543.

Clark, S., Parker, R., Prosser, B., et al., 2013. Aged care nurse practitioners in Australia: evidence for the development of their role. Aust. Health Rev. 37 (4), 594–601.

Commonwealth of Australia, 2009. Health Practitioner Regulation National Law Act. https://www.legislation.qld.gov.au/view/html/inforce/current/act-2009-045.

Commonwealth of Australia, 2010a. National health (collaborative arrangements for nurse practitioners) Determination 2010 F2010L02107. http://www.comlaw.gov.au/Details/F2010L02107.

Commonwealth of Australia, 2010b. Health Legislation Amendment (Midwives and Nurse Practitioners) Act. https://www.legislation.gov.au/Details/C2010A00029.

Cooke, H., 2006. Seagull management and the control of nursing work. Work Employ. Soc. 20 (2), 223–243.

Cooke, H., 2009. Theories of risk and safety: what is their relevance to nursing? J. Nurs. Manag. 17, 256–264.

Curtis, K., Tzannes, A., Rudge, T., 2011. How to talk to doctors – a guide for effective communication. Int. Nurs. Rev. 58, 13–20.

Dark, F., Whiteford, H., Ashkanasy, N.M., et al., 2017. The impact of organisational change and fiscal restraint on organisational culture. Int. J. Ment. Health Syst. 11, 11. doi:10.1186/s13033-016-0116-0.

Department of Health, 2016. Health workforce summaries – nursing. https://www.health.gov.au/internet/main/publishing.nsf/Content/health_workforce_data.

Department of Health, 2018. MBS arrangements for midwives and nurse practitioners. http://www.health.gov.au/internet/main/publishing.nsf/Content/D43E1F9A42656B.5ECA257BF0001D39EF/$File/MBSItems19-2.pdf.

Driscoll, A., Worrall-Carter, L., O'Reilly, J., et al., 2005. A historical review of the nurse practitioner role in Australia. Clin. Excell. Nurse Pract. 9 (3), 141–152.

Fairman, J., 2008. Making Room in the Clinic: Nurse Practitioners and the Evolution of Modern Health Care. Rutgers University Press, New Brunswick, NJ.

Francis, R., 2013. Report of the Mid Staffordshire NHS Foundation Trust Public Inquiry. The Stationery Office, London. https://www.gov.uk/government/publications/report-of-the-mid-staffordshire-nhs-foundation-trust-public-inquiry.

Friedson, E., 2001. Professionalism: The Third Logic. University of Chicago Press, Chicago.

Gardner, G., Chang, A., Duffield, C., 2007. Making nursing work: breaking through the role confusion of advanced practice nursing. J. Adv. Nurs. 57 (4), 382–391.

Gardner, G., Gardner, A., Middleton, S., et al., 2010. The work of nurse practitioners. J. Adv. Nurs. 66 (10), 2160–2169.

Garling, P., 2008. Final report of the Special Commission of Inquiry: Acute Care Services in NSW Public Hospitals: overview. NSW Government, Sydney.

Handley, C., McAllister, M., 2017. Elements to promote a successful relationships between stakeholders interested in mental health promotion in schools. Aust. J. Adv. Nurs. 34 (4), 16–25.

Harvey, C., Driscoll, A., Keyzer, D., 2011. The discursive practices of nurse practitioner legislation in Australia. J. Adv. Nurs. 67 (11), 2478–2487. doi:10.1111/j.1365-2648.2011.05650.x.

Harvey, C., Thompson, S., Pearson, M., et al., 2017. Missed nursing care as an 'art form': the contradiction of nurses as carers. Nurs. Inq. 24, e12180. doi:10.1112/nin.12180.

Horrocks, S., Anderson, E., Salisbury, C., 2002. Systematic review of whether nurse practitioners working in primary care can provide equivalent care to doctors. BMJ 324, 819–823.

International Council of Nurses (ICN), 2019. Definition of nursing. https://www.icn.ch/nursing-policy/ nursing-definitions.

Kelly, J., Garvey, D., Biro, M.A., et al., 2017. Managing medical service delivery gaps in a socially disadvantaged rural community: a nurse practitioner led clinic. Aust. J. Adv. Nurs. 34 (4), 42–49.

KPMG, 2009. Health workforce in Australia and factors for current shortages. Report prepared for the National Health Workforce Taskforce, April. https://docplayer.net/372210-Health-workforce-in- australia-and-factors-for-current-shortages.html.

Lane, R., Halcomb, E., McKenna, L., et al., 2017. Advancing general practice nursing in Australia: roles and responsibilities of primary healthcare organisations. Aust. Health Rev. 41, 127–132.

Laurant, M., Hermens, R., Braspenning, J.A., et al., 2008. An overview of patient's preference for, and satisfaction with, care provided by general practitioners and nurse practitioners. J. Clin. Nurs. 17, 2690–2698.

McGrail, M.R., Humphreys, J.S., 2009. A new index of access to primary care services in rural areas. Aust. N. Z. J. Public Health 33 (5), 418–423.

McKittrick, R., McKenzie, R., 2018. A narrative review and synthesis to inform health workforce preparation for the Health Care Homes model in primary healthcare in Australia. Aust. J. Prim. Health 24, 317–329.

Medicare Benefits Review Taskforce – Nurse Practitioner Reference Group (NPRG), 2018. Report from the Nurse Practitioner Reference Group. http://www.health.gov.au/internet/main/publishing.nsf/Content/ 58EFEA022C2B7C49CA2583960083C4EA/$File/NPRG%20Final%20Report%20-%20v2.pdf.

Meleis, A.I., 2016. Interprofessional education: a summary of reports and barriers to recommendations. J. Nurs. Scholarsh. 48 (1), 106–112.

Molina-Mula, J., Peter, E., Gallo-Estrada, J., et al., 2018. Instrumentalisation of the health system: an examination of the impact on nursing practice and patient autonomy. Nurs. Inq. 25, e12201. doi:10.1111/nin/12201.

Nelson, S., Gordon, S. (Eds.), 2006. The Complexities of Care: Nursing Reconsidered. ILR Press / Cornell University Press, Ithaca, USA.

Nelson, S., Rafferty, A.M. (Eds.), 2010. Notes on Nightingale: The Influence and Legacy of a Nursing Icon. Cornell University Press, Ithaca, USA.

Nursing and Midwifery Board of Australia (NMBA), 2016a. Registered nurse standards for practice. http:// www.nursingmidwiferyboard.gov.au/Codes-Guidelines-Statements/Professional-standards/registered- nurse-standards-for-practice.aspx.

Nursing and Midwifery Board of Australia (NMBA), 2016b. Standards for practice: enrolled nurses. http://www.nursingmidwiferyboard.gov.au/Codes-Guidelines-Statements/Professional-standards/enrolled-nurse-standards-for-practice.aspx.

Nursing and Midwifery Board of Australia (NMBA), 2016c. Registration standard for continuing professional development. https://www.nursingmidwiferyboard.gov.au/Registration-Standards/Continuing-professional-development.aspx.

Nursing and Midwifery Board of Australia (NMBA), 2016d. Safety and quality guidelines for nurse practitioners. http://www.nursingmidwiferyboard.gov.au/documents/default.aspx?record=WD16%2F19534&dbid=AP&chksum=kzFDW8ifMSFw9%2FAYl2na0A%3D%3D.

Nursing and Midwifery Board of Australia (NMBA), 2018a. Nursing and Midwifery Board of Australia: registrant data (reporting period: 1 April 2018–30 June 2018). https://www.nursingmidwiferyboard.gov.au/documents/default.aspx?record=WD18%2f26398&dbid=AP&chksum=qNWDOD2t5jceAnYCnCrL1A%3d%3d.

Nursing and Midwifery Board of Australia (NMBA), 2018b. Nurse practitioner standards for practice – effective from 1 January 2014, updated March 2018. https://www.nursingmidwiferyboard.gov.au/Codes-Guidelines-Statements/Codes-Guidelines.aspx.

Nursing and Midwifery Board of Australia (NMBA), 2018c. Code of conduct for nurses. https://www.nursingmidwiferyboard.gov.au/Codes-Guidelines-Statements/Professional-standards.aspx.

Nursing and Midwifery Board of Australia (NMBA), 2019. CATSINaM and NMBA joint statement on cultural safety. https://www.nursingmidwiferyboard.gov.au/Codes-Guidelines-Statements/Position-Statements/joint-statement-on-culturally-safe-care.aspx.

Parker, R., Forrest, L., Ward, N., et al., 2013. How acceptable are primary health care nurse practitioners to Australian consumers? Collegian 20 (1), 35–41.

Parry, Y., Grant, J., 2016. Nursing in Australia. In: Willis, E., Reynolds, L., Keleher, H. (Eds.), Understanding the Australian Health Care System, third ed. Elsevier, Sydney, pp. 245–255.

Pesce, A., 2010. President's message, 12 November. Australian Medical Association, Barton ACT. https://ama.com.au/media/ama-president-dr-andrew-pesce-speech-national-press-club-wednesday-21-july-2010.

Productivity Commission, 2005. Australia's health workforce. Research Report. Productivity Commission, Canberra.

Productivity Commission, 2017, Shifting the dial: 5 year productivity review. Report no. 84. Productivity Commission, Canberra.

Tuohy, C.J., 1999. Accidental Logics: The Dynamics of Change in the Health Care Arena in the United States, Britain, and Canada. OUP, New York.

Wand, T., White, K., Patching, J., et al., 2012. Outcomes from the evaluation of an emergency department-based mental health nurse practitioner outpatient service in Australia. J. Am. Acad. Nurse Pract. 24 (3), 149–159.

Wei, L., Gerdtz, M., Manias, E., 2016. Creating opportunities for interdisciplinary collaboration and patient-centred care: how nurses, doctors, pharmacists and patients use communication strategies when managing medications in an acute hospital setting. J. Clin. Nurs. 25, 2943–2957.

Wilson, A.J., Palmer, L., Levett-Jones, T., et al., 2016. Interprofessional collaborative practice for medication safety: nursing, pharmacy, and medical graduates' experiences and perspectives. J. Interprof. Care 30 (5), 649–654.

World Health Organization (WHO), 2006. Working together for health. World health report. http://www.who.int/whr/2006/whr06_en.pdf/.

Further Reading

Birks, M., Davis, J., Smithson, J., et al., 2016. Registered nurse scope of practice in Australia: an integrative review of the literature. Contemp. Nurse *52* (5), 522–543. doi:10.1080/10376178.2016.1238773.

Harvey, C., Thompson, S., Pearson, M., et al., 2017. Missed nursing care as an 'art form': the contradiction of nurses as carers. Nurs. Inq. 24, e12180. doi:10.1112/nin.12180.

Rankin, J., 2009. The Nurse Project: an analysis for nurses to take back our work. Nurs. Inq. 16 (4), 275–286.

Online Resources

Australian College of Nurse Practitioners (ACNP) peak national organisation for nurse practitioners: http://www.acnp.org.au

Australian Health Practitioners Regulation Agency (AHPRA) is the organisation responsible for the implementation of the Commonwealth Government National Registration and Accreditation Scheme across Australia. The scheme saw 10 health professions including nursing come under a single regulatory authority: http://www.ahpra.gov.au

Australian Nursing and Midwifery Accreditation Council (ANMAC) is the accrediting authority for nursing and midwifery under the National Registration and Accreditation Scheme. It sets standards for accreditation, accredits nursing and midwifery courses and providers and undertakes migration skill assessment of internationally qualified nurses and midwives seeking to work in Australia: https://www.anmac.org.au

Australian Primary Health Care Nurses Association represents nurses who work in primary care settings. Their website presents position statements, frameworks for working in general practices and other role related issues: https://www.apna.asn.au/profession/what-is-primary-health-care-nursing

Congress of Aboriginal and Torres Strait Islander Nurses and Midwives is the peak organisation for registered nurses and midwives who identify as Aboriginal and Torres Strait Islanders. It has now linked with the Nursing and Midwifery Board of Australia to promote culturally safe care: http://www.catsinam.org.au

International Council of Nurses (ICN) represents the interests of nursing internationally through the development of nursing health policy in areas such as ethics, professional practice and regulation: http://www.icn.ch

Joint statement on cultural safety guidelines for practice at: https://www.nursingmidwiferyboard.gov.au/Codes-Guidelines-Statements/Position-Statements/leading-the-way.aspx

Nursing and Midwifery Board of Australia (NMBA) is the national nursing and midwifery regulatory authority under the National Registration and Accreditation Scheme: http://www.nursingmidwiferyboard.gov.au

CHAPTER 24

Occupational therapy

Sandra Mortimer and Brenton Kortman

Key learning outcomes

When you finish this chapter you should be able to:

+ describe occupation and its relationship to health and well-being
+ describe the scope and organisation of occupational therapy in Australia
+ describe the application of occupational therapy across the life-span and in different contexts
+ describe the range of roles that occupational therapists may undertake within the Australian health care system
+ reflect on the likely impact of contemporary trends and health issues on the future profile of occupational therapy.

Key terms and abbreviations

Alzheimer's disease

American Occupational Therapy Association (AOTA)

Australian Health Practitioner Regulation Agency (AHPRA)

client-centred practice

continuing professional development (CPD)

National Disability Insurance Scheme (NDIS)

occupation

occupational engagement

occupational justice

occupational therapist (OT)

Occupational Therapy Board of Australia (OTBA)

speech pathologist (SP)

spinal cord injury

World Federation of Occupational Therapists (WFOT)

Introduction

This chapter will introduce the concepts and practice of occupational therapy in Australia. To be able to understand what occupational therapy is, you first need to understand the meaning of the term 'occupation'. This is what most clearly differentiates the occupational therapist (OT) from other members of an interprofessional health care team. The initial section of this chapter will discuss the concept of occupation. The second part will then outline how occupation is related to health and well-being and therefore applied as therapy, particularly in an Australian context.

Occupation and occupational engagement

Occupation is defined by the **American Occupational Therapy Association (AOTA)** as 'daily life activities in which people engage' (American Occupational Therapy Association 2014, p. S43). You can see by this definition that it is much broader than 'work', which is so often what people associate with occupation. Occupation in this context encompasses everything we do. What we do, and how and why we do these things, has a significant impact on our health and well-being.

Occupational therapy is about 'achieving health, well-being, and participation in life through engagement in occupation' (American Occupational Therapy Association 2014, p. S4). Occupational therapy intervention focuses on supporting clients, who may be individuals, groups or populations, to engage in the occupations of everyday life that support them to live meaningful lives (World Federation of Occupational Therapists (WFOT) 2012). It is important to keep in mind that what is 'meaningful' needs to be defined by the client. To do this, OTs need to be able to understand the barriers and facilitators to occupational engagement. **Occupational engagement** is the 'performance of occupations as the result of choice, motivation, and meaning within a supportive context and environment' (American Occupational Therapy Association 2014, p. S42).

The occupational therapist uses occupation as a therapeutic tool. The occupations that people choose to undertake often reflect and shape their current and future identity (Phelan & Kinsella 2014). Think about an occupation you enjoy and how you feel when you do it. Think about how that occupation reflects your sense of your self and how this may have changed over time. Occupations are central to a person's sense of competence and have particular value and meaning to that individual (American Occupational Therapy Association 2014). Engaging in occupations can influence mood, emotions, physical and cognitive capacities.

PAUSE
for
REFLECTION
...

Read the following and reflect on the influence of meaningful occupation.

Picture Maggie, a 76-year-old woman with **Alzheimer's disease** who has been living in a nursing home for 3 months following the death of her husband. She has become less and less responsive to her children, the staff and her surroundings. She sits day after day slumped over in her wheelchair.

The OT talks with Maggie's children to see what occupations have been important in her life, and discovers that Maggie used to love music and dancing. She danced as a young child right through to her 30s, and then was involved in teaching children. She loved musicals and was always singing, listening to music, working on routines and sewing costumes.

The OT suggests they bring in some examples of her former interests and start talking with Maggie about this. The OT explains how we experience our occupations through a range of our senses and how this may help Maggie access her memories.

Her children bring in photos, trophies, music, ballet costumes, Maggie's old sewing box and, becoming very creative, a pair of old, smelly tap shoes. They spread these around Maggie and gently talk to her about what they have found, showing her the items and allowing her to feel them and experience them. Slowly but surely, Maggie begins to respond and starts to talk about her dancing days as she handles the costumes and shoes. She shows interest in her environment, notices the photos and starts to smile. She then looks up at her daughter and smiles at her.

Occupational engagement is highly individualised. One person may categorise ironing as work, another as a domestic chore and yet another may find it relaxing and calming. When OTs work with clients they identify and analyse the individual elements of each occupation and consider how these support or hinder occupational engagement, the impact this has on the client's health and well-being, and their ability to participate in life as they would wish to. They match this with their understanding of the client as a whole and the factors that may impact on that person's occupational choices. These factors may include the client's values, beliefs and spirituality, body functions and body structures. The final element that OTs consider is the environmental factors that influence occupational engagement. These include cultural, personal, temporal, virtual, physical and social contexts (American Occupational Therapy Association 2014). Context and environment influence how and when an occupation is carried out. As an example, think about the occupation of swimming. You could swim in many different environments such as the beach, a river, a public indoor pool, a private backyard pool. How might these different places influence the way you swim? An indoor pool can be used any time of the year regardless of the weather. Taking a swim to cool down in summer in a backyard pool is very different to swimming laps for fitness in an indoor public pool.

PAUSE
for
REFLECTION
...

Consider how your understanding about occupation has changed since reading the above. Can you see how it encompasses much more than 'work'?

Impact of occupation on health and well-being

As well as the definitions of health already considered in this book, occupational therapy considers health as a resource to allow people to engage in meaningful occupation.

Active engagement in meaningful occupation generally promotes, facilitates and maintains health and well-being. There are cases, however, where active engagement in occupation can be harmful to health and well-being – for example, addictive occupations such as gambling. Another example is professional musicianship. The occupation of rehearsing and performing with a violin at a professional level requires the musician to hold certain parts of their body (trunk, neck, shoulders) in sustained and often awkward positions while other body parts (fingers, wrists) are engaged in fast and repetitive movements for long periods of time. The focus and concentration required to play at this level means that musicians often lose track of time. They enter a state of 'flow' which has been defined as a rare focused state of consciousness (Csikszentmihalyi 1993). This is usually considered to be a health-enhancing state, but a study of professional musicians by Guptill (2012) drew attention to the negative effects that 'flow' can have on health. Despite the fact that these musicians experienced pain and physical injury as a result of their playing, many of them still reported an enhanced sense of well-being because the occupation was so valued, reflected their sense of identity and positively influenced their mood and emotional state (Guptill 2012). This study highlights the importance of understanding an occupation and taking into consideration the person's perspective, particularly around the value or meaning of the occupation.

Occupational therapists consider that people thrive when they are able to participate in a range of occupations that match their needs, interests and capacities. A state of occupational imbalance occurs when excessive time is spent in one or more areas of life at the expense of others (Backman 2010). For example, a student could spend much of their time playing computer games at the expense of study, which impacts negatively on their goal of achieving a university education.

Supportive environments also play a crucial role in maximising participation, health and well-being. Occupational therapists consider the social determinants of health and understand that these influence opportunities to participate in occupations. This applies across all ages, but can be highlighted when considering learning and development outcomes for young children. Children learn and develop from a context of safe and secure relationships and opportunities to engage in core occupations such as playing. When working with a child presenting with a developmental delay, an OT will strive to understand the broader social, cultural and environmental influences that may be impacting on this child and family, such as access to safe and secure environments, safety, adequate shelter and food, parental well-being and mental health and financial security. The OT will be mindful of these when planning therapeutic interventions (see Case study 24.1 later in the chapter as an example).

Occupational science

Occupational science offers a knowledge base that supports occupational therapy practice with a focus on analysing and optimising knowledge about occupation (Wright-St Clair & Hocking 2014). It is important for OTs to understand people as occupational beings and to understand how occupation can influence a person's life both positively and negatively. As already discussed in this book, efficiency, effectiveness and equity are core drivers for health system performance, and in challenging economic environments there is increasing pressure from health services and other employers to apply evidence and demonstrate value.

Occupational justice

Occupational therapists also focus on the social justice agenda previously discussed in this book by considering human rights from an occupational perspective. The **World Federation of Occupational Therapists (WFOT)** *Position statement on human rights* (2006) endorses the United Nations' (1948) *Universal declaration of human rights* and adds a perspective in relation to human occupation and participation that recognises people's rights to participate in meaningful occupations consistent with their culture, context and values. Occupational justice 'is concerned with enabling, mediating and advocating for environments in which all people's opportunities to engage in occupation are just, health-promoting and meaningful' (Hocking 2017, p. 33).

A model of **occupational justice** described by Townsend and Wilcock (2004) highlights the need to consider and protect people's different priorities, needs and capacities and how they are expressed through what they do. Occupational rights include the right to:

♦ participate in a range of occupations for health, development and social inclusion

♦ make choices and share decision-making in daily life

♦ experience meaning and enrichment in one's occupations

♦ receive fair privileges for diverse participation in occupations (Wilcock & Hocking 2015, p. 407).

This approach expands possible occupational therapy intervention from an individual clinical role to one of working with people, populations and communities to advocate for and enact change at a policy or program level to address issues of occupational injustice. Occupational deprivation is one outcome of occupational injustice, and is defined as 'a state of prolonged preclusion from engagement in occupations of necessity and/or meaning due to factors which stand outside of the control of the individual' (Whiteford 2000, p. 305). Alex's situation as described in the following *Pause for reflection* is an example of occupational deprivation.

PAUSE
for
REFLECTION
...

Alex is a 23-year-old man who has experienced significant brain damage as a result of a car accident and requires high-level care. The only residential option that could provide 24-hour nursing care at the level he requires is an aged-care facility. He has lived in this facility for the past 3 years. Imagine how Alex's daily life and the occupations he wants and needs to do are affected by living in this environment. How does this impact on his occupational rights?

This is an example of occupational injustice. In this case, an occupational therapist could work as part of a team to advocate for Alex's occupational rights, could work with the aged-care facility to consider environmental and program modifications to address issues of occupational deprivation, and could support submissions to the National Disability Insurance Scheme to consider better funding options.

• Refer to the Young People in Nursing Homes National Alliance (www.ypinh.org. au) for further information on this issue.

• See also Occupational Therapy Australia's 2015 submission *Adequacy of existing residential care arrangements available for young people with severe physical, mental or intellectual disabilities in Australia*, available through their website (https://www.otaus.com.au/sitebuilder/advocacy/knowledge/asset/files/43/ senatecommuntiyaffairs-youngpeopleinrcfota.pdf).

Occupation as therapy

The use of occupation as therapy has been recorded since ancient times, with noted Greek and Roman physicians such as Hippocrates and Celsus advocating their use. A more organised form of occupational therapy emerged around 200 years ago within large mental asylums. People with mental illnesses were managed by being sent to asylums and essentially incarcerated, often with the use of shackles or other restraints. Key European physicians including Philippe Pinel (often referred to as the 'father of modern psychiatry') transformed these large asylums by removing inmates' chains and providing them with a daily structure that involved regular occupations including physical exercise, work, music, reading and farming. This change was evocatively captured by French painter Robert-Fleury in 1896 (Fig. 24.1).

From the late 1800s, occupation began to be used more in deliberately therapeutic ways, individualised to each patient and conceptualised scientifically within contemporary journals. Like many other allied health professions, however, the first formal occupational therapy educational programs emerged around World War I, with large numbers of war-wounded personnel requiring rehabilitation. From that point on, occupational therapy began to expand to focus increasingly on aspects such as physical

FIGURE 24.1 PINEL A LA SALPÊTRIÈRE BY T. ROBERT-FLEURY, 1896

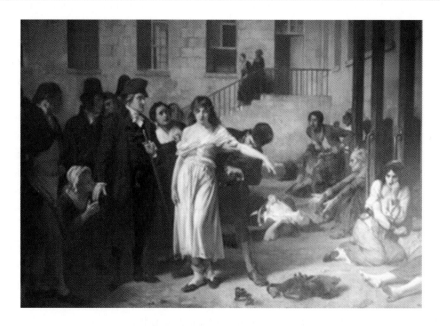

Source: Public domain

recovery and function using occupation in addition to mental health. World War II saw the development of the first Australian occupational therapy educational program in Sydney in 1942 (Bearup 1996).

How occupational therapy is organised in Australia

Educational programs for occupational therapy are at Bachelor's or Master's degree level in Australia. Some countries, such as the USA, now require a Master's or a Doctoral degree as a minimum qualification for practice. Programs in Australia need to be accredited by the Occupational Therapy Council, alongside criteria that ensure that the required competencies for entry-level therapists are met (Occupational Therapy Council 2013). An essential part of this accreditation is the requirement that occupational therapy students must have a minimum of 1000 hours of fieldwork practice in their course.

Occupational therapy is a registered profession, so to be able to practise as, and call yourself, an OT you must be registered with the **Australian Health Practitioner Regulation Agency (AHPRA)**. The **Occupational Therapy Board of Australia (OTBA)** works under the auspices of the AHPRA to set standards, regulate therapists and manage complaints against therapists. In June 2018, there were 20,975 registered OTs in Australia (Australian Health Practitioner Regulation Agency (AHPRA) 2018). Occupational therapy students are also registered by the AHPRA and have similar requirements to other therapists around aspects such as health (i.e. fitness to practise) and character (in particular, criminal history). One of the key registration requirements for OTs is the need to demonstrate the completion of **continuing professional development (CPD)** activities to renew their registration annually. The OTBA requires OTs to complete at least 30 hours of targeted education each year (Occupational Therapy Board of Australia 2013). Many people may consider that when they graduate with a university degree they would have covered what there is to know about their professional area. However, as outlined in Chapter 1, patient safety and quality in health care have become increasingly important public issues. Health professionals need to continue to develop their knowledge and skills to ensure client safety and best practice; the CPD requirements are an example of how this need has been translated into the *Health Practitioner Regulation National Law*.

In addition to the registration authority in Australia, OTs also have a professional association, Occupational Therapy Australia, which operates to promote occupational therapy and support members. Professional associations are organised and operated by members of the profession, and are therefore different to the legal authority of the registration boards. Occupational Therapy Australia is the peak professional body representing the interests of OTs and is a major provider of CPD, including national and state conferences. The association has an official journal, the *Australian Occupational Therapy Journal*, which is one of the key internationally recognised journals in the profession. Occupational Therapy Australia also provides practical support to members, such as a mentoring program for new therapists and access to professional indemnity insurance (Occupational Therapy Australia 2019).

The WFOT is the key international body for occupational therapy and sets minimum standards for occupational therapy educational programs which are used as part of course accreditation in Australia. The WFOT has enabled consistent standards for OTs across the world. The federation is recognised by the United Nations and regularly collaborates with other key international bodies such as the World Health Organization (WHO) in key projects around occupation and well-being (WFOT, 2019).

Occupational therapy practice in Australia

Occupational therapists in Australia work with people across all age-groups, from newborn babies to those very senior in years. Most OTs (90%) work in what is described as a clinical role, but some work in other roles such as administration, education, research or project work (Department of Health 2019). Within clinical roles, OTs are mostly employed with 'occupational therapist' in their job title, although some are employed in more generic positions such as case managers or lifestyle advisors. OTs work across a number of settings, including hospitals, rehabilitation centres, primary health centres, schools, aged-care facilities and people's homes or workplaces.

Occupational therapists frequently work with individuals, but may also work with groups of people or with organisations to enhance their occupational engagement. As an example of working with all of these, an OT may provide a service for an *organisation*, such as an industrial workplace, providing *education groups for workers* around body mechanics with the aim of reducing manual-handling injuries. The people that OTs work with may be called by various terms relevant to their setting, such as student, worker, patient or consumer, but typically OTs identify those they work with as *clients* (American Occupational Therapy Association 2014). The term 'client' raises a central aspect for OTs: **client-centred practice**. At the heart of occupational therapy is the collaboration between the client and the therapist in determining the scope of any occupational performance issues and in setting goals that are meaningful and relevant to the client (Schell et al. 2014). The WFOT (2012, para 1) describes occupational therapy as 'a client-centred health profession concerned with promoting health and well-being through occupation. The primary goal of occupational therapy is to enable people to participate in the activities of everyday life'. The three areas that OTs focus on to achieve this goal include aspects of the *person*, the *occupation* and the *environment*, and occupational therapy intervention is built around these aspects.

As an example of this, consider Tom, who sustained a **spinal cord injury** following a car accident. The OT assesses *personal factors* that are impacting on his occupational engagement. In this case, the injury has fully severed the connections between Tom's brain and spinal cord, meaning that there is a total loss of sensation in his legs and lower trunk and he is unable to move his lower-limb muscles. One of Tom's key goals is to regain mobility. The OT works with Tom to strengthen his upper limbs to compensate for the loss of lower-limb function, so that he can transfer from chairs and beds using his arms instead. Strengthening his upper limbs also prepares Tom for the daily rigours of using a wheelchair to mobilise.

Using a wheelchair is an example of how an OT may modify an *occupation* to enable engagement in daily life tasks. The OT carefully measures Tom for a wheelchair, taking into account his specific interests and lifestyle. For example, does the wheelchair need to be lightweight and able to be dismantled easily to go into a car? Given Tom's lack of sensation, he is at risk of skin breakdown. To address this the OT needs to provide appropriate pressure-relieving cushions as part of the wheelchair provision, and will also teach Tom routine movements to ensure that the blood flow to the areas he is sitting on is maintained.

The OT also considers the *environment* in which each occupation will be taking place:

◆ What are Tom's home and workplace like?

◆ Is access possible or are modifications to the environment needed, such as ramps at entrances?

This example shows a full range of interventions that an OT may use when considering the person, occupation and environment, and their interaction. With the ability to mobilise restored, capacity is opened up for Tom to increase his occupational engagement in other key life areas such as work, study, leisure and socialising.

The number of OTs has grown substantially over the last decade. Occupational Therapy Board of Australia (2018) data confirm the number of registered OTs increased by 58% from 2013 to 2018. Historically, the vast majority of OTs in Australia have been employed by government or non-government agencies. However, this is changing and over more recent times there has been growth in the number of therapists moving into private practice. From 2013 to 2016 the number of solo private practitioners increased by 24%, which was a higher proportion of growth than most other work settings (Department of Health 2018). Key private-practice areas include working with children, work injury prevention and management, mental health, home modifications, driver assessment, hand injuries, rehabilitation and disability. The increase in private practice reflects the fact that funding streams have also increased for private practice in many areas. As outlined in Chapter 1, Tuohy (1999) points out that the health reform agenda continues to shape the mix of private versus public provision of health care. For example, prior to the implementation of the **National Disability Insurance Scheme (NDIS)**, disability providers were mostly block-funded with government funding being given to key agencies to provide set services. The NDIS has seen a shift from block funding to funding individualised, goal-based services. The NDIS promotes a fee-for-service model that enables different agencies and also private practitioners to take advantage of direct payment.

Increasing delivery of services through programs like the NDIS potentially offers clients more choice in health practitioners. However, it could also lead to more fragmented care. OTs frequently work with other health professionals in an interdisciplinary team, as outlined in Chapter 1. Private practice can potentially make this harder and require considerable effort by practitioners to ensure that intervention is coordinated for their clients. Case study 24.1 highlights the role of occupational therapy and how interdisciplinary practice is important in meeting the needs of clients.

Case Study 24.1

Providing occupational therapy in an interdisciplinary context

Jacob is 2.5 years old and has been referred to an early childhood development team by his mother, Ruth, because he is not yet talking. Ruth and Jacob meet with two members of the interdisciplinary team, an OT and a **speech pathologist (SP)**. After a brief time where they play together, getting comfortable in the play space, the role of the service and the purpose of this initial meeting are explained.

Continued

The OT talks with Ruth and takes an in-depth developmental, medical and occupational history of Jacob and his family. She gains a sense of what has happened in this boy's life to date, and how this might be impacting on his learning and development. She establishes a relationship with Ruth that honours and respects Ruth's role as the expert in Jacob's life, and begins to build a therapeutic partnership that will underpin future interventions. She also gains a sense of the environments in which Jacob interacts (home, child care, etc.) and how these may influence his development. The questions she asks help to establish a sense of how considerations of safety, employment and financial security, nutrition, physical activity and sleep may be influencing health and well-being for this boy and his family. She also gains a sense of how Ruth is feeling and what support or challenges she has in her role as his mother and in any other key roles she plays.

During this time, the SP plays with Jacob and gains a sense of his capacities and challenges. The OT and SP then swap over and the SP develops her connection with Ruth, explaining what she has noticed about Jacob's play and communication and checking whether this is typical for him. She then asks specific questions that may shed more light on Jacob's speech and language development while the OT interacts with Jacob and gains a sense of his fine and gross motor skills, play styles and preferences and sensory responses.

Once the initial information is gathered, the OT and SP discuss with Ruth their observations, any recommendations that could be put into action straight away, and jointly develop a therapy plan. Following the session, the SP and OT write a summary which captures the family's circumstances as well as their combined assessment of Jacob's speech and language skills, fine and gross motor skills, concentration and attention, sensory responses, play styles and skills, and how he responds to his mother, the therapists and the therapy environment. This information is discussed at the weekly interdisciplinary team meeting, which includes the OT, SP, child psychologist, social worker, physiotherapist and dietitian. Jacob and his family's needs are prioritised and a service plan is agreed on. A copy of this is sent to Ruth.

Case study questions

1 What are the advantages for Ruth and Jacob of this interdisciplinary approach?
2 How does this interdisciplinary approach strengthen the occupational therapy approach and reduce costs and waiting times for occupational therapy specifically and the health service as a whole?
3 What might be some challenges of working in an interdisciplinary team?

Summary

This chapter has provided information on the occupational therapy profession, in particular:

- An in-depth understanding of occupation and how its therapeutic use underpins occupational therapy. Occupations are activities that hold meaning and value for people. Occupation influences people's health and well-being and shapes our identity.
- Occupational science is the study of human occupation and all its complexity.
- Occupational justice considers issues of rights, equity and justice from an occupational point of view, and contributes another perspective to contemporary local and global health issues.
- Occupational therapy has developed from its early days in large mental health asylums to a progressive profession working across many sectors and undertaking many roles. These include clinical, academic, managerial, advocacy and support roles.
- Educational programs within Australia are at Bachelor's or Master's degree level.
- Occupational therapy is a registered profession under the Australian Health Practitioner Regulation Agency, and therapists are required to undertake regular continuing professional development. Occupational Therapy Australia operates as the peak body representing occupational therapists across the country.
- Occupational therapists work in a client-centred framework, and specifically consider aspects of the person, the occupation and the environment in their assessment and therapy.
- The number of occupational therapy positions has grown considerably over the past decade. Therapists are increasingly finding employment in private practice, mainly because of different funding streams becoming available from the state and federal governments.

Review Questions

1 Define 'occupation', and describe how it influences health and well-being.
2 Explain how occupational science relates to occupational therapy.
3 What does an occupational perspective on health and justice contribute to the Australian health care system?
4 Why do registration boards, and many professional associations, require health professionals to provide evidence of continuing professional education?
5 Where do occupational therapists generally work, and how is this changing? What are the factors that are driving this? Apply Bacchi's analysis discussed in Chapter 1 and work through the six questions when considering how the NDIA policy is impacting on the delivery of health care services.

References

American Occupational Therapy Association, 2014. Occupational therapy practice framework: domain and process, 3rd edition. Am. J. Occup. Ther. 68 (Suppl. 1), S1–S51.

Australian Health Practitioner Regulation Agency 2018 AHPRA Annual Report 2017 / 18. www.ahpra.gov. au/annualreport/2018/national-boards.html.

Backman, C., 2010. Occupational balance and wellbeing. In: Schell, B., Gillen, G., Scaffa, M. (Eds.), Willard and Spackman's Occupational Therapy, twelfth ed. Lippincott Williams & Wilkins, Philadelphia, pp. 231–249.

Bearup, C., 1996. Occupational Therapists in Wartime. Australian Association of Occupational Therapists, Adelaide.

Csikszentmihalyi, M., 1993. Activity and happiness: toward a science of occupation. J. Occup. Sci. 1 (1), 38–42.

Department of Health, 2018. Occupational therapy 2016 fact sheet. Department of Health, Canberra. https://hwd.health.gov.au/webapi/customer/documents/factsheets/2016/Occupational%20 Therapy%20-%202016.pdf.

Department of Health, 2019. Characteristics of each occupational category. Department of Health, Canberra. http://www.health.gov.au/internet/publications/publishing.nsf/Content/mental-ba-eval-c -toc~mental-ba-eval-c-2~mental-ba-eval-c-2-1#2.1.3.

Guptill, C., 2012. Injured professional musicians and the complex relationship between occupation and health. J. Occup. Sci. 19 (3), 258–270.

Hocking, C., 2017. Occupational justice as social justice: the moral claim for inclusion. J. Occup. Sci. 24 (1), 29–42. doi:10.1080/14427591.2017.1294016.

Occupational Therapy Australia, 2015. Adequacy of existing residential care arrangements available for young people with severe physical, mental or intellectual disabilities in Australia. www.otaus.com.au/ news-events/id/311.

Occupational Therapy Australia, 2019. About us. https://www.otaus.com.au/about/about-the-association.

Occupational Therapy Board of Australia (OTBA), 2013. Continuing professional development. OTBA, Melbourne. https://www.occupationaltherapyboard.gov.au/Codes-Guidelines.aspx.

Occupational Therapy Board of Australia (OTBA), 2018. Statistics. https://www.occupationaltherapyboard. gov.au/About/Statistics.aspx.

Occupational Therapy Council (OTC), 2013. Accreditation standards for entry-level occupational therapy education programs, OTC, Perth. otcouncil.com.au/wp-content/uploads/2012/09/Accred-Standards-December-2013.pdf.

Phelan, S.K., Kinsella, E.A., 2014. Occupation and identity: perspectives of children with disabilities and their parents. J. Occup. Sci. 21 (3), 334–356.

Schell, B., Scaffa, M., Gillen, G., et al., 2014. Contemporary occupational therapy practice. In: Schell, B., Gillen, G., Scaffa, M. (Eds.), Willard and Spackman's Occupational Therapy, twelfth ed. Lippincott Williams & Wilkins, Philadelphia, pp. 47–58.

Townsend, E., Wilcock, A.A., 2004. Occupational justice and client centred practice: a dialogue in progress. Can. J. Occup. Ther. 71 (2), 75–87.

Tuohy, C., 1999. Accidental Logics: The Dynamics of Change in the Health Care Arena in United States, Britain and Canada. OUP, New York.

United Nations (UN) 1948. Universal declaration of human rights. UN, Geneva. https://www.un.org/en/ universal-declaration-human-rights/index.html.

Whiteford, G., 2000. Occupational deprivation: global challenge in the new millennium. Br. J. Occup. Ther. 63 (5), 200–204.

Wilcock, A.A., Hocking, C., 2015. An Occupational Perspective on Health, third ed. SLACK Incorporated, Thorofare NJ, pp. 390–419.

World Federation of Occupational Therapists (WFOT), 2006. Position Statement on Human Rights (CM2006). WFOT, Perth.

World Federation of Occupational Therapists (WFOT), 2012. Definition of Occupational Therapy. WFOT, Perth.

World Federation of Occupational Therapists (WFOT), 2019. Partners. https://www.wfot.org/about/partners.

Wright-St Clair, V., Hocking, C., 2014. Occupational science. In: Schell, B., Gillen, G., Scaffa, M. (Eds.), Willard and Spackman's Occupational Therapy, twelfth ed. Lippincott Williams & Wilkins, Philadelphia, pp. 82–93.

Further Reading

American Occupational Therapy Association, 2014. Occupational therapy practice framework: domain and process. Am. J. Occup. Ther. 68 (Suppl. 1), S1–S51.

Brown, T., Bourke-Taylor, H., Isbel, S., et al., 2017. Occupational Therapy in Australia: Professional and Practice Issues. Allen & Unwin, Crows Nest, NSW.

Burnett, S., 2018. Personal and social contexts of disability: implications for occupational therapists. In: Pendleton, H., Schultz-Krohn, W. (Eds.), Pedretti's Occupational Therapy: Practice Skills for Physical Dysfunction, eighth ed. Elsevier Mosby, Missouri, pp. 71–91.

Dickie, V., 2014. What is occupation? In: Schell, B., Gillen, G., Scaffa, M. (Eds.), Willard and Spackman's Occupational Therapy, twelfth ed. Lippincott Williams & Wilkins, Philadelphia, pp. 2–8.

Online Resources

Advance Healthcare Network RehabInsider for Occupational Therapy Practitioners – an informative online magazine about occupational therapy: http://rehab-insider.advanceweb.com/category/ot/.

Occupational Therapy Australia – the peak body representing occupational therapists in Australia; this website has sections for students to learn more about the profession: www.otaus.com.au.

Occupational Therapy Board of Australia – the regulatory board for occupational therapy in Australia has statistics on registered therapists, plus the guidelines and standards that are required to be met: www.occupationaltherapyboard.gov.au.

World Federation of Occupational Therapists – this website can be used to obtain information about occupational therapy internationally: www.wfot.org.

Young People in Nursing Homes National Alliance – this website contains further information about the issue of young people with significant disabilities and complex support needs being accommodated in aged-care facilities in Australia: www.ypinh.org.au.

CHAPTER 25

The continued professionalisation of paramedics and prehospital care

Louise Reynolds and Elizabeth Goble

Key learning outcomes

When you finish this chapter you should be able to:

- discuss the nature of the work of paramedics, including workload, funding and skills
- discuss the evolving models of prehospital care delivery in meeting service user demands and community expectations
- describe the interdisciplinary relationship between paramedics and other health professionals
- analyse the emergence of paramedic as a profession with focus on the way industrial and education reform facilitated these changes
- paramedic registration and how this relates to evolving professionalism.

Key terms and abbreviations

ambulance ramping
ambulance service
Australian Health Practitioner Regulation Agency (AHPRA)
community paramedicine
Council of Ambulance Authorities (CAA)
emergency department (ED)
extended care paramedics (ECPs)
handover
intensive care paramedics (ICPs)
protected title
registration
regulation
user pays

Introduction

In this chapter we will discuss the continued professionalisation and evolving role of paramedics in delivering prehospital care in Australia. Paramedics provide care in the community, both emergency and non-emergency, with an ever increasing scope of practice. This expanding scope of practice includes the ability to 'treat and not transport' or to refer patients to different health care providers or services, enabling patients to avoid or delay unnecessary hospital admission.

At the time of writing, the term of paramedic has now been deemed to be a **protected title**, meaning those eligible for registration with the **Australian Health Practitioner Regulation Agency (AHPRA)** can be called paramedic (this will be discussed later in the chapter). Despite the inclusion of 'paramedic' to the AHPRA register, paramedic care improves health outcomes

(Bjorklund et al. 2006; Quinn et al. 2009; Ranchord et al. 2009), yet are categorised by the Australian Bureau of Statistics (ABS) (2013) as a Health and Welfare Support Worker, rather than as a professional.

Employment and education

Paramedics are typically employed by a state government **ambulance service,** which is defined as a method of transporting a person to hospital or other medical care facility (*Health Care Act* (SA) 2008). However, paramedics are increasingly being employed in the defence forces, private sector for non-emergency transport, mass public events, occupational safety, and industrial and mining sites. Once qualified, paramedics can gain further specialisations in their clinical treatment: extended care, mental health, hazardous rescue and remote area wilderness.

In Australia, the minimum qualification is an Associate Degree, an Advanced Diploma or a Diploma (ABS 2013; Paramedics Australasia 2016), although in many states the only way to become and be employed as a paramedic is through firstly obtaining a 3-year undergraduate Bachelor degree (Australian Qualification Framework (AQF) Level 7). In Table 25.1, at the time of writing, is an outline of the type of education requirements for employment with state ambulance services. As you can see, most state services have pre-employment pathways with the exception of two states that retain some form of vocational pathway options.

Paramedics can be both employed full time or work in a voluntary capacity for an ambulance service. Volunteers are typically providing care in rural and remote regions. Whether employed or

TABLE 25.1 EMPLOYMENT / RECRUITMENT TYPES								
Employment	NSW	VIC	QLD	WA	SA	TAS	ACT	NT
Graduate employment	Y	Y	Y	Y	Y	Y	Y	Y
Vocational training / recruitment	Y			* employed while undertaking tertiary studies				

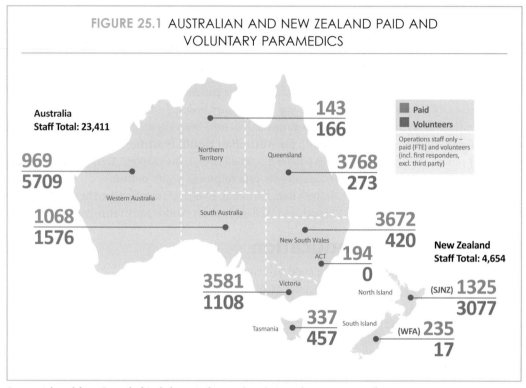

FIGURE 25.1 AUSTRALIAN AND NEW ZEALAND PAID AND VOLUNTARY PARAMEDICS

Sources: Adapted from Council of Ambulance Authorities (2018). Annual report 2017–18 (https://www.caa.net.au/images/documents/caa_annual_reports/CAA_Annual_Report_2017-18.pdf); Productivity Commission (2019). Report on government services. https://www.pc.gov.au/research/ongoing/report-on-government-services/2019/health/ambulance-services/rogs-2019-parte-chapter11.pdf

voluntary, the scope of practice, that is the range and type of medical treatment being provided, will depend on the qualification and training undertaken. As seen in Fig. 25.1, the mix of paid and volunteer paramedics varies from state to state.

In 2017–18 the Australian ambulance services:

◆ employed nearly 17,000 full-time workers
◆ had over 6500 volunteers
◆ had over 3000 first responders.

Legislation and funding of state-based ambulance services

Ambulance services are state-based organisations, with all but WA and NT being administered by state governments. In WA and NT, St John Ambulance is the principal provider (Productivity Commission, 2019). This is in part due to the historical origins of various state and territory ambulance services which were provided by non-government organisations (NGOs) such as St John Ambulance. Some of these services were later absorbed and are now administered wholly by respective state governments.

Nearly 25% of the Australian public assumes that Medicare covers ambulance services (Finder AU n.d.). The Commonwealth Government does not fund ambulance services and they are not included in Medicare or any healthcare agreements. If Medicare were to fund ambulance services, Medicare would need to increase by 0.3% to cover the costs (Livingston et al. 2007).

As you can see in Table 25.2, the funding for ambulance services comes from direct state (or territory) revenue, insurance schemes and user payments. The Productivity Commission (2019) reports that the total expenditure for the Australian ambulance industry is nearly $3.6 billion which is an annual growth of nearly 3.7% since 2013–14. Even with these different funding models, some ambulance services are provided free of charge with others requiring insurance cover making them a **user pays** service (see Table 25.2). Insurance can be purchased through the ambulance service or through private health insurance.

Nationally, 3.5 million incidents were reported to ambulance services, in which 4.4 million ambulances responded and assessed 3.3 million patients (Productivity Commission 2019). While largely experiencing growth in patients transported, some states were busier than others. In explaining these variations, Gaughan et al. (2018), Honeyford et al. (2018) Lowthian et al. (2011) and Schierholtz et al. (2018) identified a complex array of various factors: ageing population, changes in social support, accessibility of services and increased awareness. With the dual function of prehospital care being treatment and transport, the usual destination for the sick and injured is a public hospital **emergency department (ED)**.

What Fig. 25.2 (Productivity Commission 2019) also shows is the variation of activity of ambulance services across Australia. This also extends to the type of patient presented to emergency departments. In 2017–18 over 3.7 million patients were assessed, treated and transported to emergency departments by ambulance, composed of 37.3% emergency, 35.8% urgent and 26.9% non-emergency (Productivity Commission 2019). Yet, it is claimed more than 50% of these hospital transfers are avoidable (NHPA 2013).

Yet, emergency patient presentations to emergency departments are only a small proportion of workload for hospitals (<12%) (Productivity Commission 2019). Not all patients seen by paramedics are taken to hospital (Productivity Commission 2019), with a growing number of patients being able to be 'treated and not transported' or being referred to other pathways of care. Of the total patients seen by paramedics in 2017–18, 15.5% are treated and not transported (Productivity Commission 2019). Increasing, this model of treat and not transport patients means that paramedics are leaving patients at home and referring them to follow-up care from health services other than the ED.

With over seven million people attending an emergency department (AIHW 2017), many of who are later admitted, hospitals at various times are unable to cope. A chain reaction or flow on effect occurs when large numbers of people present to an emergency department at one time, say during winter. This effect causes **ambulance ramping,** which is when no suitable ED bed is available for a patient who arrives by ambulance at hospital, preventing them from being admitted to hospital (Gaughan et al. 2018; Hammond et al. 2012; Honeyford et al. 2018). With the paramedic still delivering treatment to the patient on board, the ambulance, is forced to wait outside the ED until such time as the patient can be accommodated and assessed by hospital staff.

TABLE 25.2 STATE AMBULANCE SERVICE LEGISLATION, INSURANCE AND REVENUE

State	Legislation	Insurance required	Fees	Total revenue $M
New South Wales	Health Services Act (NSW) 1997	Insurance required but free for some concession card holders and specific groups	$382.00 call out $3.44 per km	1022.9
Victoria	Ambulance Services Act (Vic) 1986	Insurance needed but concession card holders free (clinically necessary treatment & transport	$1234 (metro) $1820 (for regional)	1048.6
Queensland	Ambulance Service Act (Qld) 1991	Free service		755
Western Australia		Insurance needed Some concessions for specific groups	$967 (for life threatening-urgent conditions)	289.5
South Australia	Health Care Act (SA) 2008	Insurance needed Some concessions for specific groups	$976 call out + $5.60 per km	3.5.4
Tasmania	Ambulance Service Act (Tas) 1982	Free service		75.8
Australian Capital Territory	Emergencies Act (ACT) 2004	Insurance needed Some concessions for specific groups Free for concession card holders	$936 (treatment and transport) + $12 per km travelled outside of ACT	50.7
Northern Territory		Insurance needed Free for concession card holders	$745 call out + $5.10 per km	34.5

Sources: Productivity Commission (2019). Report on government services. https://www.pc.gov.au/research/ongoing/report-on-government-services/2019/health/ambulance-services/rogs-2019-parte-chapter11.pdf; ABC News (2018). Ambulance costs around Australia: why is it free in some states and not others? http://www.abc.net.au/news/2018-07-20/ambulance-fees-around-australia/10015172

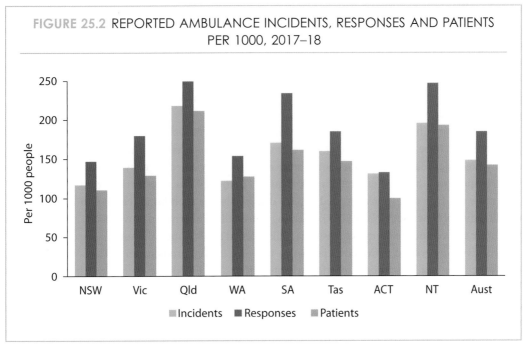

FIGURE 25.2 REPORTED AMBULANCE INCIDENTS, RESPONSES AND PATIENTS PER 1000, 2017–18

Source: Productivity Commission (2019). Report on government services. https://www.pc.gov.au/research/ongoing/report-on-government-services/2019/health/ambulance-services/rogs-2019-parte-chapter11.pdf

A root cause analysis would determine that ramping is due to ageing population, increases in co-morbid chronic conditions, changes in family structures and social support, pricing (free service), reduced access to other primary health care services (such as after hours GP services), increased health awareness and changes in community expectations, and lack of alternate services (Gaughan et al. 2018; Honeyford et al. 2018; Livingston et al. 2007; Lowthian et al. 2011).

PAUSE
for
REFLECTION
...

Thinking ahead to your future career in prehospital care, have you identified your employer of choice? Have you considered any other potential employers in the private sector? Or even overseas ambulance services?

Evolving roles to address 'problems' for service delivery

There has been a range of innovations in service delivery models in order to cope with the increased demand. One example is up skilling paramedics or expanding their scope of practice to include clinical skills such as suturing. Some ambulance services have introduced other ways to operate more efficiently by changing various aspects of their operations. This has included outsourcing their non-emergency transfer services to private providers, introducing civilian call takers into the communications centre, outsourcing major event standbys, first aid training and paramedic education to other providers. The emergence of various private providers means that the 'marketplace' of prehospital care services has now become increasingly competitive with over 122 permanent private sector employers of paramedics Australia wide (Townsend & Eburn 2014).

The tension is managing demand and community expectations for ambulance services. Often patients expect to be treated at hospital, however what is perceived as requiring urgent and immediate care by the caller may in actual fact not require attendance by an emergency ambulance paramedic nor transport to a hospital emergency department. Being able to screen triple zero (000) calls to determine the type of response needed service delivery is one such initiative used to filter demand (Audit Office of New South Wales 2017), referring those calls to alternate pathways such as the national telephone advice line Healthdirect Australia, falls referral service and other outreach services.

The evolving role of paramedics is also in response to the problem for patients being able to access their General Practitioner, particularly after hours. As noted elsewhere (see Chapter 21) and by Duckett et al. (2013), GPs who are often the first point of contact for a patient with the health care system are unevenly distributed through our community. This is even more evident in outer metropolitan, rural and remote areas, which have fewer GPs than in major cities (Duckett 2014), with the shortfall requiring to be absorbed by ambulance services.

The community paramedic has evolved to respond to the lack of health care provision in rural and remote areas of Australia (Duckett et al. 2013). The goal of **community paramedicine** is to fill the gaps in the health care system (Wingrove 2011). This is particularly evident in North America and Australia (Martin & O'Meara 2019; O'Meara 2014; O'Meara et al. 2016) facilitated by telehealth technology (Choi et al. 2016) (see Chapter 16). While community paramedicine is not a new concept, as noted by Garza (2008) who described a Canadian initiative where lengthy response times and transportation were common, community paramedics now attend to the health care needs of many frail, elderly people living with chronic co-morbid conditions requiring blood glucose monitoring, insulin administration, medication compliance, falls assessment, phlebotomy, and immunisations. All these tasks can safely be incorporated into an expanded suite of skills and treatments provided by paramedics (Martin & O'Meara 2019) and now with the evolving use of e-health technology.

In Australia, the further training and upskilling of paramedics has seen the development of **Intensive Care Paramedics (ICPs) and Extended Care Paramedics (ECPs).** ICPs have received further training to provide advanced treatment to those patients who have specific health care needs (e.g. severe trauma or medical conditions). Further up-skilling of ICPs has led to the introduction of ECPs, who are able to treat patients in their homes and reduce congestion in EDs. Various states (WA (Finn et al. 2013), NSW and SA (SA Health (n.d.); Grantham et al. 2010)) and overseas services (New Zealand) have introduced ECPs as a strategy to reduce presentations, initially as trials, but once successful on a permanent basis. An evaluation by Thompson et al. (2014a, b) reported that ECPs are a cost effective and safe alternative with savings of between $411 and $998 per patient as a result of avoiding presentation at the emergency department. Their research shows that ECPs treated 27% of patients with general symptoms (headache, fever, fainting, sick, unwell) who did not need to be transported to an ED.

PAUSE
for
REFLECTION
...

Community Paramedicine is a role very similar to that of a community health nurse, or district nurse. How might the role differ? Find out what community nursing services are provided in your state or territory and what forms of community paramedicine are also available. Is there an overlap? What potential conflicts, if any, could potentiate between these two professional groups?

Interprofessional practice

You will recall from the definition of interprofessional practice in Chapter 1, prehospital care – that is, the work of paramedics – draws heavily on interprofessional practice. This is because on arrival to the ED, paramedics '**handover**' care of the patient to the triage nurse. Paramedics can remain working alongside nurses and doctors primarily in the ED, such as in the country, rural or remote areas, and it is in this environment where succinct and thorough communications skills predominate.

In order for the continuity of care, the handover can be challenging. Between the paramedic and the receiver of the information, which could be either a Registered Nurse or a doctor, there are two separate activities: 'doing' patient care assessment and 'listening' to the information (Owen et al. 2009). The handover, as a skill, is not without complications, with US data revealing an accuracy rate of 36%; however, the authors acknowledged that this might be confounded by inexperience (Scott et al. 2003). The Australian data differs, though, as Jenkin et al. (2007) noted that paramedics needed to repeat their handover when the environment was hectic. However, Yong et al. (2007) reported that 90% paramedics' handover details for major trauma presentations were relevant.

PAUSE
for
REFLECTION
...

The nature of the paramedic work with hospital avoidance through referrals to other services highlights the interprofessional relationships required for continuity of care. This includes working with outreach services, home and community care providers for respite and aged care, palliative care, in-home nursing care and allied health professionals.

The relationship between paramedicine, nursing and medicine offers unique opportunities for collaboration for 21st-century health care. With universities offering flexible pathways into health professional education with combined nursing/paramedic degree, double degree and honours programs, there is great sharing of knowledge and skills (Box 25.1). However, many paramedic academics see the development of a specialised body of knowledge as important and further research is being undertaken to provide distinct boundaries (see Hein 2009; Madigan 2013; O'Donnell 2006;

BOX 25.1 AUSTRALIAN AND NEW ZEALAND
UNIVERSITY PROVIDERS OF PARAMEDIC
UNDERGRADUATE DEGREE PROGRAMS AND
HOMEPAGES

Australian Capital Territory (ACT)
Australian Catholic University (ACT, Vic, Qld, NSW) http://www.acu.edu.au/

New South Wales (NSW)
Charles Sturt University http://www.csu.edu.au/
University of Western Sydney http://www.uws.edu.au/

Queensland (Qld)
Griffith University http://www.griffith.edu.au/
James Cook University http://www.jcu.edu.au/
Queensland University of Technology http://www.qut.edu.au/
University of Queensland http://www.uq.edu.au/
University of Southern Queensland https://www.usq.edu.au/
University of Sunshine Coast http://www.usc.edu.au/

South Australia (SA)
Flinders University http://www.flinders.edu.au/

Tasmania (Tas)
University of Tasmania (Tas, NSW) http://www.utas.edu.au/

Victoria (Vic)
Federation University Australia http://federation.edu.au/
LaTrobe University http://www.latrobe.edu.au/
Monash University http://www.monash.edu.au/
Victoria University http://www.vu.edu.au/

Western Australia (WA)
Curtin University https://www.curtin.edu.au/
Edith Cowan University http://www.ecu.edu.au/

O'Meara 2002; Reynolds 2008; Williams 2011). Unlike nursing, paramedics are not seeking professionalisation through a separation from working 'under' medical supervision rather to working alongside. This may well be a result of the youthfulness of the profession, the close control still exercised by medicine over paramedic practice, a pragmatic response to power, or a reflection of their role. There are parallels between paramedicine, nursing (see Chapter 23) and midwifery (Chapter 22) in their relationship to medicine (Chapter 21). Consider that each of these professions draw on the same knowledge of anatomy, physiology and patient care treatment and therapies. Yet, the differences lie in how the treatment is delivered.

Case study 25.1 outlines an example of the work of paramedics as they engage in patient care.

Dorothy is an 84-year-old female living independently at home, with some supported care through her local council's Home and Community Care program. She has a number of chronic conditions such as atrial fibrillation, hypertension and hyperlipidemia. These are well managed by her local general practitioner (GP) and medication. Dorothy is a widow, and her family lives interstate.

Dorothy is an avid gardener, and has a fall in her backyard. Wearing her personal safety alarm, on a necklace pendant, she activates it by pressing the button. This raises the alarm to the state ambulance service which dispatches' a nearby crew to Dorothy's house.

Initially, the paramedic crew couldn't locate Dorothy and notify the Communication Centre to contact the police, as they may have to break into her house. However, part of the conditions of her personal alarm subscription was the installation of a key in a locked box in a location recorded on the ambulance service computer system. This information was relayed to the attending crew who were able to gain access into the property once the police was in attendance.

Dorothy was found in the rear garden complaining of pain to her left hip. The paramedic crew assessed her injuries and made a provisional diagnosis of fractured neck of femur. Along with splinting, posturing, and initial pain relief, the paramedic crew prepared Dorothy for transport to the local public hospital. However, the pain relief offered by the paramedic crew was not sufficient in easing Dorothy's pain, so the crew called for Intensive Care paramedic backup. The ICP who attended was able to give her a different type of analgesia that was more effective in relieving her pain.

The paramedic crew handed over care to the emergency department triage Registered Nurse. After a period of time, Dorothy was transferred to ward where she underwent surgery for a hip replacement. After a week, she was transferred by non-emergency ambulance to a rehabilitation hospital for ongoing treatment to help her regain her mobility.

Once she was discharged home, Dorothy had some ongoing issues with her surgical wound on her hip, which remained problematic in terms of healing. Dorothy had in-home support from the Royal District Nursing Service for her wound management. As it was after hours and her GP clinic was closed, so the RDNS RN rang the ambulance service as he was concerned about the condition of the wound heading into a weekend. The call taker in the Communications Centre through questioning the RN dispatched an Extended Care Paramedic to assess Dorothy. The ECP was able to treat and assess her wound with some other medications and made a referral that Dorothy follows up with her GP the next day.

Case study questions

1 What important information would the paramedic providing the initial handover to the Registered Nurse at the Emergency Department triage about Dorothy's social situation? Why would this be important for noting by the hospital?

Continued

2 Identify the various points where Dorothy's care has been transferred. At these points, consider the type of information that is being transferred along with her care needs.

3 Consider how with an ageing population and older people living in their homes, the types of other care providers that paramedics may come into contact with, such as the Royal District Nursing Service in caring for elderly people. Identify five (5) other providers that paramedics may come into contact with.

Hazards of paramedic practice

Because of the nature of prehospital treatment, paramedics are subject to significant stressors and potential hazards. They attend to people in distress or agitation, make critical decisions in life-threatening situations, and are continually confronted with potentially traumatic scenes (Arial et al. 2011; Holland 2011; LeBlanc et al. 2011; Shepherd & Wild 2014; van der Ploeg & Kleber 2003). Because of these factors, paramedics have one of the highest rates of burnout compared with other health professions (LeBlanc et al. 2011). More alarmingly, an Australian Senate Inquiry revealed in 2010 that, in the preceding 12-year period, 110 emergency services personnel took their own lives (Ashbury et al. 2018).

In order to combat this over the last two decades, many ambulance services have incorporated a formal Peer Support program and have occupational psychologists available for consultation. The historical stigma attached to the utilisation of such resources seems to be lessening, and when available it has been shown to reduce distress, particularly by increasing the level of perceived colleague/organisational support (Gouweloos-Trines et al. 2017).

Compounding the psychological stressors, professions such as paramedicine, that involve close contact with clients or patients, are at greater risk of being exposed to client initiated workplace violence (Brough 2005). This includes intimidation, sexual harassment, and verbal, physical and sexual abuse. In both international and Australian studies it has been found that around 80% of paramedics have experienced a form of workplace violence, most predominantly verbal abuse (Boyle & McKenna 2017; Boyle et al. 2007).

The tension is how to protect the paramedic in a workplace that is unpredictable. It is estimated that 87.5% of paramedics in South Australia and Victoria had been exposed to a range of violent assaults and 38% of paramedics claimed they had endured incidents of physical abuse (Boyle et al. 2007). The risks associated with an increasingly violent workplace have resulted in higher than average injury rates and even fatalities for Australian paramedics (Maguire et al. 2018). Alarmingly, paramedics experience injury rates seven times higher than the national average for serious injury, and six times the national average for fatality. The higher than average rate of injury can be explained by the nature of the work: lifting, falls, motor vehicle accidents, assaults, and mental stress (Maguire et al. 2018). In order to prepare students, paramedic curriculum includes topics such as physical fitness and wellbeing, manual handling and safety work practices, such as 'breakaway' training (Stephens, 2017).

PAUSE
for
REFLECTION
...
Given the high rates of injury associated with the work of paramedics, what are your thoughts about what is an acceptable risk in your workplace? You might like to refer back to Chapter 14, and consider some of the points raised about the employer and employees responsibilities in their workplace. Consider whether these risks would be acceptable in your current workplace.

Reform in the ambulance industry

Over the last 10 years, two significant industrial reforms have taken place in prehospital care / paramedicine: pre-employment education and recognition of professional remuneration. These two reforms, separate in themselves yet interrelated, both recognise the emergence of paramedics as a health professional.

The transfer of paramedic education into the higher education sector was in part a continuation of the improvements in the quality of paramedic training that began in the late 1980s, with momentum gaining traction in the mid 1990s with support of the peak employer body, the **Council of Ambulance Authorities (CAA)**. Prior to paramedics being university educated, their training was delivered in-house and primarily from on-the-job experiences. Often there were no formalised or accredited education programs available. Through various industrial campaigns highlighting the need for improved training and professionalisation of the work of paramedics, vocationally based curriculum was developed to prepare ambulance officers for the increasingly specialised clinical work and meet the requirements of a formal and recognised qualification (Reynolds 2008). Yet, in Australia, though universities have been delivering paramedic education for over 20 years, there still remain critics of whether 'paramedics need degrees' (Ludwig 2018).

In moving from competency-based training to higher education, paramedic students are required to understand two processes: the 'how' and the 'why' of patient care. In understanding the 'why' is the development of critical thinking and problem-solving approach, which is the basis for university higher education. The CAA spearheaded further reforms in paramedic education in the mid-1990s with the development of accreditation standards for the various university and VET level programs now operating in Australia. Leaders in paramedic education are engaged in paramedic research (such as O'Donnell 2006; O'Meara 2002; Reynolds 2008; Williams 2011) by questioning why paramedics undertake certain clinical actions and examined the validity of those actions in the prehospital setting through greater understanding of the operational environment. You will no doubt have in your program of studies a research topic that allows you to gain knowledge and skills of research practices. This then leads further to skilled paramedic practitioners who can question the evidence basis of many standard patient care actions (which had been adopted primarily from the disciplines of medicine and nursing) and translated to the out of hospital environment whereby its efficacy and effectiveness can be further evaluated.

As of 2019, there are over 7500 paramedic university students (Table 25.3).

PAUSE *for* REFLECTION ...

Looking at the number of student paramedics currently undertaking their studies (Table 25.3), what if any are your concerns about finding employment? With limited employment opportunities in some Australian states due to low staff turnover, what alternatives have you or would you consider?

Registration versus regulation

For some time, the term 'paramedic' was not a 'protected title'. The ability to use the title of 'paramedic', in the same way as 'nurse', 'teacher' or 'lawyer' was not yet protected through registration except in South Australia and Tasmania, along with a proposed bill for Victoria (*Health Practitioner Regulation National Law Act* (SA) 2010; Townsend & Eburn 2014). This meant that there were no unifying standards or codes of conduct to regulate those who used or practised as a paramedic.

A federal government recommendation (Parliament of Australia 2016) argued that the registration of paramedics recognised the importance of their contribution to public safety, the level of complexity of work and their public standing. This was part of a movement that argued that registration is part of the ongoing professionalisation process (Reynolds 2004), and indeed is necessary for paramedics.

A registration body is there to protect the public (Duckett 2014; Eburn & Bendall 2010; Health and Care Professions Council (HCPC) 2018) as it sets standards and codes of conduct which the

TABLE 25.3 ENROLMENTS AND UNIVERSITY PROVIDERS OF PARAMEDIC PROGRAMS

Location	Total enrolments
Australian Capital Territory	190
Queensland	2950
Tasmania	106
Western Australia	773
New South Wales	1062
South Australia	350
Victoria	2080
TOTAL	7511

Source: Productivity Commission (2019). Ambulance services. Chapter 11 in Report on government services. https://www.pc.gov.au/research/ongoing/report-on-government-services/2019/health/ambulance-services/rogs-2019-parte-chapter11.pdf; university homepages

registrant needs to uphold and maintain. These standards have been published by the Paramedicine Board of Australia (2018) and relate to continuing professional development, criminal history, English language skills, indemity insurance and recency of practice. The code of conduct covering paramedics covers various other health professions in what is expected and acceptable behaviour (Paramedicine Board of Australia 2018). However, registration may not be seen as a panacea for professionalism, as recently reported by the increasing complaints by the Health and Care Professions Council (HCPC) in the United Kingdom (UK) (van der Gaag et al. 2017). It is reported that UK paramedics are disproportionally reported to the regulatory body (HCPC), however much of the reporting is done as self referrals, with no further action being taken. In explaining this phenomena, the reasons behind the complaints may be due to the evolving nature of paramedic practice, increased pressure in the workplace and changing public expectations for what is professional behaviour (van der Gaag et al. 2017).

Prior to joining AHPRA, the standards and codes of conduct of paramedics were regulated through their individual state based services, which meant that complaints against their employees are handled internally and lacked transparency. Skill currency, maintenance and accreditation were managed through their employment by their employer, not externally. This meant those paramedics working outside emergency services (such as mining or industrial sites) might not have been able to maintain their skills.

In understanding the delay in gaining paramedic registration, we can turn to Tuohy (1999). She reminds us of the different interest groups involved in changing health care systems. By identifying the vested interests of the various parties, their position on the issue of registration becomes clear. There are two parties involved in the paramedic debate: the employer (that is the state or territory service) and the employee (represented by peak professional body). The employers are represented by the Council of Ambulance Authorities and the professional body by Paramedic Australasia. Both have issued statements (CAA 2008; Paramedics Australasia 2015) reflecting their argument. Paramedic Australasia argue for registration on the basis of risk management for service provision, safety, quality and corporate governance (Paramedics Australasia 2015), while the CAA (2008) stated that paramedics and prehospital care is already highly regulated through the safe systems put in place by employers, therefore negating the need for an external independent body. As of November 2018, AHPRA accepted applications for registration to the Paramedicine Board.

Summary

This chapter has described the funding, innovation, history, interprofessional practice and reforms for paramedics and prehospital care. Paramedics have been successful in attaining health registration with AHPRA and continue to be educated and conduct research. Paramedics have responded to the current pressures in the health care system by up-skilling and targeting their specialised services to include work in the community through expanding their scope of practice. However, alcohol- and drug-fuelled violence directed toward paramedics increasingly makes their workplace unsafe.

Review Questions

1 Identify the tiers of paramedic practitioner and the skills associated with those levels.

2 Identify the impact of registration upon the employment opportunities for paramedics

3 Volunteer ambulance officers deliver basic prehospital care in the rural and remote areas of the country. In what way might this be construed as an issue of inequity for those living in rural and remote areas?

4 List the advantages and disadvantages of shifting pre-employment education of paramedics rather than employer-based vocational training

5 What is the problem facing ambulance services with the increasing violence being experienced by paramedics?

References

ABC News, 2018. Ambulance costs around Australia: why is it free in some states and not others? http://www.abc.net.au/news/2018-07-20/ambulance-fees-around-australia/10015172.

Ambulance Service Act (Qld), 1991. https://www.legislation.qld.gov.au/view/pdf/inforce/current/act-1991-036.

Ambulance Service Act (Tas), 1982. https://www.legislation.tas.gov.au/view/whole/html/inforce/current/act-1982-105.

Ambulance Services Act (Vic), 1986. http://www.legislation.vic.gov.au/domino/Web_Notes/LDMS/LTObject_Store/LTObjSt1.nsf/DDE300B846EED9C7CA257616000A3571/0ACC3D0242728DEFCA2577610017A1D1/$FILE/86-114a036.pdf.

Arial, M., Wild, P., Benoit, D., et al., 2011. Multi-level modelling of aspects associated with poor mental health in a sample of prehospital emergency professionals. Am. J. Ind. Med. 54, 847–857.

Ashbury, E., Rasku, T., Thyler, L., et al., 2018. IPAWS: the International Paramedic Anxiety Wellbeing and Stress study. Emerg. Med. Australas. 30, 132–136.

Audit Office of New South Wales, 2017. Annual report 2016/17. https://www.audit.nsw.gov.au/annual-reports/annual-report-2016-17.

Australian Bureau of Statistics (ABS), 2013. The Australian and New Zealand Standard Classification of Occupations (ANZSCO) version 1.2 (cat. no. 1220.0). ACT, Canberra. http://www.abs.gov.au/ANZSCO.

Australian Institute of Health and Welfare, 2017. Emergency department care 2016–17: Australian hospital statistics. Health services series no. 80. Cat. no. HSE 194. AIHW, Canberra.

Bjorklund, E., Stenestrand, U., Lindback, J., et al., 2006. Pre-hospital thrombolysis delivered by paramedics is associated with reduced time delay and mortality in ambulance-transported real-life patients with ST-elevation myocardial infarction. Eur. Heart J. 27 (10), 1146–1152.

Boyle, M., Koritsas, S., Coles, J., et al., 2007. A pilot study of workplace violence towards paramedics. Emerg. Med. J. 24, 760–763.

Boyle, M., McKenna, L., 2017. Paramedic student exposure to workplace violence during clinical placements – a cross-sectional study. Nurse Educ. Pract. 22, 93–97.

Brough, P., 2005. Workplace violence experienced by paramedics – relationship with social support, job satisfaction, and psychological strain. Aust. J. Disast. Trauma Stud. 2, 1–11.

Choi, B.Y., Blumberg, C., Williams, K., 2016. Mobile integrated health care and community paramedicine: an emerging emergency medical services concept. Ann. Emerg. Med. 67 (3), 361–366.

Council of Ambulance Authorities (CAA), 2008. CAA position statement: Council of Ambulance Authorities views on the regulation of pre-hospital providers. https://www.paramedics.org/content/2009/10/caaregistrationstatement.pdf.

Council of Ambulance Authorities (CAA), 2018. Annual report 2017/18. https://www.caa.net.au/images/documents/caa_annual_reports/CAA_Annual_Report_2017-18.pdf.

Duckett, S., 2014. The need for a regulatory rethink: a perspective from Australia. Fut. Hosp. J. 1 (2), 117–121.

Duckett, S., Breadon, P., Ginnivan, L., 2013. Access All Areas: New Solutions for GP Shortages in Rural Australia. Grattan Institute, Melbourne.

Eburn, M., Bendall, J., 2010. The provision of Ambulance Services in Australia: a legal argument for the national registration of paramedics. J. Emerg. Prim. Health Care 8 (4), article 990414.

Emergencies Act (ACT), 2004. https://www.legislation.act.gov.au/a/2004-28/current/pdf/2004-28.pdf.

Finder AU, no date. Australians misusing ambulance service. https://www.finder.com.au/australians-misusing-ambulance-service.

Finn, J.C., Fatovich, D.M., Arendts, G., et al., 2013. Evidence-based paramedic models of care to reduce unnecessary emergency department attendance–feasibility and safety. BMC Emerg. Med. 13 (1), 13.

Garza, M., 2008, July 26. Beyond EMS: Community paramedics make house calls. http://www.jems.com/article/cardiac-circulation/beyond-ems.

Gaughan, J., Kasteridis, P., Mason, A., et al., 2018. Waits in A&E departments of the English NHS, 2018 International Health Congress, St Hugh's College, Oxford University, 28–30 June. http://www.globalhealthcongress.org/.

Gouweloos-Trines, J., Tyler, M.P., Giummarra, M.J., et al., 2017. Perceived support at work after critical incidents and its relation to psychological distress: a survey among prehospital providers. Emerg. Med. J. 34, 816–822.

Grantham, H., Hein, C., Elliott, R., 2010. South Australian Ambulance Service (SAAS) Extended Care Paramedic (ECP) pilot project. J. Emerg. Prim. Health Care 8 (3), 32.

Hammond, E., Shaban, R.Z., Holzhauser, K., et al., 2012. An exploratory study to examine the phenomenon and practice of ambulance ramping at hospitals within the Queensland Health Southern Districts and the Queensland Ambulance Service. Queensland Health and Griffith University, Brisbane. https://research-repository.griffith.edu.au/bitstream/handle/10072/49997/74885_1.pdf?sequence=1&isAllowed=y.

Health and Care Professions Council (HCPC), 2018. About us. http://www.hcpc-uk.co.uk/aboutus/.

Health Care Act (SA), 2008. https://www.legislation.sa.gov.au/LZ/C/A/HEALTH%20CARE%20ACT%202008/CURRENT/2008.3.AUTH.PDF.

Health Practitioner Regulation National Law (SA), 2010. https://www.legislation.sa.gov.au/LZ/C/A/HEALTH%20PRACTITIONER%20REGULATION%20NATIONAL%20LAW%20(SOUTH%20AUSTRALIA)%20ACT%202010/CURRENT/2010.5.AUTH.PDF.

Health Services Act (NSW), 1997. https://legislation.nsw.gov.au/inforce/59d71b18-59e1-693c-e068
-b6c6de1d2851/1997-154.pdf.

Hein, C., 2009. Extraglottic airway devices and the paramedic user: teaching, learning, patient safety and
device suitability. Unpublished PhD thesis, Flinders University School of Medicine.

Holland, M., 2011. The dangers of detrimental coping in emergency medical services. Prehosp. Emerg.
Care 15 (3), 331–337.

Honeyford, K., Bottle, A., Aylin, P., 2018. ED attendances: an overlooked performance metric? A
statistician's perspective, 2018 International Health Congress, St Hugh's College, Oxford University,
28–30 June. http://www.globalhealthcongress.org/.

Jenkin, A., Abelson-Mitchell, N., Cooper, S., 2007. Patient handover; time for a change? Accid. Emerg. Nurs.
15 (3), 141–147.

LeBlanc, V.R., Regehr, C., Birze, A., et al., 2011. The association between posttraumatic stress, coping, and
acute stress responses in paramedics. Traumatology 17 (4), 10–16.

Livingston, C., Condron, J., Dennekamp, M., et al., 2007. Factors in ambulance demand: options for
funding and forecasting. Australian Institute for Primary Care, Faculty of Health Sciences, Latrobe
University, Vic.

Lowthian, J.A., Jolley, D.J., Curtis, A.J., et al., 2011. The challenge of population ageing: accelerating
demands for emergency ambulance services by older patients 1995–2015. Med. J. Aust. 194 (11),
574–578.

Ludwig, G., 2018. EMS: do you need a college degree to be a paramedic? Firehouse, 1 September. https://
www.firehouse.com/careers-education/article/21013720/
do-you-need-a-college-degrees-to-be-paramedic-firehouse-gary-ludwig.

Madigan, V., 2013. Learning outcomes for human medicine derived from the examination of animal
treatment model. Unpublished PhD thesis, Charles Sturt University, New South Wales.

Maguire, B.J., O'Meara, P., O'Neill, B.J., et al., 2018. Violence against emergency medical services personnel:
a systematic review of the literature. Am. J. Ind. Med. 61 (2), 167–180.

Martin, A.C., O'Meara, P., 2019. Perspectives from the frontline of two North American community
paramedicine programs: an observational, ethnographic study. Rural Remote Health 19, 4888.

National Health Performance Authority (NHPA), 2013. Healthy communities: selected potentially avoidable
hospitalisations in 2011–12. NHPA, Sydney Australia.

O'Donnell, M.J., 2006. A study on the congruence between a baccalaureate paramedic program and
industry competency expectations. EdD thesis, Flinders University School of Education.

O'Meara, P., 2002. Models of ambulance service delivery for rural Victoria. Unpublished PhD thesis,
University of New South Wales School of Public Health and Community Medicine, Sydney.

O'Meara, P., 2014. Community paramedics: a scoping review of their emergence and potential impact. Int.
Paramedic Pract. 4 (1), 5–12.

O'Meara, P., Stirling, C., Ruest, M., et al., 2016. Community paramedicine model of care: an observational,
ethnographic case study. BMC Health Serv. Res. 16 (1), 39.

Owen, C., Hemmings, L., Brown, T., 2009. Lost in translation: maximizing handover effectiveness between paramedics and receiving staff in the emergency department. Emerg. Med. Australas. 21, 102–107. doi:10.1111/j.1742-6723.2009.01168.x.

Paramedicine Board of Australia, 2018. Code of conduct f(interim). https://www.paramedicineboard.gov.au/Professional-standards/Codes-guidelines-and-policies/Code-of-conduct.aspx.

Paramedics Australasia, 2015. Registration. https://www.paramedics.org/?s=registration+.

Paramedics Australasia, 2016. Paramedicine role descriptions. https://paramedics.org/wp-content/uploads/2016/09/PRD_211212_WEBONLY.pdf.

Parliament of Australia, 2016. Establishment of a national registration system for Australian paramedics to improve and ensure patient and community safety. https://www.aph.gov.au/Parliamentary_Business/Committees/Senate/Legal_and_Constitutional_Affairs/Paramedics/Report.

Productivity Commission, 2019. Ambulance services. Chapter 11 in Report on government services. https://www.pc.gov.au/research/ongoing/report-on-government-services/2019/health/ambulance-services/rogs-2019-parte-chapter11.pdf.

Quinn, T., Albrarran, J.W., Cox, H., et al., 2009. Pre-hospital thrombolysis for acute ST segment elevation myocardial infarction: a survey of paramedics' perceptions of their role. Acute Card. Care 11 (1), 52–58.

Ranchord, A.M., Prasad, S., Matsis, P., et al., 2009. Paramedic-administered prehospital thrombolysis is safe and reduces time to treatment. N. Z. Med. J. 122 (1302), 47–53.

Reynolds, L., 2004. Is pre-hospital care really a profession? J. Emerg. Prim. Health Care 2 (1–2), article 990086.

Reynolds, L.C., 2008. Beyond the Frontline: An interpretative ethnography of a statewide ambulance service. Unpublished PhD thesis, University of South Australia Division of Business and Enterprise, Adelaide.

SA Health, (nd). SA Ambulance fact sheet Extended care paramedics (ECPs). http://www.saambulance.com.au/LinkClick.aspx?fileticket=7dKFTy8RTL0%3d&tabid=82.

Schierholtz, T., Carter, D., Kane, A., et al., 2018. Impact of lift assist calls on paramedic services: a descriptive study. Prehosp. Emerg. Care 23 (2), 233–240. doi:10.1080/10903127.2018.1483454.

Scott, L., Brice, J., Baker, C., et al., 2003. An analysis of paramedic verbal reports to physicians in the emergency department trauma room. Prehosp. Emerg. Care 7 (2), 247.

Shepherd, L., Wild, J., 2014. Cognitive appraisals, objectivity and coping in ambulance workers: a pilot study. Emerg. Med. J. 31, 41–44.

Stephens, J., 2017. Benefits of teaching students de-escalation and breakaway skills. Nurs. Times 113 (1), 58.

Thompson, C., Williams, K., Masso, M., 2014a. HWA Expanded scopes of practice program evaluation: national synthesis. http://ro.uow.edu.au/cgi/viewcontent.cgi?article=1381&context=ahsri.

Thompson, C., Williams, K., Morris, D., et al., 2014b. HWA expanded scopes of practice program evaluation: extending the role of paramedics sub-project final report. Centre for Health Service Development, University of Wollongong.

Townsend, R., Eburn, M., 2014. Paramedics administer drugs and deliver babies, they deserve national registration. The Conversation, 13 November. http://theconversation.com/paramedics -administer-drugs-and-deliver-babies-they-deserve-national-registration-33882.

Tuohy, C., 1999. Accidental Logics: The Dynamics of Change in the Health Care Arena in United States, Britain and Canada. Oxford University Press, New York.

van der Gaag, A., Gallagher, A., Zasada, M., et al., 2017. People like us? Understanding complaints about paramedics and social workers. https://www.hcpc-uk.org/globalassets/resources/reports/people-like- us-understanding-complaints-about-paramedics-and-social-workers.pdf.

van der Ploeg, E., Kleber, R.J., 2003. Acute and chronic job stressors among ambulance personnel: predictors of health symptoms. Occup. Environ. Med. 60 (Suppl. 1), i40–i46.

Williams, B., 2011. Graduate attributes and the professionalisation of Australian paramedics: an empirical study. Unpublished PhD thesis, Monash University Faculty of Education. Centre for the Advancement of Learning and Teaching, Clayton, Vic.

Wingrove, G., 2011. International roundtable on community paramedicine. J. Emerg. Prim. Health Care 9 (1), 9–11.

Yong, G., Dent, A., Weiland, T., 2007. Handover from paramedics: observations and emergency department clinician perceptions. J. Emerg. Med. Aust. 20 (2), 149–155.

Further Reading

Bacchi, C., 2016. Problematizations in health policy: questioning how "problems" are constituted in policies. SAGE Open 6 (2), 2158244016653986.

Eburn, M., Bendall, J., 2010. The provision of ambulance services in Australia: a legal argument for the national registration of paramedics. Aust. J. Paramed. 8 (4), 4.

van der Gaag, A., Gallagher, A., Zasada, M., et al., 2017. People like us? Understanding complaints about paramedics and social workers. https://www.hcpc-uk.org/globalassets/resources/reports/people-like- us-understanding-complaints-about-paramedics-and-social-workers.pdf.

Online Resources

Hammond, E., Shaban, R.Z., Holzhauser, K., et al., 2012. An exploratory study to examine the phenomenon and practice of ambulance ramping at hospitals within the Queensland Health Southern Districts and the Queensland Ambulance Service. Queensland Health & Griffith University, Brisbane. https://research- repository.griffith.edu.au/bitstream/handle/10072/49997/74885_1.pdf?sequence=1&isAllowed=y.

The Council of Ambulance Authorities website: http://www.caa.net.au/.

CHAPTER 26

The pharmacist's unique contribution to Australia's health system

Stephen Carter

Key learning outcomes

When you finish this chapter you should be able to:

+ describe the key activities of pharmacists
+ understand the unique contribution of community pharmacies to the health system, which includes the judicious sale of medicines and the provision of health services
+ explain the extent to which pharmacists collaborate with other members of the health care system
+ using Tuohy's model of accidental logics, discuss how the Australian health system could make the most use of pharmacists' unique skillset.

Key terms and abbreviations

consultant pharmacist
community pharmacy
Community Pharmacy Agreement (CPA)
consumers
customers
dose administration aids (DAA)
general practitioner (GP)
home medicines review (HMR)
Medical Benefits Scheme (MBS)
medicines
minor ailments
opioid substitution programs
patients
Pharmaceutical Benefits Scheme (PBS)
Pharmaceutical Society of Australia
Pharmacy Guild of Australia
Quality Care in Pharmacy Program (QCPP)
quality use of medicines (QUM)
residential aged-care facility (RACF)
residential medication management reviews (RMMRs)

Introduction

This chapter provides an introduction to the profession of pharmacy. The chapter will describe range of the roles of pharmacists currently working in Australia and show how these roles are being developed, regulated and funded. It briefly looks to the history of the profession, and discusses how many pharmacists look towards a future that makes more use of their unique skills. Please also note that this chapter should be read in conjunction with Chapter 7 describing the **Pharmaceutical Benefits Scheme (PBS)**.

What do pharmacists do?

When thinking about the roles of pharmacists, it is important to consider the relationship between people and their use of medicines. This is because pharmacists are the health professionals involved in the safe custody, preparation, dispensing and provision of medicines, together with systems and information to assure quality of use (Pharmaceutical Society of Australia 2017). In Australia, pharmacists become qualified after successfully completing a Bachelor's or Master's degree in Pharmacy followed by a year-long intern training program. Pharmacists who have similar overseas qualifications may also be registered through an alternative program.

Pharmacists' training tends to cover topics such as: the physical and chemical properties of medicinal substances; how to analyse the quantity of medicines contained in formulations and in bodily samples; how to formulate raw medicines into pharmaceutical grade products; how medicines administered to the body are absorbed, distributed and eliminated; the way some medicines interact with the body to cause beneficial effects and side effects; the way medicines modify the actions of other medicines; clinical therapeutics; psychological, social and behavioural issues around using medicines; legal and ethical standards of practice; and topics in management such as human resource management. Before describing the roles of pharmacists it is helpful first to carefully consider what medicines are and how the supply of medicines is regulated.

Medicines

Medicines are used to alleviate symptoms and / or to maintain health and well-being. They form the basis for the treatment of many acute and most chronic diseases. They are widely used in Australian society, particularly among older consumers. The most recent national telephone poll demonstrated that, among persons aged 50 years and older, almost 90% had taken a medicine in the last 24 hours and more than 40% had taken four or more medicines (Morgan et al. 2012). Medicines can make a significant contribution to the health and welfare of our society. It is difficult now to imagine a world without penicillin, pain-killers, vaccinations and a plethora of other substances. Medicines are so important that the World Health Organization (WHO) maintains an Essential Medicines List, which sets out those medicines that it considers are necessary for basic health systems (World Health Organization (WHO) 2017).

The main problem with medicines is that not only do they help, but also they have the potential to cause harm. It was Paracelsus who wrote: 'All substances are poisons; there is none which is not a poison. The right dose differentiates a poison from a remedy'. The potential for harm from medicines is highlighted by the fact that, within Australia, 2%–3% of all hospital admissions are estimated to be related to problems with medicines (Roughead et al. 2013).

The need to avoid medication-related harm is also reflected in Australia's adoption of a National Medicines Policy (NMP) in 2000. (See Chapter 7 for more details.)

PAUSE
for
REFLECTION
…

Ever wondered why some medicines can be sold in a supermarket, while some are available only on the shelves of pharmacies, or you need to ask the pharmacist directly, while others need a prescription?

The laws regarding how medicines are stored and supplied are under the jurisdiction of the states and territories. For example, in NSW there is a *Poisons and Therapeutic Goods Act 1966* and its associated *Regulations*. Some medicine products are considered relatively safe and may be sold in any location (i.e. these are not scheduled). Medicine products categorised in the 'Schedules' represent a more significant risk to the consumer because of their inherent potency or because the quantity within the pack represents problems if taken in excessive doses and / or for an extended time (Box 26.1).

BOX 26.1 'THE SCHEDULES' (RELEVANT TO THE HEALTH PROFESSIONS)

- 'Pharmacy-only' medicines – must be supplied within a pharmacy where a pharmacist may be accessed if needed.
- 'Pharmacist-only' medicines – must be supplied with the active participation of a pharmacist.
- 'Prescription-only' – can be supplied on a prescription from an approved prescriber, such as medical practitioner, nurse practitioner or optometrist.

  Some 'prescription-only' medicines require an extra level of care and attention because of their potential for misuse, such as morphine-related and amphetamine-related medicines. The writing of prescriptions for and the dispensing of these medicines are tightly controlled and the medicines themselves must be stored in locked safes and each dose must be accounted for.

Workplace

While pharmacists work in a range of clinical and non-clinical settings, the majority of pharmacists in Australia are employed within community pharmacies. According to a survey in 2012 undertaken by Health Workforce Australia, around two-thirds reported their main job setting as community pharmacies. The second most frequently reported setting was within the hospital sector. (See Table 26.1.)

TABLE 26.1 PROPORTION OF AUSTRALIAN PHARMACISTS WORKING IN VARIOUS SETTINGS

Setting	%
Community pharmacy	63.1
Hospital	17.6
Community health care service	2.7
Medical centre	2.0
Other private practice	1.9
Educational facility	1.7
Other government department or agency	1.4
Pharmaceutical manufacturing	1.3
Other commercial	1.2
Residential health care facility	0.7
Defence force	0.3
Wholesale pharmacy	0.2
Correctional services	0.1
Aboriginal health service	0.1
Other – not stated	4.6

Source: Adapted from Health Workforce Australia (2014)

Roles of the pharmacist

First and foremost, the general public tends to view pharmacists' work through the lens of the supply function. This is a key role for pharmacists in community pharmacies, in hospitals and throughout the distribution chain. The pharmacist needs to ensure that the medicines are supplied in accordance with professional standards and the law and transported and stored to protect the physical and chemical properties of the medicines. In the next few sections we deal with two supply functions which most people may be familiar with: selling medicines 'over-the-counter' and dispensing medicines prescribed by a medical practitioner.

The pharmacist 'over the counter'

Australians have a deep respect for the autonomy of an individual to make their own health-related decisions. Yet there needs to be a balance between ease of access and quality use. Since pharmacists are the custodians of medicines, the physical setting for the tension between access and quality use is the **community pharmacy**. Here we consider the role of the community pharmacist.

Primary care – managing minor ailments

The pharmacist is often the first health professional that patients see for **minor ailments**. Pharmacists must be good communicators as the role of the pharmacist cannot depend on performing physical examinations. Pharmacists (or their delegated assistants) are therefore expected to initiate a dialogue with their **customers** in order to ensure that the medicines supplied are suitable, preferably evidenced-based, treatment.

The **Pharmaceutical Society of Australia** has developed and refined professional practice standards (Pharmaceutical Society of Australia 2017) which provide pharmacists with guidance about how to manage their communication with patients regarding the sale of medicines for minor ailments. It also includes structured protocols of how their delegated assistants should manage consultations with patients, and under what circumstances the assistant should refer the patient to the pharmacist. If the medicine is a 'scheduled medicine' (see Box 26.1) this means that, in order to be sold, this dialogue is expected to occur regardless of whether the customer self-selects or requests a treatment for a symptom.

The pharmacist may need to ensure that the supplied medicine is compatible with the patient's other medical conditions, other medicines and herbal (or alternative) medicines. The patient should receive instructions for use that are practical and should be provided with sufficient information to allow them to use the medicines wisely. The pharmacist also has a professional obligation to refer a patient to another health provider if he/she believes that that is in the interests of the patient. In this way, community pharmacies provide a 'triage' service.

The professional expectations of the pharmacist (and/or their delegated assistants) described above are not automatically understood by **consumers** when acting as **patients** (see definitions in the Glossary). Although some accept the pharmacist's attention to professional and regulatory obligations, others are reluctant to be questioned about their purchase of 'over-the-counter' medicines. Consumers holding these views tend to cite their own pre-existing and common-sense knowledge and believe that pharmacists undervalue patient experience. Indeed Australian research suggests that some consumers do not appear to recognise that the time that pharmacists spend with them is part of the pharmacist's role (McMillan et al. 2014).

PAUSE
for
REFLECTION
...

When purchasing medicines, which type of customer are you? Do you like to be questioned about your purchases by a pharmacist or their assistant? Do you feel reluctant to speak with the pharmacist about your needs? What would influence patients' wish to speak with the pharmacist? What would be a barrier?

The way the pharmacist or assistant converses with their customers can have a significant impact on how beneficial these encounters can be. Here, it should be noted that the lack of privacy within community pharmacies has long been recognised as a potential communication barrier.

Payments for the triage role

Within Australian community pharmacies, the vast majority of pharmacists' consultations are not paid for by governments. In addition, community pharmacies have generally not charged their customers for these relatively informal consultations. They have relied on the income derived from the mark-up from the sale of medicines, to some extent subsidised by the dispensing of prescriptions. While this strategy has worked well over the past, falling remuneration from PBS dispensing reminds pharmacists of their unfunded contribution to the health system.

Health systems overseas are tending to recognise and remunerate pharmacists for their contribution to the health system through providing structured minor ailments services. A large-scale UK cohort study found that the pharmacists' consultations lead to a high level of successful resolution of symptoms at a lower cost than would have been achieved if patients had visited medical practitioners (Watson et al. 2015). Similar findings are emerging in Canada (Rafferty et al. 2017) (Case study 26.1).

Case Study 26.1

Consider the situation: an older gentleman who lives alone has type 2 diabetes, which means that when he injures himself his wounds do not heal well. He approaches the pharmacy staff with a request for paper-based dressings. A pharmacist inspects the wound and decides to apply a more appropriate gel-based dressing. As part of the consultation, the pharmacist offers to take the gentleman's blood sugar level, which is high. The pharmacist realises that the gentleman has forgotten to take his antidiabetic medicines. The pharmacist reminds him to takes his medicines and refers him to the general practitioner (GP) for further review.

In the case study above, imagine that the pharmacy consultation takes 20 minutes, and the patient pays only for the normal cost of the dressing. If this occurred in a GP practice, the practice would also be paid a **Medical Benefits Scheme (MBS)** fee. An interesting question to consider is whether pharmacists should be paid an MBS fee for services such as this, as advocated by the Pharmaceutical Society of Australia (2016).

Dispensing medicines

To the general public, the dispensing of medicines on receipt of a prescription is probably the most familiar role of pharmacists. When dispensing, the pharmacist ensures that the supplied medicine accurately reflects the prescriber's intentions, and is consistent with the needs and safety of the patient. In order to reduce the risk of treatment-caused harm, pharmacists need to implement good systems, with continuous quality improvement coupled with a professional and patient-centred approach to dispensing. Most Australian community pharmacies subscribe to the Quality Care in Pharmacy Program (QCPP) (a quality insurance program) because the PBS provides practice incentives, which depends on maintaining QCPP accreditation. This requires each pharmacy to allocate sufficient resources, including an adequate number of pharmacists, technicians/assistants, appropriate technology, well-designed work-flow, a private or semi-private area to consult with patients and of course sufficient stock.

Prescriptions require review

It should be noted that, when dispensing prescriptions, it is not sufficient for the pharmacist to simply follow the instructions of the prescriber. Whenever a medicine is dispensed, the pharmacist is obliged to review the prescription, based on the information available to them. Using the dispensing history and information gleaned from interviewing the patient, the pharmacist needs to make several judgements regarding the appropriateness of each prescription.

These judgements of appropriateness include consideration of:

- dose, frequency and length of treatment
- whether the medicine is suitable for the condition prescribed
- the patient's past history of adverse events
- potential drug–drug interactions and drug–disease interactions
- practicality of the prescribed regimen and the likelihood of being adherent to the regimen, and
- patient preference.

In Australia, there is no legal requirement for the prescriber to include on a prescription what condition is being treated. While the pharmacist may discuss the intended purpose of the prescription with the patient or caregiver, the absence of a documented diagnosis (and other details) has tended to limit the scope of review. From 2018, the MyHealth Record (MHR) provides all health professionals with access to patient notes and event summaries, which will include diagnoses. It is expected that access to this information should fundamentally improve pharmacists' decision-making, particularly for vulnerable patients who use multiple medicines. If the pharmacist considers that the medicine may have a preventable adverse effect on the patient, it is the responsibility of the pharmacist to intervene and converse with the prescriber. Community pharmacists record these interventions and, since 2011, have been able to claim Pharmaceutical Benefit Scheme (PBS) incentive payments for doing so.

The most common reason for contact between pharmacists and medical practitioners is to sort out prescribing problems. Pharmacists tend to feel some anxiety about contacting medical practitioners regarding prescribing errors as they are also required to maintain good working relationships (Basak et al. 2015). Pharmacists therefore need to refine their communication practices with medical practitioners in order to effectively manage prescription problems in a timely fashion.

Once the pharmacist is comfortable with the prescription, the product is prepared, labelled and handed to the patient. There are certain circumstances that should prompt the pharmacist to initiate patient counselling proactively. Such circumstances may include when a new medicine is prescribed, when there is a change in the dose or frequency of administration, when the brand of medicine has changed or when the medicine is known to be particularly problematic (Pharmacy Board of Australia 2015).

Compounding

Prior to the 1950s, the majority of prescriptions were not available from wholesale manufacturers. Virtually all prescription medicines were prepared by the pharmacist according to formulae with individual ingredients using ancient techniques. Since the 1950s, however, this type of dispensing fell into decline as the 'evidence-based' pharmaceutical industry took over.

However, not all medicines, particularly creams, ointments and washes, were able to be prepared in the variety of strengths and combinations which were demanded of, for example, dermatologists. The art and science of compounding has recently undergone a minor resurgence in modern pharmaceutical practice. Using improved technology and quality processes, many community pharmacies specialise in this area in order to customise formulations to meet the specific needs of the patient and / or doctor (see http://www.pccarx.com.au/what-is-compounding).

Dose administration aids

A significant problem for people who need to use multiple medicines to treat multiple co-morbidities is their capacity to comply with the prescribed regimen. Many medicines have complicated dose regimens. In addition, many medicines should not be consumed at the same time as other medicines or must be taken at particular times in relation to other daily activities such as meals, bedtime or prior to exercise, for example. Many of these problems can be addressed by providing patients with **dose administration aids (DAAs)**. A Cochrane review concluded that DAAs modestly increased the percentage of tablets taken (Mahtani et al. 2011). DAAs are widely used by some of the most vulnerable members of our society or their caregivers.

Opiate substitution programs

Heroin and some prescribed medicines such as morphine, codeine and oxycontin are addictive and are subject to misuse. Many pharmacists working in community pharmacies, clinics and hospitals are involved in opiate substitution programs and needle exchange programs. These programs are consistent with Australia's National Drug Strategy. While some consumers can be eligible for entirely free state government-provided **opioid substitution programs,** a majority access programs through community pharmacies. In this setting, state governments pay for the cost of the opiate substitution *medicines,* but patients may pay around (AU)$30 per week for the provision of the *service.*

Vaccination

An interesting and quite recent development is that legislative changes have allowed pharmacists to provide vaccinations for influenza and other conditions. Pharmacists must be especially accredited to do vaccination and do so in a private space. The widespread role-out of pharmacist-provided vaccination has triggered numerous press releases from the medical practitioner groups such as the Australian Medical Association (AMA) and the Royal Australian College of General Practitioners (RACGP), who advocate against this and other expanded clinical roles for pharmacists (Dow 2018).

This is an example of the so-called 'turf-wars' and the thinking behind it is subject to professional bias. What is relevant to the current discussion is whether this particular turf-war may have a detrimental effect on interprofessional collaboration between GPs and pharmacists, which is discussed later.

PAUSE
for
REFLECTION
...

To what extent do you think the technology platforms such as the National Immunisation Register and the MyHealth Record will improve collaboration between community pharmacists and other members of the health care team?

Hospital pharmacy

Hospital pharmacists are involved in a range of activities aimed at improving the **quality use of medicines (QUM)** within the hospital and beyond. Some of the activities are quite specialised. Pharmacists, particularly senior pharmacists, may work on medicine and therapeutics committees where they have a role in advising the hospital on which medicines should be included on lists of medicines that are readily available in the hospital. The benefits of having these 'formularies' are that they can decrease errors and reduce costs. Pharmacists contribute to the evaluation of new and expensive medicines that specialist medical practitioners wish to use. Hospitals are often the site where clinical trials are conducted and pharmacists are often involved in this area of research.

Hospital pharmacists may be employed in medicines and / or poisons information centres. These centres provide information for consumers and health professionals and pharmacists in these areas use their skills in therapeutics, risk communication, literature searching and data management.

Focus on clinical activities in hospital pharmacy

Hospital pharmacists may be involved in a broad range of clinical activities. In hospitals, pharmacists tend to have access to the complete patient record. Records include diagnoses, reasons for admission, pathology reports, medical and paramedical opinions. Pharmacists may have direct contact with the patient and their caregivers. Similar to that mentioned above, research in the UK (Morecroft et al. 2015) and in the Netherlands (Borgsteede et al. 2011) suggests that some patients do not expect hospital pharmacists to speak with them or to provide them with advice, which acts as a communication barrier within this setting. The close proximity to other health professionals working on ward rounds facilitates interprofessional communication. Pharmacists may have the opportunity to advise the multidisciplinary teams on their opinion of, for example: the most appropriate medicines and combinations of medicines to use, the best method to administer the medicines, the optimal doses and timing of doses; and ways to monitor for adverse effects.

The focus on clinical activities makes hospital pharmacy a very attractive career option for pharmacy interns, despite the high level of competition for positions (Shen et al. 2014). The competition is thought to be high because graduating pharmacy students perceive that the role of the hospital pharmacist is particularly patient focused and that their skills can have a direct contribution to patient care.

An emerging role for hospital pharmacists is to work within accident and emergency departments. Here the pharmacist performs medication reconciliation using a systematic process to obtain an accurate and complete list of all medications taken prior to admission to hospital. The pharmacist's knowledge of the appearance of the various brands and formulations of medicines and the way consumers use and describe them is particularly useful. Medication reconciliation is recommended by the Australian Commission on Safety and Quality in Health Care whenever patients are transferred between settings, both within the hospital and in the transition between hospital and the home or **residential aged-care facility (RACF)**. Evidence suggests that having pharmacists perform medication reconciliation reduces the chances of medication errors (Cheema et al. 2018).

Pharmacists working interprofessionally

Home medicines review (HMR)

Home medicines review is an interesting model for examining how interprofessional collaboration between pharmacists and GPs can work in practice. Further, the HMR model is useful for examining how Tuohy's model of accidental logics helps us to understand how we can plan for improving patients' access to pharmacist-provided services.

An HMR is initiated with a request from the patient's GP to a pharmacist, who may be their preferred community pharmacist or a **consultant pharmacist** who works independently. Pharmacists who perform HMR must be accredited by an approved credentialling body. The pharmacist generally visits the patient and caregiver(s) at their home for an extended interview regarding medication management issues. Following the visit, the pharmacist sends a written report documenting medication review findings and recommendations to the GP, who then formulates a revised medication management plan with the patient (see Case study 26.2).

Case Study 26.2

HMR and interprofessional practice

Consider Margaret, a 72-year-old woman who has osteoarthritis, thyroid insufficiency, type 2 diabetes, mild kidney failure and recently post-herpetic neuralgia (persistent pain after shingles). At a regular visit, Margaret's GP notes that Margaret has a lot of sedation from something her specialist prescribed (amitriptyline) for shingles pain but Margaret can't recall what that was.

Dr George Abbas suggests that Belinda arrange for a home medicines review. At the home visit, Belinda (the accredited pharmacist) and Margaret spend about 40 minutes discussing Margaret's medication history, her understanding and use of her medicines and her therapeutic goals. Since starting the amitriptyline for shingles, she has been very tired in the mornings and complained of a very dry mouth. The pharmacist believes that, although the initially prescribed dose of amitriptyline is sometimes used for her type of pain, the dose may have been too high in her case.

Belinda asks Margaret about her use of over-the-counter medicines and herbal / traditional medicines. Margaret has also been taking ibuprofen, an anti-inflammatory that she purchased from the supermarket for shingles pain. The problem for Margaret is that anti-inflammatory medicines can be harmful for people with mild kidney failure. Belinda needs to write a HMR report to Dr Abbas, but because she is quite concerned about Margaret's excessive sedation she calls him at the end of the interview. Dr Abbas agrees with Belinda's suggestion to reduce the dose and asks Margaret to see him in a week's time. Margaret then meets with Dr Abbas and discusses the content of Belinda's HMR report. In addition to dealing with the dose of amitriptyline, Belinda's report highlights the problems with Margaret's use of ibuprofen (kidney problems) and suggests some alternatives. Margaret and Dr Abbas agree on a revised medication plan, a copy of which is given to Margaret and another sent to Margaret's regular pharmacy.

PAUSE
for
REFLECTION
...

HMR is highly regarded by patients (Carter et al. 2015) who are very willing to receive the service and HMR improves health outcomes (Jokanovic et al. 2015). Can you think of any reason why implementation of the program in Australian GP practices remains low (Costa et al. 2015)?

Consider the physical, social and psychological needs that are required for pharmacists and doctors to collaborate.

Pharmacists in residential aged-care facilities (RACFs)

Pharmacists have a role in improving medication safety within RACFs. Here, consultant pharmacists may provide medication management services and / or services designed to improve the quality use of medicines (QUM) (Department of Health and Ageing 2011).

Consultant pharmacists have been remunerated to perform **residential medication management reviews (RMMRs)** since 1997 as part of the PBS. RMMRs are comprehensive reviews of the residents' medications. The pharmacist collaborates with nursing and support staff, medical practitioners and the community pharmacist who supplies the residents' medicines. The RMMR aims to ensure that residents are receiving appropriate medication therapy, including monitoring.

A QUM service is separate to a RMMR service and has a focus on improving the quality use of medicines by influencing practices and procedures. When performing QUM services, the pharmacist provides medication advisory activities, quality assurance and continuous improvement activities and education for nursing and support staff.

Reducing sedative prescribing in residential aged-care facilities

An area of particular focus on both RMMR and QUM activities in aged-care facilities is to reduce the overall use of medicines that are particularly harmful for the oldest old. One class of medicines that are potentially harmful include antipsychotic medications that are used to manage behavioural and psychological symptoms of dementia. There is increasing concern among government and consumer groups that there is overuse of medicines to control behaviour. The RedUSe program was a multi-site multidisciplinary project, aiming to reduce reliance on such sedatives (Westbury et al. 2018). In this program, consultant pharmacists analysed prescription patterns and provided feedback to doctors, nurses and other staff. Following this, each care facility had a high-level review of practices designed to manage the behavioural and psychological symptoms of dementia without medications. The program demonstrated significant reductions in sedatives and is an example of a model of interprofessional collaboration. It is expected this program will feature in future updates of Reeve's Cochrane review of interprofessional collaboration to improve professional practice and health care outcomes.

PAUSE
for
REFLECTION
...

How do you feel about older persons with dementia being provided with sedative medicines to control challenging behaviours? What do you think would be the impact on the residential care facilities' workload if sedatives were reduced?

Funding non-supply services – Tuohy's accidental logics

This brings us to the issue of funding for HMRs and RMMRs. Note that payments made to pharmacists are provided through the PBS, while payments to medical practitioners for their input are provided through the Medical Benefits Scheme (MBS).

Recall that the PBS (see Chapter 7) began in the 1950s and was centred on remunerating pharmacists for '*supplying*' medicines. The terms of payments have been negotiated between the Commonwealth and pharmacy owners through **Community Pharmacy Agreements**. Yet, since 1997, the Commonwealth would only remunerate '*services*' such as RMMR and HMR through the PBS. These '*services*' can be provided outside pharmacies by pharmacists who do not own a pharmacy. Tuohy might describe this an 'accident' of history and would note the logic of the decisions that followed.

An interesting and seemingly unpredicted consequence of this occurred in 2013–14. In previous agreements, payments for HMR were significantly below those budgeted. As of 2009, across Australia nearly 2000 pharmacists had achieved accreditation to be consultant pharmacists, yet the number of HMRs claimed for annually was only around 50,000. At that stage, payments for HMR were made to the community pharmacy owners, who either acted as the consultant pharmacist themselves or employed one. Under the influence of lobbying from *independent* consultant pharmacists prior to the fifth agreement (in 2010), changes to the agreement subsequently allowed for payments for HMRs and RMMRs directly to the independent consultants, effectively bypassing community pharmacies.

This change saw many consultant pharmacists being able derive a decent income solely by performing HMRs. Indeed many pharmacists had begun to see this as an attractive and seemingly sustainable career path. By 2013, the increase in HMR provision resulted in an unpredicted and significant shortfall in PBS funds which had been allocated to the service. This was managed in negotiations between the **Pharmacy Guild of Australia** and the Commonwealth by limiting the number of HMRs that an individual pharmacy or pharmacist could claim for each month. The 'capping' of the service had little effect on overall payments to community pharmacies, but clearly had a detrimental effect on payments to independent (consultant) pharmacists who were trying to make a career in this area. The 'capping' of services was criticised publicly by many pharmacist groups and consumer groups, both of whom highlighted that patients in need were left without access to this highly regarded service. Note that there was no concomitant 'cap' placed on MBS payments to general practitioners, despite the fact that medical practitioners initiate the service.

Pharmacists in medical centres

An interesting development in the career options for pharmacists is pharmacists working in general practice surgeries (Christopher Freeman 2016). In this role, pharmacists have clinical roles in performing medication reviews and supporting GPs with prescribing advice. It is easy to imagine that pharmacists could use more of their skills through having greater access to medical records. Collaboration with doctors and practice nurses is facilitated and leads to significant health care improvements for patients. GP practice pharmacists also provide non-clinical roles, similar to the work in RACFs. Here pharmacists may conduct prescribing audits with feedback to prescribers. The concept of the GP practice pharmacist is supported by the PSA, the Consumers Health forum and some GPs. An economic analysis suggests that, for every $1 spent on GP practice, pharmacists would return $1.55 in health care savings (Delloites Access Economics 2015). At present, the biggest barrier to having pharmacists working in GP practices is the lack of a sustainable funding mechanism (Freeman 2016).

Summary

The emerging role of pharmacists as members of the health care team is at a critical stage in history. Australian pharmacists and the health system in general will benefit by finding new and equitable ways to make better use of pharmacists' unique skills. When reviewing the content of this chapter, we can reflect on how:

- consumers, governments and other third-party payers may not have formed clear expectations about the emerging role of the clinical pharmacist
- the Community Pharmacy Agreement, which was originally conceptualised and designed to fund *supply* through the PBS, has become the major source of funding for *services*. The PBS has, on the one hand, supported the pharmacist's role in the health system through funding access to medicines. At the same time, community pharmacy's reliance on the PBS has arguably stymied an emerging role because most of the funds paid to the owners of pharmacies relate to supply
- pharmacists working within medical practices and clinics may become commonplace. This concept has the in-principle support of medical groups
- the Pharmaceutical Society of Australia advocates that pharmacists should be provided with Medicare provider numbers for payments through the MBS, similar to most other health professionals (Pharmaceutical Society of Australia 2016)
- specialisation in pharmacy practice is currently emerging.

Review Questions

1 Describe the range of activities that a community pharmacist provides within a community pharmacy.

2 Compare the opportunities for interprofessional collaboration with other members of the health care team for hospital pharmacists with those of a community pharmacist.

3 Considering the training and skills of pharmacists, and reflecting on your own experience with pharmacists, to what extent are Australians making most use of pharmacists' expertise?

4 How could we use Touhy's accidental logics to help Australia make better use of pharmacist's skills?

5 How could we use Carol Bacchi's model to redefine the problem of sedative use in residential aged-care facilities?

References

Basak, R., Bentley, J.P., McCaffrey, D.J., et al., 2015. The role of perceived impact on relationship quality in pharmacists' willingness to influence indication-based off-label prescribing decisions. Soc. Sci. Med. 132, 181–189.

Borgsteede, S.D., Karapinar-Çarkit, F., Hoffmann, E., et al., 2011. Information needs about medication according to patients discharged from a general hospital. Patient Educ. Couns. 83, 22–28.

Carter, S.R., Moles, R., White, L., et al., 2015. The impact of patients' perceptions of the listening skills of the pharmacist on their willingness to re-use Home Medicines Reviews: a structural equation model. Res. Social Adm. Pharm. 11, 163–175.

Cheema, E., Alhomoud, F.K., Kinsara, A.S.A., et al., 2018. The impact of pharmacists-led medicines reconciliation on healthcare outcomes in secondary care: a systematic review and meta-analysis of randomized controlled trials. PLoS ONE 13, e0193510.

Costa, D., Van, C., Abbott, P., et al., 2015. Investigating general practitioner engagement with pharmacists in home medicines review. J. Interprof. Care 29 (5), 469–475. doi:10.3109/13561820.2015.1012253.

Delloites Access Economics, 2015. Analysis of non-dispensing pharmacists in general practice clinics. Australian Medical Association, Canberra. www2.deloitte.com/au/en/pages/economics/articles/analysis-non-dispensing-pharmacists-general-practice-clinics.html.

Department of Heath and Ageing, 2011. Quality use of medicines (QUM). http://www.health.gov.au/internet/main/publishing.nsf/Content/nmp-quality.htm.

Dow, A., 2018. Pharmacists and doctors trade jabs over the best time to get flu shot. Sydney Morning Herald. 29 March. https://www.smh.com.au/healthcare/pharmacists-and-doctors-trade-jabs-over-the-best-time-to-get-flu-shot-20180328-p4z6ne.html.

Freeman, C.D.R., Aloizos, J., Williams, I., 2016. The practice pharmacist: a natural fit in the general practice team. Aust. Prescr. 39, 211–214.

Health Workforce Australia (HWA), 2014. Pharmacists in focus. Australia's Health Workforce Series. https://www.hwa.gov.au/sites/default/files/HWA_Australia-Health-Workforce-Series_Pharmacists%20in%20focus_vF_LR.pdf.

Jokanovic, N., Tan, E.C.K., Van Den Bosch, D., et al., 2015. Clinical medication review in Australia: a systematic review. Res. Social Adm. Pharm. 12, 384–418.

Mahtani, K.R., Heneghan, C.J., Glasziou, P.P., et al., 2011. Reminder packaging for improving adherence to self-administered long-term medications. Cochrane Database Syst. Rev. (9), CD005025, doi:10.1002/14651858.CD005025.pub3.

McMillan, S.S., Kelly, F., Sav, A., et al., 2014. Consumer and carer views of Australian community pharmacy practice: awareness, experiences and expectations. J Pharm. Health Serv. Res. 5, 29–36.

Morecroft, C.W., Thornton, D., Caldwell, N.A., 2015. Inpatients' expectations and experiences of hospital pharmacy services: qualitative study. Health Expect. 18, 1009–1017.

Morgan, T.K., Williamson, M., Pirotta, M., et al., 2012. A national census of medicines use: a 24-hour snapshot of Australians aged 50 years and older. Med. J. Aust. 196, 50–53.

Pharmaceutical Society of Australia, 2016. Review of pharmacy remuneration and regulation submission: a discussion paper. http://www.health.gov.au/internet/main/publishing.nsf/Content/review-pharmacy-remuneration-regulation-submissions-cnt-10/$file/481-2016-29-09-pharmaceutical-society-of-australia.pdf.

Pharmaceutical Society of Australia, 2017. Professsional practice standards, version 5. https://www.psa.org.au/practice-support-industry/professional-practice-standards/.

Pharmacy Board of Australia (PBA), 2015. Guidelines for dispensing of medicines. PBA, Canberra. https://www.pharmacyboard.gov.au/Codes-Guidelines.aspx.

Poisons and Therapeutic Goods Act 1966 No. 31. (NSW). https://www.legislation.nsw.gov.au/inforce/1b61875d-cae0-c9b2-aa52-aa46cc0a14ed/1966-31.pdf.

Rafferty, E., Yaghoubi, M., Taylor, J., et al., 2017. Costs and savings associated with a pharmacist's prescribing for minor ailments program in Saskatchewan. Cost Eff. Resour. Alloc. 15, 3.

Roughead, L., Semple, S., Rosenfeld, E., 2013. Literature Review: medication safety in Australia. ACSQHC, Sydney.

Shen, G., Fois, R., Nissen, L., et al., 2014. Course experiences, satisfaction and career intent of final year pre-registration Australian pharmacy students. Pharm. Pract. 12, 392.

Watson, M.C., Ferguson, J., Barton, G.R., et al., 2015. A cohort study of influences, health outcomes and costs of patients' health-seeking behaviour for minor ailments from primary and emergency care settings. BMJ Open 5 (2), e006261. doi:10.1136/bmjopen-2014-006261.

Westbury, J.L., Gee, P., Ling, T., et al., 2018. RedUSe: reducing antipsychotic and benzodiazepine prescribing in residential aged care facilities. Med. J. Aust. 208, 398–403.

World Health Organization (WHO), 2017. WHO model list of essential medicines 20th list. http://www.who.int/medicines/publications/essentialmedicines/en/.

Further Reading

Health Workforce Australia (HWA), 2014. Pharmacists in focus. Australia's Health Workforce Series. http://iaha.com.au/wp-content/uploads/2014/03/HWA_Australia-Health-Workforce-Series_Pharmacists-in-focus_vF_LR.pdf.

For an international perspective on workforce development. https://www.fip.org/workforce.

Online Resources

Advanced practitioner framework for pharmacists: www.advancedpharmacypractice.com.au.

Australian Commission on Safety and Quality in Healthcare – medication safety: http://www.safetyandquality.gov.au/our-work/medication-safety/.

Fifth Community Pharmacy Agreement: http://5cpa.com.au/.

National Drug Strategy: http://www.nationaldrugstrategy.gov.au/internet/drugstrategy/publishing.nsf/Content/home.

Pharmaceutical Society of Australia: http://www.psa.org.au/.

Pharmacy Board of Australia: http://www.pharmacyboard.gov.au/.

Pharmacy Guild of Australia: http://www.guild.org.au/.

Society of Hospital Pharmacists of Australia: http://shpa.org.au/.

CHAPTER 27

Health profession regulation: the case of physiotherapy

Matthew Sutton and Adam Govier

Key learning outcomes

When you finish this chapter you should be able to:

- ◆ provide a brief history of the physiotherapy profession in Australia
- ◆ understand the roles and purpose of the physiotherapy profession
- ◆ outline the different clinical fields in which physiotherapists work in the Australian health care system and the career structure in the public and private sectors
- ◆ define the roles of the relevant regulatory bodies for the physiotherapy profession in Australia
- ◆ describe the requirements for registration as a physiotherapist
- ◆ discuss the advantages and ways in which physiotherapists may work in a multidisciplinary environment
- ◆ discuss the challenges facing the physiotherapy profession and the opportunities for further development.

Key terms and abbreviations

Australian Health Practitioner Regulation Agency (AHPRA)

Australian Physiotherapy Association (APA)

Australian Physiotherapy Council (APC)

chronic disease management (CDM)

continuing professional development (CPD)

emergency department (ED)

extended-scope physiotherapist (ESP)

interprofessional collaboration (IPC)

Physiotherapy Board of Australia (PBA)

primary-contact practitioners (PCPs)

primary-contact status

World Confederation for Physical Therapy (WCPT)

Introduction

The **World Confederation for Physical Therapy (WCPT)** provides the following definition of the roles of physiotherapy:

> Physical therapy [physiotherapy] provides services to individuals and populations to develop, maintain and restore maximum movement and functional ability throughout the lifespan. This includes providing services in circumstances where movement and function are threatened by ageing, injury, pain, diseases, disorders, conditions or environmental factors. Functional movement is central to what it means to be healthy. *(World Confederation for Physical Therapy 2017, p. 1)*

The terms 'physical therapy' and 'physiotherapy' are used interchangeably and are dependent on the country of practice. In Australia, the term 'physiotherapy' is the accepted nomenclature for the profession.

While the WCPT definition above provides some clarity around the purpose of physiotherapists, the following definition from the **Australian Physiotherapy Council (APC)** provides further insight into the role of the profession:

> The practice of physiotherapy incorporates assessment, interpretation and analysis of findings, planning, intervention and evaluation of pain, physical dysfunction and movement disorders. *(Australian Physiotherapy Council 2006, p. 9)*

The profession of physiotherapy focuses on the assessment and management of human movement. Physiotherapists have a role across the entire life-span, from neonatal intensive-care units working with premature babies through to assisting function and quality of life in elderly and palliative care environments at the end of life. Physiotherapists work across a range of health care settings, with the primary aim of improving the quality of life of the people, or clients, they are treating. The scope of the roles of the profession is illustrated in Fig. 27.1.

History

The physiotherapy profession has evolved significantly over time. Physiotherapy in Australia developed from a massage-based profession (the Society of Trained Masseuses (STM)) established by British-trained nurses in 1894 (Fig. 27.2). The society, now known as the Chartered Society of Physiotherapists, was initially formed to legitimise what was at the time considered a practice of questionable morality by the medical profession, with the lines between legitimate massage and prostitution being at times unclear (Calvert 2002, p. 101). The membership of this society was limited to females, with males being allowed access to treatment only via a referral from a doctor. Although the society lacked professional autonomy, it did establish two extremely important historical moments in the history of physiotherapy. First, it legitimised the practice of massage, a key intervention for the physiotherapy profession for decades to come; second, it established a formal teaching pathway to obtain registration to be eligible for membership of the STM (Nicholls & Cheek 2006). Indeed, in 1906 the Australian Massage Association was formed by Teepoo Hall, an Indian immigrant with significant education and training in the

FIGURE 27.1 THE CLIENT-CENTRED APPROACH IN PHYSIOTHERAPY

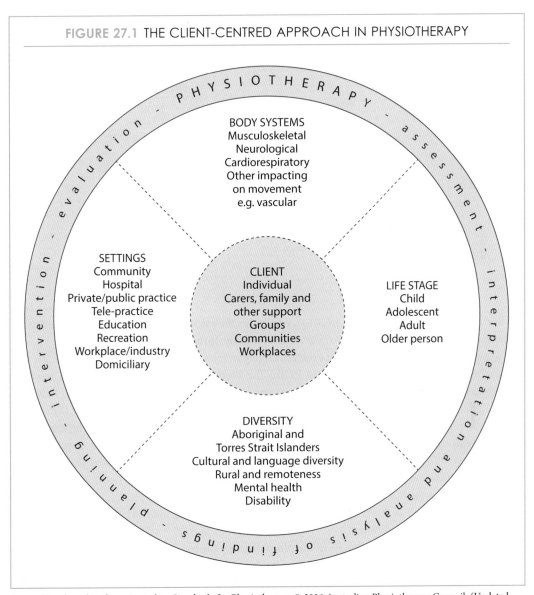

Source: Based on data from Australian Standards for Physiotherapy © 2006 Australian Physiotherapy Council. (Updated standards were released in 2015. Please see Physiotherapy practice thresholds in Australia and Aotearoa New Zealand. https://physiocouncil.com.au/media/1020/physiotherapy-board-physiotherapy-practice-thresholds-in-australia-and-aotearoa-new-zealand-6.pdf for further information)

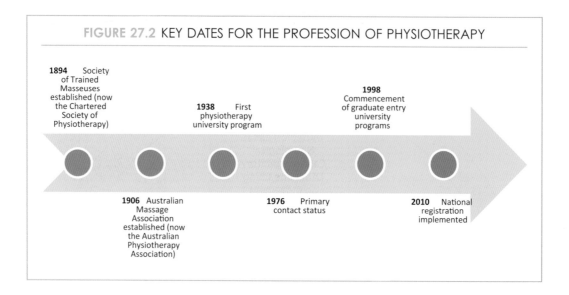

FIGURE 27.2 KEY DATES FOR THE PROFESSION OF PHYSIOTHERAPY

medical and science fields (McMeeken 2014), which was the association that is now recognised as the professional body for Physiotherapists, the **Australian Physiotherapy Association (APA)**.

The role of the physiotherapist has evolved, largely in relation to societal demands, with the title 'physiotherapist' being adopted in the mid 1920s. The World Wars (1914–18 and 1939–45) resulted in mass casualties returning from service, requiring a greater emphasis on rehabilitation following injury. In between these wars, the poliomyelitis epidemic resulted in a further demand for the services of physiotherapists (Forster 1969). Historically, poliomyelitis had been treated by immobilising affected limbs through splinting. However, Elizabeth Kenny, who obtained the nursing title of 'sister' through her involvement in the Australian Army Nursing Service in World War I, promoted the use of heat and joint mobilisation – a role to which physiotherapists were highly suited (Ross 1983). The role of the physiotherapist has been shaped in more recent times by the emphasis on evidence-based practice (EBP), as well as the rise in prevalence of chronic diseases such as osteoarthritis, diabetes and cardiorespiratory conditions.

One of the most significant events in the physiotherapy profession in Australia occurred in 1976 (Chipchase et al. 2006) – the establishment of **primary-contact status**. This allowed people to be treated by a physiotherapist without referral by a doctor and provided the profession with significantly increased autonomy. Australia was the first country to enact this change, which resulted in significant debate among the global physiotherapy community. Whereas some countries continue to require a doctor's referral to be treated by a physiotherapist, many other countries (such as the UK and USA) now have a primary-contact practice model of care.

Registration pathway and requirements

The first university course to provide an educational pathway for the physiotherapy profession was established at the University of Queensland in 1938. This was a 3-year diploma program (Forster

1969). The WCPT has since established the minimum duration of education required to become a physiotherapist to be 4 years. Australia has incorporated this guideline into all national curricula, and all physiotherapy Bachelor's programs are now of 4 years duration (Australian Qualifications Framework Council 2013). In the late 1990s, the APA endorsed the introduction of graduate-entry physiotherapy programs (Chipchase et al. 2006). These programs are typically 2 years in duration for a Master's degree and 3 years for a Doctoral degree qualification. There are currently 20 universities across Australia offering physiotherapy programs, with undergraduate, graduate entry masters and doctoral programs available (Australian Health Practitioner Regulation Agency (AHPRA) 2018).

In Australia, the professional title of 'physiotherapist' is protected by legislation. This means that only those that have graduated from an APC-accredited program can bestow this title upon themselves. Additionally, in order to practise as a physiotherapist, registration must be renewed annually. Prior to 2010, this process was state/territory based, but in July 2010 a national registration body, the Australian Health Practitioner Regulation Agency, was introduced. Physiotherapy was one of 10 health professions that established this registration board. One of its key purposes is to protect public safety by ensuring that all health practitioners registered comply with all registration requirements. These requirements can be viewed on the **Australian Health Practitioner Regulation Agency (AHPRA)** website. Subsequently, any physiotherapist registered with the AHPRA is eligible to practise across Australia. To maintain registration, physiotherapists must participate in ongoing education, referred to as **continuing professional development (CPD)**. The minimum requirement for CPD is 20 hours per year of relevant educational activities.

Despite registration being a nationally administered process, legislation remains state/territory based. Legislation provides the framework by which physiotherapists are able to practise. For example, according to most state legislation in Australia, physiotherapists are able to use acupuncture as a treatment. However, there are other treatments that are prohibited by legislation. For example, physiotherapists are unable to prescribe medications in Australia. Each state has legislation defining which health professionals are able to prescribe, order and administer medications, most commonly referred to the Drugs and Poisons Act although the exact name differs from state to state. Physiotherapists are not identified in any state-based legislation as health practitioners able to prescribe medications, with doctors, nurses, optometrists and podiatrists being the professionals most commonly identified in the relevant legislation. However, it is important to note that other countries such as the UK have introduced limited prescribing rights for physiotherapists.

Relevant professional and regulatory bodies

The **Physiotherapy Board of Australia (PBA)** is one of the most important regulatory organisations for the physiotherapy profession, and exists as a sub-branch of the AHPRA. The role of the PBA is to administer and manage the registration of physiotherapists and students, and develop the code of conduct by which registered physiotherapists must abide as part of professional practice. This code is based on the four ethical principles of autonomy, beneficence (providing a positive health outcome), non-maleficence (doing no harm) and justice. It is also the role of the PBA to manage complaints and notifications made against physiotherapists. Further detail on the roles of the PBA can be found online.

The APA is the national professional body that represents physiotherapists, and plays a key role in advocating for the rights and progression of the physiotherapy profession. While membership of the APA is voluntary, it plays an important role in the establishment of CPD programs. The APA has national special-interest groups – for example, acupuncture and dry needling, animal, aquatic, cardiorespiratory, palliative care, disability, **emergency department (ED)**, gerontology, mental health, musculoskeletal, neurology, occupational health, paediatric, pain, rural, sports, and women's health. A full list of the special interest groups is available via the APA website. Through an APA-administered process, physiotherapists are able to develop professional expertise and recognition within each of these health areas to receive specialist recognition through the APA specialisation pathway. This allows the physiotherapist to use a specialist title – for example, specialist sports physiotherapist or specialist neurological physiotherapist. However, the specialist title is not regulated by the PBA as its role is to provide general registration only.

> **PAUSE**
> *for*
> **REFLECTION**
> ...
>
> As can be seen, the profession of physiotherapy is quite tightly regulated. There are a number of health care industries or areas that do not have such regulation in place. Can you think of some of the advantages of having such regulations? Are there any disadvantages to having such a high level of regulation? What are some possible challenges to enforcing these regulations?

Current status of physiotherapy

Physiotherapists most commonly pursue a pathway into clinical practice. There are three core clinical areas in which entry-level Australian physiotherapists are commonly trained: musculoskeletal, neurological and cardiorespiratory physiotherapy. However, physiotherapists also develop expertise in many other areas such as the APA national specialty areas listed above. Physiotherapists work in private, public and non-government organisations (NGOs) or community organisations and across rural, regional and metropolitan settings. In this context, community organisations are health care organisations that are financed by a mixture of public and private income sources to provide health care services to the community.

The introduction of the AHPRA in 2010 enabled for the first time the collection of reliable demographic and epidemiological data across Australia for the profession of physiotherapy. In 2014, Health Workforce Australia (HWA, 2014) released a report outlining information on Australia's physiotherapy workforce, using data collected over the years 2011–12. Since then, the National Health Workforce Data Set (NHWDS) has provided this information through a combination of survey and registration renewal data. These data showed that in 2016 there were 24,271 registered and employed physiotherapists. The workforce had seen a yearly growth rate of 5%, increasing by 4046 since 2013 (Australian Government, 2018). Of the physiotherapy workforce, 92% worked primarily in a clinical role, with 53% of these reporting their principal scope of practice as musculoskeletal, followed by 14% working in aged care.

There has been a trend of increased participation in the private workforce, with a corresponding decrease in the public sector. From 2013 to 2016, there was a reduction of just over 2% of the workforce reporting working in the public sector, with a corresponding increase in private-sector participation of nearly 3% (Australian Government, 2018). The majority of physiotherapists work in metropolitan areas, with 81% of Australian physiotherapists working in a major city and 13% working in inner regional locations.

Working in the public health care system

Physiotherapists working in the public health care system in Australia do so predominantly in a hospital environment. This provides the opportunity to work across a range of clinical areas. In the hospital setting, early-career physiotherapists will gain experience in the core clinical areas of musculoskeletal, cardiorespiratory and neurological physiotherapy and may also be introduced to other areas such as paediatrics, orthopaedics, gerontology and women's health. It is through this pathway that many physiotherapists develop a broad range of skills and gain experience in a variety of clinical areas.

Physiotherapists in the public system may also work in primary care as community-based physiotherapists. In these roles, they may work in a community health service or supported residential facility (SRF), or visit people's places of residence to assist with optimising functional abilities and quality of life.

While the physiotherapy profession has a national registration structure, salaries and awards are state / territory based. These are negotiated between employers and the relevant unions through the enterprise bargaining process, which occurs around every 3 years. Although wages and conditions differ across states and territories, there exist some general consistencies. The first band or grade of physiotherapists generally has less than 4–5 years of post-registration clinical experience and works across a range of clinical areas. Physiotherapists working in the second band are starting to develop expertise in a particular clinical area and are expected to work with less direct supervision. It is not uncommon for second-band physiotherapists to also continue to work in a range of fields. Band three physiotherapists are considered to have developed expertise in their clinical area and provide supervision to staff and consultation in this area. More recently, with the development of advanced-practice and extended scope of practice roles, physiotherapy is seeing the development of clinical roles in bands four and five, when previously these bands were largely restricted to management positions.

Working in the private health care system

The majority of physiotherapists working in the private sector do so in private-practice clinics as **primary-contact practitioners (PCPs)**, predominantly in the area of musculoskeletal physiotherapy (Health Workforce Australia 2014). Other clinical specialties in which physiotherapists work privately include women's health, paediatrics and aged care. Physiotherapists also work in private hospitals and undertake occupational health roles for private companies.

Private-practice physiotherapists regularly treat people without first getting a referral from a doctor. This model provides a significant degree of autonomy, but it carries a greater degree of risk. Consider that many people will see a physiotherapist for lower-back pain without first visiting their local doctor. In an extremely small percentage of people, lower-back pain may be caused by a serious health condition such as cancer, an aortic aneurysm or a deep infection. Consequently, physiotherapists must have adequate training and expertise to be able to recognise signs of serious pathology and refer to a doctor or ED for appropriate management. Additionally, physiotherapists need to have the expertise to identify other serious pathologies such as fractures after trauma – for example, an ankle injury sustained while playing sport. To facilitate this, physiotherapists are able to order X-rays that are partly funded by the federal government through Medicare.

So who pays for services provided by the private health sector? For physiotherapists, this is no different to many other health care professionals: they use a fee-for-service system. The fees charged by physiotherapists are largely driven by market forces. In contrast to the Australian Medical Association (AMA), the APA does not provide a recommended fee schedule. In 2012, the average fee for an initial consultation in Victoria was around $64 for a standard consultation (Australian Physiotherapy Association 2013), paid by users of the service. If users have private health insurance cover, they will be reimbursed a percentage of the total fee. Since 2000, many private practices have become 'preferred providers' for private health insurers. In return for the private health insurer recommending the services of a particular practice, the user will pay a smaller gap between the consultation fee and the rebate from the insurer. There has been considerable debate among the profession regarding the advantages of being involved in such a system, as while it potentially increases the number of people seen by a practice it also reduces revenue per customer. The APA has concerns that such preferred-provider arrangements will potentially lead to an imbalance of power between small physiotherapy practices and private health insurers in Australia. The insurance company, not the physiotherapist, sets the fees and potentially reduces revenue per client. Additionally, there is no obvious justifiable reason for assigning a higher rebate to preferred providers with respect to either improved health outcomes or greater clinical expertise. This practice also has the potential to drive prices down across the entire industry in order for practices to compete at a financial level. Consequently, physiotherapy practices are investing in other means to improve services. It is now not uncommon for practices to have purpose-built gymnasiums, including aquatic physiotherapy facilities, which were rare prior to 2000. Physiotherapy practice business models have also undergone significant change in this time. Historically, private practices were largely managed by a sole practitioner but Australia has recently seen the emergence of franchise-style practices.

Private practices often provide services for what are termed 'compensable' clients. These clients have generally incurred an injury at their place of work, or been involved in a motor vehicle accident. In most instances, a general practitioner (GP) will need to initiate the process of establishing a management plan and which health care professionals are to be involved in the client's treatment. Once a claim has been approved by either WorkCover or the relevant insurance body, any services provided will be funded by the insurer. The fees are set by the insurer, and are generally at a lower level than the standard practice scheduled fee. Additionally, because the insurers (including WorkCover) are state/territory based, fees vary between states and territories. (See Chapter 13 for a discussion on the workers' compensation health care system.)

In 1999, the federal government, via Medicare, introduced the Enhanced Primary Care (EPC) scheme in recognition of the increased prevalence of chronic disease. This was renamed the Chronic Disease Management (CDM) schedule in 2005. Through this scheme, private-practice physiotherapists were able to receive funding for services from the federal government for the first time. A GP is required to initially assess a client with a chronic condition such as diabetes or osteoarthritis and implement a team care arrangement (TCA), which may include services from a physiotherapist or other allied health professional. To be eligible for a TCA, at least three health care professionals (including the GP) need to be involved in the management of the client. A maximum of five visits to allied health professionals in a single year is funded. While this scheme was widely acknowledged as a positive step towards addressing chronic disease through a multidisciplinary approach, there has been criticism that the number of visits funded is insufficient to significantly improve health outcomes in a population with complex health needs (Foster et al. 2008). This can be illustrated by considering an elderly person with both diabetes and osteoarthritis. There is strong evidence to support interventions provided by physiotherapists, occupational therapists (OTs), dietitians, podiatrists and exercise physiologists (Huang et al. 2010; Pittet et al. 1999; Rannou & Poiraudeau 2010). However, with only a total of five visits allowed in a single year across all allied health professionals, there would obviously be considerable rationalisation of which services to select. Indeed, the client might be able to see a physiotherapist only once or twice under such circumstances. A therapist's ability to provide a meaningful and effective intervention may be impaired, potentially compromising the patient outcome.

Recently the introduction of My Aged Care and the National Disability Insurance Scheme in Australia have created a new client-centred approach to distribution of federal funding for health services. Clients or their families eligible for funding through these schemes establish goals and develop care plans with assistance from a planner. The service providers are then engaged to provide the services on a fee for service model. This has created opportunities for the development of new services through the private and NGO sectors, but has also challenged both sectors to adapt their business models.

PAUSE
for
REFLECTION
...

Physiotherapists work within the public and the private health care systems. Consider whether working in one system or another would potentially influence your working practice. Things you could consider include the client profile, the type of specialty areas you would be working in and the effect of varying resources on the quality of care able to be provided. How could the different funding models within the private sector affect the type of services provided? Consider a compensable client (a client who has their services paid for by an insurance company following an injury related to their place of work or in a motor vehicle accident) versus a client on a TCA.

Interprofessional collaboration – the role of physiotherapy

There is growing acknowledgement within the health care sector of the importance of effective interprofessional teams to deliver high-quality care. As a result, there is increasing emphasis on physiotherapists working in interprofessional models of care, alongside doctors, nurses and other allied health professionals. **Interprofessional collaboration (IPC)** is 'the process in which different professional groups work together to positively impact health' (Zwarenstein et al. 2009, p. 2). As its name suggests, a multidisciplinary team is one in which a number of health care professionals are involved in a client's care. The distinction for an interprofessional collaborative model of care is that this involves a model in which all health professionals associated with a client's care work collaboratively, with effective communication, common goal-setting and a client-centred approach. The members of an interprofessional care team vary widely. For example, a physiotherapist working in women's health in a hospital will collaborate with gynaecologists, midwives and nurses; in a neurological rehabilitation facility managing people with stroke the health care team might include doctors, occupational therapists, speech therapists, dietitians and nurses. Health outcomes are optimised when these health care professionals work effectively through clear communication, common goal-setting and a strong understanding of both the roles they are providing and those provided by the health care professionals they are working with (Satterfield et al. 2009). Case study 27.1 provides a detailed example of an IPC model of care.

Case Study 27.1

Interprofessional models of care

Joan is a 78-year-old woman living alone in her own single-level home. She is relatively fit and active despite a history of diabetes and has no community supports in place. While out shopping, Joan sustains a fall injuring her back and sustaining a laceration to her head. She is taken by ambulance to hospital where she is assessed by a physiotherapist in the ED. Joan is diagnosed with a crush fracture of her lumbar spine.

After her immediate care needs are met in the ED with analgesia, suturing and dressing of her laceration and a thorough assessment, the focus of her care turns to discharge. Joan is struggling to walk and concerned about how she will manage on her own at home. In consultation with the other members of the team, her physiotherapist organises for Joan to be admitted to the short-stay medical unit, which admits patients for up to 48 hours. The short-stay unit has a multidisciplinary team to facilitate safe discharge of patients home.

Case study questions

1 What are some of the key problems or issues that need to be addressed by the health professionals involved in Joan's care?

2 Which health professions will need to be involved in the initial acute care of Joan in the ED?

3 What are the key challenges for safely discharging Joan home?

4 What professionals will need to be involved in Joan's care in the short-stay unit?

5 What types of home services and follow-up will be required?

Drivers for change – expanding the scope of practice

There is growing international recognition that, to deliver sustainable health care into the future, new and innovative models of care need to be developed requiring a shift in traditional professional boundaries by changing current scopes of practice (Duckett et al. 2014; Nelson et al. 2014; Queensland Department of Health 2014). This shift in boundaries includes both the development of **extended-scope physiotherapist (ESP)** roles, allowing health professions to take on roles previously undertaken by other professions, and the shifting of tasks from qualified physiotherapists to physiotherapy assistants.

The role of the physiotherapist has evolved considerably over the years, driven by factors such as the demand for rehabilitation of injured returning servicemen and servicewomen, the introduction of primary-contact status and a shift in focus to EBP. Another key driver for the change faced by the Australian health care system is the shift in focus from treating acute conditions such as infections and other short-term conditions to treating chronic conditions such as osteoarthritis, diabetes and cardiovascular disease, with half of all Australians estimated as having a chronic health condition such as arthritis, back pain, asthma and diabetes (Australian Institute of Health and Welfare (AIHW), 2018, p. 96). As physiotherapists, a different approach is required to manage chronic conditions. For example, when treating someone with chronic breathing problems such as emphysema as a cardiorespiratory physiotherapist, a key goal is to maximise the client's ability to manage the disease on their own as the condition will be affecting them for the rest of their life. This is in contrast to an acute condition such as pneumonia, in which a physiotherapist will play an active role in improving the condition of the client with the aim of returning to full pre-sickness function.

An increasing aged population in Australia has contributed to medical services struggling to meet demand. Two examples of how this is influencing the health system are an increase in waiting times to see medical specialists and increasing demands on EDs. These two issues have been a key driver for the development of new roles for physiotherapists in Australia over the past 15 years. Physiotherapists have expanded their scope of practice to take on roles traditionally undertaken by the medical profession in order to cost-effectively improve productivity in an increasingly strained health care system. An example of an advanced- or extended-practice role is the use of physiotherapists in the ED. Physiotherapists in these roles are able to manage a cohort of patients presenting to hospital EDs without a doctor needing to assess them. Presentations suitable to be managed by a physiotherapist are most commonly minor trauma involving soft-tissue injuries, lower-back pain, uncomplicated bone fractures or vestibular disorders. Studies have consistently shown that people managed by a physiotherapist are seen faster and spend significantly less time in the hospital than if they had been seen by a doctor (Bird et al. 2016; Sutton et al. 2015). Physiotherapists have, additionally, expanded into roles that reduce waiting times for specialist outpatient appointments – for example, assessing people waiting to see an orthopaedic specialist due to hip, knee, shoulder or back problems and providing an appropriate management plan. Health services that have implemented these services have shown reductions in their waiting times to see a specialist (Stanhope et al. 2012).

The development of ESP roles presents several challenges for the profession. Developing appropriate training pathways is extremely complex and requires collaboration and cooperation across many different sectors, including tertiary institutions, all relevant professional bodies and both state and federal governments. Formal university qualifications to support ESP roles, including the ordering and interpretation of imaging and the prescribing of medications, have been trialled, but the sustainability of these types of postgraduate program is uncertain.

The blurring of roles does not only apply to the physiotherapy profession in expanding its scope of practice. In 2014, an Australian health report recommended that 25% of the tasks performed by physiotherapists in an acute care hospital could potentially be carried out by physiotherapy assistants (Duckett et al. 2014). A physiotherapy assistant has more limited qualifications and works under the supervision of a physiotherapist, taking on work of a less complex nature such as supervising exercise programs or assisting clients to mobilise once it is assessed as safe to do so by a physiotherapist. With increasing demands on health services, rising costs and the increasing prevalence of chronic diseases driving the need for change to the way health care services are delivered, the shifting of professional tasks to assistants is likely to have a positive cost impact (see Box 27.1). Additionally, such a shift would potentially free up physiotherapists to focus on roles utilising their full scope of practice, including the developing ESP roles.

BOX 27.1 EXPANDING THE SCOPE OF PRACTICE

People referred to spinal surgeons with back problems often have to wait long periods of time before they are seen in the public health care system. As experts in managing back pain, appropriately experienced physiotherapists have been effective in reducing this wait in many hospitals across Australia. Additional skills that these physiotherapists must develop include the ability to understand complex investigations such as magnetic resonance imaging (MRI) and computed tomography (CT) scans, as well as an appreciation of people that would benefit from having spinal surgery.

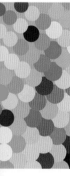

Summary

This chapter has provided a broad outline of the role of the physiotherapy profession within the Australian health care system:

- Physiotherapists play an important role in the delivery of health care services in Australia.
- There are many clinical fields in which physiotherapists work, including musculoskeletal, cardiorespiratory, neurological, paediatric, women's health, occupational health, community and palliative care.

- The roles of physiotherapists have evolved significantly in the 20th century, owing to factors such as the World Wars, poliomyelitis, the introduction of evidence-based practice, the advent of primary-contact status and the increase in prevalence of chronic diseases.
- Physiotherapy accreditation and registration are overseen by the Australian Physiotherapy Council and the Australian Health Practitioner Regulation Agency.
- Physiotherapists work in many different health environments, including public, private and non-government organisations.
- The roles of physiotherapists will very likely continue to evolve, with a greater focus on managing chronic conditions as well as expanding their scope of practice into areas such as emergency medicine and orthopaedics.
- The profession of physiotherapy is likely also to be influenced by the introduction and progression of physiotherapy assistants undertaking roles traditionally conducted by physiotherapists.

Review Questions

1 Outline the process by which the title and roles of a physiotherapist are protected.
2 Outline some of the key differences in the roles performed by a public and a private physiotherapist (in the same clinical field, e.g. musculoskeletal).
3 What possible changes to the roles of a physiotherapist would you anticipate if the trend of an increased privately funded workforce continues?
4 What are some of the drivers for change relating to the roles of physiotherapists in the past 30 years?
5 Consider a person who has arthritis in both knees and is overweight. Currently, such a person could access five government funded visits per year to an allied health professional, including a physiotherapist. Discuss both advantages and disadvantages with this strategy to manage this chronic condition. What implications would this have on how the client is treated by a physiotherapist?

References

Australian Government, 2018. Health workforce data. Data tool, Department of Health, Canberra. http://hwd.health.gov.au/datatool.html.

Australian Health Practitioner Regulation Agency (AHPRA), 2018. Approved programs of study. AHPRA. Melbourne. http://www.ahpra.gov.au/Education/Approved-Programs-of-Study.aspx?ns=1.

Australian Institute of Health and Welfare (AIHW), 2018. Australia's health 2018. Cat. no. AUS 221. AIHW, Canberra. https://www.aihw.gov.au/reports/australias-health/australias-health-2018/contents/table-of-contents.

Australian Physiotherapy Association (APA), 2013. Review of TAC Victoria schedule of fees for physiotherapy services (private). APA, Camberwell, Vic.

Australian Physiotherapy Council (APC), 2006. Australian standards for physiotherapy, APC, Camberwell, Vic.

Australian Qualifications Framework Council., 2013. Australian qualifications framework. Australian Qualifications Framework Council, Brisbane, SA.

Bird, S., Thompson, C., Williams, K.E., 2016. Primary contact physiotherapy services reduce waiting and treatment times for patients presenting with musculoskeletal conditions in Australian emergency departments: an observational study. J. Physiother. 62 (4), 209–214.

Calvert, R.N., 2002. The History of Massage: An Illustrated Survey From Around the World. Inner Traditions / Bear & Co., Rochester, VT.

Chipchase, L.S., Galley, P., Jull, G., et al., 2006. Looking back at 100 years of physiotherapy education in Australia. Aust. J. Physiother. 52 (1), 3–7.

Duckett, S., Breadon, P., Farmer, J., 2014. Unlocking Skills in Hospitals: Better Jobs, More Care. Grattan Institute, Melbourne.

Forster, A., 1969. Physiotherapy in Australia. Aust. J. Physiother. 15 (3), 96–99.

Foster, M.M., Mitchell, G., Haines, T., et al., 2008. Does Enhanced Primary Care enhance primary care? Policy-induced dilemmas for allied health professionals. Med. J. Aust. 188 (1), 29.

Health Workforce Australia (HWA)., 2014. Australia's health workforce series – Physiotherapists in focus, HWA, Adelaide.

Huang, M., Hsu, C., Wang, H., et al., 2010. Prospective randomized controlled trial to evaluate effectiveness of registered dietitian-led diabetes management on glycemic and diet control in a primary care setting in Taiwan. Diabetes Care 33 (2), 233–239.

McMeeken, J., 2014. Celebrating a shared past, planning a shared future: physiotherapy in Australia and New Zealand. N. Z. J. Physiother. 42 (1), 1.

Nelson, S., Turnbull, J., Bainbridge, L., et al., 2014. Optimizing Scopes of Practice: New Models for a New Health Care System, Canadian Academy of Health Sciences, Ontario, Canada.

Nicholls, D.A., Cheek, J., 2006. Physiotherapy and the shadow of prostitution: the Society of Trained Masseuses and the massage scandals of 1894. Soc. Sci. Med. 62 (9), 2336–2348.

Pittet, D., Wyssa, B., Herter-Clavel, C., et al., 1999. Outcome of diabetic foot infections treated conservatively: a retrospective cohort study with long-term follow-up. Arch. Intern. Med. 159 (8), 851–856.

Queensland Department of Health., 2014. Ministerial taskforce on health practitioner expanded scope of practice: final report, Allied Health Professions' Office of Queensland, Brisbane, p. 112.

Rannou, F., Poiraudeau, S., 2010. Non-pharmacological approaches for the treatment of osteoarthritis. Best Pract. Res. Clin. Rheumatol. 24 (1), 93–106.

Ross, P., 1983. Kenny, Elizabeth (1880–1952), Australian Dictionary of Biography. National Centre of Biography, Australian National University, Canberra. http://adb.anu.edu.au/biography/kenny-elizabeth-6934/text12031, published first in hardcopy 1983.

Satterfield, J., Spring, B., Brownson, R., et al., 2009. Toward a transdisciplinary model of evidence-based practice. Milbank Q. 87 (2), 368–390.

Stanhope, J., Grimmer-Somers, K., Milanese, S., et al., 2012. Extended scope physiotherapy roles for orthopedic outpatients: an update systematic review of the literature. J. Multidiscip. Healthc. 5, 37.

Sutton, M., Govier, A., Prince, S., et al., 2015. Primary-contact physiotherapists manage a minor trauma caseload in the emergency department without misdiagnoses or adverse events: an observational study. J. Physiother. 61 (2), 77–80.

World Confederation for Physical Therapy (WCPT), 2017. Policy statement: description of physical therapy. WCPT, London.

Zwarenstein, M., Goldman, J., Reeves, S., 2009. Interprofessional collaboration: effects of practice-based interventions on professional practice and healthcare outcomes. Cochrane Database Syst. Rev. (3), CD000072.

Further Reading

Australian Health Practitioner Regulation Agency – codes and guidelines: www.physiotherapyboard.gov.au/Codes-Guidelines.aspx.

Australian Physiotherapy Association – NDIS resources: http://www.physiotherapy.asn.au/APAWCM/Resources/Clinician_resources/DisabilityNDIS/APAWCM/Advocacy/NDIS_Resources.aspx?hkey=f3d995ed-e314-48b0-b200-21216a125390.

Australian Physiotherapy Council – Australian standards for physiotherapy: http://www.physiotherapy.asn.au/DocumentsFolder/Resources_Private_Practice_Standards_for_physiotherapy_practices_2011.pdf.

Physiotherapy Board of Australia (PBA) 2014. Physiotherapy Regulation at Work in Australia, 2014/15, Australian Health Practitioner Regulation Agency, PBA, Canberra. https://www.physiotherapyboard.gov.au/News/2016-04-08-physiotherapy-regulation.aspx.

Online Resources

Australian Physiotherapy Association (APA): www.physiotherapy.asn.au.

Centre for the Advancement of Interprofessional Education (CAIPE): caipe.org.uk.

Physiotherapy Board of Australia: http://www.physiotherapyboard.gov.au/.

World Confederation for Physical Therapy – practice resources: https://www.wcpt.org/practice.

CHAPTER 28

Speech pathology and audiology: assessment and intervention for communication impairment

Chris Brebner, Christopher Lind, Jane Bickford and Lisa Callahan[a]

Key learning outcomes

When you finish this chapter you should be able to:

- identify common communication difficulties that occur over the life-span, arising from speech, language and/or hearing difficulties, and the impact of communication impairments on everyday life
- identify some major clinical intervention activities undertaken by speech pathologists and audiologists
- contrast patterns of public and private service provision in speech pathology and audiology
- identify political, commercial and professional forces that have shaped current models of speech pathology and audiology services
- identify the purpose and impact of, and delivery models for, addressing communication impairment.

Key terms and abbreviations

acquired acute difficulties	communication access
audiology	communication impairment
auditory processing disorders (APDs)	complex communication needs
Australian Hearing	conductive hearing loss
autism spectrum disorder (ASD)	degenerative neurological conditions
biopsychosocial model	developmental disabilities
Child and Family Health Service (CaFHS)	dysphagia
Commonwealth Acoustics Laboratories (CAL)	ear, nose and throat (ENT) specialist

[a]We acknowledge the contributions by Lisa Jane Moody and Catherine Olssen to the chapter in the 3rd edition of this book.

expressive communication impairments
International Classification of Function (ICF)
intervention services
National Disability Insurance Agency (NDIA)
National Disability Insurance Scheme (NDIS)
noise-induced hearing loss
otitis media (OM)

presbycusis
professional development
receptive communication impairment
rubella
speech pathology
tinnitus
universal neonatal hearing screening (UNHS)

Introduction

This chapter outlines service delivery models for two allied health professions that together play key roles in assessing and alleviating **communication impairment** in today's Australian health care system. Despite commonality of purpose, the two professions – **speech pathology** and **audiology** – are practised in very different ways. The interplay of forces influencing current care models presented to the general public in speech pathology and audiology include:

♦ relative emphasis on public versus private practice
♦ introduction of the National Disability Insurance Scheme (NDIS) for service provision to people with long-term needs related to disability
♦ the balance between service delivery and supply of devices / equipment
♦ the role of government in service delivery (Duckett 2014)
♦ the availability of services to various sectors of the Australian community (Tuohy 1999).

Communication and communication impairment

Communication is a basic human right (United Nations 1948) and is fundamental to how people relate to each other across their life-span. Babies begin to develop their communication skills from birth. Their early experiences start with development of eye contact with their caregiver. They play with taking turns and making sounds and experimenting with attempts at words. From infancy, children use communication skills to develop interpersonal relationships, which shapes their social skills and personalities. These skills enable learning of spoken language, which facilitates later development of reading and writing. Children develop language and communication skills as they grow, with most children reaching adult language competence by about 16 years of age. As adults, we use communication skills to establish and maintain relationships as well as to plan, work and interact within our communities. Through communication we solve problems, converse with others, tell stories and argue points. Communication enables us to recall and share memories, to predict and look forwards and to reflect. It shapes our image of ourself and of others. In fact, communication is a critical yet subtle human behaviour that facilitates everyday participation in our community.

To communicate, spoken and / or written messages need to be formulated and understood. In this process, there are many points when communication can be compromised or interrupted, resulting in communication impairment (Denes & Pinson 1993; Humes & Bess 2014). **Expressive communication impairments** occur when delivery of a message is disrupted. This can result from cognitive, intellectual, motor or physiological processes that are immature / delayed or impaired, impacting on intelligibility or meaning of a spoken message. **Receptive communication impairments** occur when understanding of another's message is disrupted. This may include impairments of hearing or decoding spoken or written language, which may impact on an individual's participation in everyday interaction.

Expressive and receptive impairments of speech, hearing, language and communication are often 'invisible' until the person who is affected by them interacts with others. They are more prevalent than is often realised. People who have communication difficulties may experience limitations to their participation in everyday life.

The World Health Organization's **International Classification of Function (ICF)** (World Health Organization (WHO) 2001) is a **biopsychosocial model** that has influenced allied health practice. The ICF provides a framework for the relationship between structure and function, activity and participation and has influenced understanding and treatment of communication disorders internationally. Historically, clinic-based intervention dominated speech pathology and audiology practices, but the ICF has increased awareness of the impact of communication disorders on everyday participation, bringing these services into the community. In addition to the social stigma related to communication disorders (Simmons-Mackie & Damico 2007; Southall et al. 2010), visible signs of communication difficulty such as facial palsy associated with neurological damage, or hearing aids worn to reduce the impact of hearing loss, may influence one's social identity. More recently, models of intervention based on patient- and family-centred care have become more frequent in both professions. This has changed the balance between clinically measured outcomes commonly addressing impairment and psychosocial assessment of everyday participation and quality of life.

Speech pathology – speech, language and swallowing

Difficulties understanding and / or producing speech are relatively common, and arise from developmental disabilities, acquired acute difficulties or degenerative neurological conditions. **Developmental disabilities** can have known or unknown causes, and may be of genetic origin. Developmental disabilities include disorders such as **autism spectrum disorder (ASD)**, intellectual disability and cerebral palsy. **Acquired acute difficulties** arise from traumatic brain injury (TBI) or cerebral vascular accident (CVA) / stroke, and **degenerative neurological conditions** such as dementia or motor neurone disease. Speech pathologists also work with people experiencing swallowing problems or **dysphagia**. Dysphagia often occurs after stroke or brain injury, and can result in food or liquid entering the airways or lungs, causing respiratory problems, increasing health risks such as dehydration and resulting in longer hospital stays (Serra-Prat et al. 2012). People with lifelong disabilities such as cerebral palsy may also experience dysphagia. In fact, dysphagia in children with developmental disorders has been estimated to be between 30% and 80% (Arvedson 2008; Brackett et al. 2006; Lefton-Greif 2008; Manikam & Perman 2000). In this population, dysphagia may be associated with inadequate nutrition and hydration, respiratory problems leading to increased morbidity, and increased choking risk. Dysphagia also co-occurs with dementia, with conservative estimates suggesting that 15% of the elderly population is affected (Barczi et al. 2006).

Speech Pathology Australia, the national peak body for speech pathologists, recently estimated that around 5% of Australians have some form of communication impairment and a further 5%

have difficulty in swallowing (Speech Pathology Australia 2014a). Exact figures are difficult to establish owing to coexistence across disorders; for example, people with hearing impairment commonly also experience other communication impairments. Prevalence measures vary across ages and by area of difficulty; for example, 10% of preschool children have difficulty with speech (Skeat et al. 2013), 20% of 4-year-old children have difficulty with language skills (Australian Government 2013; Reilly et al. 2010) and 25% of adults over 85 years have dementia (Speech Pathology Australia 2014b).

There are effective **intervention services** for communication and swallowing issues, and recent international studies demonstrate their clinical cost–benefit (Speech Pathology Australia 2014b). The need for early intervention for children with communication impairment is well established. Difficulties with speech, language and communication impact on children's social and emotional well-being and on acquisition of literacy skills, with children with communication impairments having a higher incidence of difficulty learning to read and write (Reilly et al. 2010; Skeat et al. 2013). These difficulties often continue to impact negatively on social and emotional well-being, educational and employment outcomes into adulthood (Mustard 2008; del Zoppo et al. 2015).

Case study 28.1 examines the management of complex health needs after surgery.

Case Study 28.1

Complex health needs managed over long distances

Ron is 64 years old and lives in a large regional town 250 kilometres from the capital city. Four months ago he was diagnosed with advanced laryngeal cancer and underwent surgery to remove his larynx (laryngectomy) and radiation treatment. The surgery has resulted in him needing to breathe through a hole in his neck (stoma) and has affected his ability to talk and eat. Ron's treatment took place in the capital city at a major hospital with a specialist multidisciplinary team. Since his treatment he has been experiencing some problems with swallowing, communication and breathing. Ron lives alone and is socially isolated. He has a brother living in the city and knows a few other men who go to the same pub. Ron stopped work as a labourer a few years ago owing to a back problem.

When Ron was in hospital he received support from specialist doctors, nurses and allied health professionals. He was encouraged to look after his stoma and have softer foods to manage his swallowing problems. Until recently, he could communicate only by writing messages or using an electronic device with a synthetic sound.

Since his laryngectomy, Ron has had difficulty adjusting to the changes to his life. Communicating has been challenging and he has avoided using his electronic device. Due to the seriousness of his illness and treatment he has to travel to the city for specialist appointments. These visits cost a lot in travel and accommodation expenses. They also exacerbate his back pain. A few weeks ago he had another surgical procedure so he can now use a voice prosthesis to help him talk. Ron has to get his voice prosthesis changed every few months by a speech pathologist. He mentions to his specialist team that for financial and physical reasons he finds it difficult to come to the city for appointments.

Continued

Ron's hospital-based speech pathologist gets in touch with the local speech pathologist in his regional town's health service. She finds out that this speech pathologist is a new graduate with no direct experience supporting people who have had a laryngectomy. This is a common scenario as there is often little local expertise with laryngectomy. She recommends that the speech pathologist comes to a study day for community-based speech pathologists in 1 month and provides links to online recourses to help her to familiarise herself with voice rehabilitation after laryngectomy.

The local speech pathologist attends the study day and is able to practise the management of a voice prosthesis under the supervision of the hospital speech pathologist. The local speech pathologist arranges a telehealth session with the hospital speech pathologist so that she can supervise her when she changes Ron's voice prosthesis for the first time. The session takes extra time for the speech pathologists involved with Ron's care but it reduces the need for Ron to visit the capital. Initially, the local speech pathologist is able to see Ron weekly and she builds a strong working relationship with him. She identifies that he is quite isolated and links him with a local community support group. This appears to help him with his communication proficiency and acceptance of his situation.

Case study questions

1 What issues does the local-based speech pathologist face in supporting Ron with his voice rehabilitation in his local community?

2 How might the hospital speech pathologist further support the local speech pathologist to support Ron?

3 Outline what other benefits Ron may experience from having his care needs being managed locally.

Audiology – hearing and related disorders

The overall prevalence of hearing loss in the Australian community has been reported to be as high as 16%–20% (Chia et al. 2007; Wilson et al. 1999). Further, the prevalence of hearing loss is substantially skewed, particularly by age and gender. Approximately 33% of the Australian population aged over 48 are reported to have some degree of age-related hearing loss, with significantly more men than women under 80 years of age experiencing this type of hearing loss (Gopinath et al. 2009).

Children are also commonly affected by hearing loss. **Otitis media** (OM), a condition affecting the middle ear (and thus causing a **conductive hearing loss**), is the most common cause of hearing loss in children, which has its highest prevalence among children up to the age of 6–7 years (Jervis-Bardy et al. 2014). OM is a fluctuating condition that typically results in mild–moderate hearing loss and, at worst, results in a moderate degree of hearing loss. The prevalence of childhood OM is influenced by the child's anatomy, exposure to infectious agents and access to primary health care. Rates of chronic middle ear infections among Indigenous children, particularly those who live in rural and remote Australia, are much higher than among urban non-Indigenous children, which is primarily due to social and environmental factors (Jervis-Bardy et al. 2014). Hearing health is critical to quality of life, yet many children do not have access to the appropriate primary health care either through a general practitioner (GP) or a local audiologist.

Sensorineural (and most commonly, permanent) hearing loss occurs when the cochlea or hearing nerve is damaged or malformed. Between two and three babies in every thousand live births have a detectable level of sensorineural hearing loss in one or both ears (National Institute on Deafness and Other Communication Disorders 2015). In Australia, up to 12 babies in every 10,000 will have moderate or greater loss in both ears, and a further 23 will acquire hearing loss requiring hearing aids by the age of 17 years (Australian Hearing 2015). If left unmanaged, any type of hearing loss in childhood has the potential to impact on speech and language development, communication, learning and quality of life, and may result in lifelong disability.

While there are a number of known risk factors for permanent congenital hearing loss, including family history, ototoxic medications, craniofacial abnormalities and **rubella** or cytomegalovirus (CMV) infection in the baby, many children born with permanent hearing loss do not have these risk factors. Currently, although **Universal Neonatal Hearing Screening (UNHS)** screening protocols vary between states and territories, these programs report hearing screening of more than 95% of all live births in Australia (Leigh 2010). Since the introduction of newborn hearing screening programs in Australia, the average age for diagnosis of congenital hearing loss has dropped from 2.5 years to 3 months, meaning more children are able to access early-intervention services for hearing loss.

Early diagnosis by 3 months of age, and early intervention (often comprising a hearing aid fitting and speech/language therapy program) by 6 months of age may potentially decrease or avoid some of the negative impacts of congenital hearing loss. Audiologists and speech pathologists work closely with families and other service providers such as the **Child and Family Health Service (CaFHS)** to implement evidence-based strategies supporting language and communication development.

Early-intervention programs for children with sensorineural hearing loss have different perspectives on sign language (such as Signed English or Auslan) and the use of visual speech cues (such as lip-reading and cued articulation). Signed English is a signed version of English where there is a one-to-one correspondence between the spoken or written word and the sign. Auslan (Australian sign language) is a unique language with its own grammar and syntax. The ideologies behind various early-intervention models of practice require that parents be supported in their selection of the services that best suit their child.

The most commonly occurring causes of adult-onset hearing loss are (a) **noise-induced hearing loss (NIHL)**, which has its effect largely on adults working in industry, in the armed forces or in the music industry, results in permanent damage to the inner ear and is most commonly bilateral; and (b) age-related hearing loss (or **presbycusis**), which has its greatest effect on those over 55–60 years of age and is also a permanent bilateral condition.

Audiological practice may be divided according to its diagnostic and rehabilitative focus. By far the more common practice of the two in audiology today is rehabilitation, particularly the selection and provision of hearing aids to adults who have acquired hearing loss. Interventions direct clinical effort towards addressing the needs of the patient in their everyday communicative environment and by extension on the impact of the individual's hearing impairment on their family members. These patient- and family-centred care models emphasise functional clinical outcomes as the ultimate goals of hearing rehabilitation.

Audiologists also deal with hearing-related disorders such as **tinnitus** (ringing in the ears), **auditory processing disorders** (APDs – problems with the way individuals process what they hear) and some cases of vertigo (dizziness) arising from pathologies of the ear and / or along the pathways from the ear to the brainstem.

PAUSE
for
REFLECTION
...

Together, speech pathologists and audiologists assess and treat communication impairment (as outlined in the text) and ultimately support the participation of the individual in everyday activities. As such, the work of audiologists and speech pathologists moves beyond impairment to consider issues of participation. In what ways may their clinical work be considered to fit within a biopsychosocial model of health?

Case study 28.2 examines the management of newborn hearing impairment.

Case Study 28.2

Navigating referral pathways: communication and the case of newborn hearing impairment

Anna is one of four paediatric audiologists at a community health service in metropolitan Adelaide who performs hearing assessments for babies who don't pass their newborn hearing screenings. These tests allow for early diagnosis of permanent hearing impairment and referral to other service providers to help manage the hearing loss, including ear, nose and throat (ENT) specialists, speech pathologists and audiologists who specialise in fitting hearing aids and cochlear implants.

Anna receives a referral to see 2-month-old Andrew, who did not pass his newborn hearing screenings. The referral documentation from the nurse states that Andrew's family has recently immigrated to Australia from Italy and speaks little English. Andrew was unwell for several weeks at birth and requires the ongoing use of an oxygen tank. The family was reported to have missed several earlier appointments because of difficulty arranging care for their two older children and arranging transport.

Case study questions

1 What are the positive aspects of communication in this case study?

2 What things will Anna need to consider when contacting the family to make a hearing assessment appointment for Andrew?

3 How might Anna manage these concerns before and during the appointment?

4 If Andrew is found to have permanent hearing loss, what will be the important aspects of the style and content of communication between Anna and the service providers who help to manage hearing loss?

Education, employment and registration

Speech pathology

Speech pathology is a university-level professional entry allied health qualification. There are currently 17 universities across Australia offering 13 undergraduate and 12 postgraduate degree programs. In 2018, 18 programs had full professional accreditation with Speech Pathology Australia. There are no registration requirements for speech pathologists.

There were over 8500 speech pathologists working in Australia in 2018 (Speech Pathology Australia n.d.). It is a young, feminised profession with nearly half of Speech Pathology Australia's practising membership in 2015 under 35 years of age and with less than 3% men (Speech Pathology Australia 2016).

Speech pathologists assess and treat people who have communication and swallowing impairments. These encompass speech, language, swallowing, voice, fluency (i.e. stuttering) and multimodal communication (i.e. using additional means of communicating such as sign language). They work with people across the life-span in a variety of private and public settings, including kindergartens, schools, aged-care facilities and hospitals, rehabilitation and mental health services, community health centres, maternal and child health services and private practices. Speech pathologists provide consultative and individual therapy, work in small groups and educational settings, provide home-based services and work in communities to build **communication access**.

Speech pathologists are employed in a range of sectors. Recent employment growth in the private sector now sees 62.5% of Speech Pathology Australia members working in private practice. Other sectors include government services (37.6%) and non-government organisations (5.3%). Nationally, speech pathologists predominately work in urban areas, with only 4.5% of speech pathologists in rural locations (Speech Pathology Australia 2016). Speech pathologists often work part-time. In 2011 the average number of hours worked was 30.3 (Health Workforce Australia 2014).

There is an unmet need for speech pathology services in early-childhood and school settings, aged-care and disability sectors, the juvenile justice system and acute and subacute hospital and rehabilitation settings (Speech Pathology Australia 2016). Policy changes and new funding arrangements in disability, education, health and aged care, including the NDIS, Commonwealth home support packages and activity-based funding, influence speech pathology service delivery and practice. Technology enhancements are enabling innovations such as telepractice to meet service demands in regional locations (Speech Pathology Australia 2018).

Audiology

Audiology in its current form is a relatively young profession. Audiology commenced in Australia as professional training by the (then) Commonwealth Acoustics Laboratories (CAL) for psychology graduates in the 1960s (Upfold 2008), and became a graduate diploma course in the mid 1970s and a Master's degree program in 1996. There are currently six Australian university programs for audiology. Australian audiology graduates are required to demonstrate clinical competency in order to be eligible for membership of Audiology Australia on the basis of their having graduating from an accredited course and having met competency standards, which are assessed while on clinical placement during their study. Audiologists are not required to be registered in order to practise in Australia, nor do they need to be members of a professional body. Employment in Australia requires only eligibility for membership to Audiology Australia. However, for some time membership of the professional body has been required for the practitioner to undertake clinical activities on behalf of the Federal Government's Office of Hearing Services. More recently, membership has also been required in order to provide audiology services under the NDIS (see Chapter 12).

Much of the audiological practice we know today grew out of two important world events – the first inflicted on adults and the second arising among children. First, at the end of World War II, audiological services were offered to servicemen and servicewomen who had returned from their military service with hearing loss arising from chronic and acute noise exposure (Upfold 2008). In North America, veterans' medical institutions such as the Walter Reed Army Hospital published much early research in rehabilitative audiology, primarily on the outcomes of supplying hearing aids to veterans. Second, in the 1940s many of the currently used paediatric audiology practices were developed in response to the children affected by the rubella epidemics that occurred between 1939 and 1941 (Upfold 2008). It is of note that the incidence of hearing loss in newborns dropped largely as a result of the community health vaccination programs to prevent rubella (Gelfand 2009). Now, among children who have hearing loss, close to 50% of permanent sensorineural hearing losses occurring prior to 3 years of age are genetic in origin (Gorlin & Toriello 2013).

Diagnostic audiology services are undertaken primarily by public hospitals for inpatient or outpatient clients, commonly provided in conjunction with ENT, oncology, paediatric, geriatric or surgical referrals. More recent hospital-based audiological practices have included the assessment of newborns, leading to the UNHS programs around Australia that were established in 2000. Recent developments in the analysis of genetic sites of hearing disorders, and the instigation of the UNHS programs, have greatly increased the sensitivity of diagnosis and identification of the causes of hearing loss in young children (Shearer et al. 2013).

Practice within the Australian health care system

This section highlights how funding models impact on service delivery to the Australian community for communication impairment. Although the issues outlined are often particular to speech pathology or audiology, the case studies and questions raise matters for consideration, and we encourage you to look behind the detail to the broader issues. In many cases these issues are pertinent to other areas of health practice.

Speech pathologists and audiologists share the goal of alleviating the impact of communication impairment via a number of service delivery models. Speech pathologists provide services in a range of settings (e.g. acute (public) hospital, community centre, home, school, etc.) and within a number of different structures (e.g. consultative, individual, small treatment group, group training and information sessions for clients and/or their communication partners).

In contrast, few private-practice audiologists work in interdisciplinary settings. Note that audiology is heavily reliant on technology for its practice in both diagnosis and intervention. The supply of hearing aids raises some of the most interesting and contentious issues in the conduct of health services in the Australian health system. The fundamental issue is one of equity of access to increasingly expensive and sophisticated hearing aids and devices. Two issues around the delivery and pricing of technology-driven services, addressed in previous editions of this book (Lind & Olsson 2012; Lind et al. 2016), remain central to models of service delivery among private-practice audiology clinics. The first involves aggregation of service and device costs, which typically results in offers of 'free' hearing tests where the cost of the test is actually built in to the cost of supplying a hearing device. The second involves the acceptance of direct and indirect inducements to favour the supply of a particular company's devices.

The majority of publicly funded audiology hearing-aid provision services today are available to eligible members of the general public through the federal government's hearing-aid voucher scheme provided by **Australian Hearing** or by registered providers in private clinics. As a result, Medicare rebates for these hearing services are of limited relevance. Those not eligible for government-funded services may seek relief from commercial hearing aid costs via private health insurance. Private health insurers may fund a portion of the cost of an eligible hearing-aid fitting every 3–5 years. The federal government acknowledged the need for a substantial restructuring of Australian Hearing's services in its 2014 Budget, but at the time of writing no announcement on the nature of any change has been made.

Ethical clinical practice in a complex and challenging environment

Complexities and challenges face health care clinicians in all workplace environments (e.g. health care, education, disability) where demand and supply diverge, where distance impacts on service delivery, where vulnerable client groups (especially those with **complex communication needs**) are disadvantaged, where emerging technologies prompt clinicians to re-examine and change practice, where client issues are diverse, where chronic and long-term care and management are required, where organisations are uncertain about funding levels, where program direction and organisational structure are changing and where there is increasing legislation and compliance required at federal and state/territory level.

With particular reference to the supply of devices (e.g. hearing aids), the pressures to meet standards of accountability simultaneously to government, shareholders, employers and professional bodies have brought great tension to hearing heath care service providers. The premise that the health provision model will operate as a free-market economy fails when the service and the device supplied to the client are sufficiently complex to prevent consumers from acting on the basis of informed choice in these purchases. Selection of devices is thus an 'expert' decision, and may sometimes mask incentive-driven practice which potentially limits client access to the full range of available devices.

The contemporary approach to problem-solving in ethical service delivery is to inform, educate and discuss with clinicians the integration of decision-making into everyday practice, how to view ethical dilemmas as they arise and what approaches clinicians can use to resolve and even anticipate such dilemmas (Audiology Australia 2014; Speech Pathology Australia 2010). In addition to a set of shared clinical values, each clinician brings a unique set of underlying perspectives and beliefs to each event. For newer graduates, it may be that these perspectives cannot clearly be articulated, but ethical enquiry allows clinicians to make explicit the decision-making processes they undertake.

The National Disability Insurance Scheme

In health service delivery for those eligible for government support, short-term funding responses have often been applied to long-term intervention needs for those with communication impairment. To address this, and to give people with disability a greater say in the services they receive, the *National Disability Insurance Scheme Act 2013* was passed into legislation, establishing the **National Disability Insurance Scheme** (NDIS) and the agency responsible for delivering the scheme, the **National Disability Insurance Agency** (NDIA).

As you may recall from Chapter 12, the NDIA was chartered to fund reasonable and necessary support to help participants (i.e. individuals with disability, their families and carers) to reach their goals, objectives and aspirations, and undertake activities that enable the participant's social and economic participation. The NDIS has resulted in a transition from block-funding of disability service provider organisations to individualised funding for participants in the NDIS. Access to the NDIS for children with a range of communication difficulties has had a significant impact on paediatric service provision, with a proliferation of private practitioners providing services to these children.

Children with developmental difficulties and long-term intervention needs may also experience limitation on activity in other developmental areas such as gross motor or cognitive development. They will often require support relating to technology or therapeutic support aiming to reduce the impact of communication difficulties (e.g. direct intervention, provision of assistive technology such as electronic speech output devices, hearing aids or cochlear-implant speech processors for individuals with hearing impairment). They may also need support such as assistance with personal care, social skills development, and technology intended to address other support needs (such as independent mobility) (Horn & Kang 2012).

In conjunction with the NDIS, the health and education sectors are expected to maintain provision of services and support to people with speech and/or hearing disabilities (Department of Human Services, n.d.). Historically, access to services with a medical or educational focus for people with these disabilities has been limited. The best outcomes for people with speech, language and/or hearing disabilities are achieved through coordinated person-centred services (Smith-Merry & Gillespie, 2016; Smith-Merry et al., 2018). Implementation of the NDIS provides an opportunity to develop a set of principles and protocols to assist in determining roles and responsibilities across and between sectors (Smith-Merry et al., 2018). However, there are significant challenges in creating a consistent national approach.

A final word

Inequality of access to services has critical social consequences. Many people are not eligible for government support and cannot afford to attend for diagnosis and possible amelioration of the barriers they face to communication participation. This limited access to services impacts on the individuals themselves, and those who wish to communicate with them. There is current and clear evidence of the effects of changes to government regulation and funding models on the provision of speech and / or hearing services, particularly to low-income earners and others who are disenfranchised in the community. Changes in the profile and funding of service provision impacts on clinical governance, such as clinicians' access to **professional development**, with particular emphasis on the identification and provision of services that are more clinically complex. Thus there are potential risks for quality of service delivery. In response, professional bodies tend to step in to ensure that minimum practice standards are being met, via continuing professional development in some cases and by professional regulation in others (Tuohy 1999). It remains a balancing act to maintain and develop knowledge and skills across a workforce, while recruiting large numbers of professionals to meet increased demand.

Summary

In this chapter we have outlined:

- the practice of two professions whose major focus is remediation of motor, sensory, cognitive and behavioural impairments influencing everyday communication: speech pathology and audiology
- the similarities and differences in their modes of practice, particularly in (a) the balance of diagnostic and intervention activities, (b) the emphasis on technological versus communication-based intervention, and (c) the government regulation applied to the two professions' activities
- some of the ethical issues in delivering care to clients, with particular focus on the National Disability Insurance Scheme (NDIS)
- the impact of federal government funding for speech pathology and audiology services via the NDIS.

Review Questions

1 What impact on the relationship between the state, providers and the private system may flow from the roll-out of National Disability Insurance Scheme funding?

2 What is problematic about being allowed to diagnose clients' hearing loss as well as recommend and supply their hearing aids?

3 Discuss the issues raised in the *Pause for reflection* box and the case studies in the light of arguments that health is a human right, not a commodity.

4 Compare and contrast the examples of Tuohy's (1999) interplay of regulatory / commercial / professional pressures model from within speech pathology and audiology, with respect to their effects on client access and outcomes.

5 Discuss the types of speech pathology services that might be more likely to be provided in acute care versus rehabilitation contexts. Why might there be a difference in the services provided in different contexts?

References

Arvedson, J., 2008. Assessment of pediatric dysphagia and feeding disorders: clinical and instrumental approaches. Dev. Disabil. Res. Rev. 14 (2), 118–127.

Audiology Australia, 2014. Ethics guidelines. http://www.audiology.asn.au.

Australian Government, 2013. A Snapshot of Early Childhood Development in Australia 2012 – AEDI National Report. Australian Government, Canberra.

Australian Hearing, 2015. Hearing loss. Australian Hearing, North Ryde. www.hearing.com.au/category/about-hearing.

Barczi, S., Sullivan, P.A., Robbins, J., 2006. How should dysphagia care of older adults differ? Establishing optimal practice patterns. Semin. Speech Lang. 21 (4), 347–361.

Brackett, K., Arvedson, J.C., Manno, C.J., 2006. Pediatric feeding and swallowing disorders: general assessment and intervention. Perspectives on Swallowing and Swallowing Disorders (Dysphagia) 15 (3), 10–14.

Chia, E.M., Wang, J.J., Rochtchina, E., et al., 2007. Hearing impairment and health-related quality of life: the Blue Mountains Hearing Study. Ear Hear. 28, 187–195.

del Zoppo, C., Sanchez, L., Lind, C., 2015. A long-term follow-up of children and adolescents referred for assessment of auditory processing disorder. Int. J. Audiol. 54 (6), 368–375.

Denes, P.B., Pinson, E.N., 1993. The Speech Chain: The Physics and Biology of Spoken Language. Worth, New York.

Department of Human Services, n.d. People with disability. Australian Government, Canberra. https://www.humanservices.gov.au/individuals/people-disability.

Duckett, S. 2014. Is Medicare sustainable? and, Is the question helpful or not? Presentation to Grattan Institute AHHA roundtable, Canberra. grattan.edu.au/wpcontent/uploads/2014/05/540_presentation_duckett_medicare_anniversary_140130.pdf.

Gelfand, S.A., 2009. Essentials of Audiology, third ed. Thieme, New York.

Gopinath, B., Rochtchina, E., Wang, J.J., et al., 2009. Prevalence of age-related hearing loss in older adults: Blue Mountains Study. Arch. Intern. Med. 169 (4), 415–418.

Gorlin, R.J., Toriello, H.V., 2013. Genetic hearing loss – a brief history. In: Toriello, H.V., Smith, S.D., (Eds.), Hereditary Hearing Loss and its Syndromes, third ed. OUP, New York, pp. 1–3.

Health Workforce Australia (HWA), 2014. Australia's Health Workforce Series: Speech Pathologists in Focus. HWA, Canberra.

Horn, E.M., Kang, J., 2012. Supporting young children with multiple disabilities: what do we know and what do we still need to learn? Topics Early Child Spec. Educ. 31 (4), 241–248.

Humes, L.E., Bess, F.H., 2014. Audiology and Communication Disorders, second ed. Walters Kluwer Health, Philadelphia.

Jervis-Bardy, J., Sanchez, L., Carney, A.S., 2014. Otitis media in indigenous Australian children: review of epidemiology and risk factors. J. Laryngol. Otol. 128 (Suppl.S1), S16–S27.

Lefton-Greif, M., 2008. Pediatric dysphagia. Phys. Med. Rehabil. Clin. N. Am. 19, 837–851.

Leigh, G., 2010. Early identification of hearing loss in Australia: well begun is not all done! The 2010 Libby Harricks Memorial Oration. Conference paper, Sixth Australian National Deafness Sector Summit,

Sydney, Australia. https://www.researchgate.net/publication/281630822_Early_identification_of
_hearing_loss_in_Australia_Well_begun_is_not_all_done_The_2010_Libby_Harricks_Memorial_
Oration.

Lind, C., Olsson, C., 2012. Speech pathology and audiology: service delivery and technology in
communication disorders. In: Willis, E., Reynolds, L., Keleher, H. (Eds.), Working in the Australian Health
Care System, second ed. Elsevier, London, pp. 291–304.

Lind, C., Olsson, C., Brebner, C., Moody, L-J., 2016. Speech pathology and audiology: assessment and
intervention for communication impairment. In: Willis, E., Reynolds, L., Keleher, H. (Eds.), Understanding
the Australian Health Care System, third ed. Elsevier Australia, Chatswood NSW, pp. 345–348.

Manikam, R., Perman, J.A., 2000. Pediatric feeding disorders. J. Clin. Gastroenterol. 30 (1), 34–46.

Mustard, F., 2008. Early childhood development: the best start for all South Australians. Report
commissioned for the Department of Education and Children's Services, South Australia. http://
parliament.wa.gov.au/parliament%5Ccommit.nsf/(Evidence+Lookup+by+Com+ID)/042B5F88C1D95F8
148257831003C11C1/$file/ef.aar08.aqton.Education.attachment.pdf.

National Disability Insurance Scheme Act 2013 (Cwlth) www.comlaw.gov.au/Details/C2013A00020.

National Institute on Deafness and Other Communication Disorders (NIDCD), 2015. Quick statistics.
NIDCD, Bethesda, MD. www.nidcd.nih.gov/health/statistics/pages/quick.aspx.

Reilly, S., Wake, M., Ukoumunne, O.C., et al., 2010. Predicting language outcomes at 4 years of age:
findings from Early Language in Victoria Study. Pediatrics 126 (6), e1530–e1537.

Serra-Prat, M., Palomera, M., Gomez, C., et al., 2012. Oropharyngeal dysphagia as a risk factor for
malnutrition and lower respiratory tract infection in independently living older persons: a population-
based prospective study. Age. Ageing 41 (3), 376–381.

Shearer, A.E., Hildebrand, M.S., Sloan, C.M., et al., 2013. Genetic diagnosis and gene discovery for hearing
loss using massively parallel sequencing. In: Toriello, H.V., Smith, S.D. (Eds.), Hereditary Hearing Loss
and Its Syndromes, third ed. OUP, New York, pp. 91–97.

Simmons-Mackie, N.N., Damico, J.S., 2007. Access and social inclusion in aphasia: interactional principles
and applications. Aphasiology 21, 81–97.

Skeat, J., Wake, M., Ukoumunne, O.C., et al., 2013. Who gets help for pre-school communication problems?
Data from a prospective community study. Child Care Health Dev. 40 (2), 215–222.

Smith-Merry, J., Gillespie, J., 2016. Flexible funding for effective, individualised, integrated care. 4th World
Congress on Integrated Care (WCIC4). International Foundation for Integrated Care (IFIC), Wellington.

Smith-Merry, J., Hancock, N., Gilroy, J., et al., 2018. Mind the Gap: the National Disability Insurance Scheme
and psychosocial disability. Final report: Stakeholder identified gaps and solutions.

Southall, K., Gagné, J.P., Jennings, M.B., 2010. Stigma: a negative and a positive influence on help-seeking
for adults with acquired hearing loss. Int. J. Audiol. 49, 804–814.

Speech Pathology Australia: 2010. Code of ethics. https://www.speechpathologyaustralia.org.au/SPAweb/
Members/Ethics/Code_of_Ethics/SPAweb/Members/Ethics/HTML/Code_of_Ethics.
aspx?hkey=1a179303-f14a-49c8-be12-eb9ac73f565c.

Speech Pathology Australia: 2014a. Communication impairment in Australia. http://www.
speechpathologyaustralia.org.au/library/2013Factsheets/Factsheet_Communication_Impairment_in_
Australia.pdf.

Speech Pathology Australia: 2014b. Submission to the inquiry into the prevalence of different types of speech, language and communication disorders and speech pathology services in Australia (submission 224). https://www.aph.gov.au/Parliamentary_Business/Committees/Senate/Community_Affairs/Speech_Pathology/Submissions.

Speech Pathology Australia, 2016. Understanding the Landscape – a Stimulus Paper. SPA, Melbourne.

Speech Pathology Australia. (2018). Clinical education in Australia: building a profession for the future. https://www.speechpathologyaustralia.org.au/SPAweb/Resources_For_Speech_Pathologists/Clinical_Education/SPAweb/Resources_for_Speech_Pathologists/Clinical_Education/Clinical_Education.aspx?hkey=fbbaa348-9422-4bc4-87f1-7ebac62aba97.

Speech Pathology Australia (n.d.) Find a certified practising member of Speech Pathology Australia. https://www.speechpathologyaustralia.org.au/SPAweb/Resources_for_the_Public/Find_a_Speech_Pathologist/SPAweb/Resources_for_the_Public/Find_a_Speech_Pathologist/All_Searches.aspx?hkey=0b04c883-80b2-43e7-9298-7e5db5c75197.

Tuohy, C.J., 1999. Accidental Logics: The Dynamics of Change In the Health Care Arena in the United States, Britain, and Canada. Oxford University Press, New York.

United Nations (1948) Universal Declaration of Human Rights. http://www.un.org/en/udhrbook/pdf/udhr_booklet_en_web.pdf.

Upfold, L., 2008. A History of Australian Audiology. Phonak Australia, Sydney.

Wilson, D.H., Walsh, P.G., Sanchez, L., et al., 1999. The epidemiology of hearing impairment in an Australian adult population. Int. J. Epidemiol. 28, 247–252.

World Health Organization (WHO), 2001. International classification of functioning, disability and health: ICF. WHO, Geneva. http://www.who.int/iris/handle/10665/42407.

Further Reading

Access Economics: 2006. Listen hear! The economic impact and cost of hearing loss in Australia, Access Economics. http://www.audiology.asn.au/public/1/files/Publications/ListenHearFinal.pdf.

Couzos, S., Metcalf, S., Murray, R., 2008. Ear health. In: Couzos, S., Murray, R. (Eds.), Aboriginal Primary Health Care: An Evidence-Based Approach, third ed. OUP, Melbourne, pp. 308–354.

Online Resources

Audiology Australia – ethics guidelines: www.audiology.asn.au/index.cfm/resources-publications/professional-resources.

Beaton, G.R. 2010. Why professionalism is still relevant. George Beaton: www.beatonglobal.com/why-professionalism-is-still-relevant.

Department of Health – Medicare primary care items: www.health.gov.au/mbsprimarycareitems.

National Disability Insurance Scheme: http://www.ndis.gov.au/.

Department of Health Hearing Services Program: www.hearingservices.gov.au.

Speech Pathology Australia – Code of ethics: www.speechpathologyaustralia.org.au/about-spa/code-of-ethics.

Speech Pathology Australia – Scope of practice: www.speechpathologyaustralia.org.au/professional-standards-ps/scope-of-practice.

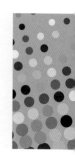

Glossary

1967 Referendum A landmark vote to change the Australian Constitution to allow the Commonwealth Government to make special laws intended to be for the benefit of Indigenous Australians that led to certain legislation such as land rights, antidiscrimination and cultural heritage protection. Sometimes mistakenly considered the point when citizenship was awarded to Indigenous Australians.

ableist or abelism Discrimination against people living with disability. The 'ableist' world-view is that able-bodied are the norm in society, and that people living with disability must strive to become that norm. The ableist view holds that disability is a mistake or tragedy rather than a simple consequence of human diversity, akin to ethnicity, sexual orientation or gender.

Aboriginal and Torres Strait Islander Australia's First Peoples.

acceptability Social and cultural factors that influence a client's preference for a service (Levesque et al. 2013).

access The degree of 'fit' between the characteristics of providers and health services and the ability of the clients (potential access) (Penchansky & Thomas 1981).

acquired acute difficulties A disability contracted as a result of an accident or disease, acquired brain disorder as a result of a head injury.

active ageing policy This term underlies health promotion campaigns that encourage physical activity and social involvement in old age.

activities of daily living (ADL) The things we normally do most often daily to live, including activities such as eating, bathing, dressing, grooming, work, homemaking and leisure.

activity-based funding (ABF) A hospital financing system whereby funding is to a state or private hospital based by on the number of episodes of care or activity which is undertaken. (See also Casemix.)

acute care The care provided to patients when they are very ill, which often lasts for a short term.

advanced practice A state of professional maturity in which the individual demonstrates a level of integrated knowledge, skill and competence that challenges the accepted boundaries of practice (McGee & Castledine 2003).

adverse events Adverse events are unintended and sometimes harmful occurrences associated with the use of a medicine, vaccine or medical device (Therapeutic Goods Administration https://www.tga.gov.au/reporting-adverse-events).

affordability Financial and time costs related to using the service (Levesque et al. 2013).

ageing in place The ability to live in one's own home or room within a residential aged care home safely, independently and comfortably, regardless of age, income or level of capacity. Ageing in the right place extends this concept to the ability to live in the place with the closest fit with the person's needs and preferences – which may or may not be one's own home (WHO 2015).

allocative efficiency A condition achieved when resources are allocated in a way that allows the maximum possible net benefit from their use. When an efficient allocation of the resources has been attained, it is impossible to increase the well-being of anyone person without harming another person. Therefore, the allocation of resources is able to achieve the best possible result in relation to the outlay (Bentley et al. 2008).

allopathy A philosophy of medicine that cures with opposites. The action of the pharmaceutical drug is the direct opposite to the effects of the illness, e.g. codeine phosphate, the primary effect of which is to cause constipation, used to treat diarrhoea.

Alzheimer's disease The most common form of dementia, affecting up to 70% of all people with dementia. Alzheimer's disease damages the brain, resulting in impaired memory, thinking and behaviour.

ambulance ramping When an ambulance presents to an emergency department and no bed is available, forcing the patient to remain under the care of ambulance personnel.

ambulance service A method of transporting a person to hospital or other medical care facility (*Health Care Act (SA) 2008*).

ambulatory services Services provided on a walk-in or short-term basis such as outpatient services, clinics and day programs.

Anangu The Ngaanyatjarra, Yankunytjatjara, Pitjantjatjara Women's Council term for people, which has come to imply Aboriginal people.

antimicrobial stewardship Governance structures that ensure judicious use of antibiotics, given the dangers of over-prescribing.

approachability Identifying that a service exists, that it can be used and can change a client's health status (Levesque et al., 2013).

appropriateness The fit between a client's health care needs and the timeliness and care spent trying to provide the correct treatment and care (Levesque et al., 2013).

assessment The action of assessing a patient for the required diagnosis and care planning needs.

asylum An older term for hospitals for people who are mentally ill.

audiologist A health-care professional with postgraduate training in hearing sciences and human communications who test, diagnose, and manage hearing loss, tinnitus, and balance problems across the life-span.

auditory processing disorder (APD) A problem with the way an individual processes what they hear.

Australian Health Practitioner Regulation Agency (AHPRA) The government agency which manages the registration and renewal processes for health practitioners on behalf of 15 national health bodies.

Australian Hearing The largest provider of the Australian Government Hearing Services Program to children and young adults under the age of 26, veterans, Indigenous adults, pensioners and people with complex hearing needs.

authority-required benefit A medicine which is included on the Schedule of Pharmaceutical Benefits only when specific patient criteria are fulfilled, and which requires a number to appear on the prescription as confirmation.

autonomy of practice The capacity to work without interference from any other group in terms of what is done, and the resources used.

availability The existence and geographical location of a service and appropriately skilled personnel that can potentially be reached by clients (Levesque et al. 2013).

'Baby Boom' generation Those born in the post-war period (1946–64). (This definition often differs between countries.)

bed block A situation that arises where a patient requires admission to a hospital bed but there are no beds available.

benefits Financial payments made to a sick person such as an injured worker, or to health care and other providers on behalf of the sick or injured person. These may include health care, income replacement, lump sums or other payments subject to the provisions of the workers' compensation legislation.

big data Very large sets of data that are produced by people using the internet, and that can only be stored, understood, and used with the help of special tools and methods (Cambridge English Dictionary 2018).

bioequivalence Demonstration that one brand behaves in a similar manner to another brand in relation to the concentration of the medicine in the blood at different times after a patient takes a dose.

biopsychosocial model An approach to health care that sees illness and health as the interaction between the biological, the psychological and the social.

bipartisan agreement in health An agreement involving two parties finding enough common ground to support core principles of health reforms.

Birthing on Country (BoC) Maternity services designed and delivered for First Peoples women that are community based and governed, allow for incorporation of traditional practice, involve a connection with land and country, incorporate a holistic definition of health, value First Peoples' knowledge, are culturally safe, and developed by, or with, Indigenous people (Kildea et al. 2012 cited in Kildea et al. 2016).

blame game Tactic whereby different levels of government shift blame to each other for problems within the health system.

blame-shifting Tactic of trying to blame another level of government if policies are not working well (NHHRC 2008).

block funded Refers to non-individualised funds whereby consumers purchase goods or services directly from a service provider, rather than a portable package of funds given to an individual to choose services.

block grant In a fiscal federal form of government, a block grant is a large sum of money granted by government or provider to the supplier of the service with only general provisions as to the way it is to be spent.

brand equivalence The status granted by the TGA to a generic brand of a medicine where evidence has been provided that it has a similar effect in the body to the effect of the originator brand.

brand premium The additional cost paid by a patient for a particular (usually originator) brand of a PBS item when a less expensive generic brand is available.

bulk-billing A payment option within Medicare (national health insurance) where the health service provider (such as a GP) is paid a percentage of the scheduled fee directly by the government as full payment for their service, which leaves no other payment or contribution from the patient. The key purpose of bulk-billing is to provide an economic constraint on medical fees and charges.

bureaucracy The organisation of government departments into many divisions.

capacity When an individual is able to make their own decisions because they have the ability to understand the information given to them, retain information, weigh up the choices and then be able to communicate their decision and choice.

carer A person whose life is affected by having a close relationship with a person with mental illness, disability or chronic illness.

casemix funding A method of allocating funds based on the activities hospitals perform, and on the types and number of patients treated. Funding is allocated on the basis of relative cost of patients treated and to reward improved performance and efficiency (Victoria State Government 2018).

chronic mental illness Someone who is experiencing long-term residual symptoms of mental illness.

chronological age The time lived since birth.

claim An application for injury compensation made by an injured person to a compensation authority, sometimes through a third-party insurer.

claims management organisation The organisation responsible for managing workers' compensation claims on behalf of the system regulator. In some jurisdictions this is the regulator and in others this is a private sector insurer.

claims manager The professional responsible for managing a compensation claim, including reviewing and approving payments for health care and rehabilitation expenses.

client A person or organisation using a service. In the case of pharmacy, a client is a customer who uses the community pharmacy regularly.

client-centred practice An 'approach to service that incorporates respect for and partnership with clients as active participants in the therapy process' (Schell et al. 2014, p. 1230).

clinical nurse A registered nurse and/or midwife with advanced nursing skills, usually with a minimum of 3 years post registration experience. The role is predominantly clinical in nature.

clinical stream A series of processes that provide integrated medical care to a patient in order to determine and execute a specific care plan.

Close the Gap Australian government policy which focused on improving the well-being of Indigenous Australians. Also a policy directive of the World Health Organization.

Closing the Gap A policy that aims to improve the lives of First Peoples by eliminating the gap in health and social outcomes between Indigenous and non-Indigenous Australians.

Closing the Gap co-payment scheme A scheme designed to improved access to medicines by Aboriginal and Torres Strait Islander peoples through provision of additional subsidies under the PBS.

code of conduct Good medical/health care practice (the code) describes what is expected of all health professionals registered to practise in Australia. It sets out the principles that characterise good practice and makes explicit the standards of ethical and professional conduct expected of the health professional by their professional peers and the community.

commissioning The process of planning, purchasing and monitoring services for a geographically defined population or sub-population that takes account of the needs of individual client (Harris et al. 2015).

Commonwealth Ombudsman A government agency that assists members of the public with disputes.

communication access Activities aimed at creating a world where people who have speech and hearing difficulties are able to communicate successfully with everyone.

communication impairment Umbrella term covering all limitations in expressive and/or receptive communication, and arising in speech, language, literacy, voice, fluency and/or social communication (Speech Pathology Australia 2014).

community control The local community having control of issues that directly affect their community. Implicit in this definition is the clear statement that Aboriginal people must determine and control the pace, shape and manner of change and decision-making at local, regional, state and national levels.

community health services (CHS) State-funded services which provide primary health care, focusing on people with, or at risk of, poorer health, under a social model of health.

community paramedicine A model of care which expands the scope of practice of paramedics to include the delivery of primary health care, substitution and/or coordination of care.

community pharmacy A pharmacy business which is owned by pharmacist(s), operates within a single store, and normally has a retail component and a dispensary.

Community Pharmacy Agreement (CPA) An agreement between the Australian Government and the Pharmacy Guild of Australia. It provides funding to around 5400 community pharmacies for dispensing PBS medicines and providing pharmacy services and to pharmaceutical wholesalers.

complex communication needs People with complex communication needs have communication problems associated with a wide range of physical, sensory, cognitive and environmental causes which restrict/limit their ability to participate independently in society. Hearing loss affecting the outer ear and/or middle ear and thus limiting the conduction of sound to the inner ear (or cochlea). Most commonly conducive hearing losses are amenable to medical or surgical intervention.

concession card holders Individuals and families who are eligible for welfare or social security support, including the age pension, disability support, unemployment or low-income support.

conductive hearing loss Hearing loss caused by a blockage in the middle or outer ear which halts the transmission of sound waves to the inner ear.

constructivist learning Encouraging students to use active techniques (experiments, real-world problem-solving) to create more knowledge and then to reflect on and talk about what they are doing and how their understanding is changing.

consultant pharmacist A pharmacist who has done additional training and is accredited to perform home medicine reviews and residential medication management reviews.

consumer A term used by advocacy groups which refers to a person who receives services such as mental health care or care for their chronic condition or pharmacy products.

consumer-directed care (CDC) A model of service delivery designed to give consumers more choice.

contextual learning Learning takes place when teachers are able to present information in a way that students are able to construct meaning based on their own experiences.

continuity of midwifery care (caseload) (CoC) A maternity service model in which women receive continuity of care from a known midwife throughout pregnancy, during birth and across the early parenting journey (usually to 6 weeks postpartum).

contracting out A process where another party external to the organisation is paid to undertake services instead of the contracting organisation.

co-option A term used by practitioners of techniques, therapies and equipment devised by another profession without adopting the knowledge base of that profession or acknowledging its origins, e.g. the use of acupuncture by medical doctors.

co-payment/gap payment Contribution to the cost of a medicine made by the patient. The difference between what is charged by the doctor, hospital or health professional for the service and what the client receives in reimbursements by Medicare or a private insurer.

corporatised To be subject to corporate ownership or control. In medicine, medical practices are increasingly being bought out by organisations that then re-employ the doctors to work in their clinics for a salary.

cost-shifting Activities aimed at making a health care service eligible for funding by a different level of government than is currently involved (NHHRC 2008).

cultural awareness The initial awareness of cultural difference between groups that is usually based on the overt differences such as language, food preferences, history, dress, etc. An awareness of difference is the first step toward cultural safety and competence.

cultural competence A diversity of definitions exist – one defines cultural competence as 'the ability of systems to provide care to patients with diverse values, beliefs and behaviours, including tailoring delivery to meet patients' social, cultural and linguistic needs' (Betancourt et al., 2002, p. v).

cultural safety Both a philosophy and way of working that is mindful of cultural difference, defined by the NZ Nursing Council as the effective care 'of a person or family from another culture, and is determined by that person or family. Culture includes, but is not restricted to, age or generation; gender; sexual orientation; occupation and socioeconomic status; ethnic origin or migrant experience; religious or spiritual belief; and disability.' (Nursing Council of New Zealand 2011).

customer Someone who, regardless of whether the visit is for health- or medicine-related reasons, interacts with a community pharmacy or service provider with the intention of purchasing products and/or using the service.

day hospital A hospital providing services for patients who then return home or to another facility at night.

degenerative neurological conditions Progressive conditions affecting the brain and causing deterioration over time (e.g. motor neurone disease, Parkinson's disease).

de-institutionalisation The process of moving long-term residents from institutional (hospital) care into the community.

dementia A chronic and progressive condition characterised by memory loss and other cognitive deficits.

dental decay/dental caries Disease of the teeth.

dental practitioner Registered dental practitioners are described in detail in Table 15.2 on pp. 251–2.

developmental disabilities Developmental physical, sensory, cognitive or psychological problems that are generally severe and chronic and impact on everyday life.

Diagnosis Related Groups A patient classification scheme that provides a means of relating the numbers and types of patients treated in a hospital to the resources required by the hospital (AIHW 2001, p. 148). Usually measured through length of stay and resource allocation.

dietitian An expert in human nutrition and dietetics with tertiary qualifications in both nutrition education/promotion and medical nutrition therapy.

digital divide Digital divide describes the divide between urban and regional/rural populations in access to the internet and digital infrastructure. It can also refer to the gaps in access to digital infrastructure even within urban populations.

digital health Digital health is connecting different points of care electronically, so health information is shared securely.

Digital Inclusion Index An index which measures three vital dimensions of digital inclusion: access, affordability and digital ability.

disability A social construct that results from barriers experienced in the environment in which a person lives and interacts and is not inherent within the person. It reflects the interaction between features of a person's body and features of the society or environment in which he or she engages.

diversity An understanding that each individual is unique and recognising our individual differences. These can be along the dimensions of race, ethnicity, gender, sexual orientation, socio-economic status, age, physical abilities, religious beliefs, political beliefs or other ideologies (Associated Students of the University of Oregon 1999).

dose administration aid (DAA) A device that allows individual medicine doses to be organised into spaces for each dose time.

dynamic efficiencies The ability of a system to adapt and adjust to change to create effective provision of services.

dysphagia A neuromuscular condition which causes difficulties in swallowing.

economic rationalism A term used to describe a range of economic policies which aim to reduce the extent of government intervention in the economy and to increase reliance on markets to direct economic activity. Some policies which are associated with 'economic rationalism' include outsourcing, reducing government spending, privatisation and deregulation.

effectiveness In health this refers to care that results in positive outcomes.

efficiency 'The relationship between the cost of various inputs and the output produced' (National Health Ministers' Benchmarketing Working Group, 1996).

elective surgery Surgery that is not medically required within 24 hours (AIHW 2013).

electronic health record (HER) A system where health information about individuals or populations is compiled electronically over time.

endorsed midwife A midwife who can prescribe scheduled medications approved by the PBS and order diagnostic and screening tests.

enrolled nurse (EN) A second-level nurse who provides nursing care under the direct or indirect supervision of a registered nurse, and must hold enrolled nursing registration with the Nursing and Midwifery Board of Australia. This group is also known as a Division 2 nurse in the State of Victoria.

evidence-based medicine (EBM) An approach to medicine holding that all clinical practice should be based on evidence from randomised control trials to ensure treatment effectiveness and efficacy.

evidence-based practice The incorporation of the best research evidence to inform clinical treatment decisions and patient values.

expressive communication impairments Reduced ability to convey spoken, gestural/sign language or written information.

extended care paramedic Highly trained and skilled paramedic who is able to independently manage and treat patients, which includes referral and alternate care pathways.

extended scope of practice Health professional whose scope of practice adopts knowledge, skills and abilities that traditionally belong in the expert domain of another profession (e.g. nurse practitioners).

federalism States coming together under a national government with responsibility for services divided between the state and national government.

fee for service A payment model where services are unbundled and paid for separately. In health care, it gives an incentive for physicians to provide more treatments because payment is dependent on the quantity of care, rather than quality of care.

feminisation of care A theory which suggests the majority of unpaid care of people with a mental illness, the elderly or those with a disability is done by women.

First Peoples The original inhabitants of a country.

food insecurity Whenever people do not at all times have physical, social and economic access to sufficient, safe and nutritious food (Gallegos et al. 2017).

formal services Services provided by government and non-government services wherein care is delivered by trained staff.

Framework for Quality Maternal and Newborn Care (QMNC) The Framework describes the essential care and services for childbearing women and newborn infants in all settings that strengthen women's capabilities in the context of respectful relationships, is tailored to their needs, and focuses on promotion of normal reproductive processes.

gap fee The difference between what is charged by the doctor, hospital or health professional for the service and what the client receives in reimbursements by Medicare or a private insurer.

gate-keeper A service provider who controls access to higher levels of medical care.

general patients Individuals and families who are not eligible for a concession card.

generic brand A brand of a medicine which is produced after the patent on that medicine has expired, and which is an alternative to the originator brand.

generic substitution Replacement of one brand of a medicine by another which is considered to be brand equivalent.

geographical classification system The use of physical location data that can be used to inform policy and/or resource allocation (McGrail & Humphreys 2009).

Gross Domestic Product (GDP) The overall value of a country's economy measured by the value of all goods and services.

handover A verbal report which includes the transfer of information such as clinical treatment/s and responsibility of patient care.

health As defined by World Health Organization (WHO 1946), it is a 'state of complete physical, mental, and social well-being, and not merely the absence of disease or infirmity'.

health care delivery system System consisting of an array of clinicians, hospitals and other health care facilities, insurance plans, and purchasers of health care services, all operating in various configurations of groups, networks, and independent practices.

health care system Activities and institutions in a society that deliver health care services to the population. These comprise health departments, hospitals, clinics, services (medical, nursing, dental, traditional health care, homeopathy) etc.– all being distinguishable systems of health care or parts thereof (van Rensburg 2012).

health care system performance The quality, accuracy, speed and cost at which health services are provided measured by present standards and indicators on health system effectiveness, appropriate use of services provided and improvement of health outcomes for patients and the wider community.

health determinant See social health determinants.

health equity The rights of people to have equitable access to services on the basis of need, and the resources, capacities and power they need to act upon the circumstances of their lives that determine their health (Keleher & MacDougall 2015).

health for all A program goal of the World Health Organization (WHO), which seeks to secure the health and wellbeing of people around the world.

health inequity Difference in the health status between population groups that can be linked to potentially modifiable social or economic factors and deemed to be unfair or stemming from some form of injustice.

health sector reform The sustained and purposeful change to improve efficiency, equity, productivity and effectiveness of the health sector.

health system This includes the entire national health care system as well as all those extraneous matters which are either directly or indirectly associated with health especially the surrounding environment of the health care system and the population served (van Rensburg 2012).

health workforce shortage Shortage of skilled health care workers.

healthy ageing The process of developing and maintaining the functional ability that enables well-being in older age (WHO 2015).

high-risk strategy A strategy that targets the right patients at high risk of developing a serious condition, such as pregnant women or overweight men who are smokers.

holistic An approach to healing which recognises a person as a unique totality; mind, body and spirit.

horizontal equity When people with the same needs have the access to the same resources (Starfield, 2011).

hospital separation A complete episode of care from admission to discharge, death, transfer or change to different type of care.

human rights model A model for addressing disability or disadvantage to go beyond legal requirements to policy and practices.

hybrid system Health care system with a combination of public and private services; often medically necessary services are provided via the public system and funded through taxation, co-existing with a private system for people who pay through self-financing.

iatrogenic A term referring to further illness conditions that result from medical treatment. For example, when older people are hospitalised for treatment, they may become disoriented, fall, acquire infection or be afflicted by drug interactions.

impairment Any loss or abnormality of psychological, physiological or anatomical structure or function.

individualised funding A portable package of funds allocated to a particular individual that facilitates their control over how they purchase support for their needs.

informal care Informal care of persons with a disability or chronic condition or an elderly person that is undertaken by unpaid workers such as family and friends. Informal care is an integral part of community-based care.

information asymmetry In health care, this often refers to the information or knowledge difference between patients and health care providers, but it can also describe inequalities in the availability of information or knowledge about, for instance, private and public services.

inpatient A patient receiving treatment as an admitted patient in a hospital, generally staying in hospital on an overnight basis or longer.

institutional mix An assessment of what institutions are involved in an issue.

institutionalisation The management of people with mental illness in institutions (psychiatric hospitals), or those in other institutions such as orphanages or residential aged-care homes.

insurance Financial cover taken out to protect oneself against future misfortune such as illness, loss of life, or loss of goods.

integrated care This involves services working together to meet care needs to improve access and equity and ensure all consumer needs are met. This may involve joint service planning.

interprofessional education (IPE) 'An intervention where the members of more than one health or social care profession, or both, learn interactively together, for the explicit purpose of improving interprofessional collaboration or the health / well-being of patients / clients, or both' (Reeves et al. 2013, p. 2).

interprofessional practice (IPP) When two or more health care professionals, work as a team with a common purpose, commitment, mutual respect in a complementary manner to achieve health care delivery and improved patient outcome (Health Workforce Australia (HWA) 2013).

intersectoral collaboration Work across sectors such as health, education, justice, sport and recreation, and agriculture, to achieve an outcome that a single sector could not achieve alone.

intervention services Services that target development of specific skills (e.g. speech pathology services for children with delayed speech or language, audiology services for adults with hearing loss or tinnitus or applied behaviour analysis therapy for autism spectrum disorders).

involuntary care The enforced care provided when the person is believed to have a mental illness and deemed a risk to themselves or others and requires either further assessment or inpatient / community care by mental health professionals.

key worker The clients' contact person within a mental health team.

knowledges The knowledge and belief systems of a particular cultural group.

life expectancy The average number of years that a newborn would be expected to live if they are subject to the age-specific mortality rate during a given period.

mainstream General term for Western biomedical health care; usually denotes majority or dominant government-controlled services.

mandatory price disclosure A policy which requires manufacturers to report (disclose) the actual prices they charge pharmacists for each generic brand of a medicine, including any discounts.

market failure A situation where the market does not provide a service to those without capacity to pay; the government may step in and provide these services.

market-based A system based on private enterprise, goods and services whereby government control is generally limited.

market-driven health care system A situation whereby a service or good must be paid for, and it is sold for a profit, in this case when individuals pay for their own health care, often to private providers of health care.

medical dominance A situation where the profession of medicine has the majority of the power over health care decisions, including over the work of other health professionals.

medical model A model that sees normal human conditions such as childbirth, ageing or disability as requiring medical intervention. Disability is viewed as a problem of the person, directly caused by disease, trauma, or other health condition, which therefore requires sustained medical care provided in the form of individual treatment by professionals. In the medical model, management of the disability is aimed at a 'cure'.

medical nutrition therapy The specific nutritional management of a range of health conditions and associated symptoms involving the application of current nutrition practice.

Medicare The Australian public health insurance scheme.

Medicare Benefits Schedule (MBS) Health care services subsidised by the Australian government.

Medicare levy A component of personal income taxation used to partially fund the Australian health care system.

Medicare Levy Surcharge (MLS) An additional surcharge on the Medicare levy paid by higher income earners who do not have sufficient private health insurance.

medicines Chemical or biological substances which are used to prevent and / or treat health conditions.

minor ailment A medical condition which may be managed without necessarily accessing medical services.

mixed system A system of health care or education that has both public (and free) services as well as services that can be purchased.

mobile-driven health service delivery Health service delivery utilising the functionality of mobile devices to collect, share, record and deliver health data or services.

modalities Distinct areas of complementary and alternative health practice, e.g. naturopathy, massage.

moral hazard An economic term referring to a lack of incentive to protect oneself against risk because others will pay for the consequences; in health care it refers to the additional care patients may receive because it is paid for by insurance.

morbidity Illness, disease.

mortality Deaths. The mortality rate is a measure of the number of deaths in a given population.

national competency standards Benchmark skills and knowledge set by accrediting agencies.

National Disability Insurance Scheme (NDIS) A scheme for provision of support services to people with disabilities where people are given a budget to purchase the services that they require.

national health insurance (NHI) model Model using private-sector providers, but payment comes from a government-run insurance program that every citizen pays into.

national health model Also known as the Beveridge model, it is characterised by universal health care coverage of all citizens by a central government and financed through general tax revenues.

national health system Health sector of a society or country; it encompasses policies, programs, institutions and actors that provide health care-organised efforts to treat and prevent disease. Note that beyond the official or mainstream health care as a country's health care system, the non-official, unorthodox health practices and care traditions also constitute part of a country's health care system (van Rensburg 2012).

National Law Refers to the *Health Practitioner Regulation National Law Act* that is in force in each state and territory.

National Medicines Policy (NMP) A national framework for the provision of medicines in Australia which covers appropriate access and quality.

national standard Knowledge, skills and level of care that all states and services must reach.

neoliberalism A liberal political philosophy that argues the economy is best controlled by the private sector rather than by government (Mazurek et al. 2017).

new public health An explicitly social and political approach to health development that emphasises knowledge to action on the social determinants of health, intersectoral action to support health, healthy public policy, environments for health, sustainable development and equity in health (Keleher & MacDougall 2015).

new public management (NPM) The principles of the market applied to public institutions and as a consequence to the working conditions of those employed in these institutions (Cairney 2002).

Ngangkari Healer who promotes the health and well-being of primarily Anangu people.

noise-induced hearing loss (NIHL) Hearing loss affecting the inner ear (i.e., cochlear or auditory nerve) as a result of either long-term exposure to high levels of noise or exposure to explosive noise such as rifle fire. NIHL most commonly arises from occupational noise exposure but also may arise from the use of personal amplification systems.

non-government organisation (NGO) A private organisation that is independent of the government.

nurse practitioner (NP) A registered nurse whose registration has been endorsed by the Nursing and Midwifery Board of Australia as a nurse practitioner under Section 95 of the National Law, and holding a Master's level qualification. Nurses in this group can apply to have access to the PBS by the Commonwealth Health Minister.

Nursing Midwifery Board of Australia (NMBA) The legally constituted body in Australia charged with the regulation of nursing and midwifery professional practice with an aim to protect the public through ensuring nurses and midwives demonstrate acceptable standards of practice.

nutritionist An expert in human nutrition, usually with tertiary qualifications in nutrition education / promotion.

obesity epidemic A term used to illustrate the increase in severity and rapid expansion of the prevalence of obesity in many nations globally, including Australia.

obesogenic environment A term that includes all features of the environment in which people live out their lives which can contribute to obesity for both individuals and whole populations. This includes the built, physical, food and social environment which encourages overconsumption, unhealthy food choices, sedentary behaviour and reduced physical activity.

occupation The day-to-day activities of life.

occupational engagement The 'performance of occupations as the result of choice, motivation, and meaning within a supportive context and environment' (American Occupational Therapy Association (AOTA) 2014, p. S42).

occupational justice 'Access to and participation in the full range of meaningful and enriching occupations afforded to others, including opportunities for social inclusion and the resources to participate in occupations to satisfy personal, health and societal needs' (AOTA 2014, p. S35).

occupational rehabilitation Rehabilitation activities focused on returning an injured person to the workplace, rather than treating the underlying health condition.

old public health A social movement of the 19th century that worked to improve living conditions through the development of physical infrastructure, including water, sanitation and housing, as well as policy and legislation to support and drive change (Keleher & MacDougall 2015).

opioid substitution programs The provision of medicines which are intended to reduce or eliminate illicit opioid use, along with support and advice on substance abuse.

oral health therapy practitioner A practitioner qualified as a dental therapist and dental hygienist.

organisational politics The ways in which individuals and groups within an organisation get and use power or influence, usually to protect or enhance their position.

originator brand The brand of a medicine which is first made available for patient use, usually while a patent is in operation.

out-of-pocket model A model of health care where the patient has to pay for the services of the health professional from their own income or wage.

outpatient A patient receiving treatment where they are not required to be admitted to a hospital bed, such as when visiting a medical specialist for the regular review of a chronic health condition or accessing an emergency department for short-term treatment.

patent A legally enforceable right for a device, substance, process or method which gives the owner or inventor exclusive commercial rights for a specified period of time.

patient A person who interacts with a specific health provider for health or medicine-related reasons.

payment for performance Payment closely linked to activity-based funding model, where health care systems are paid for the amount of throughput, rather than outcomes.

performance management A situation where an employee has ongoing meetings with their supervisor to monitor and improve their performance.

perinatal Usually defined as the period from the 20th week of gestation and ends 1– 4 weeks after birth.

periodontal disease Disease of the gums and supporting structures of the teeth.

person-centred care Care derived from an assessment of a resident's or patient's abilities as well as impairments. It includes attention to psychosocial needs and is based on a care plan that where possible, includes residents' input and choices.

person-centred planning/approach An approach, service philosophy and range of processes that aims to discover and act on what is important to a person. It involves continual listening and learning, focusing on what is important to someone now and in the future, and acting on this in consultation with their family and their friends. The individual and their aspirations and goals are at the centre of decision-making.

perverse incentives An incentive to shift the cost of providing health care to another party (another level of government or different part of the health system).

Pharmaceutical Benefits Scheme (PBS) A scheme designed to provide necessary subsidised medicines to Australians at a cost that individuals and the community can afford.

Pharmaceutical Society of Australia The peak national professional pharmacy organisation representing Australia's 28,000 pharmacists working in all sectors and across all locations.

Pharmacy Guild of Australia The national peak body representing the owners of Australia's 5400 community pharmacies.

population health An approach to service delivery and provision that is about improving the health of the whole population, as well as addressing the inequities in health status between different groups.

population strategy A strategy that attempts to control the incidence of the determinants of health, and thus to shift the distribution of exposure across the whole population.

practice nurse A registered or enrolled nurse employed in a general practice setting (not a registered group, like the nurse practitioner, but so named because they work in general practice).

presbycusis Bilateral (and most commonly) sensorineural hearing impairment that occurs as people age.

prevention paradox Interventions that achieve large overall health gains for whole populations as opposed to those that offer small advantages to individuals at high risk. In other words, preventing small risks in large populations leads to greater health outcomes than avoiding large risks in a smaller number of high-risk individuals.

primary care An episode of care for diagnosis, treatment of illness or disease management, as well as an entry point into the health system for people who are seeking help. In Australia, general practice is seen as part of primary care.

primary carer Person who takes primary responsibility for provision of unpaid care.

primary contact practices People who are able to make contact with a service without a referral from a GP.

primary contact status The status by which an individual has first contact with a service provider.

Primary Health Network (PHN) A government-funded organisation that plans and purchases primary care services for a region.

primary mental health care The activity of a health care professional who acts as a first point of contact for patients with mental health issues.

primary prevention Prevention of illness or disease before it occurs through interventions such as health education, screening and immunisation.

private for-profit Where an organisation operates a service or product that is sold for a profit.

private health insurance (PHI) Health insurance provided by industry rather than government-run insurance.

private health insurance model A term referring to health insurance plans marketed by the private health insurance industry, as opposed to government-run insurance programs. It is characterised by employment-based or individual purchase of private health insurance financed by individual and employer contributions. It allows the insuree to be treated in a private or public hospital as a private patient; it also provides cover for services not covered by national or social health insurance.

private health insurance rebate A means-tested contribution through the taxation system to individuals and families towards the cost of private health insurance.

private hospital Hospital owned by a for-profit or not-for-private entity, with services paid for by patients themselves, insurance companies, or agreements with governments.

private prescription Prescription for medicines which are not eligible for subsidy under the PBS.

privatisation The transfer of previously public services or products to the private sector.

proceduralist A physician or surgeon who is skilled at diagnostic or therapeutic procedures, or whose work consists largely of carrying out such procedures, e.g. an endoscopist.

productivity The relationship between the mix of inputs and outputs (NHMBWG 1996: 34).

professional closure A profession closes ranks to ensure that other groups or occupations cannot have access to practise. This might be done through preventing those who have not passed examinations from practising or through legislation that limits practice.

professional development Ongoing education and training taken by professionals to increase and extend their skill and knowledge.

professional monopoly A situation where a profession controls a particular service.

professionalisation The social process of becoming a professional.

programmatic assessment An approach in which routine information about the learner's competence and progress is continually collected, analysed and, where needed, complemented with purposively collected additional assessment information, with the intent to both maximally inform the learner and their mentor and allow for high-stakes decisions at the end of a training phase.

progressive tax Taxes based on a generic notion of 'ability to pay'. They vary according to how much money an individual / family earns – lower earnings equal a lower level of tax paid whereas higher earnings result in higher tax paid.

prophylactically A therapy used to prevent an illness or disease, e.g. giving a patient antibiotics to prevent an infection.

protected title A designated professional title which is protected by law. Making claims of and acting as a registered health professional when not registered is an offence under National Law.

public dental services Dental services funded by governments and provided to eligible people through public and community sector agencies.

public health The art and science of preventing disease and injury, prolonging life and promoting health through the organised efforts of society.

public health nutrition A branch of nutrition practice with a focus on promoting good health and the primary prevention of disease at the population level utilising policy, research and interventions which highlight healthy eating.

public health system The system of health care delivered by the government.

public–private partnership (PPP) 'An arrangement where the private sector supplies assets and services that traditionally have been provided by the government. In addition to private execution and financing of public investment, PPPs have two other important characteristics: there is an emphasis on service provision, as well as investment, by the private sector; and significant risk is transferred from the government to the private sector' (World Bank, 2014, pp. 17–18) although governments are usually required to pay back the funds used to provide the service.

quality-adjusted life-year (QALY) A value, measured in years, that takes into account both the quality and quantity of life and is a measure of the benefit to a patient that results from taking a new medicine or treatment.

quality use of medicines (QUM) The rational choice of medicines which are suitable for particular conditions and patients, and ensuring their safe and effective use. One of the four tenants of Australia's National Medicine Policy and means the safe, efficacious, judicious and appropriate use of medicines.

receptive communication impairment Reduced ability to understand another person's communication (spoken, gestured / signed or written).

reciprocal health care agreement (RHCA) A formal written agreement with another country which allows access to the PBS and Medicare for their citizens while visiting Australia, and some health care benefits to Australians when they are visiting the other country.

recovery A situation where the person no longer has the illness and is well.

reference pricing Setting the price of a PBS medicine by comparing it with the price of the other brands (originator and / or generic) of that medicine or the cost paid for the medicine in other countries.

reflective learning A way of allowing students to step back from their learning experience to help them develop critical thinking skills and improve on future performance by analysing their experience.

registered nurse (RN) A nurse with a minimum 3-year training certificate and postgraduate qualifications who must be registered with Nursing and Midwifery Board of Australia. A registered nurse works without supervision and is accountable for providing nursing care. This group is also known as a Division 1 nurse in the State of Victoria.

registration A process by which a professional is registered with an external agency having verified their capacity to act to an agreed standard.

regulation The act of being regulated, which means being subject to laws, principles or rules that control or govern.

regulator The government authority responsible for oversight and management of the workers' compensation system.

relative health status Defining one's health in relationship to others.

repatriation beneficiaries Eligible war veterans, former members of the Australian Defence Force and their widows/widowers and dependents.

repeats Additional supplies of a medicine which are allowed on a prescription and which can be provided to a patient after the initial prescription supply has been used.

residential aged-care facility (RACF) A facility that provides residential care for the older person. The facility in Australia can be either public, not for profit or for profit. Each facility is funded according to the dependency of its residents (not all who are over 65).

residential services Government-regulated facilities that house and provide long-term medical and social care to frail elderly people. These facilities also offer short-term respite care.

restricted benefit A medicine which is included on the Schedule of Pharmaceutical Benefits only when specific patient criteria are fulfilled but which does not require a number to appear on the prescription as confirmation.

restrictive practices A group of professionals arrange to limit access to their profession or to limit the activities of some practitioners.

retirement The action of leaving one's job and ceasing to seek out paid employment.

risk management The process of forecasting risks or planning and organising in order to prevent possible risks.

rubella A virus (also known as German measles) that can cause birth defects or death of an unborn fetus if contracted during pregnancy. Sensorineural (inner ear) hearing loss in a newborn baby is a common consequence of maternal rubella.

rural workforce incentives Initiatives aimed at attracting and retaining health professionals in non-metropolitan areas (Commonwealth Department of Health 2018).

Safety Net scheme A scheme under the PBS and Medicare which provides additional financial assistance to families with high medicines or health costs.

Schedule of Pharmaceutical Benefits The list of medicines which have been approved for government subsidy under the PBS.

school dental services A government service providing free general dental care to eligible school-aged children.

scope of practice The boundaries of practice for a health profession.

secondary care Health care that is provided by a specialist upon referral from a primary health provider.

secondary prevention Timely treatment that seeks to arrest or slow existing conditions to minimise complications as well as maintaining health.

selective primary health care A limited form of primary health provision that is disease focused and limited in scope, hence it is a form of selective service provision rather than comprehensive.

self-determination The ability or right to make one's own decisions without interference from others.

self-regulate The capacity of individuals, organisations or professions to rule or govern themselves without outside interference.

sentinel events Sets of adverse events, agreed upon by the health ministers, which result in death or serious harm to a patient, such as medication errors, maternal deaths, suicide of an inpatient, or procedure involving the wrong patient or body part, resulting in death or major permanent loss of function (Australian Commission for Safety and Quality in Health Care, 2017).

shared care Health care that is shared between two or more health practitioners.

social capital The resource capacity derived from the network of individual or group social relationships of people who live and work in a particular society, which enables that society to function effectively.

social contract An agreement between the individual and the state over what the state will provide for the citizen, e.g. financial support when sick.

social determinants of health (SDH) The fundamental structures of social hierarchy and the social, economic and politically determined conditions that result in good health, ill health or disease, and in which people grow, live, work and age.

social gradient The patterns that emerge from inequality in the health status of populations that mirror inequality in socio-economic status.

social health insurance (SHI) One of the mechanisms for raising and pooling funds to finance health services, along with tax-financing, private health insurance, community insurance and others. Typically, working people and their employers, as well as the self-employed, pay contributions that cover a package of services available to the insuree and their dependents.

social inclusion Process that reduces disadvantage through greater access to opportunities to participate fully in society.

social insurance model Also known as the Bismarck model, it is characterised by compulsory coverage that is funded by employer, individual and private insurance funds.

social model of disability A model that sees 'disability' as a socially created problem and not an attribute of an individual, but rather a complex collection of conditions many of which are created by the social environment. Effective management requires social action and is the collective responsibility of society to make the environmental modifications necessary to facilitate full participation of people living with impairment in all areas of life. From this perspective, equal access for someone living with impairment / disability is a human rights issue.

social model of health A model oriented to a holistic understanding of a client, patient or resident. This model promotes social participation and self-fulfillment despite the effects of disease and impairment.

socio-economic status The social and economic position of a given individual, or group of individuals, within the larger society. It is usually, but not always, conceived of as a relative concept and can be measured for the individual, family, household or community / area.

speech pathologist (SP) Tertiary qualified professional who works with people with communication and / or swallowing difficulties.

spinal cord injury A disruption of the nervous tissue in the spinal cord, generally following trauma, which impairs sensation or movement control.

stepped care 'An evidence-based, staged system comprising a hierarchy of interventions, from the least to the most intensive, matched to the individual's needs' (Department of Health 2016).

stigma A feeling of being devalued when you are mentally ill, have a disability or belong to a stigmatised group (e.g. race, sexual preferences), because of negative stereotypes about the condition.

structural/power balance The balance of influence across key categories including, in the case of health care, the balance across the state, the medical profession and private finance.

system A group of elements or components that are interrelated, interdependent and interact. Together they form a complex whole, which develops patterns over time.

systematic literature review (SLR) A highly structured literature review that deals with a particular research question.

telehealth The delivery of health services using information and communication technologies (WHO 2009).

tertiary care Care for more-complex and/or acute conditions requiring intensive support and treatment, usually provided in hospitals.

the State The government, the opposition, the public service, the military and the legal system of judges, and public employed lawyers and the police.

theory An intellectual tool for understanding a situation.

tinnitus The experience of buzzing or ringing in the ears. In most cases, the cause is unknown.

transdisciplinary Approaches that require team members to share roles and systematically cross discipline boundaries. Primarily to pool and integrate the expertise of team members so that efficient and comprehensive assessment and intervention may be provided. Professionals from different disciplines teach, learn, and work together to accomplish a common set of intervention goals for an individual. The role differentiation between disciplines is defined by the needs of the situation rather than by discipline-specific characteristics.

treatment order A legal order that can be made by a medical practitioner or authorised health professional for the treatment of a person if the person has a mental illness; and the person requires treatment for the person's own protection from harm or for the protection of others.

universal access The principle that all citizens have equal access to health services.

universal health coverage/universalism Principle of ensuring that all people have access to needed health services (including prevention, promotion, treatment, rehabilitation and palliation) of sufficient quality to be effective while also ensuring that the use of these services does not expose the user to the financial hardship (WHO 2018).

universalism An approach to centrally funded services such that they are available to everyone, on the basis of need.

unlicensed health care worker A person who performs care duties under supervision but is not granted a licence under formal registration, e.g. nursing registration. This group is trained to provide care or other duties either through further education sector or in-house training at their place of work. They do not have the right to use the title of the profession.

user involvement Situation where users of services are involved in planning service delivery.

user pays Economic principle whereby consumers pay a fee for goods and/or services.

utilisation The act of accessing health care (also *realised* access) (Penchansky & Thomas 1981).

vertical equity Situation where people with more needs are provided with more resources (Starfield, 2011).

weighted average disclosed price (WADP) The weighted average of the actual prices charged to pharmacists for each generic brand of a medicine, as disclosed by all manufacturers of a particular PBS item, and which is used to set the government price.

welfare state A society in which the government provides for the welfare of citizens in terms of health care and other social services (e.g. education, unemployment, etc.).

woman-centred care In midwifery, the woman is at the centre of her care and the midwife has a relationship with the woman who has a relationship with the baby. In this relationship, each woman is seen as an individual with different needs, values and cultural beliefs.

work disability The inability to participate in employment due to a health condition, such as an injury or illness.

work disability duration The amount of time taken away from work due to injury or ill health.

References

American Occupational Therapy Association (AOTA), 2014. Occupational therapy practice framework: domain and process, third ed. Am. J. Occup. Ther. 68 (Suppl. 1), S1–S51.

Associated Students of the University of Oregon, 1999. Summer Diversity Initiative: definition of diversity. http://gladstone.uoregon.edu/~asuomca/diversityinit/definition.html.

Australian Commission for Safety and Quality in Health Care (ACSQHC), 2017. Australian safety and quality framework for health care: putting the framework into action. ACSQHC, Sydney. https://www.safetyandquality.gov.au/wp-content/uploads/2011/01/ASQFHC-Guide-Healthcare-team.pdf.

Australian Institute of Health and Welfare (AIHW), 2001. National health data dictionary. Version 10. Cat. no. HWI 30. AIHW, Canberra.

Australian Institute of Health and Welfare (AIHW), 2013. National definitions for elective surgery urgency categories: proposal for the Standing Council on Health. https://www.aihw.gov.au/reports/hospitals/national-definitions-for-elective-surgery-urgency/contents/summary.

Bentley, T., Effros, R., Palar, K., et al., 2008. Waste in the US health care system: a conceptual framework. Milbank Quarterly 86 (4), 629–659.

Betancourt, J.R., Green, A.R., Carrillo, J.E., 2002. Cultural competence in health care: emerging frameworks and practical approaches. The Commonwealth Fund, New York. http://www.commonwealthfund.org/usr_doc/betancourt_culturalcompetence_576.pdf.

Cairney, P., 2002. New public management and the Thatcher healthcare legacy: enough of the theory, what about the implementation? Br. J. Polit. Int. Relat. 4 (3), 375–398.

Cambridge English Dictionary, 2018. 'big data'. https://dictionary.cambridge.org/dictionary/english/big-data.

Commonwealth Department of Health, 2018. Stronger rural health – recruitment and retention – workforce incentive program. http://www.health.gov.au/internet/budget/publishing.nsf/Content/budget2018-factsheet28.htm.

Department of Health, 2016. PHN Primary mental health care flexible funding pool implementation guidelines: stepped care. Commonwealth of Australia, Canberra. http://www.health.gov.au/internet/main/publishing.nsf/Content/2126B045A8DA90FDCA257F6500018260/$File/1PHN%20Guidance%20-%20Stepped%20Care.pdf.

Gallegos, D., Booth, S., Cleve, S., et al., 2017. Food insecurity in Australian households from charity to entitlement. In: Germov, J., Williams, L. (Eds.), A Sociology of Food and Nutrition, fourth ed. OUP, Melbourne, Chapter 4.

Harris, M., Gardner, K., Powell Davies, G., et al., 2015. Commissioning primary health care: an evidence base for best practice investment in chronic disease at the primary–acute interface: an Evidence Check rapid review brokered by the Sax Institute (www.saxinstitute.org.au) for NSW Health, 2015.

Health Care Act (SA), 2008. https://www.legislation.sa.gov.au/LZ/C/A/HEALTH%20CARE%20ACT%202008/CURRENT/2008.3.AUTH.PDF.

Health Workforce Australia (HWA), 2013. Health professionals prescribing pathway (HPPP) project, final report. HWA, Adelaide.

Keleher, H., MacDougall, C. (Eds.), 2015. Glossary. In: Understanding Health, fourth ed. OUP, Melbourne.

Kildea, S., Lockey, R., Roberts, J., et al., 2016. Guiding principles for developing a Birthing on Country service model and evaluation framework, phase 1. Mater Medical Research Unit and University of Queensland, Brisbane.

Levesque, J.F., Harris, M.F., et al., 2013. Patient-centred access to health care: conceptualising access at the interface of health systems and populations. Int. J. Equity Health 12 (18), 1475–9276.

Mazurek Melnyk, B., Fineout-Overholt, E., Giggleman, M., et al., 2017. A test of the ARCC C model improves implementation of evidence-based practice, healthcare culture, and patient outcomes. Worldviews Evid. Based Nurs. 14 (1), 5–9.

McGee, P., Castledine, G., 2003. Advanced Nursing Practice, second ed. Blackwell Science, Oxford.

McGrail, M.R., Humphreys, J.S., 2009. Geographical classifications to guide rural health policy in Australia. Aust. New Zealand Health Policy 6, 28. doi:10.1186/1743-8462-6-28.

National Health Ministers' Benchmarking Working Group (NHMBWG), 1996. First national report on health sector performance indicators: public hospitals – the state of play. AIHW, Canberra. https://www.aihw.gov.au/getmedia/a6bff00a-d7d8-45d6-8dd0-42ace859d4b8/fnrhspi-c00.pdf.aspx.

National Health and Hospitals Reform Commission (NHHRD), 2008. National Health and Hospitals Reform Commission terms of reference (online), Commonwealth of Australia, Canberra. nhhrc.org.au/terms-ofreference.

Nursing Council of New Zealand, 2011. http://pro.healthmentoronline.com/assets/Uploads/refract/pdf/Nursing_Council_cultural-safety11.pdf.

Penchansky, R., Thomas, J.W., 1981. The concept of access: definition and relationship to consumer satisfaction. Med. Care 19 (2), 127–140.

Reeves, S., Perrier, L., Goldman, J., et al., 2013. Interprofessional education: effects on professional practice and healthcare outcomes (update). Cochrane Database Syst. Rev. (3), CD002213.

Schell, B., Gillen, G., Scaffa, M. (Eds.), 2014. Willard and Spackman's Occupational Therapy, twelfth ed. Lippincott Williams & Wilkins, Philadelphia, p. 1230.

Speech Pathology Australia, 2014. Communication impairment in Australia. http://www.speechpathologyaustralia.org.au/library/2013Factsheets/Factsheet_Communication_Impairment_in_Australia.pdf.

Starfield, B., 2011. The hidden inequity in health care. Int. J. Equity Health 10 (1), 15.

van Rensburg, H., 2012. Health and Health Care in South Africa. Van Schaik, Pretoria.

Victoria State Government, 2018. Casemix funding. https://www2.health.vic.gov.au/hospitals-and-health-services/funding-performance-accountability/activity-based-funding/casemix-funding.

World Bank, 2014. Public–private partnerships: reference guide. Version 2.0. World Bank Group, Washington, DC. http://documents.worldbank.org/curated/en/2014/01/20182310/public-private-partnerships-reference-guide-version-20/.

World Heath Organization (WHO), 1946. Preamble to the constitution of the World Health Organization (WHO) as adopted by the International Health Conference, New York 19–22 June 1946. WHO, Geneva.

World Heath Organization (WHO), 2009. Telemedicine: opportunities and developments in member states. WHO, Geneva.

World Health Organization (WHO), 2015. World report on ageing and health. WHO, Geneva.

World Health Organization (WHO), 2018. Universal health coverage and health financing. WHO, Geneva. http://www.who.int/health_financing/universal_coverage_definition/en//.

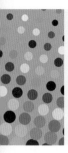

Abbreviations

AAC	augmentative and alternative communication.
AASW	Australian Association of Social Workers.
ABF	activity-based funding.
ABS	Australian Bureau of Statistics.
ACA	*Affordable Care Act*.
ACAS	Aged Care Assessment Service.
ACCHO	Aboriginal Community Controlled Health Organisation.
ACCHS	Aboriginal Community Controlled Health Services.
ACCN	Australian College of Critical Care Nurses.
ACFI	Aged Care Funding Instrument.
ACHSM	Australasian College of Health Service Management.
ACM	Australian College of Midwives.
ACN	Australian College of Nursing.
ACNP	Australian College of Nurse Practitioners.
ACSQHC	Australian Commission on Safety and Quality in Health Care.
ADG	Australian Dietary Guidelines.
ADHA	Australian Digital Health Agency.
ADL	activities of daily living.
AEP	Accredited Exercise Physiologist.
AES	Accredited Exercise Scientist.
AHMAC	Australian Health Ministers Advisory Council.
AHP	allied health professional.
AHPA	Allied Health Professions Australia.
AHPRA	Australian Health Practitioner Regulation Agency.
AHRC	Australian Human Rights Commission.
AHW	Aboriginal health worker.
AIDS	acquired immune deficiency syndrome.
AIHW	Australian Institute of Health and Welfare.
AMA	Australian Medical Association.

AMC	Australian Medical Council.
AMS	Aboriginal-controlled Medical Service.
ANMAC	Australian Nursing and Midwifery Accreditation Council.
AOD	alcohol and drugs.
AOTA	American Occupational Therapy Association.
APA	Australian Physiotherapy Association.
APAC	Australian Psychology Accreditation Council.
APC	Australian Physiotherapy Council.
APD	accredited practising dietitian / auditory processing disorder.
APP	advanced practice physiotherapist.
APRA	Australian Prudential Regulation Authority.
ARIA	Accessibility / Remoteness Index of Australia.
ARN	Access Relative to Need index.
AROH	Australian Register of Homoeopaths.
ARONAH	Australian Register of Naturopaths and Herbalists.
ASD	autism spectrum disorder.
ASGC-RA	Australian Standard Geographic Classification – Remoteness Areas.
ATSI	Aboriginal and Torres Strait Islander.
BoC	Birthing on Country.
BOiMHC	Better Outcomes in Mental Health Care.
CAAC	Central Australian Aboriginal Congress.
CaFHS	Child and Family Health Service.
CAL	Commonwealth Acoustics Laboratories.
CAM	complementary and alternative medicine.
CAPHIA	Council of Academic Public Health Institutions of Australia.
CDC	consumer-directed care.
CDM	chronic disease management.
CEO	chief executive officer.
CFO	chief financial officer.
CHP	community health program.
CHS	community health service.
CHSP	Commonwealth Home Support Program.
CIO	chief information officer.
CLP	Cleft Lip and Palate.
CNA	comprehensive needs assessment.
CNC	clinical nurse consultant.
CNS	clinical nurse specialist.
COAG	Council of Australian Governments.
CoC	continuity of midwifery care (caseload).

COO	chief operating officer.
COPD	chronic obstructive pulmonary disease.
CPA	Community Pharmacy Agreement.
CPD	continuing professional development.
CPHC	comprehensive primary health care.
CPI	Consumer Price Index.
CS	caesarean section.
CSDH	Commission on the Social Determinants of Health.
CSIRO	Commonwealth Scientific and Industrial Research Organisation.
CTG	Closing the Gap.
CVA	cerebral vascular accident.
DAA	Dietitians Association of Australia / dose administration aid.
DALYS	disability adjusted life-years.
DE	developmental educator.
DEAI	Developmental Educators Australia Incorporated.
DH	dental hygienist.
DRG	Diagnosis Related Group.
DVA	Department of Veterans' Affairs.
EBM	evidence-based medicine.
ECP	extended-care paramedic.
ED	emergency department.
EHO	environmental health officer.
EHR	electronic health record.
EN	enrolled nurse.
ENT	ear, nose and throat.
ESP	extended-scope physiotherapist.
ESSA	Exercise & Sports Science Australia.
GDP	gross domestic product.
GFC	global financial crisis.
GP	general practitioner.
GPMP	general practitioner management plan.
HAC	hospital-acquired condition.
HACC	Home and Community Care Program.
HAI	hospital-acquired infection.
HCH	health care home.
HCP	home care package.
HIM	health information manager.
HIV	human immunodeficiency virus.
HMR	home medicines review.

HWA	Health Workforce Australia.
IAHP	Indigenous Australians' Health Programme.
ICF	International Classification of Function.
ICM	International Confederation of Midwives.
ICN	International Council of Nurses.
ICP	intensive care paramedic.
IHPA	Independent Hospital Pricing Authority.
IMA	independent medical assessment.
IPC	interprofessional collaboration.
IPE	interprofessional education.
IPP	interprofessional practice.
IRSAD	Index of Relative Socio-economic Advantage and Disadvantage.
LHN	Local Hospital Network.
MaCCS	Models of Maternity Care Classification System.
MBS	Medicare Benefits Schedule.
MDT	multidisciplinary teams.
MGP	midwifery group practice.
MHR	My Health Record.
MLS	Medicare levy surcharge.
MMM	Modified Monash Model.
MPH	Master of Public Health.
NACCHO	National Aboriginal Community Controlled Health Organisation.
NACCHS	National Aboriginal Community Controlled Health Services.
NASRHP	National Alliance of Self Regulating Health Professionals.
NBN	National Broadband Network.
NCD	non-communicable disease.
NCMHCD	National Community Mental Health Care Database.
NDIA	National Disability Insurance Agency.
NDIS	National Disability Insurance Scheme.
NDS	National Disability Services.
NFP	not-for-profit.
NGO	non-government organisation.
NHI	national health insurance.
NHMRC	National Health and Medical Research Council.
NHPA	National Health Priority Area.
NMBA	Nursing and Midwifery Board of Australia.
NMP	National Medicines Policy.
NP	nurse practitioner.
NPM	new public management.

NPYWC	Ngaanyatjarra, Pitjantjatjara, Yankunytjatjara Women's Council.
NRHA	National Rural Health Alliance.
NSA	Nutrition Society of Australia.
NSQHS	National Safety and Quality Health Service.
OECD	Organisation for Economic Co-operation and Development.
OHS	Office of Hearing Services.
OHT	oral health therapist.
OM	otitis media.
OT	occupational therapist.
OTBA	Occupational Therapy Board of Australia.
PBA	Physiotherapy Board of Australia.
PBAC	Phamaceutical Benefits Advisory Committee.
PBS	Pharmaceutical Benefits Scheme.
PCEHR	personally controlled electronic health record.
PCMH	patient-centred medical home.
PCO	primary care organisation.
PCP	primary-contact practitioner.
PHC	primary health care.
PHCAP	Primary Health Care Access Program.
PHI	private health insurance.
PHN	Primary Health Network.
PHOFA	Public Health Outcome Funding Agreement.
PII	professional indemnity insurance.
PPACA	*Patient Protection and Affordable Care Act.*
PPP	public–private partnership.
QALY	quality-adjusted life-year.
QCPP	Quality Care in Pharmacy Program.
QMNC	quality maternal and newborn care.
QOL	quality of life.
QUM	quality use of medicines.
RACDS	Royal Australian College of Dental Surgeons.
RACF	residential aged-care facility.
RACMA	Royal Australasian College of Medical Administrators.
RAD	refundable accommodation deposit.
RCT	randomised controlled trial.
RHCA	reciprocal health care agreement.
RMMR	residential medication management review.
RMO	resident medical officer.
RN	registered nurse.

RNutr	registered nutritionist.
RRMA	Rural, Remote and Metropolitan Areas.
RTW	return to work.
SARRAH	Services for Australian Rural and Remote Allied Health.
SARS	severe acute respiratory syndrome.
SDH	social determinants of health.
SLR	systematic literature review.
SP	speech pathologist.
SPA	Speech Pathology Australia.
SPHC	selective primary health care.
TAFE	Technical and Further Education.
TBI	traumatic brain injury.
TCA	team care arrangement.
TGA	Therapeutic Goods Administration.
TMO	trainee medical officer.
UCC	urgent care centre.
UNHS	universal neonatal hearing screening.
UNICEF	United Nations Children's Fund.
VBHC	value-based health care.
VET	Vocational Education and Training.
VHC	Veteran's Home Care.
WADP	weighted average disclosed price.
WCPT	World Confederation for Physical Therapy.
WFOT	World Federation of Occupational Therapists.
WHO	World Health Organization.
WTP	What's the problem?

496

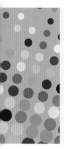

Index

Page numbers followed by "*f*" indicate figures, "*t*" indicate tables, and "*b*" indicate boxes.